ESSENTIALS OF NURSING CHILDREN AND YOUNG PEOPLE

T0315430

ESSENTIALS OF NURSING CHILDREN AND YOUNG PEOPLE

2ND EDITION

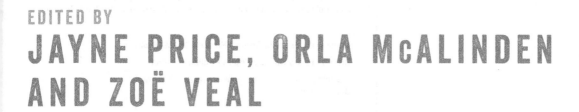

EDITED BY

JAYNE PRICE, ORLA McALINDEN AND ZOË VEAL

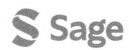
Sage

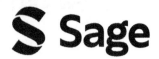

1 Oliver's Yard
55 City Road
London EC1Y 1SP

2455 Teller Road
Thousand Oaks
California 91320

Unit No 323-333, Third Floor, F-Block
International Trade Tower,
Nehru Place, New Delhi-110 019

8 Marina View Suite 43-053
Asia Square Tower 1
Singapore 018960

Editor: Martha Cuneen
Assistant editor: Sahar Jamfar
Production editor: Sarah Sewell
Copyeditor: Elaine Leek
Proofreader: Clare Weaver
Marketing manager: Ruslana Khatagova
Cover design: Sheila Tong
Typeset by: C&M Digitals (P) Ltd, Chennai, India
Printed in the UK

Introduction and editorial arrangement © Jayne Price, Orla McAlinden and Zoë Veal 2024

Chapter 1 © Nicola Mitchell, Joanna Smith and Jackie Vasey 2024
Chapter 2 © Orla McAlinden 2024
Chapter 3 © Rebecca Saul and Alison Twycross 2024
Chapter 4 and Chapter 20 © Mary Brady and Linda Moore 2024
Chapter 5 © Georgina Green 2024
Chapter 6 © Jane Hughes, Amanda Kelly, Tracey Jones and Orla McAlinden 2024
Chapter 7 © Gareth Jones, Sarah Jones, Orla McAlinden and Jacqui Scrace 2024
Chapter 8 © Marc Cornock 2024
Chapter 9 © Cameron Cox and Zoe Clark 2024
Chapter 10 © Gill Langmack and Elisabeth O'Brien 2024
Chapter 11 © Orla McAlinden 2024
Chapter 12 © Melanie Robbins and Cilla Sanders 2024
Chapter 13 © Mandy Brimble and Sarah Reddington-Bowes 2024
Chapter 14 © Rachael Bolland 2024
Chapter 15 © Nicky Varley and Elena Higginson 2024
Chapter 16 © Karen Pattrick 2024
Chapter 17 © Zoë Veal, Orla McAclinden and Doreen Crawford 2024
Chapter 18 © Jo Bailey and Zoë Veal 2024
Chapter 19 © Stuart Hibbins 2024
Chapter 21 © Kate Davies 2024
Chapter 22 © Katie Warburton 2024
Chapter 23 © Julia Judd 2024
Chapter 24 © Lizzy Hoole 2024
Chapter 25 © Shirin Pomeroy 2024
Chapter 26 © Zoë Veal and Colin Veal 2024
Chapter 27 © Zoë Veal, Rebekah Overend and Doreen Crawford 2024
Chapter 28 © Elizabeth Gillespie and Jayne Price 2024
Chapter 29 © Usha Chandran and Fiona Lynch 2024
Chapter 30 © Kathleen Mangahis and Catharine Grob 2024
Chapter 31 © Jayne Price and Suzanne Coulson 2024
Chapter 32 © Antoinette Menezes, Tracie Lewin-Taylor and Jayne Price 2024
Chapter 33 © Jayne Price and Melissa Heywood 2024
Chapter 34 © Trish Griffin and Jane Lopez 2024
Chapter 35 © Laurence Baldwin and Ann Cox 2024
Chapter 36 © Melanie Hayward 2024
Chapter 37 © Claire Anderson 2024
Chapter 38 © Lorraine Highe 2024

Apart from any fair dealing for the purposes of research, private study, or criticism or review, as permitted under the Copyright, Designs and Patents Act, 1988, this publication may not be reproduced, stored or transmitted in any form, or by any means, without the prior permission in writing of the publisher, or in the case of reprographic reproduction, in accordance with the terms of licences issued by the Copyright Licensing Agency. Enquiries concerning reproduction outside those terms should be sent to the publisher.

Library of Congress Control Number: 2023936152

British Library Cataloguing in Publication data

A catalogue record for this book is available from the British Library

ISBN 978-1-5297-6734-6
ISBN 978-1-5297-6733-9 (pbk)

At Sage we take sustainability seriously. Most of our products are printed in the UK using responsibly sourced papers and boards. When we print overseas we ensure sustainable papers are used as measured by the Paper Chain Project grading system. We undertake an annual audit to monitor our sustainability.

DEDICATION

Jayne: In memory of David J. Thomas, an inspirational children's nurse whose impact on the care of children with cancer/palliative care needs and their families will never be forgotten.

Orla: To Alex and Sharon, thank you for all that you do. I am ever grateful for the care and love you show for children with complex needs.

Zoë: For the previous and current undergraduate children's nursing students at UWE Bristol – you are my inspiration.

CONTENTS

ONLINE RESOURCES

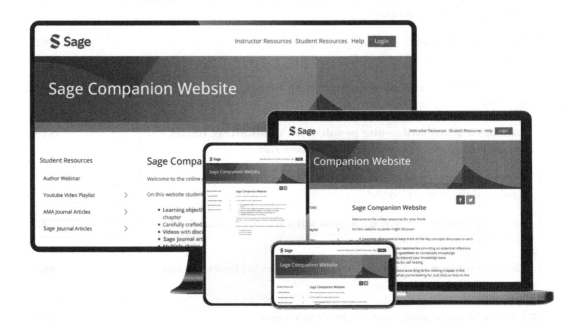

Visit **https://study.sagepub.com/essentialchildnursing2e** to find a range of additional resources for both students and lecturers, to aid study and support teaching.

For students

Additional case studies and scenarios to give you even more insight into how theory works in the real world.

Suggestions for textbook activities to test and compare your knowledge.

For lecturers

Lecturer's guide that outlines the key learning objectives covered in each chapter and provides you with suggested activities/examples to use in class or for assignments.

Testbanks containing questions related to the key concepts in each chapter can be downloaded and used in class, as homework or exams.

ABOUT THE EDITORS AND CONTRIBUTORS

ABOUT THE EDITORS

Jayne Price is Professor of Children's Nursing at Kingston University London. She qualified as a general nurse in 1991 (Belfast) and as a children's nurse (Leeds) in 1995. Her clinical background within children's nursing includes a strong focus on oncology and palliative care. Having taught as a Senior Lecturer (Education) at Queen's University Belfast since 2001, Jayne moved to Kingston University in 2014. In her current role, Jayne teaches and facilitates student learning from foundation degree through to PhD level and has received a number of awards for teaching/educational developments. Throughout her career to date Jayne has made stringent efforts to enhance care for children requiring a palliative approach and their families, through practice, education and research. She is a Trustee of Martin House Children's Hospice and is also involved in the work of Shooting Star Children's Hospices. Jayne has published and presented widely nationally and internationally.

Orla McAlinden has been an adult nurse since 1979 (Royal Victoria Hospital Belfast, Northern Ireland, working through the period of civil and political turbulence known as 'the Troubles') and a children's nurse since 1986 (Queen Mary's Hospital Carshalton) and a Lecturer in Children's Nursing at Queen's University Belfast in Northern Ireland since 1992. Her clinical background with children includes medical/surgical nursing, education and clinical experience in PICU and NICU (Lewisham & Evelina Children's Unit at Guy's Hospital London). Orla's clinical and professional interests lie in ethical, legal and professional aspects of children's nursing, with a particular interest in infant mental health, emotional/mental health and wellbeing, complex needs and CAMHs-related issues.

Currently, Orla works in the Criminal Justice System in Northern Ireland in a Category A Prison, and as a Teaching Assistant at Queens University Belfast, Northern Ireland. She is a member of the Editorial Advisory Panel for the *Nursing Children and Young People's Journal*, an ex-Specialist Advisor with the Care Quality Commission (CQC), an ex- Steering Group member for RCN Community & Continuing Care Forum, and a Social Media Moderator for that Forum's Facebook/Twitter pages. She is a keen participant with the @WeCYPNurses community on Twitter and an advocate for professional social media use and is also a member of the CYP Nurse Academic Network.

Zoë Veal is a senior lecturer in children's and young people's nursing at the University of the West of England (UWE), Bristol and has been a registered children's nurse since 1995. Her clinical background has predominately focused on surgical specialties, having worked in both short-stay and long-stay surgical units, cardiology and cardiac surgery (Bristol Royal Hospital for Children), burns and reconstructive surgery and neurology and neurosurgery (Frenchay Hospital, Bristol). In her current role, Zoë teaches and facilitates student learning from foundation year through to master's level in both theory and practice modules (clinical skills) and has a particular interest in the history of nursing and the use of fiction in nurse education. Zoë has undertaken a number of roles within the university, including programme leadership, and she was professional lead for children and young people's nursing at UWE Bristol during the COVID pandemic. She is currently the admissions tutor for the undergraduate children and young people's nursing degree programme and is also a member of the CYP Nurse Academic Network. Alongside her nursing degree and professional registration as a children's nurse, Zoë also holds degrees in literature and teaching, and is currently working towards a professional doctorate in education (EdD).

ABOUT THE CONTRIBUTORS

Dr Claire Anderson EdD, MSc, PGCHE, BSc, Senior Fellow HEA, Head of Work Force Development, University of West London.

Jo Bailey RN (Child), BSc(Hons), Assistant Cardiac Nurse Specialist, Bristol Royal Hospital for Children.

Dr Laurence Baldwin is currently an Assistant Professor at Coventry University where he is Course Director for the pre-registration MSc in Mental Health Nursing and runs a CYPMHS module.

Rachael E. Bolland RGN, RSCN, MA, MSc, PGCert Ed, Fellow of HEA.

Mary P. Brady RGN, RSCN, BSc (Hons.), CHSM, PGCLT HE, MSc, Senior Fellow HEA.

Dr Mandy Brimble Senior Lecturer in Children and Young People's Nursing at the School of Healthcare Sciences, Cardiff University and Senior Fellow of Advance HE.

Usha Chandran Senior Lecturer Children's Nursing Kingston University.

Zoe Clark RN Adult, SCPHN (HV), BSc (Hons), PGDip, MSc, Fellow of HEA, Associate Professor Quality and Accreditation.

Marc Cornock academic lawyer and Senior Lecturer in the Faculty of Wellbeing, Education and Language Studies at The Open University.

Suzanne Coulson RSCN, BHSc (Hons), PG Cert Clinical Education, Fellow of HEA, Clinical Educator, Children & Young People's Haematology & Oncology, Leeds Children's Hospital, Leeds Teaching Hospitals NHS Trust.

Dr Ann Cox is a Consultant Mental Health Nurse and Clinical academic with research interests in children's rights.

Cameron Cox RN Child, SCPHN (SN), BA (Hons), PG, Fellow of HEA Kings College London.

Doreen Crawford MA, PGCert Ed, BSc (Hons) SRN, RSCN, now retired was a Fellow Royal Society Medicine, Fellow Academy Higher Education, previously a Consultant Nurse Editor for *Nursing Children and Young People*, Nurse Advisor Crawford-McKenzie Health Care Consultancy.

Kate Davies RN (Child), DipHE, BSc (Hons), MSc, NMP, PGCert Ed, Fellow of HEA, Senior Lecturer in Children's Nursing.

Georgina Green RN (Child) , SCPHN, Bsc (Hons) PG Cert Child Protection, PG Cert HE. Lecturer in Child Nursing at the University of Hull.

Elizabeth Gillespie RGN, RSCN, Specialist Practitioner Community Children's Nursing, MSc, PGCert Ed, Fellow of HEA.

Trish Griffin Associate Professor Learning Disabilities Nursing Kingston University London.

Catharine Grob Senior Lecturer Children's Nursing Kingston University London.

Melanie Hayward RN (Child), SCPHN (SN), CPNP, RNT, MAEd, PG Cert Ed, BSc Hons, Grad Cert, Dip HE, Fellow HEA, Fellow RSA is an Associate Professor in the Institute for Health and Social Care at Buckinghamshire New University.

Melissa Heywood Clinical Nurse Consultant for the Victorian Paediatric Palliative Care Program (VPPCP) at the Royal Children's Hospital (RCH), Melbourne, Australia.

Stuart Hibbins RGN, RSCN, MSc, PGCAP, Senior Lecturer, London South Bank University.

Elena Higginson BSc Hons Nursing (Child), Associate Fellow of HEA, Lecturer at University of Central Lancashire.

Lorraine Highe MA, PGCert Ed, BSc(Hons), RN (Adult), RN(Child). BSc Course Director Children's Nursing at London South Bank University.

Lizzy Hoole Senior Lecturer in Children and Young People's Nursing University of West of England.

Jane Hughes RN (Adult and Child), MA (Econ), BSc Hon, Dip N, PGDip, Fellow HEA, Senior Lecturer in Children and Young People's Nursing, The University of Manchester.

Gareth Jones RN Child, BSc (Hons) Health and Community Practice (Community Children's Nurse). Senior Manager, NHS England.

Sarah Jones RN Child, BSc (Hons) Health and Community Practice (Community Children's Nurse). Head of Nursing, The Lifetime Service, Sirona.

Tracey Jones RN Child, BSc, MSc, PGDip in HE, Senior Fellow of the HEA, Lecturer in Nursing, University of Manchester.

Julia Judd RSCN, RGN, MSc. Advanced Nurse Practitioner, Children's Orthopaedics.

Amanda Kelly RN Child, MSc, Senior Specialist Nurse for Looked After Children, Manchester University Foundation Trust, Manchester.

Gill Langmack BSc (Hons), PGCHE, FHEA, Lecturer in Child Health Nursing, University of Nottingham.

Tracie Lewin-Taylor Shooting Star Chase's Symptom Care Team.

Jane Lopez MA, BEd(Hons), RNT, RNLD, Dip N.

Fiona Lynch RGN, RSCN, BSc (Hons), MSc (Adv Pract) MSc (Health Res) PICU Consultant Nurse, Evelina London.

Kathleen Mangahis RGN, BSc, Grad Cert Neo, MSc, PGCCE, NMC Teacher, FHEA. Senior lecturer Children's Nursing and Pathway Lead for the Neonatal Modules in Kingston University.

Antoinette Menezes PhD, MSc, PGCert HE, RGN.

Nicola Mitchell RNC, Adv. DPSN, MSc, PG Cert HPE, FHEA Lecturer in Children's Nursing, University of Leeds.

Linda Moore RGN, RSCN, BSc(Hons), PGDip Ed, MSc, Senior Fellow HEA.

Elisabeth O'Brien BSc (Hons), MEd, RGN, RHV, PGCHE, FHEA, Lecturer, Child Health and Safeguarding Lead, School of Health Sciences, University of Nottingham.

Rebekah Overend leads the Faculty of Children's Nurse Education at the Bristol Royal Hospital for Children and is an active member of the Paediatric Critical Care Society Education group.

Karen Pattrick RN (Child), BSc Hons, MSc, FHEA. Lecturer in Children's Nursing and Programme Director for the BSc Nursing (Child) at the University of Hull.

Shirin Pomeroy RN (Child), BA (Hons), MSc, PGCert Burn Care.

Sarah Reddington-Bowes Vice Chair CPHVA Executive and PT Health Visitor.

Melanie Robbins RGN, RSCN, RHV, DNCert, RNT, BSc, MSc, Fellow of HEA, Professional Lead for Nursing (Child).

Katie Warburton (Rowson) RN Child, BSc, MSc, NMP, RNT, FHEA. Senior Lecturer at University of Central Lancashire.

Cilla Sanders RGN, RN (Child), BSc(Hons) Nursing, BSc (Hons) Specialist Practitioner Children's Community Nursing, PG Cert Clinical Education, MEd. Programme Lead for Child Nursing at the University of Leeds.

Rebecca Saul RGN, RSCN, MSc, PGCE, PGCert, Clinical Nurse Specialist, Pain Control Service, Great Ormond Street Hospital for Children NHS Foundation Trust, London, UK.

Jacqui Scrace RN Child, BSc (Hons) (Community Children's Nursing), MA, QN. Interim Assistant Director of Nursing for Children and Young People, NHS England South West.

Jean Shapcott SRN, RSCN, PGCEA, MSc, retired Senior Lecturer in Children's Nursing, Kingston University.

Joanna Smith PhD, MSc, BSc (Hons), RSCN, RGN, Professor of Nursing in Child Health at Sheffield Children's NHS Foundation Trust/Sheffield Hallam University.

Alison Twycross RGN, RMN, RSCN, MSc, DMS, Cert Ed(HE), PhD, Previously Deputy Dean and Lead Nurse and Professor of Children's Nursing at London South Bank University.

Nicky Varley teaches across a range of subjects for both the Pre and Post Registration Nursing programmes.

Dr Jackie Vasey RGN, RSCN, BSc (Hons), PGDip HPE, Doctor of Nursing formerly of the University of Huddersfield.

Colin Veal RN (Child), BSc, MSc Advanced Practice, Senior Lecturer in Children and Young People's Nursing, University of the West of England (UWE) Bristol.

FOREWORD

BERNIE CARTER

THE MORE PLACES YOU'LL GO

This second edition of *Essentials of Nursing Children and Young People* provides the building blocks for a lifetime of learning about nursing children, young people and their families. Education is often talked of as a gift that provides the platform for growth, transformation, enabling the person to achieve and to be an asset to their community and then to share their knowledge with others. Those learning about the essentials of how to nurse children, young people and their families are at the start of an exciting, challenging and ultimately highly rewarding journey that will support them to become the future expert practitioners, innovators, managers, leaders, educators, researchers and policy-makers within their field.

As someone nearer the end of a lifetime involved with nursing children and young people, I am still learning and critically reflecting on what I know and what I still need to better understand. The never-ending nature of education and learning could seem daunting, but it is both crucial for the children and young people who are the focus of our professional attention, and it is also an adventure in curiosity that can lead to improvements in care, innovation and the ways we can provide skilled compassionate care.

Nursing children and young people requires nurses to have an extensive knowledge base and skill set that allows them to engage with and care for children and young people in an increasingly unpredictable world. Nurses who work with children and young people practise in a wide variety of settings, ranging from the very highly technological tertiary settings such as critical care through to primary care settings and the home. Each setting and every individual engagement with a child or young person and their family requires us to draw on the skills and knowledge we gained from education and learning to meet their particular and unique needs.

Nurses work in a world that does not stay still so the skills and knowledge we learn on our journey to become a registered nurse who is qualified to care for children and young people are essential elements to be drawn on as well as questioned and challenged. The education of nurses who care for children, young people and their families increasingly accommodates and responds to changes in the epidemiology of childhood illness and the increasing complexity of need, as well as changes in demographics. What we know now will not be sufficient to meet future needs; hence, the need for us to continue to read, learn, question our assumptions, and add to the evidence base for our practice.

Educators have a major part to play in creating the leaders, managers and innovators of the future; they light the flame, inspire and nurture. Nursing children and young people requires nurses to think boldly and think how they can inspire change and make changes that will improve care. We need to have our eyes on the horizon. Leadership, mentorship and being a change agent is not something that should be left to the more or most experienced people. Nurses who care for children and young people need to be encouraged, and encourage others, to share ideas and to propose, implement, manage and sustain change. Leadership is not a role, it is a way of thinking, being and acting in partnership with colleagues, children, young people, and families and other stakeholders. Leadership is about being adaptable and flexible in your thinking, inspiring others to ensure best practice. We should all aspire to be leaders, even if only in a small way.

Nurses who care for children and young people often say or are taught that they are the child's advocate. This is true, but too often this is a narrow view of advocacy where we speak up for one child or one situation; this is important as it can make a real change for the child or young person or that situation. However, true child-centred advocacy comes when we become more politically aware and active around the challenges that children and young people face. Child poverty and health inequalities exert malign effects on children's health and wellbeing and even in wealthy countries with good health systems progress against poverty and its impacts on children is precarious. Children and young people live with these impacts and nurses see these impacts every day in their practice. Asthma is one example where our knowledge, skills and experience need to reach out beyond delivering the best possible care to encompass political activism in demanding that the causes of asthma such as air pollution should be addressed. Nursing children and young people activism needs to be based on social justice and we need to be engaged.

Activism is also vital to protect the pre-registration education of children and young people's nurses. Looking back over the history of children's nursing education, it has been threatened with marginalisation and there is almost always an underlying rumbling threat to withdraw pre-registration child nurse training. For those who want to protect pre-registration training, activism is one of the ways in which we can fight future threats.

I come back to the point made at the start: education is a gift we should treasure and should never take for granted. The better educated we are as nurses, the better we can serve the children and young people we care for and the better we can shape the future of children and young people's nursing.

I'll leave you with words from Dr Seuss which perhaps sum things up more aptly than even the best-written textbook or academic paper:

> The more that you read,
> the more things you will know.
> The more that you learn,
> the more places you'll go.

Professor Bernie Carter
Professor of Children's Nursing, Faculty of Health, Social Care and Medicine
Edge Hill University

PUBLISHER'S ACKNOWLEDGEMENTS

The editors and Sage would like to thank all the students, patients/service users and nurses who contributed their stories to the book and online resources. The book is much richer for your contribution. We would also like to thank all the students, lecturers and practitioners who helped to review this book's content, design, and online resources to ensure it is as useful as possible.

VOICES

We would like to give special thanks to all the families who contributed their voices to this book, the book is richer for your contributions. We would also like to thank the students and nurses who also contributed their voices. All voices have been anonymised to protect privacy unless otherwise requested.

PUBLISHER'S ACKNOWLEDGEMENTS

The authors and publisher are grateful to the following parties for permission to reproduce their material:

Case Study 1.1 with thanks to Amy Ward, Health Visitor.

Case Study 1.2 with thanks to Sarah Dawson, Alex's mother.

Case Study 1.3 with thanks to Georgia Long, Third year nusing student at time of writing.

Figure 3.2 Revised FLACC Scale. Reproduced with kind permission, © The Regents of the University of Michigan.

Figure 3.3 Faces Pain Scale. Reproduced with kind permission, © 2001, International Association for the Study of Pain.

Figure 9.1 MASH, Multi Agency Working and Information Sharing Project: Final Report. London: Home Office © Crown copyright.

Table 9.1 A MASH team comprises five core elements, London Safeguarding Children Board London MASH Project: The Five Core Elements. © Crown copyright.

Table 9.2 Different types of FGM. Reproduced with permission of the World Health Organization (WHO).

Table 9.3 Overall effects of FGM, NHS Choices (2014) *Female Genital Mutilation*. Used with permission under the terms of the Open Government Licence www.nationalarchives.gov.uk/doc/opengovernment-licence.

Table 11.1 Baby bonds, adapted from Moulin, S., Waldfogel, J. and Washbrook, E. (2014) *Baby Bonds: Parenting, Attachment and a Secure Base for Children*. London: The Sutton Trust. Reproduced with kind permission of The Sutton Trust.

Figure 12.1 The Assessment Framework (HM Government, 2015, p.22). © Crown copyright.

Table 12.1 Percentage of children classified as obese in the UK. Adapted from House of Common Library briefing paper Number 3336. © Crown copyright.

Table 13.1 4, 5, 6 health visiting model (DH, 2015). Used with permission under the terms of the Open Government Licence www.nationalarchives.gov.uk/doc/opengovernment-licence.

Table 14.1 Summary of symptoms and signs suggestive of specific diseases (NICE, 2013). Reproduced with permission of the National Institute for Health and Care Excellence.

Table 14.2 Sites and devices to be used when measuring body temperature in infants and children (NICE, 2013). Reproduced with permission of the National Institute for Health and Care Excellence.

Table 14.3 Management according to risk of serious illness (NICE, 2013). Reproduced with permission of the National Institute for Health and Care Excellence.

Table 14.4 Assessing dehydration in children under 5 years (NICE, 2009). Reproduced with permission of the National Institute for Health and Care Excellence.

Table 14.6 Risk stratification tool for a 7-year-old with suspected sepsis (adapted from NICE, 2016a). Reproduced with kind permission of the UK Sepsis Trust.

Table 14.7 Emergency department Red Flag Sepsis criteria for children aged 5–11 years. Reproduced with kind permission of the UK Sepsis Trust.

Table 14.8 Example of Paediatric Sepsis 6 chart: Complete all elements within one hour. Reproduced with kind permission of the UK Sepsis Trust.

Figure 14.1 Poster from the UK Sepsis Trust. Reproduced with kind permission of the UK Sepsis Trust.

Table 21.1 Conditions seen in paediatric endocrinology, Raine, J.E., Donaldson, M.D.C., Gregory, J.W. & van Vliet, G. (2011) *Practical Endocrinology and Diabetes in Children*, 3rd edn. Chichester: Wiley-Blackwell. Reproduced with kind permission of John Wiley and Sons Inc.

Page 334 Hypoglycaemia or 'hypos', bullet point list, adapted from Hanas, R. (2015) *Type 1 Diabetes in Children, Adolescents and Young Adults*, 6th edn. Somerset, Class Health. Reproduced with kind permission of Class Publishing.

Table 21.2 How diabetes interferes with normal adolescence, Dmitri, P. (2012) 'Endocrine and Metabolic Disorders', in *Illustrated Textbook of Paediatrics*, 4th edn (Lissauer, T. and Clayden, G., eds). Edinburgh: Mosby/Elsevier. Reproduced with permission of Elsevier under STM Guidelines: www.stm-assoc.org/copyright-legal-affairs/permissions/permissions-guidelines/.

Figure 21.2 Correct measurement of head circumference. Photo reproduced with kind permission of Lee Martin.

Figure 21.3 Measuring a child. Photo reproduced with kind permission of Lee Martin.

Table 21.4 Causes of short stature, Laing, P. (2014): 'Growth failure and hormone therapy'. *British Journal of Nursing* 23, S3-9. Reproduced with kind permission, © 2015 MA Healthcare Ltd.

Figure 23.3 Pavlik harness. Reproduced with permission from Clarke, S. and Santy-Tomlinson, J. *Orthopaedic and Trauma Nursing: An Evidence-based Approach to Musculoskeletal Care*, 2014, Wiley–Blackwell.

Figure 23.5 Left club foot. Reproduced with permission from Clarke, S. and Santy-Tomlinson, J. *Orthopaedic and Trauma Nursing: An Evidence-based Approach to Musculoskeletal Care*, 2014, Wiley–Blackwell.

Figure 24.1 X-linked inheritance. Reproduced with kind permission of the Genetic Support Foundation.

Figure 25.1 Image created from: St Helens and Knowsley Teaching Hospitals NHS Trust (2010–13) *Mersey Burns*. Reproduced with kind permission of *Mersey Burns*.

Figure 25.2 Lund and Browder chart, Harwood-Nuss A., Wolfson, A. and Linden, C. *The Clinical Practice of Emergency Medicine*. Philadelphia: Wolters Kluwer; 2015. Reproduced with permission.

Table 26.3 Assessing dehydration in children under 5 years, National Institute for Health and Clinical Excellence (2009) *CG84 Diarrhoea and Vomiting Caused by Gastroenteritis in Under 5s: Diagnosis and Management*. London: NICE. Reproduced with permission.

Table 26.4 Treatment of clinical dehydration and clinical shock based on NICE guidelines, National Institute for Health and Clinical Excellence (2009) *CG84 Diarrhoea and Vomiting Caused by Gastroenteritis in Under 5s: Diagnosis and Management*. London: NICE. Reproduced with permission.

Figure 31.1 Symptoms of childhood cancer, Ped-Onc Resource Center (2015) *Signs of Childhood Cancer*. Reproduced with permission.

Figure 33.1 End-of-life care pathway, Widdas, D., McNamara, K. and Edwards, F. (2013) *A Core Care Pathway for Children with Life-limiting and Life-threatening Conditions*, 3rd edn. Bristol: Together for Short Lives. Reproduced with permission.

Figure 33.2 Paediatric Pain Profile, Hunt, A., Goldman, A., Seers, K., Crichton, N., Mastroyannopolou, K., Moffat, V. et al. (2003) 'Clinical validation of the paediatric pain profile', *Developmental Medicine & Child Neurology*, 46(1): 9–18. Reproduced with permission of UCLB.

Figure 36.2 The nine dimensions of the NHS Healthcare Leadership Model. Reproduced with kind permission © NHS Leadership Academy.

Figure 37.2 Driscoll's model of reflection, Driscoll, J. (2007) *Practising Clinical Supervision: A Reflective Approach for Healthcare Professionals*, 2nd edn. Edinburgh: Bailliere Tindall/Elsevier. Reproduced with permission of Elsevier under STM Guidelines: www.stm-assoc.org/copyright-legal-affairs/permissions/permissions-guidelines/.

INTRODUCTION

JAYNE PRICE, ORLA McALINDEN AND ZOË VEAL

This book has been written for nurses everywhere who look after children and young people with a healthcare need.

Whilst the book is primarily aimed at children's nursing students in years 2 and 3 of their degree programme, it also presents a solid foundation of relevant material for any nurse and in particular those registered nurses (RNs) who may be working in a children's area which is not familiar to them. It should serve as an excellent source of reference material throughout your degree and beyond.

This book was developed by a dedicated team of lecturers, practitioners, students and, of course, by children and their families/carers to support your study, practice and future continuing lifelong learning. All contributors have been keen to be involved because they know how important good nursing care is and are aware of the challenges you will face in providing quality care. Everyone involved in this book is passionate about providing you with the knowledge, skills and confidence to be the type of children's nurse who inspires and provides best evidence-based care to children and their families. In addition, we aim to enable you to create an environment for practice that prevents the negative situations you may see in the media from time to time.

The care of the child is first and foremost in all considerations; you will notice that the design and content of the book promote listening to what children tell us as well as signposting further information for you to read widely and deeply around topics. We recognise that no one text or resource can meet all your learning needs and for that reason this textbook uses a variety of features to lead you towards other evidence and learning opportunities, not least of which is respecting the needs, views and wishes of children, young people and their families at all times.

Eight key themes underpin the entire text:

1. Child- and family-centred care
2. Critical thinking and depth of theoretical thinking
3. Integration of acute and community care
4. Interprofessional working and collaboration
5. Evidence-based nursing
6. Preparation for practice placements
7. Health promotion
8. Safeguarding

These themes have been selected in consultation with a large number of course leaders in children's nursing degree programmes, and represent what they feel are essential areas of focus to be a successful children's nursing student. Keep these in mind and reflect on how you might develop your skills in these areas as you read through the text, and throughout your degree programme and practice placements.

Becoming a competent children's nurse is a long journey, and as students you are at the start. The contributors are all companions, and are at different stages of that journey. Their insight, experience and skills are freely shared with you to make you the best you can be as a children's nurse. The voices of children, young people and their families will serve as a reminder to keep them always at the heart of decisions and interventions. To care for children and young people is both a privilege and a big responsibility which will require you to be honest, transparent, inclusive and willing to be open to challenge and change. Advocacy and accountability are needed alongside excellent interpersonal and clinical skills.

A note on terminology: throughout the text we have usually referred to 'children' in place of the longer 'children and young people', and, in some cases, infants too. This is for the reason of brevity and to prevent repetition; however, in most cases (unless specified), the shorter term should be understood to refer to both children *and* young people. In the same way, the term 'family' should be understood to refer to family and/or carers.

We hope that this book will give you a great start in the practice of children's nursing. We wish you much joy and success in this wonderful field of nursing.

Professor Jayne Price
Orla McAlinden, RN Adult and Child
Zoë Veal, RN Child

PART 1   PRINCIPLES OF NURSING CHILDREN AND YOUNG PEOPLE

INVOLVING CHILDREN, YOUNG PEOPLE AND FAMILIES IN CARE

NICOLA MITCHELL, JOANNA SMITH AND JACKIE VASEY

1

THIS CHAPTER COVERS

- Social and political contexts underpinning the nursing care of children, young people, and families
- Involving children and young people, and families in care
- Family-centred care
- Child-centred care
- Key skills required when involving children, young people, and families in care

---

> "Historically, involving children and young people, as appropriate, and parents in care has not been embedded into everyday practice. In the 1990s parental participation in care was described as 'one of paediatric nursing's most amorphous and ill described concepts."
>
> **Darbyshire, 1993, p.1672.**

INTRODUCTION

Evidence suggests that involving children, young people and parents in care improves satisfaction with care and may have a positive impact on health outcomes for children and young people (Shields et al., 2012; Arabiat et al., 2018). Historically, involving children and young people, as appropriate, and parents in care has not been embedded into everyday practice. In the 1990s parental participation in care was described as 'one of paediatric nursing's most amorphous and ill described concepts' (Darbyshire, 1993, p.1672). A key role of the children's nurse includes supporting children, young people, and their families to be involved in care and care decisions; yet long-standing challenges to the implementation of family-centred care persist (Coyne, 2015; Arabiat et al., 2018; Kokorelias et al. 2019), which have been confounded by the COVID pandemic (Al-Motlaq et al., 2021; Goga et al., 2021).

While involving the whole family in the child's care is widely advocated, children have not always been encouraged to contribute to decisions about their care (Royal College of Paediatrics and Child Health (RCPCH), 2011). Children's nurses are in an ideal position to advocate on behalf of the child and enable children's views to be heard. While children's nurses will be familiar with the concept of family-centred care, a move towards a child-centred model of care could support children's nurses to foster a collaborative approach to working with children and young people. This chapter will explore both family-centred and child-centred care, and help you develop a critical approach when considering how to involve children, young people and families effectively in care.

ACTIVITY 1.1: CRITICAL THINKING

Research exploring parent-professional interactions found that the way information is communicated is not always conducive to involving families in care and care decisions (Smith, Cheater et al., 2015), highlighted in the followed extracts:

> I needed to know what was happening so I could let family know back at home. I was just having to guess because nobody told me anything. (*Admission 7, dad*)
> There is so much conflicting information really. They [doctors and nurses] do not seem to take on board what you are saying, that is my feeling. No, they really have their own agenda and that is what we are on now - their agenda. (*Admission 2, mum*, Smith, Cheater et al., 2015, p.1308)

- How can nurses ensure parents are fully informed about all aspects of their child's condition and care?
- What can nurses do to involve parents in care and care decisions?

Involvement in care and care decisions enables parents, children, and young people to contribute to choosing care interventions that meet their needs, and empowers them to contribute to the child's care (Shields et al., 2012). While both parents and health professionals expect to work in partnership, they often have different expectations and priorities, with parents often perceiving their contribution is not prioritised (Smith and Kendal, 2018). Furthermore, parents perceive their knowledge, experience, and expertise relating to their child is not always valued (Smith et al., 2015). Similarly, children and young people want to be part of decisions about them (Garnett et al., 2016). Giving children a voice enables them to develop a sense of self and improves their confidence and communication skills. In contrast, lack of involvement can lead to children and young people being fearful and anxious, and unprepared for procedures, and reduces their self-esteem (Coyne and Cowley, 2007).

SOCIAL AND POLITICAL CONTEXTS UNDERPINNING THE NURSING CARE OF CHILDREN, YOUNG PEOPLE AND FAMILIES

Understanding the historical and political contexts that influence children's nursing, and service and care delivery will help you to contextualise the changing role of the children's nurse in optimising the health and wellbeing of children. Care delivery is influenced by a range of factors, including: societal norms and values; national and international health policy and the allocation of health resources; changing disease profiles; technological advancements; and the impact of lifestyle choices on health. Children's health and wellbeing are often viewed as an important marker of a nation's wellbeing and prospects. Proportionally, children are high users of health services, yet the development of health services for children has historically been inconsistent.

One of the first hospitals specifically for children opened in Paris in 1802, with London's Great Ormond Street Hospital opening in the 1850s. Prior to this, children were often cared for alongside adults. Care specifically aimed at children began with dispensaries offering advice to mothers from poor backgrounds, who could not pay for medical care, and provided medicines for children, based on the belief that treatments for children would be best achieved by mothers caring for ill children at home. Despite promising developments during the early and mid-20th century, many children were admitted to hospital for extensive periods of time, often to recuperate from infectious diseases or minor surgery. Many wards nursed both adult patients and children, with restricted visiting for parents, and few nurses were trained in the specific needs of children.

Greater understanding about the impact of separating children from their families and reduced in-patient and institutional care influenced the approach to caring for children. The seminal work of Bowlby (1953) and Robertson (1958), a psychiatrist and psychoanalyst respectively, highlighted the emotional trauma of children when separated from their mothers. Although Bowlby's and Robertson's classical theories on young children's responses when separated from their mother have been criticised, they were a catalyst for change (Alsop-Shields and Mohay, 2001). The plight of children in hospital was highlighted in *The Welfare of Children in Hospital* report (Ministry of Health, 1959), commonly known as the 'Platt Report', which was heralded as one of the most influential documents of its time. Key messages included staff caring for children should understand child development, recognise the family's role when a child is in hospital and provide unrestricted visiting for parents (Smith and Long, 2002). Increased parental presence in hospital contributed to the impetus for parents to become more involved in their child's care.

In recent times, ensuring children and families can be together during hospital admissions has been threatened by the safety measures required during the COVID-19 pandemic. Guidance for visiting inpatient settings set by NHS England (2020) recognises parents as essential visitors, but healthcare organisations had greater discretion in how they implemented visiting polices. During the pandemic the many Trusts, including specialist children's hospitals, limited visiting to one parent. These measures focus on safety of COVID-19 transmission, but do not take account of the benefits of parental presence for both child and parent (Goga et al., 2021). Every attempt should be made to keep children, particularly neonates, and their families together (Tscherning et al., 2020; Goga et al., 2021).

Children with life-limiting conditions and complex health needs are now surviving into adulthood. The profile of childhood diseases, particularly in developed countries, significantly changed during the latter part of the 20th century, with a decline in the incidence and outcome of previously fatal communicable infectious diseases and an increase in long-term conditions. The management of children with long-term conditions, complex needs and those dependent on advanced technologies primarily takes place in the home environment, with the responsibility for monitoring symptoms and responding to changes in the child's condition becoming primarily the role of parents (Wang and Barnard,

2004). Consequently, the role of the nurse shifts from care provider to one of educator, supporter and advocate. Case study 1.1 outlines Amy's experience as a health visitor of supporting a family at home to care for their baby, Aisha, who had a life-limiting condition.

CASE STUDY 1.1: AISHA

While on the postnatal ward, establishing Aisha's feeding was challenging, causing her parents anxiety about taking Aisha home as they perceived there would be lack of support to ensure her nutritional needs would be met. In my role as health visitor, I ensured all members of the multidisciplinary team (hospital, community and hospice) along with Aisha's parents were aware of Aisha's needs, and established a plan of care and schedule of visits; a priority was for Aisha to spend as little time as possible in hospital and the number of home visits not to be intrusive.

As Aisha's parents became more confident in caring for her and learned her behavioural cues they were able to share this knowledge with nursing and medical staff and provided supportive care, with Aisha at the centre of all decisions. Health professionals were able to work collaboratively and in partnership with Aisha's parents; they did not initially want to carry out invasive procedures such as passing a nasogastric tube, which was respected. There was a gradual transition from professionals making most decisions about Aisha's care to transferring almost all care to parents as their skills and confidence grew. Right to the end of Aisha's life her parents were fully involved in all discussions and decisions about her care, with consideration to her siblings' needs throughout.

Aisha died at 4 months of age. At bereavement visits provided following Aisha's death her mother spoke with pride about Aisha's life and her amazement at the care that had been wrapped around her; her worries of being forgotten after leaving hospital were unfounded.

- What contributed to the success of the team in involving Aisha's parents in her care?
- Reflect on any similar experiences you have – what were the challenges and facilitators to involving the family in care?

INVOLVING CHILDREN AND YOUNG PEOPLE IN CARE AND CARE DECISIONS

The social constructs of childhood influence how children are viewed and beliefs about the abilities of children to participate in care decisions. Traditionally, society has been divided into two broad groups, namely childhood and adulthood, with the passage into adulthood synonymous with rights, privileges and obligations (Franklin, 1995). The concept of 'agency' is particularly relevant to the children's nurse and can be thought of in terms of the child's ability to reflect and act on information and an understanding that any decisions made have consequences (Mayall, 2002). The concept of child agency is complicated because children are often perceived as lacking adult reasoning and the cognitive capacity to participate in complex decisions.

The philosophical perspectives of paternalism, interventionalism and libertarianism can offer explanations about how individuals view the child's ability to participate in decisions and the rights bestowed on them (Franklin, 1995). Paternalists make choices on behalf of the child because they perceive that children are vulnerable and not capable of making autonomous rational decisions.

Interventionists assume it is the responsibility of the decision-maker to act in a child's best interests and while like paternalism, the power balance has shifted to the health professional. Evidence suggests that children want to be heard but view health professionals as interventionists who do not support their involvement in care decisions (O'Quigley, 2000).

Unlike paternalists, libertarians advocate that children can make informed choices and through experience would learn to contribute to decision-making processes (Franklin, 1995). Intuitively, a libertarian approach for a young child, who is unlikely to have the cognitive capacity to make complex healthcare decisions, seems inappropriate. However, young children can be involved in some choices about their care, which may depend on the relative importance of the decision. A more pragmatic approach to involving children and young people in care decisions is to be mindful of the differences in the way children think and process information. Children and young people should be supported to make decisions as appropriate and their participation in care valued, whilst recognising that the level of agency will evolve as the child matures (Mayall, 2002). Ravi Mistry, the Youth Advisory Panel Member at the Royal College of Paediatrics and Child Health (RCPCH), who actively promotes the inclusion of young people in healthcare, stated:

> Participation encourages integration and inclusion, lets youth feel valued and leads to progress. It is a right and should not be tokenistic, where services merely ask youth for their views just so they fit in with a trend. I would urge all to include the views of children and young people wherever possible, the benefits are clear. (Ravi Mistry, Youth Advisory Panel Member, RCPCH, 2011, p.3)

NICE (2021) guidance on babies, children and young people's experience of healthcare advocates that all who wish to be, are involved in decisions about their care. Children enjoy being involved in care decisions (Garnett et al., 2016), and it improves the relationship between children and health professionals because issues important to children are more likely to be addressed (RCPCH, 2011). Children and young people should be provided with age and developmentally appropriate information to help them be involved in decisions about them (NICE, 2021). Involvement in decisions is particularly important in the context of childhood long-term conditions, where the young person will be preparing to make the transition to adult services. Case study 1.2 highlights how Sarah perceived her son was involved in care on a Teenage Cancer Unit.

SEE ALSO
CHAPTERS 8
AND 12

CASE STUDY 1.2: ALEX

We were asked at the time of Alex's diagnosis, 'What do you want to tell Alex?' Al was 14-and-a-half years old, sensible, able to verbalise emotions and debate the rationale for decisions made. So we took the view he should be included in everything – nothing to be hidden from him. We did not want to have discussions in secret or whisper behind closed doors. Al could consent to everything himself, although we were all involved in the discussions about whether he would go on a drug trial treatment protocol or offered alternative options, and what the pros and cons for all care and treatments were so he (and we) could make informed decisions. Al was the one who knew how he was feeling and Al was the one to live with the consequences of decisions made so it seemed right he should be involved.

- How can nurses communicate effectively with children, young people and their families when breaking bad news or negotiating care?

SEE ALSO
CHAPTER 2

A shift from a paternalistic model of involving children and young people in care was reflected in the 1989 United Nations Convention on the Rights of the Child. Articles 12 and 13 are particularly relevant to children's nurses as they focus on children's right to participation, right to articulate an opinion and right to freedom of expression. For example, Article 12 states that 'the child who is capable of forming his or her own views has the right to express those views freely in all matters affecting the child: the views of the child being given due weight in accordance with age and maturity of the child' (United Nations, 1989). Children's nurses are often faced with a range of dilemmas in relation to involving children and young people in care. This may occur when the adults involved have differing opinions to children and young people about their care.

SAFEGUARDING STOP POINT

SEE ALSO
CHAPTER
34

The views of children or young people with a learning disability have not always been actively sought or valued (Council for Disabled Children, 2018). Yet these children are particularly vulnerable members of society.

FAMILY INVOLVEMENT IN CARE

Evidence suggests that parents want and expect to be involved in their child's care, share care decisions and work in collaboration with health professions but want choices about their level of involvement (Power and Franck, 2008; Smith et al., 2015). Parents who manage their child's care at home perceive that their expertise is not valued when their child is admitted to hospital (Smith et al., 2015). Involving parents in care can reduce their anxiety and feelings of helplessness when their child is acutely ill (Twycross and Stinson, 2014), and is essential when the child has a long-term condition and parents have responsibility for delivering treatments and care at home (Smith et al., 2015). Parental involvement in care is particularly salient for the pre-verbal child and children who have difficulties with communicating where parents' unique understanding of their child must be incorporated into care.

SEE ALSO
CHAPTER 2

WHAT'S THE EVIDENCE?

Research continues to identify that involving parents in their child's care is challenging, as highlighted in the evidence presented in Table 1.1; you may wish to discuss with peers and practice supervisors the reasons why implementing research about involving families in care in practice is challenging.

Table 1.1   Findings from studies about involving parents in their child's care

Author	Study aim	Key findings
Arabiat et al. (2018) Australia	Cross-sectional survey to understanding of how parents experience family-centred care	• Parents defined family-centred care as the family being included in the child's care, and health professionals supporting the whole family. • Although 85% of parents reported positive experiences of family-centred care, some parents did not perceive their contribution to care was valued or important.

Author	Study aim	Key findings
Smith and Kendal (2018), England	Qualitative study exploring parent and healthcare professionals' views of collaboration in care in the management of childhood long-term conditions	• Although parents and professionals agree that collaboration is needed, parents perceived their needs are often unmet. • Health professionals' expectations are influenced by their knowledge, experience, and relative objectivity. • Relationship-building and good communication are central components of collaboration.
Coyne (2015), Ireland	Qualitative study exploring children, their parents and health professionals' perspectives and expectations of family-centred care	• Family-centred care reduces children's distress when in hospital and improve the quality of care. • Nurses perceived that family-centred care was central to care delivery but the roles and boundaries between parent and nurse were unclear. • Family-centred care operated in the context of minimal collaboration or negotiation with parents.
Coyne et al. (2013), Ireland	Survey of nurses' perceptions and practices of family-centred care	• Family-centred care was central to valuing family individuality. • Family is a resource in providing information about the unique needs of the child. • Although nurses supported the philosophy of family-centred care they struggled to apply the principles to practice.
Macdonald et al. (2012), Canada	Observational study that explored the family's experience of family-centred care	• Embedding family-centred care into practice is challenging; differences exist in the way family-centred care operated between families and professionals. • Care practices should not solely rely on better information exchange but require health professionals to consider reducing the barriers to involving the family in care.
Sousa et al. (2013), Portugal	Survey of parents' perspectives about being involved in their child's care	• Gaining information about their child's condition was an overwhelming priority for parents. • Parents wanted to participate in their child's care but did not want to disrupt nursing routines. • Being present during their child's hospital stay was thought to be essential to their child's safety and wellbeing.
Uhl et al. (2013), USA	Mixed methods study exploring parents' experiences of family-centred care following their child's admission to hospital	• A child's admission to hospital is a stressful event, associated with uncertainty, fear and lack of control in relation to meeting their child's needs; involving parents in care can ameliorate their emotions, anxiety and stress • Characteristics valued by parents in health professionals included treating them with dignity, being courteous and actively listening to their concerns. • Information sharing was identified as central to involving parents in care.

Despite the development of a range of models and frameworks that aim to foster the family's involvement in care over the past two decades, concepts such as 'parental participation', 'partnership with parents' and 'family-centred care' remain poorly defined and are often used interchangeably (Hutchfield, 1999; Franck and Callery, 2004; Coyne et al., 2013; Smith, Swallow et al., 2015). Lack of clarity and understanding of terminology have contributed to poor implementation of these concepts into practice; how nurses develop effective partnerships with the child and their family. Establishing the level of involvement in care and decisions about care that children, young people and parents are willing and/or able to undertake is fundamental to working in partnership with the family. At times parents may have minimal involvement in their child's care – for example, on first contact with services or during emergency care, while at the opposite end of the spectrum parents may lead care – for example, in the context of childhood long-term conditions (Smith et al., 2010). However, being valued, experiencing effective information exchange and, if desired, being supported to undertake usual childcare activities, should be the minimal involvement parents can expect (Hutchfield, 1999). Individual family needs and preferences are unique and may change over time, reflecting changing levels of involvement in care. Table 1.2 highlights the relationship between the terminology associated with involving parents in care and levels of involvement.

Table 1.2 Levels of parental involvement in care

Hierarchy of care (Hutchfield, 1999)	Level of involvement (Smith et al., 2010)
Family-centred care • Parents lead care and are fully involved in all decision-making as equal partners. • Parents are expert and knowledgeable in all aspects of care for their child, which is respected. • The nurse's role is one of consultant and counsellor. • The child and other family members are involved in care.	**Parent, and child as appropriate, lead care** Family leads care with support from health professionals.
Partnership with parents • Parents have equal status as caregivers, are knowledgeable and have skills required to deliver care. • Parents are empowered to give care; parents and nurses negotiate roles parents undertake. • Parents are primary, but not total, caregivers. • Nurses support, advise and facilitate parents to care for their child.	**Parents and nurses work in partnership** Parents and nurses have equal status for care and in decisions about care delivery.
Parental participation • Parents participate in usual childcare and through negotiation undertake some aspects of nursing care. • Nurses remain responsible for ensuring all care is given, and often act as gatekeepers for the care parents undertake. • Nurses act as primary caregivers, but support and teach parents how to provide care as appropriate.	**Involvement of parents in care** The nurse involves parents in care but retains responsibility for care and leads care delivery.
Parental involvement • Nurses respect parents as a constant in the child's life and their unique knowledge of their child. • Nurses provide care and support parents to undertake usual childcare and emotional support to their child. • Nurses ensure parents have appropriate information and are advocates for the child and family.	**No/minimal involvement of parents in care** The nurse leads and delivers care.

Partnership in care

You may be familiar with the 'partnership in care model of paediatric nursing', widely adopted within the UK, as the underpinning philosophy for the care of children (Casey, 1995). Central to the model was the interconnected relationship between the four dimensions associated with nursing: person (or in this case child and family), health, environment, and nursing. The model emphasised that care is best undertaken by the family with support from skilled health professionals by empowering parents, and children and young people as appropriate, to contribute to care (Casey, 1995). However, there were concerns that a shift from parent involvement to one of partnership occurred in the absence of the essential component of negotiation, and that parents may not have been empowered to become responsible for delivering treatments and care, but expected to undertake new roles delegated to them by the nurse (Coyne, 1996).

Parent participation in care has been widely researched in hospital settings with key findings suggesting: a coercive system of involving parents exists that hinders the development of effective parent–professional partnerships (Corlett and Twycross, 2006); parents being disempowered with care delegated to them by health professionals, resulting in anxiety when undertaking complex care tasks (Coyne and Cowley, 2007); and different perspectives about what constitutes collaboration and participation between parents and health professionals (Power and Franck, 2008). For participation to be meaningful, health professionals need to understand parents' perspectives (Power and Franck, 2008), which can be challenging because healthcare is increasingly varied with patients' expectations, experiences, knowledge of health and health-related issues, and the degree they wish to participate in care, being highly diverse. Although partnership in care has been positioned as a philosophy underpinning the care of children and young people (Casey, 1995), there is increasing consensus that partnership in care is a central component of family-centred care (Shields et al., 2012; Smith, Swallow et al., 2015).

Family-centred care

The Institute for Patient- and Family-Centered Care (2017, p.2) defines family-centred care as 'an approach to the planning, delivery, and evaluation of healthcare that is grounded in mutually beneficial partnerships among healthcare providers, patients, and families'. Family-centred care both guides care based on recognising the importance of the family in optimising the child's health and wellbeing and is a philosophy that shapes policy and health services (Shields et al., 2012). The eight core elements central to family-centred care developed by the American Association for the Care of Children's Health (Harrison, 2010, p.336) are:

SEE ALSO
CHAPTER 6

1. Recognition that the family is the constant in a child's life is incorporated into child health policy.
2. Facilitating family/professional collaboration at all levels of hospital, home, and community care.
3. Exchanging complete and unbiased information between families and professionals.
4. Honouring cultural diversity, strengths, and individuality within and across all families, including ethnic, racial, spiritual, social, economic, educational, and geographic diversity.
5. Recognising and respecting different ways of coping and providing developmental, educational, emotional, environmental, and financial supports to meet diverse needs.
6. Encouraging and facilitating family-to-family support and networking.
7. Ensuring that hospital, home, and community service and support systems for children needing specialised health and developmental care and their families are flexible, accessible, and comprehensive in responding to diverse family-identified needs.
8. Recognising families have strengths, concerns, emotions, and aspirations beyond their need for specialised health and developmental services and support.

Embracing family-centred care requires that nurses caring for children view the family as an integral part of the child's life (Smith et al., 2010), which is reflected in the way care is organised, planned, delivered, and evaluated around the whole family (Shields et al., 2012; Coyne et al., 2013). While many children's nurses endorse family-centred care and are passionate about involving families in care, evidence suggests that family-centred care is not consistently and effectively embedded into practice (Shields et al., 2012; Coyne et al., 2013). Furthermore, there is a lack of robust evidence to support the impact of family-centred care on the health of children and the impact on the child and family experiences (Shields et al., 2012). Consequently, family-centred care has been criticised for being espoused rather than embedded into care delivery (Coyne et al., 2013). Lack of understanding of how to implement and embed family-centred care into practice hinders parental involvement in care. Nurses need to adopt the principles of empowerment, negotiation, and participation, to actively involve parents in their child's care (Smith et al., 2010).

Activity 1.2 helps you to consider ways to work in partnership with children, young people, and families.

ACTIVITY 1.2: CRITICAL THINKING

- What is meant by the term 'family'?
- What is patient- and family-centred healthcare?
- What is family nursing and how does this differ from family-centred care?
- How does family-centred care relate to nursing and nursing practice?

Think about the questions above and discuss with peers.

KEY SKILLS REQUIRED WHEN INVOLVING CHILDREN, YOUNG PEOPLE AND FAMILIES IN CARE AND CARE DECISIONS

Valuing children's, young people's and parents' contribution is central to their involvement in care decisions. The relationship between the family and health professional must be based on developing mutual trust and respecting each other's skills, experiences, and perspectives. Facilitating partnership working requires nurses to move away from a paternalistic approach and work to actively reduce the power imbalance between them and parents. Involving parents as partners in care requires health professionals to recognise and embrace parents' unique knowledge of their child and incorporate that knowledge into clinical decisions (Smith, Cheater et al., 2015). The principles of involving children, young people and families in care and care decisions include:

- Developing a trusting relationship with the child and family by getting to know the family, and valuing their knowledge and experiences.
- Respecting and being sensitive to the individual family context.
- Focusing on problem-based communications by listening and responding to the child and family's concerns and drawing on their expertise.
- Providing regular opportunities for a mutual exchange of information that is meaningful and delivered in a way that meets the child and family's needs.
- Facilitating children and parents to be involved in the child's care; clarifying and negotiating roles to reach a mutual agreement about care responsibilities.
- Including children and parents as members of the interdisciplinary care team and valuing their contribution.
- Collaborating and sharing decisions about care; maintaining contact and offering ongoing support (Smith, Cheater et al., 2015; Smith, Swallow et al., 2015).

Effective communication with children and families enables them to make informed choices about their involvement in care and the delivery of treatments (Smith et al., 2010).

SEE ALSO
CHAPTER 2

CHILD-CENTRED CARE

Children's nurses must advocate for children and young people and ensure they have opportunity to participate in care, and that they and their families are central to care decisions. Child-centred care is an approach to care that places the child and their interests at the heart of healthcare practice and reflects the rights of children to participate in care and care decisions (Carter et al., 2014). The concept of child-centred care has been gaining international momentum because of widespread acknowledgement that children should be included and participate in decisions about them (Ford, Campbell et al., 2018). Child-centred care is not mutually exclusive with family-centred care but can be thought of as being complementary to family-centred care (Carter et al., 2014). Both models recognise the social and cultural contexts that shape children's lives and influence their health and wellbeing. However, child-centred care differs from family-centred care in that there is greater emphasis on the concerns of the child and young person, which may not be the same as those of their parents or health professionals (Soderback et al., 2011) and acknowledges children as having agency (Carter et al., 2014), as previously outlined. Family-centred care is typically framed around collaboration between parent/s and health professionals, with the child or young person often the passive partner even when they have capability to make decisions (Ford, Campbell et al., 2018). In contrast, in child-centred care the child's concerns and needs are the primary focus of care.

The core principles of family-centred care, previously outlined, such as complete and unbiased information sharing, valuing the family as constant, facilitating parent–professional collaboration, and empowering the family to be partners in care, and respecting the cultural diversity of families (Smith, Swallow et al., 2015) are equally important when adopting a child-centred philosophy of care. However, the values underpinning child-centred care include:

- Placing children's needs and their best interests at the centre of all care decisions.
- Recognising children and young people as individuals, albeit part of a wider family.
- Listening to and supporting children, irrespective of age and ability to express their views.
- Recognising that children's views are not always the same as those of their parents/carers.
- Understanding children and young people's perspectives of health and illness.
- Positioning the child or young person as the central member of the family–health professional partnership.
- Supporting and providing opportunities and space to enable children and young people to be active participants in their care and involving them in decision-making processes.
- Respecting children and young people's privacy and dignity.

(Soderback et al., 2011; Carter et al., 2014)

Children and young people need support to develop the confidence and communications skills to participate in decisions about their health in consultation with health professionals. Interventions to promote participation in consultations and support young people to develop communication skills when interacting with health professionals are emerging with positive outcomes (Milnes et al., 2014). The extent to which children can be fully involved in care depends on their age and developmental stage. Young children have the capacity to make complex decisions about the management of their condition, but many children want to share decisions with parents (Garnett et al., 2016). Although children want to be involved in decisions that impact on them, a UK national survey of almost 19,000 children's experiences of being in hospital identified that 43% of 12-year-olds felt they were not fully involved in decisions about their care (Care Quality Commission, 2015). Involving children and young people to participate in care and care decisions requires health professionals to hear, value and appreciate their views, which can be achieved by:

- Providing age-appropriate information for the child to express their views.
- Allowing children to tell the 'whole story' without interrupting.
- Remaining open-minded and non-judgemental.
- Viewing children's abilities and competencies as being different rather than of less importance to those of adults.
- Being alert to signs of distress in the child.
- Being aware of the impact of developmental and cultural factors, and that some children will not want to be involved in care and care decisions.
- Assuring or clearly identifying limits of confidentiality.

(O'Quigley, 2000)

Below, Georgia, a 3rd-year student nurse at the time of writing, shares her experience of implementing child-centred care for a young person.

CASE STUDY 1.3: GEORGIA

Throughout my child nursing degree, I gained theoretical learning around a range of aspects of nursing practice, including mental health and psychology when caring for children and young people. While working in practice, I was able to implement my knowledge and understanding of the recognition, management, and treatment of children with mental health illness. During my second year I undertook a placement within the Children and Adolescent Mental Health Service (CAMHS), where support and care is provided to children, young people with their mental health illness and their families. While working within the CAMHS service I learned the importance of understanding the child as a whole and not focusing just on their mental health illness. In one episode of care, I accompanied a consultant psychiatrist who was reviewing a young person with a history of self-harm and suicidal ideations and struggled to communicate their feelings and emotions, finding it difficult to open to health professionals. Whilst talking to the young person, I was able to introduce normal conversation that did not focus solely on their mood that day or their mental health, but a chance to talk about day-to-day things and find out more about them as a person. Building this relationship enabled the young person to become comfortable to share some of their experiences of living with their mental health and its impact on their daily life. During this experience, I learned the importance of gaining insight about the person as an individual, as well as understanding the impact of their mental health illness. It is essential when caring for children and young people to help them to manage their emotions, thoughts and feelings and provide tools that work for the individual, and tailored coping strategies.

- Georgia outlines useful strategies to develop therapeutic relationships with young people. Consider how you may do this with children of other age groups, for example preschool children or early adolescence.

FUTURE DIRECTIONS

While family-centred care has evolved and developed over time, implementation remains problematic (Shields, 2015; Kokorelias et al., 2019), which has been attributed to unclear roles and boundaries between parents and health professionals, entrenched professional practices and attitudes towards working with families, and lack of organisational or managerial guidelines aimed at supporting the implementation of patient-centred care (Smith, Swallow et al., 2015). In addition, although there is an extensive amount of literature, and research on family-centred care, evidence in relation to health outcomes for the child and family is limited (Shields, 2015). Research has primarily focused on obser-vations of parent–nurse interactions, perspective of parents or family caregivers, and perspective of health professionals, and primarily in hospital settings (Harrison, 2010). While family-centred care is multifaceted and the complexity of attributing improved health outcomes specifically to family-centred care makes undertaking intervention studies challenging, additional research is needed to explore the outcomes for families, children and healthcare professionals, across care contexts, of family-centred care.

Child-centred care is a relatively new concept, and therefore children's nurses and child-focused researchers could work together to ensure child-centred care has a sound and robust evidence base and does not succumb to the criticisms of family-centred care. Current research is focusing on defin-ing child-centred care and identifying its conceptual boundaries (Ford, Campbell et al., 2018), and researchers are already developing measures of child-centred care such as a self-reported psychosocial, physical, and emotional needs questionnaire for children in hospital (Foster et al., 2019).

Globally, healthcare delivery is shifting from treating acute illness to supporting people who man-age with long-term conditions, necessitating health professionals to move from a position of care prescriber to one of collaborator, working in partnership with individuals and their families. Shared decision-making has gained prominence in clinical practice and is based on the premise that the patient has unique experiences and insights, while health professionals have experiences and knowl-edge of care in similar situations, with the aim that treatment and care decisions are mutually agreed (Entwistle, 2009). Empowering patients to self-manage their care has the potential to improve health outcomes; patients are more likely to respond and act on illness symptoms, use medicines and treat-ments more effectively, have greater understanding of the implications of professional advice and are better able to cope with their condition (Coulter et al., 2008). Shared decision-making has relevance for individuals with long-term conditions because the day-to-day care and management of their condi-tion becomes primarily their responsibility and/or their families' responsibility.

———————— CHAPTER SUMMARY ————————

- Involving and supporting children and young people, as appropriate, and their families in care and care decisions should be embedded within children's nursing
- The models and frameworks to support children's nurses to work effectively with children, young people and families appear difficult to embed into everyday practice
- However, the underpinning principles of involvement are essential to effective care delivery and include: valuing parents' expertise and knowledge about their child; forming effective partner-ships with the child and family; facilitating the child and family to participate in care delivery
- Successful involvement as highlighted in this chapter can be achieved through the process of negotiation, empowerment, and shared goal-setting, and ensuring effective information provi-sion to enable the child and family to collaborate in care decisions

BUILD YOUR BIBLIOGRAPHY

Books

FURTHER
READING

- Carter, B., Bray, L., Dickinson, A., Edwards, M. and Ford, K. (2014) *Child Centred Nursing: Promoting Critical Thinking*. London: Sage.

  Provides varied and contemporary perspectives on involving children and young people in their care.

- Smith, L. and Coleman, V. (eds) (2010) *Child and Family-Centred Healthcare: Concept, Theory and Practice*. 2nd ed. Basingstoke: Palgrave Macmillan.

  This book provides a useful introduction to the concept of child and family-centred care from a range of perspectives against the backdrop of child healthcare in the UK.

Journal articles

FURTHER
READING:
ONLINE
JOURNAL
ARTICLES

These articles will help you to explore some key concepts of child and family involvement in care and decision-making.

- Arabiat, D., Whitehead, L., Foster, M., Shields, L. and Harris, L. (2018) 'Parents' experiences of Family Centred Care practices'. *Journal of Pediatric Nursing*, 42: 39–44.

- Coyne, I. (2015) 'Families and health-care professionals' perspectives and expectations of family-centred care: hidden expectations and unclear roles'. *Health Expectations*, 18 (5): 796–808.

- Ford, K., Dickinson, A., Water, T., Campbell, S., Bray, L., and Carter, B. (2018) 'Child centred care: challenging assumptions and repositioning children and young people'. *Journal of Pediatric Nursing*, 43, e39–e43.

Weblinks

FURTHER
READING:
WEBLINKS

- www.nice.org.uk/guidance/ng204 NICE guideline making recommendations on providing a good patient experience for babies, children, and young people.

- www.ipfcc.org – Institute for Patient- and Family-Centered Care Website designed for health professionals, children, and families as a resource to highlight the importance of child and family participation in healthcare decisions and delivery. The Institute for Patient- and Family-Centered Care (IPFCC) is an American-based non-profit organisation founded in 1992 and aims to enhance understanding and practice of patient- and family-centred care. IPFCC serves as a central resource for policy-makers and patient and family leaders.

- https://incfcc.weebly.com/ – website detailing the work of The International Network for Child and Family Centred Care (INCFCC). The International Network for Child and Family Centred Care is a collaboration of experts from around the world who work together in research, practice development and education on the topic of child- and family-centred care.

REFERENCES

Al-Motlaq, M., Neill, S., Foster, M. J., Coyne, I., Houghton, D., Angelhoff, C., Rising-Holmström, M. and Majamanda, M. (2021) 'Position Statement of the International Network for Child and Family Centred Care: Child and Family Centered Care during the COVID19 Pandemic'. *Journal of Pediatric Nursing*, 61: 140–3.

Alsop-Shields, L. and Mohay, H. (2001) 'John Bowlby and James Robertson: theorists, scientists and crusaders for improvements in the care of children in hospital'. *Journal of Advanced Nursing*, 35 (1): 50–8.

Arabiat, D., Whitehead, L., Foster, M., Shields, L. and Harris, L. (2018) 'Parents' experiences of Family Centered Care practices'. *Journal of Pediatric Nursing*, 42: 39–44.

Bowlby, J. (1953) *Child Care and the Growth of Love*. Harmondsworth: Penguin.

Care Quality Commission (2015) *Children and Young People's Inpatient and Day Case Survey 2014 – Key Findings*. London: Care Quality Commission.

Carter, B., Bray L., Dickinson, A., Edwards, M. and Ford, K. (2014) *Child-Centered Nursing: Promoting Critical Thinking*. London: Sage.

Casey, A. (1995) 'Partnership nursing: influences on involvement of informal carers'. *Journal of Advanced Nursing*, 22: 1058–62.

Corlett, J. and Twycross, A. (2006) 'Negotiation of parental roles within family-centered care: a review of the literature'. *Journal of Clinical Nursing*, 15: 1308–14.

Coulter, A., Parsons, S. and Askham, J. (2008) *Where Are the Patients in Decision-Making about Their Own Care?* Copenhagen: WHO.

Council for Disabled Children (2018) Barriers to Participation: A Transforming Care Partners Resource. Available at: https://councilfordisabledchildren.org.uk/resources/all-resources/filter/information-and-advocacy-families/barriers-participation (accessed 11 January 2023).

Coyne, I. (1996) 'Parent participation: a concept analysis'. *Journal of Advanced Nursing*, 23: 733–40.

Coyne, I. (2015) 'Families and health-care professionals' perspectives and expectations of family-centered care: hidden expectations and unclear roles'. *Health Expectations*, 18 (5): 796–808.

Coyne, I. and Cowley, S. (2007) 'Challenging the philosophy of partnership with parents: a grounded theory study'. *International Journal of Nursing Studies*, 44: 893–904.

Coyne, I., Murphy, M., Costello, T., O'Neill, C. and Donnellan, C. (2013) 'A survey of nurses' practices and perceptions of family-centered care in Ireland'. *Journal of Family Nursing*, 19: 469–88.

Darbyshire, P. (1993) 'Parents, nurses and paediatric nursing: a critical review'. *Journal of Advanced Nursing*, 18: 1670–80.

Entwistle, V. (2009) 'Patient involvement in decision-making: the importance of a broad conceptualization'. in A. Edwards and G. Elwyn (eds), *Shared Decision-Making in Health Care: Achieving Evidence-Based Patient Choice*. Oxford: Oxford University Press. pp. 17–22.

Ford, K., Campbell, S., Carter, B. and Earwaker L. (2018) 'The concept of child-centered care in healthcare: a scoping review protocol'. *JBI Database of Systematic Reviews and Implementation Reports*, 16 (4): 845–51.

Foster, M., Whitehead, L. and Arabiat D. (2019) 'Development and validation of the needs of children questionnaire: an instrument to measure children's self-reported needs in hospital'. *Journal of Advanced Nursing*, 75 (10): 2246-58.

Franck, L.S. and Callery, P. (2004) 'Re-thinking family-centered care across the continuum of children's healthcare'. *Child: Care, Health and Development*, 30 (3): 265–77.

Franklin, B. (1995) *The Handbook of Children's Rights: Comparative Policy and Practice*. London: Routledge.

Garnett, V., Smith, J. and Ormnady, P. (2016) 'Child–parent shifting and shared decision-making for asthma management – a qualitative interview based study'. *Nursing Children and Young People*, 28 (4): 16–22.

Goga, A., Feucht, U., Pillay, S., Reubenson, G., Jeena, P., Mahdi, S., Mayet, N.T., Velaphi, S., McKerrow, N., Mathiva, L.R. and Makubalo, N. (2021) 'Parental access to hospitalised children during infectious disease pandemics such as COVID-19'. *South African Medical Journal*, 111 (2): 100–5.

Harrison, T.M. (2010) 'Family-centered pediatric nursing care: state of the science'. *Journal of Pediatric Nursing*, 25: 335–43.

Hutchfield, K. (1999) 'Family-centered care: a concept analysis'. *Journal of Advanced Nursing*, 29: 1178–87.

Institute for Patient- and Family-Centered Care (IPFCC) (2017) *Advancing the Practice of Patient and Family-Centered Care in Hospital Settings*. Bethesda, MD: Institute for Patient- and Family-Centered Care. Available at: www.ipfcc.org/resources/getting_started.pdf (accessed 19 June 2017).

Kokorelias, K.M., Gignac, M.A.M., Naglie, G. and Cameron, J.I. (2019) 'Towards a universal model of family centered care: a scoping review'. *BMC Health Services Research*, 19: 564.

Macdonald, M.E., Liben, S., Carnevale, F.A. and Cohen, S.R. (2012) 'An office or a bedroom? Challenges for family-centered care in the pediatric intensive care unit'. *Journal of Child Health Care*, 16: 237–49.

Mayall, B. (2002) *Towards a Sociology of Childhood: Thinking from Children's Lives*. Buckingham: Open University Press.

Milnes, L.J., Mcgowan, L., Campbell, M. and Callery, P. (2014) 'A qualitative evaluation of a pre-consultation guide intended to promote the participation of young people in asthma review consultations'. *Patient Education and Counselling*, 91: 91–6.

Ministry of Health and Central Health Services Council (1959) *The Welfare of Children in Hospital. Platt Report*. London: HMSO.

National Institute for Health and Care Excellence (NICE) (2021) *Babies, Children and Young People's Experience of Healthcare*. Available at: www.nice.org.uk/guidance/ng204 (accessed 23 January 2023).

NHS England (2020) Visiting healthcare inpatient settings during the COVID-19 pandemic: principles. Available at: www.england.nhs.uk/coronavirus/publication/visitor-guidance/ (accessed 18 February 2021).

O'Quigley, A. (2000) *Listening to Children's Views*. York: Joseph Rowntree Foundation.

Power, N. and Franck, L. (2008) 'Parent participation in the care of hospitalised children: a systematic review'. *Journal of Advanced Nursing*, 62 (6): 622–41.

Robertson, J. (1958) *Young Children in Hospital*. London: Tavistock Publications.

Royal College of Paediatrics and Child Health (RCPCH) (2011) *Involving Children and Young People in Health Services*. London: Royal College of Paediatrics and Child Health.

Shields, L. (2015) 'What is "Family-Centered Care"?' *European Journal of Person Centered Healthcare*, 3 (2):139–44.

Shields, L., Zhou, H., Pratt, J., Taylor, M., Hunter, J. and Pascoe, E. (2012) 'Family-centered care for hospitalised children aged 0–12 years'. *Cochrane Database of Systematic Reviews*, DOI:10.1002/14651858.CD004811.pub3.

Smith, J. and Kendal, S. (2018) 'Parents' and health professionals' views of collaboration in the management of childhood long-term conditions'. *Journal of Pediatric Nursing*, 43: 36–44.

Smith, J. and Long, T. (2002) 'Confusing rhetoric with reality: achieving a balanced skill mix of nurses working with children'. *Journal of Advanced Nursing*, 40 (3): 258–66.

Smith, J., Cheater, F., Bekker, H. and Chatwin, J. (2015) 'Are parents and professionals making shared decisions about a child's care on presentation of a suspected shunt malfunction? A mixed method study'. *Health Expectations*, 18 (5): 1299–315.

Smith, L., Coleman, V. and Bradshaw, M. (2010) 'Family-centered care: A practice continuum', in L. Smith and V. Coleman (eds), *Child and Family-Centered Healthcare: Concept, Theory and Practice*, 2nd ed. Basingstoke: Palgrave.

Smith, J., Swallow, V. and Coyne, I. (2015) 'Involving parents in managing their child's long-term condition – a concept synthesis of family-centered care and partnership-in-care'. *Journal of Pediatric Nursing*, 30 (1): 143–59.

Soderback, M., Coyne, I. and Harder M. (2011) 'The impact of including both a child perspective and the child's perspective within health care settings to provide truly child-centered care'. *Journal of Child Health Care*, 15 (2): 99–106.

Sousa, P., Antunes, A., Carvalho, J. and Casey, A. (2013) 'Parental perspectives on negotiation of their child's care in hospital'. *Nursing Children and Young People*, 25: 24–8.

Tscherning, C., Sizun, J. and Kuhn, P. (2020) 'Promoting attachment between parents and neonates despite the COVID19 pandemic'. *Acta Paediatrica*, 109 (10): 1937–43.

Twycross, A. and Stinson, J. (2014) 'Physical and psychological methods of pain relief in children', in A. Twycross, S. Dowden and J. Stinson (eds), *Managing Pain in Children: A Clinical Guide for Nurses and Healthcare Professionals*, 2nd ed. Chichester: Wiley Blackwell.

Uhl, T., Fisher, K., Docherty, S.L. and Brandon, D.H. (2013) 'Insights into patient and family-centered care through the hospital experiences of parents'. *Journal of Obstetric, Gynaecologic and Neonatal Nursing*, 42: 121–31.

United Nations (1989) *Convention on the Rights of the Child (UNCRC)*. Available at: www.unicef.org.uk/what-we-do/un-convention-child-rights (accessed 6 June 2023).

Wang, K. and Barnard, A. (2004) 'Technology dependent children and their families: a review'. *Journal of Advanced Nursing*, 54 (1): 36–46.

EFFECTIVE COMMUNICATION WITH CHILDREN AND YOUNG PEOPLE

2

ORLA McALINDEN, ADAPTED FROM JEAN SHAPCOTT

THIS CHAPTER COVERS

- Developmental aspects of communication
- Communication in the context of family-centred care – the triad of communication
- Play as a means of communication
- Communicating with children in difficult circumstances
- Communicating using technology and social media

> " "When I told my parents that I was going to try to get into children's nursing (I was already a qualified adult nurse), my mother's response was classic – 'You're only doing that so that you can play all day and get paid for it'! In many ways she wasn't far wrong – OK, not every minute of every day is spent playing, but there is an element of play in almost every interaction that a nurse has with a child or young person and that is what makes every situation encountered by a children's nurse different."
>
> **Sadia, children's nurse** "

INTRODUCTION

Children have a right to be involved in all decisions that involve them and their healthcare (United Nations, 1989; Clarke, 2015; Kennan et al., 2019). Children must therefore receive adequate and appropriate information in order to enable them to make sense of their situation. Inability to fully understand does not justify lack of discussion with a child who wishes to be involved in their care. Opportunities for interactions provided by undertaking assessments, providing advice and information, and facilitating the expression of feelings can only be successful if children's nurses fully understand how communicative abilities develop in children and use developmentally appropriate language (Hayes and Keogh, 2012; Dryden and Greenshields, 2020). In addition, for successful and effective communication with children it is necessary to establish a good relationship with them, even when the healthcare encounter is short, since the development of therapeutic relationships between nurses, children and their families is a fundamental principle of children's nursing, especially in a rapidly changing world with new challenges as well as old (Clarke, 2015, 2022; Roberts et al., 2015; Shack et al., 2020; Charney and Camarata, 2021).

Working with children requires imperative active engagement with families in order to help them cope with the reality of illness and its consequences. Communication occurs both formally and informally in healthcare settings. While adults frequently communicate in a neutral and objective manner while gathering or imparting facts as they seek to find solutions, children are more likely to communicate when they are engaged and busy with another activity (Lambert et al., 2011; Coyne et al., 2018). Children respond better to nurses who display warm, caring, engaging and trusting behaviours as well as clear and developmentally appropriate verbal language. Children themselves have individual characteristics that are expressed both verbally and non-verbally in the way they speak, use gestures and apply and respond to touch. This can be observed in their play as well as other formal and informal interactions and is an important element of child-centred care (Coyne et al., 2018).

This chapter will enable you to explore a range of aspects of communicating with children and their families. Developmentally appropriate communication is essential if interactions with children and young people are to be effective (Coyne, 2015), but it is also important to consider the role of the child when those interactions are triadic (three-way). The quotation from a practitioner at the start of the chapter shows how some lay people might see play simply as a means of occupying a child, but it is, in fact, a really important communication tool for the children's nurse (Diaz-Rodriguez et al., 2021). Not all communication with children and families is easy – for many reasons it is often complex and sometimes difficult; one aspect often seen as particularly challenging, breaking bad news, will be explored in the chapter. Finally, it is impossible to consider communication in 21st-century children's nursing without addressing technology and social media, which can be very useful but may also create problems, as noted in the safeguarding concern identified within the chapter.

DEVELOPMENTAL ASPECTS OF COMMUNICATION

In order to maximise opportunities presented by interactions with children and young people it is essential that children and young people's nurses understand child development, as communication techniques vary according to the age and developmental stage a child has reached (Hayes and Keogh, 2012; Boyd and Bee, 2019). The psychosocial conflicts and type of thinking (Mooney, 2013) which are present in every stage of development influence the way in which children perceive healthcare encounters, which can lead to age-specific fears, misconceptions and other psychosocial issues, all of

SEE ALSO
CHAPTER 12

which can have an impact on communication (Desai and Pandya, 2013). In recent years this can be seen when looking at how children and young people experience care interventions and novel critical healthcare crises such as COVID-19 (Charney and Camerata, 2021).

Development of language and communicative ability

SEE ALSO
CHAPTER 11

Optimal development of communication skills in infancy depends on a range of intrinsic and extrinsic factors in the life of a child. Intrinsic factors are those 'pre-programmed', often biological, influences that arise from within the children themselves and about which very little can be done. Extrinsic factors include issues such as mother-to-child attachment and the social environment in which the child grows up (Prior et al., 2008; Boyd and Bee, 2019).

One of the very first forms of social interaction involves crying, through which the infant seeks to gain the attention of others to have their needs met. In their first months, infants rapidly learn that the gaze and looking behaviour of others contains vital information from which relationships with others can begin to form. In addition, they can also recognise the emotions of those close to them through facial expression. Around the age of 6 or 7 months, infants begin babbling and using vocal utterances, in addition to crying, to gain the attention of others (Boyd and Bee, 2019).

Typically, children pass through three phases of communication development (Brown and Elder, 2014; Boyd and Bee, 2019). The first of these is known as intentional communication and involves the use of vocalisation. The very early stage of this is seen in the final months of infancy when babies begin to gesture to express their needs or wants.

The second stage is symbolic communication, where toddlers and young children begin to use early language to interact with others, gain attention and meet needs. Children at this age engage in three types of behaviours that assist in the development of communication: social and language skills, namely participation in motor imitation; joint attention; and symbolic play. Joint attention is the capacity to engage in coordinated social interaction (Beuker et al., 2013; Boyd and Bee, 2019). This includes sharing attention, for example, through the use of alternating gaze, following the attention of others by, for example, following where another person is pointing, and directing the attention of another.

A sophisticated phase of communication development is linguistic communication, in which children and young people can engage in full discourse with another person using many forms of communication, which is seen in late childhood and adolescence. Whatever a child or young person's stage of communication development, children's nurses need to be able to communicate effectively with those in their care. This final phase may be seen by many as the point where communication becomes easier, but other phases of development must also be addressed, as can be seen in Table 2.1, adapted from Brown and Elder (2014).

Table 2.1 Communication and development

Early communication skill	Description	Development
Sharing attention	A triadic interaction involving the infant alternating their gaze between the adult and an object with the intention of integrating attention to the person and the object into one interaction	Sharing attention emerges around 9 months of age

Early communication skill	Description	Development
Following attention	Following the direction of the gaze or manual pointing gesture of an adult to an external object	6 months: following the head movement of an adult with their eyes or turning their head in the appropriate direction Until 12 months: fixating on the first object along the path being followed by the infant's gaze, even if it is not the target object 12-18 months: more and longer joint attention and is now able to follow attention to objects outside their visual feed Following a manual pointing gesture tends to emerge before following a gaze
Directing attention	By showing, giving, reaching and/or pointing with a clear imperative or declarative intention, the infant directs the attention of others towards objects or situations	The first declarative and imperative gestures with or without gaze alternation emerge around 9 months and become more frequent between 12 and 15 months
Language	Making sounds, speaking and understanding words to become a system of communication	First year of life: babbling and cooing 12 months: first simple words 18 months: productive vocabulary of 10-20 words 2 years: words represent or symbolise actions, objects and thoughts; productive vocabulary grows to around 100 words

Developmentally appropriate communication

Children's nurses need to be able to adapt their communication to the developmental needs of the children in their care. Crying is a powerful pre-verbal signal that infants use to communicate and gain an immediate response. Even at this very early age, it is important to be aware of cultural and family norms for responding to crying, noting how parents respond to their baby's crying behaviour, but generally nurses should respond to crying in a timely manner. A soothing and calming tone when talking to a baby helps to allay their anxiety (and that of their parents) and can be effective in stopping them crying. All children and young people's nurses are expected to have excellent communication strategies with children throughout the lifespan and time spent perfecting this skill is well spent, and will certainly not go unnoticed by familes and their children; it is also a key competency for all children and young people's nurses (NMC, 2018b).

Toddlers (1–3 years) should be approached carefully as they are often fearful of strangers. Time spent observing a toddler with their parent is time well spent as they become used to the nurse's presence and gradually accept them into their communicative world. Children of this age often have their own particular words for objects and actions and it is important for the nurse to familiarise him/herself with these so that the toddler feels heard and understood.

Children between the ages of 3 and 5 years like to establish good relationships with adults and peers. They are curious and love to explore and create, so play (which will be addressed later in this chapter) is an important means of communication with this age group. It is important to be honest with children of this age and use simple connected terms when talking to them since, despite their growing vocabulary, the ability to understand complex sentences should not be assumed.

School-age children can utilise material presented in the form of age-appropriate diagrams, illustrations and books. Third-party stories can be used effectively to gather information, such as asking, 'How might you …?' or 'Do you think that …?', particularly when direct questioning, careful observation or informal chatting are not working. This less direct approach can enable children to voice concerns or ask questions they may not otherwise have felt able to do.

Communications with children who cannot verbalise or read or who have any cognitive or sensory deficit, for whatever reason, poses immense issues for the child and family. Excellence in communication is no less a right for these children and families (United Nations, 1989) and will involve the best of child- and family-centred care (Coyne, 2015, 2018) to ensure optimum alternative strategies are used appropriately as needed and that all information resources and needs are pitched to meet the needs of the child and young person (Makaton, British Sign language, visual and audio enhancements, Story Boards and using advanced novel technologies) (Vinales, 2013; Holt et al., 2017; Franklin and Goff, 2019; Phulwari et al., 2021).

CASE STUDY 2.1: TONI

Toni is 6 years old. She has a chronic renal condition whereby she has only recently started gaining bladder control and, even now, when she needs to pass urine, she has to go straight away. As a result of this, Toni has had many hospital admissions with urinary tract infections (UTIs). Her perineal area is also prone to becoming very sore when she has little 'accidents' and has to wear slightly wet underwear.

Toni's school was reluctant to take her at the outset, believing that she could and should be dry at the age she started with them. Her parents were forced to get medical evidence before the school would take her in and, even now, some staff refuse to allow her to leave the classroom to go to the toilet, resulting in soreness and embarrassment as well as frequent UTIs.

In hospital, Toni is very clingy to whichever parent is present. Although she is generally a very bubbly and confident little girl, when she enters any healthcare environment she changes and becomes very quiet. When asked what makes a good nurse, Toni gave two answers – 'the one who hasn't got a needle in her hand' and 'the one who plays with me and doesn't just talk to mummy or daddy'.

- Why do you think Toni changes so much when she enters hospital?
- How could nurses improve Toni's experience of healthcare through effective communication?

ACTIVITY 2.1: CRITICAL THINKING

The development of communication in children with autistic spectrum disorder (ASD) follows a very different pattern to that of normally developing children (Brown and Elder, 2014). A minority will not develop any form of functional communication, while those who do often display atypical communication styles. It is likely that these develop because the children have limited understanding of the meanings and interactions of symbolic forms of language. These children may have the vocabulary and may even have learned sufficient syntax to pass standardised language screening, but they struggle in real world communication settings because they lack true understanding of meaning.

- How might children's nurses communicate effectively with children with ASD?

When answering this question, think creatively and reflect on ways that you have seen other healthcare professionals communicate in difficult circumstances.

COMMUNICATION IN THE CONTEXT OF FAMILY-CENTRED CARE - THE TRIAD OF COMMUNICATION

Many interactions in the care of children are 'triadic', that is they involve at least three parties – the child, the parent/carer and the nurse. Involvement can increase significantly where multi agency or disciplines become involved in the care of the child and family (Brenner et al., 2018). Interactions primarily occur between two parties at any one time, with the other person as an observer, therefore nurse–parent interaction is just one of the dyads that can occur. These dyads interact to form the triadic relationship which itself has features of a therapeutic alliance, whilst also possessing the potential for both cooperation and conflict in each of these alliances.

ACTIVITY 2.2: REFLECTIVE PRACTICE

On your placement take the time to observe the interactions between nurses, other staff, children and families in the clinical areas.

- What do you notice about the focus of these interactions?
- Who are most involved in the interactions?
- How satisfying do you think the interactions were for (a) the nurse, (b) the parent and (c) the child? And why?

It is important to develop a positive parent–nurse relationship since this is the key to the successful development of alliances within the triad which will ultimately improve the quality of care provided to the child. Nurse–parent interactions take place in the context of the parent's expectations, motivation and health beliefs (Callery and Milnes, 2012; Coyne, 2018; Clarke, 2022). Taking the time to listen to a parent, being attentive, validating their perspective and providing comfort ensures that parents feel supported. Children's nurses need to be aware of the importance of attitude and approach as facilitators of communication (Fisher and Broome, 2011). Ammentorp et al. (2005) note that the two factors identified by parents as having the highest priority are the need to get answers to their questions and the behaviours of nurses caring for their child, including expressing warmth, being kind, caring and taking parents' experiences seriously. Kennan et al. (2019) highlight the legal and ethical imperative in ensuring that all communication is effective (United Nations, 1989).

CASE STUDY 2.2: JOSH

Josh is a 2-year-old boy. He lives with his mother, Kelly, older sister, Jemma, and baby sister, Jasmine. Josh has recently started attending a local nursery. Four weeks ago Kelly noticed that Josh's left leg seemed very swollen and he was not putting any weight on it. The local hospital said that there was no fracture, but the leg remains swollen and painful, so Kelly took him back to the Children's Emergency Department (CED). The first nurse they encountered was very abrupt, but reluctantly agreed to book them into the department. Another nurse came into the cubicle and told Kelly that she had to take the bandage off. Josh immediately started to cry and became more and more distressed as the nurse cut away the bandage and pulled it off his leg. She told him to be quiet and made Kelly hold on to his toy rabbit as it was getting in her way.

(Continued)

Kelly and Josh were then left alone in the cubicle until another nurse, Melanie, arrived to take them off to X-ray. Seeing Josh on the trolley, she very gently picked him up and put him in his mother's arms. Seeing how upset both Kelly and Josh were, she stayed with them throughout the X-ray, gently stroking Josh's hair and putting a comforting arm around Kelly's shoulders. When the X-ray was completed, Melanie stayed with Kelly and Josh while the doctor gave them the news that Josh's leg was, in fact, fractured and that the initial diagnosis had been wrong.

- Who demonstrated more effective communication skills?
- Give reasons for your answer and reflect on your own experiences to date.

SEE ALSO CHAPTER 4,5,8 AND 9

Children's nurses generally seek to involve children in the interactions, but it is important to recognise that a child's willingness to participate cannot be assumed. Some children simply do not wish to be involved and would prefer to be 'passive bystanders' in any interactions (Lambert et al., 2011). Others may wish to be active participants at all times but, most commonly, a child's desire to be involved in any given interaction is dependent on its nature and the context within which it is taking place (Brenner et al., 2018). Competence and assent or consent are also powerful influencing factors in communicating with children and families (Cornock and McAlinden, 2018).

Children's nurses want to hear from the children themselves, not just parents speaking on their behalf, and most parents value nurses' communication with their children. As well as putting the child at ease, parents see that communication between nurses and children could uncover information that might not otherwise have been available (Callery and Milnes, 2012; Clarke, 2015, 2022; Coyne, 2015, 2018; Brenner et al., 2018). Children's nurses can employ a number of strategies to structure interactions with children, including direct questions to the child, making it clear that they are the person expected to speak next, and tacitly selecting the child by limiting eligible respondents through using phrases such as 'your diabetes', 'your medication'.

There are some situations in which the nurse–child dyad may not be effective, when, for example, younger children do not possess sufficient vocabulary to participate and situations in which children may defer to their parents or parents may respond on the child's behalf. While the majority of parental interventions during nurse–child interactions aim to supplement or clarify information provided by the child, parents might sometimes contradict their child or answer a question directed at the child, reflecting their own concerns about balancing protection (from hearing things that are too frightening or that the child may not understand) and encouraging independence.

Young people's contribution to triadic consultations is often limited despite them frequently having both the desire to participate and feelings of competence to be regarded as partners in their own care (van Staa, 2011; Cornock and McAlinden, 2018; NMC, 2018a). The most common reasons for this are considered to be the way in which the nurse controls turn-taking in the interaction and the way in which parents tend to 'jump in' to fill the gaps in information given by the young person. As a consequence, the young person is more likely to act as a 'passive bystander' because their participation has been neither requested nor encouraged.

This children's nurse recalls the experience she had with a 14-year-old boy named Rashid:

Rashid's father was killed in a road accident when he was 5 years old and he now lives with his mother and younger sisters. Despite having quite severe asthma, as the oldest child and the only boy, Rashid has taken on many of the male roles in the family. He went to see the practice nurse with his mother for his routine review and throughout the consultation, the nurse focused on his mother. Never once did she look at Rashid or direct a question to him. When he tried to speak up, the nurse cut him short and once again focused on his mother. As he left the consultation Rashid was heard to say, 'Next time, come without me. It is pointless me being here because you and the nurse seem to believe you know about my asthma better than me, so you don't need me.'

WHAT'S THE EVIDENCE?

Lambert et al. (2008) coined the term 'visible-ness' to reflect a continuum on which children's communication with nurses lies between 'being overshadowed' and 'being at the forefront'. Those children considered to be 'overshadowed' are marginal to the communication process as interactions were primarily between their parents and the healthcare professional. However, those 'at the forefront' of communication were the focal point of communication, holding a leading position in interactions as healthcare professionals communicated directly with them as well as their parents. Children's 'visible-ness' in communication is contingent on three factors:

- The child themselves in terms of their ability to articulate their thoughts and ideas or desire to participate in interactions
- Healthcare professionals' and parents' recognition of the child as part of the communication process, as well as their perception of the child's need to be involved
- The nature of the healthcare environment

In a second paper, Lambert et al. (2011) used their earlier findings to develop the Child Transitional Communication Model which explains children's roles in healthcare interactions. Within their model the authors recognised a number of conflicting perspectives:

- Child as family member versus child as independent entity
- Child as powerless versus empowered child
- Child as immature, incompetent and dependent versus child as mature, competent and independent
- Child as having the right to protection versus child as having the right to liberation
- Child as becoming versus child as being

How might a better understanding of the communicative position of a child (as opposed to that of their parent/carer) improve the quality of the care they receive?

PLAY AS A MEANS OF COMMUNICATION

Play is a central activity in the lives of most children (Hayes and Keogh, 2012; Al-Yateem and Rossiter, 2017), providing a context for communication, understanding and catharsis. Symbolic or object play in childhood helps to develop symbol representation and is critical to the development of language skills. Pretend play with objects develops naturally in most children, becoming more complex over time with the understanding of symbols during play contributing to the comprehension of language (Brown and Elder, 2014; Al-Yateem and Rossiter, 2017; Jones, 2018). Children and young people's nurses should remember that play is a specified right of the child, coupled as it is with the concept of education and learning (United Nations, 1989).

ACTIVITY 2.3: REFLECTIVE PRACTICE

On every placement, observe children at play and ask yourself the following questions:

- Are they playing alone, with an adult or another child or children?
- What communication skills are they employing within their play?
- Does their play tell you anything about them or how they are feeling?

Ask to spend a day or two with the play specialists and observe their work with the children. Discuss with them how they utilise play to assist children in that particular care setting.

Developmental aspects of play

At first sight, play may appear to be simple and enjoyed only for its entertainment value. However, beneath its apparent simplicity lies a complexity in which ideas, understanding, exploration and communication are pursued with enthusiasm and developing skill (Binns and Hicks, 2012) Through play children can experience, connect and interact with the world in order to make sense of their experiences, practise for their future life and communicate feelings they may not be able to verbalise. Have a look at the different type of play identified and described in Table 2.2.

Table 2.2 Six different types of play

Type of play	Description
Unoccupied	The child is not playing, just observing. A child may be standing in one spot or performing random movements
Solitary (independent) play	The child is alone and maintains focus on its activity. Such a child is uninterested in or is unaware of what others are doing – most common in younger children (age 2–3)
Onlooker play (behaviour)	The child watches others at play but does not engage in it themselves – also more common in younger children
Parallel play (adjacent play)	The child plays separately from others but close to them, mimicking their actions. This type of play is seen as a transitory stage as a child moves to a more socially mature associative and cooperative type of play
Associative play	The child is interested in the people playing but not in coordinating their activities with those people, or when there is no organised activity at all
Cooperative play	The child is interested both in the people playing and in the activity they are doing. The activity is organised, and participants have assigned roles. There is also increased self-identification with a group, and a group identity may emerge

The importance of play in children's nursing

Observing children at play can give children's nurses insight into how the child is thinking and dealing with experiences and new situations. When a child is unwell or in a healthcare setting for the first time, play has a particular role in helping them to understand and cope with what is happening to them. An example of this is the way in which play can help to address the negative consequences of being in hospital, which include:

- Decreasing stress
- Providing an outlet for anxiety
- Offering a diversion from unpleasant procedures and treatments
- Bringing meaning to the chaos of the experience
- Keeping memories of home and everything that is important to the child alive

Playing with dolls, books and equipment prior to a procedure can help to ease fear of the unknown and help children to become familiar with medical routines. Such carefully planned play opportunities allow children to express their feelings and promote positive coping strategies. Most play can be adapted to meet the needs of different children, but it takes time and planning as well as a real regard for play. Play specialists can provide advice on how best to create interesting play opportunities for children and develop exciting play and learning environments (Hayes and Keogh, 2012; Boyd and Bee, 2019; NAHPS, 2023) and children's nurses should work closely with play specialists and others to ensure that opportunities provided by play can be used to maximise the effectiveness of both communication and treatment. One example of how this can be achieved is through the use of distraction therapy, which aims to take the child's mind off a procedure by concentrating on something else that is happening. Distraction can be as simple as the children's nurse who has a pen shaped in the form of an animal which can be used as a puppet to distract the child or as sophisticated as projections of space scenes or a princess castle on the walls and ceiling of a treatment room. Increasing use of technology can also provide novel ways of the child or young person distracting themselves from noxious stimuli (streaming music, movies, creating and using video gaming, and use of social media tools to communicate with their friends or peer group). Cautions may be advised in some situations and settings with the use of technology, especially social media, to ensure safe and ethical use at all times. Children's nurses should also be 'media savvy' and aware of confidentiality and harm reduction, as well as observing local policy for social media use (NMC, 2022).

Therapeutic play utilises play as a means of communication as well as a mode of therapy (Binns and Hicks, 2012; NAHPS, 2023). At times play may simply be a means for a child to express their needs and desires, but at others it may be used to affect a positive therapeutic outcome, with these often being closely linked since developing a means of communication can be therapeutic in itself. Therapeutic play can be categorised as non-directive and directive, both of which can be facilitated effectively by children's nurses. Non-directive play occurs when the practitioner assumes the role of an observer whilst the child plays freely, and directive play involves the nurse becoming actively engaged and directing the child's play in order to achieve a specific aim.

Play is a very important means of communication for children and cannot be ignored by children's nurses. While it is often seen as one of the more enjoyable aspects of nursing children, it is important to recognise its value as a therapeutic tool, not simply as a means of keeping children occupied. The National Association of Health Play Specialists (NAHPS.org.uk) raises awareness of the benefits of play for ill children across the UK and Starlight Children's Foundation (starlight_uk) within NAHPS has an excellent 2022 Report on Play in Hospital and effects of COVID-19 on play and children. Within the 'Resources' section of the NAHPS website you can access literature reviews on various topics and events, including the annual NAHPS Play in Hospital Week.

COMMUNICATING WITH CHILDREN IN DIFFICULT CIRCUMSTANCES

Inevitably, these aspects of care evoke many emotional issues and reactions, but they are also care situations where effective communication is even more important than normal. All the communications skills that a children's nurse possesses are required, including supporting, observing, interviewing and listening. In addition, it is essential that the nurse has self-awareness, emotional maturity, empathy and sensitivity. Children and families often note a link between inadequate or ineffective communication and an increase in their confusion and distress. Listening to the experiences of children, young people and their families is essential to ensure quality interactions and relevance of content. This 'co-production' should be encouraged and facilitated in all situations where children and young people are the recipients of attention or care (United Nations, 1989; Brenner et al., 2018); this includes policy, curricula, information resources and evaluation of services and care given.

Breaking bad news

Barriers to communication in these situations include those related to the care environment, for example the multiple distractions inherent in a busy children's ward, physical factors and emotional issues inherent in the situation. Knowing that a child is very unwell or approaching the end of their life is inevitably stressful for their family. They may be afraid of what the future holds or even angry and frustrated with healthcare staff who they feel have 'given up' on their child. Family members often experience these situations in different ways leading to tensions within the family, while different healthcare professionals approach breaking bad news and the end of a child's life in their own individual ways (Kapur 2021, updated 2023).

ACTIVITY 2.4: CRITICAL THINKING

If you have been present when a child and family have received bad news, or even if you have not, consider how best the children's nurse might support them after their meeting with the doctor. What aspects of communication are going to be the most useful at this crucial time? What do children and parents need in order to absorb and assimilate the information they have just received?

Breaking bad news is often considered one of the most complex and challenging aspects of communication in children. While any discussion of this aspect of communication emphasises the need for appropriate, honest communication with both the child and the family, it has already been noted that the child often feels peripheral to such interactions. One of the reasons often quoted for this is lack of certainty regarding what children will understand in relation to the words 'death' and 'dying'. A number of approaches to breaking bad news to children have been noted (Kopchack Sheehan et al., 2014; Brouwer, 2021). Many adults choose to tell the truth to children while adjusting the content and timing of the message to their age and physical condition. Others 'skirt around' the facts, telling the truth but in an indirect or ambiguous way or in a way that is devoid of emotion, focusing instead on practical issues. A minority choose not to tell the child the full truth at any time during their illness.

While there is no strictly right or wrong way to break bad news to children and families, the level of satisfaction reported by children decreases with their perception of the honesty of those involved. However, each situation is unique, with every child and family experiencing it through the lens of their own beliefs, values and knowledge. Breaking bad news must occur within a partnership approach to care. While the children's nurse is often the healthcare professional who has developed a therapeutic relationship with the child and family, often over a number of years, breaking bad news is traditionally seen as the remit of the doctor. The role of the children's nurse in this situation includes facilitation, support, counselling, educating and advocating for the child and their family (Price et al., 2006; Brouwer, 2021; Kapur, 2021, updated 2023).

"I was on a long placement on a children's ward. I got to know a young man with a rare progressive genetic condition very well and his family always said that the best days on the ward were when I was looking after him. On this admission he had come in with a chest infection, but, despite several changes of antibiotics, he wasn't getting any better. The doctors told us [the nurses] that it was likely that he was going to die and asked who would accompany them when they told his parents. My mentor immediately said that I should be there, as I had a good relationship with them, and she would go with me. I wasn't so sure as I was only in my second year, but she persuaded me. It was really, really hard and I couldn't hold back the tears at one point, but I was glad I was there. His mother kept looking at me and, in the end, I just took hold of her hand, just to reassure like … Once the meeting was over, I wanted to run away, but my mentor said to me, 'Stay with them for a while. Don't worry if you don't talk, just be there for them', so I sat with them for about 15 minutes until they decided they could face going back into the ward. I didn't want to be in that meeting, but I am so glad my mentor changed my mind."

Asha, children's nursing student

"Our son Mikey has a very rare condition and the children's ward is his second home. We got to know a nursing student (Asha) very well over his last three admissions. She kept telling us that she was only in her second year, but you would not have thought it. She just seemed to know what Mikey needed and how to make me feel better too. I remember the day we were told that he was going to die. Although we always knew it would happen, we were not ready for it yet. It was a great relief to have Asha there when the doctor told us. I don't remember much of what was said, but I did feel that the doctors and nurses there really cared, not just about Mikey, but about us too. When Asha cried I just knew how much she cared about my son and then she just reached across and took my hand – I'm not usually a great one for touch, but that just felt right. I expected the nurses to leave when the doctor had finished talking to us, but Asha stayed, in silence, and somehow her presence gave me the courage to go back to see Mikey. Thank you Asha!"

David, parent

ACTIVITY 2.5: CRITICAL THINKING

Read carefully both voices above.

Why do you think Mikey's parents valued Asha and the care she provided so highly?

List the essential and desirable skills and prerequisites you feel are required by a nurse in order to deliver bad news.

COMMUNICATING USING TECHNOLOGY AND SOCIAL MEDIA

In today's society one of the most influential factors on children of all ages is technology. With this increase in technology comes an increase in skills as well as social benefits, but also the potential for harm from 'sexting', cyberbullying and Internet addiction (Donnerstein, 2012). There is clearly a need for nurses working with children, young people and families to have a fully informed evidence base with regard to the possible benefits and drawbacks of communication technology (Jones et al., 2013; National Bullying Helpline, 2023; NSPCC, 2023).

Communicating via technology occupies a unique middle ground between using spoken and written language for communication. Electronic discourse, as used in emails, text messages, etc., may in fact represent an entirely new language register and, with children and young people increasingly communicating through this new form of language, have implications for communication skills. Conversational language rules are generally adhered to online which may enhance pragmatic language skills, for example the need to provide contextual information. Users are highly aware of the social context in which they are communicating and adapt their relational tone, personal language, sentence complexity and message composition time according to the target recipients. Interestingly, quite often the technological skills of young people exceed those of adults; this can mean missed oppotrunity for direct relevant communications.

Ongoing advances in technology may facilitate child-centred approaches to care and establish interactive communication that may not have been possible previously. Use of smartphones and other devices may empower children to communicate directly with healthcare professionals, enabling them to be more involved in decisions regarding their care instead of relying on parents, particularly as they transition into young adulthood. Young people may be reluctant to visit a healthcare professional, so the use of text messaging can even provide an effective means of communicating regarding symptoms, appointments and other aspects of nursing care. Many children and young people turn to apps, websites and social media as a natural first solution to their need for information and to connect with others (Jones et al., 2013). Children and, in particular, young people are technologically adept and active on social media (Wysocki, 2015). The increase in the use of social media has been so rapid and their presence in children's everyday life is now so pervasive that, for some children and young people, it is the primary way they interact socially (McBride, 2011; National Bullying Helpline, 2023; NSPCC, 2023).

However, there are concerns regarding the increased use of communication technologies, including social media. These include the potential to encourage social isolation, which may have a negative impact on language skills. In addition, the lack of face-to-face interaction means that many contextual and non-verbal language cues may be lost. The Internet is always available and can be easily accessed by children, often with little parental supervision. Content is often unregulated and children may be exposed to extreme forms of violence, while the sexual content of the Internet is more prevalent than on other popular media. Participation in online activities is private and anonymous, which allows children to search for materials that they would not normally access through traditional media. The opportunity to access such a range of materials plays an important role in cyberbullying and child sexual exploitation. Potential victims are readily available and the identity of the aggressor is frequently unknown (CEOP, 2023; NSPCC, 2023). Your local Safeguarding Gateway can also assist if you have concerns about a child or young person's welfare; be sure you know the policy and procedure for your area to report safeguarding concerns.

SAFEGUARDING STOP POINT

While the use of technology in communication is clearly important, bullying and its impact on the lives of children are longstanding concerns for child healthcare professionals. Cyberbullying is a more recent phenomenon resulting from the blurring of the lines between aggressor and target as well as perceived imbalances of power in the online environment. It consists of any behaviour performed through electronic or digital media by individuals or groups that repeatedly communicate hostile or aggressive messages intended to inflict harm and includes spreading rumours about someone, making inflammatory comments about another person in public discussion areas, leaving abusive messages about the victim on social media pages and sending the victim pornography or other knowingly offensive graphic material.

Warning signs that children are experiencing cyberbullying include displaying numerous negative feelings, school grades beginning to drop, lack of eating or sleeping, all of which are very similar to those seen in other forms of bullying. Specific signs associated with cyberbullying include avoiding their computer, smartphone or tablet, appearing stressed when receiving an email or personal message and avoiding conversations about computer use. Children's nurses are well placed to observe these signs in those they care for and to report any suspicions as this is fast becoming a serious safeguarding concern for the 21st century.

Effective communication is crucial in children's nursing. In order to be successful in communicating with children and young people, nurses must be cognisant of the child's communicative development and use appropriate verbal and non-verbal skills.

CHAPTER SUMMARY

- Children may be overshadowed by their parents or other adults in healthcare interactions, which are generally triadic in nature
- Children's nurses need to be constantly aware of the presence of the child and involve them in communication and decisions, but only to the point that that child wishes to participate. Individuality in communicative style and preferences must always be respected. There is no better demonstration of the importance of effective communication than when it is utilised in difficult situations such as breaking bad news
- Play is an important means of communication with children. Although frequently seen as the domain of younger children, play can be used across the spectrum of childhood as a means of engaging young patients, preparing them for procedures and treatments, distraction and as a means of exploring feelings and concerns
- An important member of the interprofessional team in this regard is the play specialist who can guide nurses as to the most effective way to use play in particular situations
- While many children use electronic devices for play and recreational purposes, the Internet, texting and social media have an important and continually developing role in contemporary healthcare. While there are clear advantages of using these media in this way, it is important to remember that there are risks and potential dangers, particularly in social media and texting, which can escalate into safeguarding concerns if not addressed

It is beyond the scope of this chapter to give anything other than an overview on what is an enormous and many-faceted topic. Signposting and activities along with reflection on your own clinical practice will enhance your knowledge and awareness of this topic. We wish you many happy experiences!

BUILD YOUR BIBLIOGRAPHY

Books

FURTHER
READING

- Lambert, V., Long, T. and Kelleher, D. (2012) *Communication Skills for Children's Nurses*. Maidenhead: McGraw Hill.

  A comprehensive text exploring models of communication used by children and the associated skills.
- LeFevre, M. (2018) *Communicating and Engaging with Children and Young People*. Bristol: Policy Press.
- Smith, J. (2020) *How to Get Your Kids to Listen to You*. London: Jessica Kingsley Publications.

  This book guides parents and others in the best ways to engage with, and obtain the required information from children.
- Shapcott, J. (2016) 'Communicating with children, young people and families', in I. Gault, J. Shapcott, A. Luthi and G. Reid (eds), *Communication in Nursing and Healthcare: A Guide for Compassionate Practice*. London: Sage.

  This chapter provides an overview of some aspects of communicating with children in the context of mindful professional communication.

Journal articles

FURTHER
READING:
ONLINE
JOURNAL
ARTICLES

- Coyne, I (2015) 'Families and healthcare professionals' perspectives and expectations of family centred care: hidden expectations and unclear roles'. *Health Expectations*, 18 (5): 796–808.
- Coyne, I., Holmstrom, I. and Soderback, M. (2018) 'Centredness in healthcare: a concept synthesis of family centred care, person centred care and child centred care'. *Journal of Pediatric Nursing*, 42: 45–56.
- Kennan, D., Brady, B. and Forkan, C. (2019) 'Space, voice, audience and influence: the Lundy model of participation (2007) in child welfare practice'. *Practice*, 31 (3): 205–18.

  Ensuring children are engaged in healthcare consultations and that accurate information is obtained can be challenging, so this article outlines some useful strategies that might be employed.

Weblinks

FURTHER
READING:
WEBLINKS

- UNICEF, Communicating with Children www.unicef.org/cwc (accessed 16 March 2023) This website provides principles and guidance for children's nurses to facilitate their ongoing development of communication skills. Child development and its importance to communication are addressed alongside the rights of children to effective communication and the influence of the media on children.
- Child Development Institute, *Communication Disorders in Children and Adolescents* https://childdevelopmentinfo.com/child-psychology/children_with_communication_disorders/#.WJwxpW-LTIU (accessed 16 March 2023)
- NAHPS (National Association of Health Play Specialists) www.nahps.org.uk (accessed 5 July 2023) Although aimed at parents, this section of the website gives an insight into the nature and incidence of these disorders and provides useful links to other relevant sites.
- NICE, *Child Maltreatment: When to Suspect Maltreatment in Under 18s* www.nice.org.uk/guidance/cg89/ifp/chapter/communicating-with-and-about-children-or-young-people (accessed

16 March 2023) This page forms part of a larger set of guidance regarding safeguarding children. It reminds children's nurses of the importance of communication with and about children and young people in such situations.

REFERENCES

Al-Yateem, N. and Rossiter, R. (2017) 'Unstructured play for anxiety in pediatric inpatient care'. *Journal for Specialists in Pediatric Nursing, 22* (1): e12166.

Ammentorp, J., Mainz, J. and Sabroe, S. (2005) 'Parents' priorities and satisfaction with acute pediatric care'. *Archives of Pediatrics and Adolescent Medicine, 159*: 127–31.

Boyd, D. and Bee, H. (2019) *Lifespan Development*, 8th edn. Harlow: Pearson.

Beuker, K.T., Rommelse, N.N., Donders, R. and Buitelaar, J.K. (2013) 'Development of early multidisciplinary language: communication skills in the first two years of life'. *Infant Behavior and Development, 36* (1): 71–83.

Binns, F. and Hicks, P. (2012) 'Using play and technology to communicate with children and young people', in V. Lambert, T. Long and D. Kelleher (eds), *Communication Skills for Children's Nurses*. Maidenhead: McGraw-Hill.

Brenner, M., Kidston, C., Hilliard, C., Coyne, I., Eustace-Cook, J., Doyle, C., Begley, T. and Barratt, M.J. (2018) 'Children's complex care needs: a systematic concept analysis of multidisciplinary analysis'. *European Journal of Pediatrics, 177*: 1641–52.

Brouwer, M., Maeckelberghe, E.L.M., van der Heide A., Heim, I.M. and Verhagen, E.A.A.E. (2021) 'Breaking bad news: what parents would like you to know'. *Archives of Disease in Childhood, 106* (3): 276–81.

Brown, A.B. and Elder, J.H. (2014) 'Communication in autism spectrum disorder: a guide for pediatric nurses'. *Pediatric Nursing, 40* (5): 219–25.

Callery, P. and Milnes, L. (2012) 'Communication between nurses, children and their parents in asthma review consultations'. *Journal of Clinical Nursing, 21* (11–12): 1641–50.

CEOP Child Exploitation Safety Centre. www.ceop.police.uk/Safety-Centre/ (accessed 6 June 2023).

Charney, S.A. and Camerata, S.M. (2021) 'Potential impact of the Covid-19 pandemic on communication and language skill in children'. *Otolaryngology Head and Neck Surgery, 165* (1): 1–2.

Clarke, S. (2015) 'A child's rights perspective: the right of children and young people to participate in healthcare research'. *Issues in Comprehensive Pediatric Nursing, 38* (3): 161–80.

Clarke, S. (2022) 'An exploration of the child's experience of staying in hospital from the perspectives of children and children's nurses using child centred methodology'. *Comprehensive Child and Adolescent Nursing, 45* (1): 105–18.

Cornock, M. and McAlinden, O. (2018) 'Law and policy for children and young people's nursing', in J. Price and O. McAlinden (eds), *Essentials of Nursing Children and Young People*. London: Sage.

Coyne, I. (2015) 'Families and healthcare professionals' perspectives and expectations of family centred care: hidden expectations and unclear roles'. *Health Expectations, 18* (5): 796-808.

Coyne, I., Holmstrom, I. and Soderback, M. (2018) 'Centredness in healthcare: a concept synthesis of family centred care, person centred care and child centred care'. *Journal of Pediatric Nursing, 42*: 45–56.

Desai, P.P. and Pandya, S.V. (2013) 'Communicating with children in healthcare settings'. *Indian Journal of Pediatrics, 8* (12): 1028–33.

Diaz-Rodriguez, M., Alcantara-Rubio, L., Aguilar-Garcia, D. et al. (2021) 'The effect of play on pain and anxiety in children in the field of nursing: a systemic review'. *Journal of Pediatric Nursing, 61*: 15–22.

Donnerstein, E. (2012) 'Internet bullying'. *Pediatric Clinics of North America, 59* (3): 623–33.

Dryden, P. and Greenshields, S. (2020) 'Communicating with children and young people'. *British Journal of Nursing, 29* (20): 1164–6.

Fallon, D. (2012) 'Communicating with young people', in V. Lambert, T. Long and D. Kelleher (eds), *Communication Skills for Children's Nurses*. Maidenhead: McGraw-Hill.

Fisher, M.J. and Broome, M.E. (2011) 'Parent–provider communication during hospitalization'. *Journal of Pediatric Nursing, 26* (1): 58–69.

Franklin, A. and Goff, S. (2019) 'Listening and facilitating all forms of communication: disabled children and young people in residential care in England'. *Child Care in Practice, 25* (1): 99–111.

Hayes, N. and Keogh, P. (2012) 'Communicating with children in early and middle childhood', in V. Lambert, T. Long and D. Kelleher (eds), *Communication Skills for Children's Nurses*. Maidenhead: McGraw-Hill.

Holt, S. and Yuill, N. (2017) 'Tablets for two: how dual tablets can facilitate other-awareness and communication in learning disabled children with autism'. *International Journal of Child-Computer interaction, 11*: 72–82.

Jones, M. (2018) 'The necessity of play for children in healthcare'. *Pediatric Nursing, 44* (6):303–5.

Jones, R., Cleverly, L., Hammersley, S., Ashurst, E. and Pinkney, J. (2013) 'Apps and online resources for young people with diabetes: the facts'. *Journal of Diabetes Nursing, 17* (1): 20–6.

Kapur, S. (2021, updated 2023) 'Breaking bad news'. Don't Forget the Bubbles doi.org/10.31440/ DFTB.31906 (accessed 16 March 2023).

Kennan, D., Brady, B. and Forkan, C. (2019) 'Space, voice, audience and influence: the Lundy model of participation (2007) in child welfare practice'. *Practice, 31* (3): 205-18.

Kopchak Sheehan, D., Burke Draucker, C., Christ, G.H., Murray Mayo, M., Heim, K. and Parish, S. (2014) 'Telling adolescents a parent is dying'. *Journal of Palliative Medicine, 17* (5): 512–20.

Lambert, V., Glacken, M. and McCarron, M. (2008) '"Visible-ness": the nature of communication for children admitted to a specialist children's hospital in the Republic of Ireland'. *Journal of Clinical Nursing, 17* (23): 3092–102.

Lambert, V., Glacken, M. and McCarron, M. (2011) 'Communication between children and health professionals in a child hospital setting: a Child Transitional Communication Model'. *Journal of Advanced Nursing, 67* (3): 569–82.

McBride, D.L. (2011) 'Risks and benefits of social media for children and adolescents'. *Journal of Pediatric Nursing, 26* (5): 498–9.

Mooney, C.G. (2013) *Theories of Childhood: An Introduction to Dewey, Montessori, Erikson, Piaget & Vygotsky*. St Paul, MN: Redleaf Press.

NAHPS (National Association of Health Play Specialists) (2023) www.nahps.org.uk (accessed 5 July 2023)

National Bullying Helpline. www.nationalbullyinghelpline.co.uk (accessed 16 March 2023).

NMC (Nursing and Midwifery Council) (2018a) *The Code: Professional Standards of Practice and Behaviour for Nurses, Midwives and Nursing Associates*. London: NMC. Available at: www.nmc.org. uk/standards/code/.

NMC (Nursing and Midwifery Council) (2018b) *Future Nurse: Standards of Proficiency for Registered Nurses*. London: NMC.

NMC (Nursing and Midwifery Council) (2022) *Social Media Guidance*. London: NMC.

NSPCC (National Society for the Preventon of Cruelty to Children). https://learning.nspcc.org.uk/ (accessed 16 March 2023).

Phulwari, P.R., Kumar, D. and Goyal, P. (2021) 'From a systematic literature review to a conceptual framework for consumer disposal behaviour towards personal communication devices'. *Journal of Consumer Behaviour, 20* (5): 1353–70.

Price, J., McNeilly, P. and Surgenor, M. (2006) 'Breaking bad news to parents: the children's nurse's role'. *International Journal of Palliative Nursing, 12* (3): 115–20.

Prior, M., Bavin, E.L., Cini, E., Reilly, S., Bretherton, L., Wake, M. and Eadie, P. (2008) 'Influences on communicative development at 24 months of age: child temperament, behaviour problems, and maternal factors'. *Infant Behavior and Development, 31* (2): 270–9.

Roberts, J., Fenton, G. and Barnard, M. (2015) 'Developing effective therapeutic relationships in children, young people and their families'. *Nursing Children and Young People, 27* (4): 30–5.

Shack, A.R., Arkush, L. Reingold, S. and Weisner, G. (2020) 'Masked paediatricians during the COVID-19 pandemic and communications with children'. *Journal of Paediatrics and Child Health, 56* (9): 1475–6.

United Nations (1989) *Convention on the Rights of the Child (UNCRC)*. Available at: www.unicef.org.uk/what-we-do/un-convention-child-rights (accessed 6 June 2023).

van Staa, A.L. (2011) 'Unravelling triadic communication in hospital consultations with adolescents with chronic conditions: the added value of mixed methods research'. *Patient Education and Counselling, 82* (3): 455–64.

Vinales, J.J. (2013) 'Evaluation of Makaton in practice by children 's nursing students'. *Nursing Children and Young People, 25* (3): 14–17.

Wysocki, R. (2015) 'Social media for school nurses'. *NASN School Nurse, 30* (3): 180–8.

ASSESSMENT AND MANAGEMENT OF PAIN IN CHILDREN AND YOUNG PEOPLE

3

REBECCA SAUL AND ALISON TWYCROSS

THIS CHAPTER COVERS

- Why it is important to assess and manage pain in children
- Different strategies for assessing and managing pain in children and young people
- How to use validated pain assessment tools for children of all ages
- The pharmacology of conventional analgesic drugs
- Non-pharmacological management of pain

“Access to pain management is a fundamental human right.”

(International Association for the Study of Pain (IASP), 2015)

“I guess I would have wanted those pain medications more often, but I did not always dare to ask for them, and sometimes I was ashamed to press the call button since it made such a loud noise, and my roommate was sleeping. I would have liked it if the nurses would [come] round every hour so that I would not have to suffer from the pain because I didn't dare to use the call button. I could have told my father, but it was already eleven o'clock and he wasn't with me anymore.”

(Polkki et al., 2003, pp.39–40)

INTRODUCTION

The quotations above suggest that pain management in children is still not as good as it could be. This chapter starts by explaining the reasons it is important to assess and manage children's pain effectively in your practice and provides details of current best practice guidelines. The stages of pain management are described, followed by a discussion of the different strategies that children's nurses can use to assess a child's pain. Several commonly used pain assessment tools are described. Pharmacological strategies for managing a child's pain are explained, as are several non-pharmacological methods of pain relief.

WHY IS IT IMPORTANT TO ASSESS AND MANAGE PAIN IN CHILDREN?

Unrelieved pain has several undesirable physical and psychological consequences that affect the child in the short and longer term, including needle-fear (Eccleston et al., 2020). Pain activates potentially harmful physiological changes, including: increases to heart rate, blood pressure and myocardial oxygen demands that may affect those with underlying cardiac conditions; reduction in gastric motility that may prolong an ileus; suppression of cough in children with severe thoracic or abdominal pain may precipitate respiratory problems; and pain-induced changes to protein breakdown and glucose metabolism which may affect wound healing (Australian and New Zealand College of Anaesthetists and Faculty of Pain Management, 2020). Pain in early life can affect behavioural responses to subsequent painful procedures (Taddio et al., 1997), and pain in very premature neonates is associated with altered brain development and stress hormone (cortisol) regulation, involving pathways that are not fully understood (Grunau, 2020). There is also evidence that acute (postoperative) pain can result in chronic pain in a small but significant number of children (Lauridsen et al., 2014). Therefore, the need to manage children's pain effectively is clear.

Ongoing challenges to the implementation of pain scales in clinical practice have been observed (Andersen et al., 2017), and guidelines and frameworks have been developed to assist health professionals in assessing and managing children and young people's pain, including:

- Royal College of Nursing (RCN) (2009) *The Recognition and Assessment of Acute Pain in Children.*
- Association of Paediatric Anaesthetists of Great Britain and Ireland (APAGBI) (2012) *Pediatric Anesthesia: Good Practice in Postoperative and Procedural Pain Management*, 2nd edn.
- Australian and New Zealand College of Anaesthetists and Faculty of Pain Medicine (ANZCA&FPM) (2020) *Acute Pain Management: Scientific Evidence*, 5th edn.
- Delivering transformative action in paediatric pain: a *Lancet Child & Adolescent Health Commission* (Eccleston et al., 2020) *The Lancet Child & Adolescent Health*, Vol. 5, No. 1 (Video abstract) Available at: https://youtu.be/akN0PFeiAmQ
- Royal College of Nursing (RCN) (2015) *Pain Knowledge and Skills Framework for the Nursing Team.*

———————— SAFEGUARDING STOP POINT ————————

The Declaration of Montréal (IASP, 2015) identifies that access to pain management is a fundamental human right. However, pain in children and young people is commonly under-recognised and undertreated. This has led to calls for transformational change in all aspects of paediatric pain management to ensure pain is a key issue in healthcare and society in general, including improvements in our understanding of pain through research and its dissemination, use of effective pain assessment strategies to recognise pain, and ensuring children and young people's access to effective treatments (Eccleston et al., 2020).

STRATEGIES FOR ASSESSING PAIN IN CHILDREN

Current best practice guidelines indicate that we should:

- Carry out pain assessment routinely, alongside other physiological observations such as temperature, respiratory rate, and heart rate.
- Ensure the assessment tool chosen is validated, and developmentally appropriate.
- Ask the child about their pain using a self-report pain tool. Where this is not possible, employ an appropriate behavioural (e.g., FLACC) or combined (e.g., COMFORT) pain assessment tool.
- Involve parents/carers, and where appropriate teach them how to use pain assessment tools.
- Document pain assessments.
- Reassess pain following the implementation of pain-relieving interventions.
  (RCN, 2009)

Pain assessment and management: the basics

The stages of pain management are outlined in Figure 3.1. Pain assessment is the first step in ensuring children's pain is managed effectively. If pain is not assessed, it is difficult to evaluate the effectiveness of interventions and decide whether further action is needed.

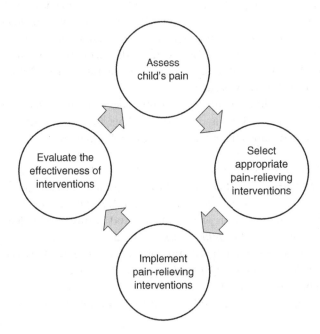

Figure 3.1 The stages of pain management (Twycross et al., 2014)

Self-report of pain

Self-report tools should normally be used with children who are:

- Old enough to understand and use a self-report scale (e.g., 3 years of age and older)
- Not overtly distressed
- Not cognitively impaired (Stinson et al., 2006)

Behavioural indicators of pain

Children can exhibit behavioural cues indicating they are in pain (Table 3.1). Where self-report is not possible and in infants, toddlers, pre-verbal, cognitively impaired and sedated children, behavioural pain assessment tools should be used (APAGBI, 2012). There is evidence that children's self-reports of pain do not correlate strongly with their behaviour (Nilsson et al., 2008) and behavioural cues may only provide an *estimate* of how much pain a child is experiencing.

Table 3.1 Behavioural indicators of pain

Changed behaviour	Increased clinging
Irritability	Unusual quietness
Flat affect	Loss of appetite
Unusual posture	Restlessness
Screaming	Whimpering
Reluctance to move	Sobbing
Aggressiveness	Lying 'scared stiff'
Disturbed sleep pattern	Lethargic

Physiological indicators of pain

Physiological parameters can form part of a child's pain assessment (Table 3.2).

WHAT'S THE EVIDENCE?

When used alone, physiological indicators are not a reliable clinical measure of pain as they can be affected by other factors such as pyrexia or anxiety, therefore a pain assessment strategy that incorporates physiological and behavioural indicators as well as self-report is preferred (APAGBI, 2012).

Table 3.2 Physiological cues

Heart rate	Increases immediately following a pain stimulus and declines as pain diminishes (whereas in infants an initial decrease is followed by a rise in heart rate) (McGrath et al., 2014)
Respiratory rate and pattern	There is conflicting evidence about whether this increases or decreases, but there is a significant shift from baseline. Breathing may become rapid and/or shallow
Blood pressure	Increases when a child is in acute pain
Oxygen saturation	Decreases when a child is in acute pain

HOW TO USE VALIDATED PAIN ASSESSMENT TOOLS FOR CHILDREN OF ALL AGES

No single pain assessment method is recommended for use in all clinical settings (APAGBI, 2012) and more than one pain assessment tool is required in a clinical area to cater for all patients. Guidance on pain assessment tools that have been developed and validated for use with children of different ages and cognitive abilities are available (RCN, 2009; ANZCA&FPM, 2020). In this chapter we will discuss the tools used most frequently.

The pain tool for neonates that has been tested most often is the Premature Infant Pain Profile (PIPP) (Stevens et al., 1996) (Table 3.3) and has evidence of reliability, validity, and ability to detect change (Stevens et al., 2010). One of the most frequently recommended behavioural pain assessment tools is the FLACC observational pain tool, (Face, Legs, Activity, Cry, Consolability), which has been validated for children from 2 months to 7 years (Merkel et al., 1997). It has been modified for use with children aged 4–12 with cognitive impairment (Revised FLACC tool) (Figure 3.2) undergoing elective surgery (Malviya et al., 2006), allowing for individualised behaviours to be included.

For verbal children, the Numerical Rating Scale (NRS-11) from 0 (no pain) to 10 (worst pain) is commonly used to measure pain intensity in procedural, postoperative, disease-related, and chronic pain and has been validated for use in children 8 years or older (Castarlenas et al., 2017).

Where self-report in younger children is required (Table 3.4), the Wong and Baker (1988) FACES Pain Rating Scale (WBFPRS) has been tested in young people aged 3–18 years and is most preferred by patients and nurses in comparison to other faces scales; however, tools with smiling (no pain) and crying (worst pain) anchors may be difficult to interpret for users under 5 years of age. The Faces Pain Scale-Revised (Hicks et al., 2001) (see Figure 3.3) is validated for measuring pain intensity in 4–12-year-olds. It employs neutral anchors and is a recommended tool for use in research studies involving young people. Both tools have been validated for use in procedural, postoperative, emergency, intensive care, and disease-related pain settings. They have both been translated into numerous languages, require minimal patient instruction, are quick to use, and are available free of charge for clinical purposes (Tomlinson et al., 2010).

Table 3.3 The Premature Infant Pain Profile (PIPP) (Stevens et al., 1996)

Indicators used	Considerations
Postmenstrual age Behavioural state Heart rate Oxygen saturation Brow bulge Eye squeeze Nasolabial furrow	• Preterm and term infants (e.g., 28-40 weeks' gestation) • Initially developed for procedural pain, requires further evaluation with very low birthweight neonates and with non-acute and post-surgical pain populations • Includes contextual indicators (e.g., postmenstrual age and behavioural state) • Indicators are scored on a four-point scale (0, 1, 2, 3) for a total score of 0 to 21 based on the gestational age of the infant • A score of 6 or less generally indicates minimal or no pain, while scores greater than 12 indicate moderate to severe pain • Pain assessments take one minute • In the revised version (PIPP-R) postmenstrual age and behavioural state indicators are only applied if other variables indicate pain

Table 3.4 Self-report pain assessment tools for verbal children

Pain assessment tool	Age range
Faces Pain Scale-Revised (FPS-R) (Figure 3.3)	• Children 4-12 years old • Has been used in young people up to 18 years (Hicks et al., 2001)
Wong-Baker FACES Pain Scale	• Children aged 3-18 years (Wong and Baker, 1988)
Numerical pain rating (NRS) scale (see Figure 3.4)	• Children aged over 8 years and adolescents for acute pain

Table 3.5 Instructions for using faces pain scales (Hockenberry et al., 2005)

Explain to the child that each face is for a person who feels happy because there is no pain (hurt) or sad because there is some or a lot of pain

Face 0 is very happy because there is no hurt at all

Face 1 hurts just a little bit

Face 2 hurts a little more

Face 3 hurts even more

Face 4 hurts a whole lot more

Face 5 hurts as much as you can imagine, although you do not have to be crying to feel this bad

Ask the child to choose the face that best describes how he/she is feeling

| Name: | Hosp No: | | Great Ormond Street NHS |
| DOB: | NHS no: | | Hospital for Children |

| | Scoring | | |
Categories	0	1	2
Face Individual Behaviours	No particular expression or smile	Occasional grimace or frown, withdrawn, disinterested *appears sad or worried*	Frequent to constant frown, clenched jaw, quivering chin *Distressed looking face; expression of fright or panic*
Legs Individual Behaviours	Normal position or relaxed; *usual tone and motion to limbs*	Uneasy, restless, tense; *occasional tremors*	Kicking, or legs drawn up; *marked increase in spasticity, constant tremors or jerking*
Activity Individual Behaviours	Lying quietly, normal position, moves easily; *Regular, rhythmic respirations*	Squirming, shifting back and forth, tense or *guarded movements; mildly agitated (eg. head back and forth, aggression); shallow, splinting respirations, intermittent sighs*	Arched, rigid, or jerking; *severe agitation, head banging, shivering (not rigors); breath-holding, gasping or sharp intake of breaths; servere splinting*
Cry Individual Behaviours	No cry/verbalisation (awake or asleep)	Moans or whimpers, occasional complaint: *occasional verbal outburst or grunt*	Crying steadily, screams or sobs, frequent complaints; *repeated outbursts, constant grunting*
Consolability Individual Behaviours	Content, relaxed	Reassured by occasional touching, hugging, or being talked to, distractable	Difficult to console or comfort; *pushing away caregiver, resisting care or comfort measures*

(Adapted from Malviya et al. 2006)

Revised FLACC-Instructions for Use

- **Individualize the tool:** The nurse should review the descriptors within each category with the child's parents or carers. Ask them if there are additional behaviours that are better indicators of pain in their child. Add these behaviours to the tool in the appropriate category.
- Each of the five categories (F) Face; (L) Legs; (A) Activity; (C) Cry; (C) Consolability is scored from 0–2, which results in a total score between zero and ten.
- **Patients who are awake:** Observe for at least 1–3 minutes. Observe legs and body uncovered. Reposition patient or observe activity, assess body for tenseness and tone. Initiate consoling interventions if needed.
- **Patients who are asleep:** Observe for at least 5 minutes. Observe body and legs uncovered. If possible reposition the patient. Touch the body and assess for tenseness and tone.

| Version No: 1.0 | Version date: 15/04/2010 | Document development lead: Jude Middleton | I:\Pain Control Service\Assessment\Revised FLACC\Revised FLACC Paperwork.doc |

Figure 3.2   Revised FLACC Scale

© The Regents of the University of Michigan. Reproduced with permission.

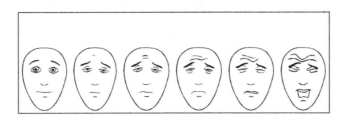

Figure 3.3   Faces Pain Scale – Revised (FPS-R) (Hicks et al., 2001)

Reproduced with permission and available at: www.iasp-pain.org/resources/faces-pain-scale-revised/?itemnumber=1519

| No pain | 0 | 1 | 2 | 3 | 4 | 5 | 6 | 7 | 8 | 9 | 10 | Most Pain |

Figure 3.4   Numerical Rating Scale (NRS)

ACTIVITY 3.1: CRITICAL THINKING

Taking into account the information above, how would you assess pain in children of the following ages:

- Newborn infant
- Baby aged 6 months
- Child aged 6 years
- Adolescent aged 14 years
- Child aged 11 years with severe cognitive impairment

ACTIVITY 3.2: REFLECTIVE PRACTICE

- Based on your experiences on clinical placement to date, how well integrated with practice are current pain assessment and management guidelines?
- How might you change your practice to ensure you are practising evidence-based nursing?

CASE STUDY 3.1: JENNY

Jenny is 9 years old and has been admitted via Accident and Emergency to the ward with a facial laceration. Angela is a newly qualified staff nurse and has been asked to assess Jenny's current level of pain before analgesia is prescribed. Angela accesses the hospital's online pain assessment form and finds herself presented with a bewildering array of self-report and behavioural pain assessment tools. How might Angela choose the right assessment tool?

ACTIVITY 3.3: REFLECTIVE PRACTICE

- Do you think a child's self-report of pain (using tools as mentioned above) should always be the primary consideration when assessing their pain? What other factors might you consider?
- How well do you think pain scores are recorded in practice?

PHARMACOLOGICAL MANAGEMENT OF PAIN: THE PHARMACOLOGY OF CONVENTIONAL ANALGESIC DRUGS

Role of multimodal analgesia

Multimodal analgesia is the use of analgesic pharmacological techniques in a complementary manner, targeting different aspects of the pain pathway, to achieve balanced analgesia, thus minimising the doses required and the potential side effects associated with each agent and maximising drug efficacy

(McGrath et al., 2014). It is recommended in paediatric postoperative (APAGBI, 2012), emergency (Maurice et al., 2002), procedural (Eccleston et al., 2020) and oncology (Raphael et al., 2010) settings.

The World Health Organization (WHO, 2012) advocates a *two-step strategy* for the pharmacological treatment of pain for conditions such as cancer, sickle cell disease, burns and trauma, based on the selection of analgesic drugs in relation to pain severity. The *first step* recommends the use of paracetamol and ibuprofen for mild pain; the *second step* includes the addition of low doses of strong opioids for the treatment of moderate pain, which may be increased if pain is severe.

Non-steroidal anti-inflammatory drugs

The NSAIDs most commonly used in young people within the UK are non-selective COX inhibitors (ibuprofen, diclofenac and mefenamic acid) (Neubert et al., 2010). Non-steroidal anti-inflammatory drugs (NSAIDs) act both centrally and peripherally and have analgesic and antipyretic actions. NSAIDs work by inhibiting the action of the enzyme cyclooxygenase (COX), active during the inflammatory process (Figure 3.5). Cyclooxygenase exists in two forms (COX-1 and COX-2) and the key side effects (outlined in Table 3.6) associated with NSAIDs are related to the inhibition of the enzyme COX-1, which is responsible for homeostatic properties, such as gastric mucosa function, platelet activation and renal blood flow (Neal, 2016). Ibuprofen and naproxen are thought to be weakly COX-1-selective (Dale and Haylett, 2009) and ibuprofen is associated with fewest side effects (APAGBI, 2012).

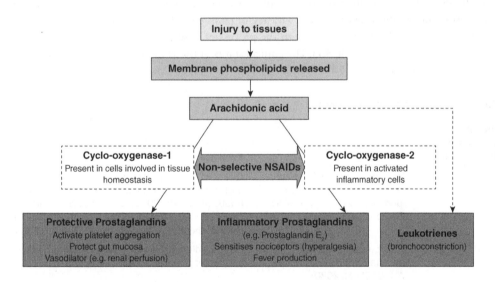

Figure 3.5 Action of non-selective NSAIDs

Adapted from www.medscape.com

Table 3.6 Common side effects of non-selective NSAIDs (Neal, 2009; APAGBI, 2012)

Side effect	Description and evidence
Gastric irritation	Prostaglandins protect the gastric mucosa by stimulating bicarbonate and mucous secretion. NSAIDs should be avoided where there is a history of peptic ulcer disease. The short-term use of NSAIDs (1-3 days) is associated with low risk of gastric side effects (especially if ibuprofen is used).

(Continued)

Table 3.6 (Continued)

Side effect	Description and evidence
Reduces renal blood flow	Prostaglandin acts on the glomerulus and renal medulla, causing vasodilation and increasing the flow of blood to the kidney; their inhibition by NSAIDs may reduce renal blood flow, cause retention of sodium and renal impairment. This effect may be increased in children who are dehydrated, have renal failure or are being administered drugs known to affect renal function.
Exacerbation of asthma	The inhibition of prostaglandins may increase the conversion of arachidonic acid to leukotrienes, which may potentially induce bronchospasm in some asthmatic children. Therefore, it may be continued short-term where uneventful previous NSAID use has been confirmed.
Disrupts platelet function	NSAIDs reduce the production of thromboxane involved in platelet aggregation and should be avoided in children with coagulation disorders or those receiving anticoagulant agents.

Paracetamol

Paracetamol has similar properties to NSAIDs but lacks their anti-inflammatory action. Paracetamol and NSAIDs used in combination produce better analgesia than either drug alone (APAGBI, 2012). The mechanism of action of paracetamol is not clearly understood but may be linked to the inhibition of the synthesis of prostaglandin (Electronic Medicines Compendium, 2022) which excites nociceptive (pain sensing) nerve fibres. The analgesic efficacy of paracetamol is based on it reaching an optimal plasma concentration in the blood through the process of absorption, which may be influenced by the route of administration (Table 3.7). The clinical status of the child may also have a bearing on the administration of paracetamol (Table 3.8).

Table 3.7 Absorption of paracetamol

Route of paracetamol administration	Comments	Evidence
Oral	Dependent on gastric emptying and the transit of the drug to the duodenum, where it is rapidly absorbed	Children under 3 months may have variable rates of gastric emptying and in neonates this may be slow and erratic (Anderson, 2008). Similarly, delayed gastric emptying may affect the absorption of paracetamol in the postoperative child (van der Westhuizen et al., 2011)
Rectal	Absorption may be less predictable and slower (ANZCA&FPM, 2020)	Initial loading doses may be needed to achieve satisfactory analgesia (APAGBI, 2012)
Intravenous	Alternative route of administration when enteral absorption is reduced (Anderson and Palmer, 2006)	Intravenous administration has been demonstrated to achieve superior analgesia to rectal (Prins et al., 2008) or oral routes (van der Westhuizen et al., 2011)

Table 3.8 Paracetamol use in children with specific clinical conditions

Condition	Evidence for the use of paracetamol
Neutropenia	Although recommended for management of acute cancer pain (Raphael et al., 2010), paracetamol is contraindicated in the neutropenic patient because of its potential to mask pyrexia, which may be a key indicator of potentially life-threatening infection. However, paracetamol may be considered if the child is receiving broad-spectrum antibiotics (Johnson, 2013)

Condition	Evidence for the use of paracetamol
Asthma	The proposed association between paracetamol use during infancy or pregnancy and later development of asthma is lost when confounding factors such as childhood respiratory infections are considered (ANZCA&FPM, 2020)

Opioids

Pain-sensing first-order neurones (nociceptors) transmit painful stimuli to the dorsal horn of the spinal cord where a neurotransmitter (glutamate) is released, causing second-order neurones to carry pain information via the thalamus to the sensory cortex. Opioid agents (such as morphine and tramadol) mimic the effect of endogenous opioids. Opioid receptors respond to endogenous opioid release, by reducing calcium ion entry to the nerve-cell, suppressing the release of neurotransmitter; they also act on the postsynaptic membrane to enhance potassium ion outflow making the nociceptor less excitable (hyperpolarisation), thus reducing transmission at the synapse (Figure 3.6) (Neal, 2016).

Potential side effects of opioids are outlined in Table 3.9.

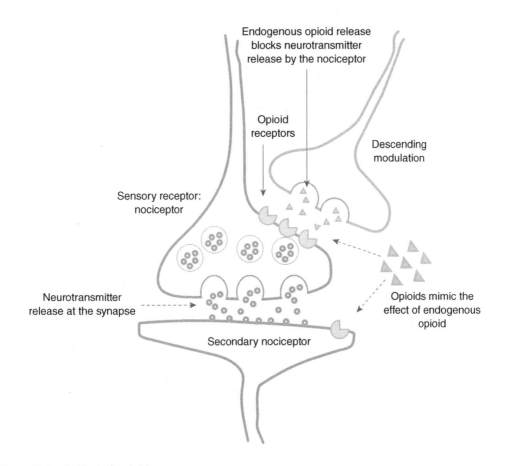

Figure 3.6 Action of opioids

Adapted from www.biology-pages.info/D/Drugs.html

Tramadol

Since the withdrawal of codeine from use in children under 12 years of age (Medicines and Healthcare products Regulatory Agency, 2013) following fatalities after administration post-adenotonsillectomy to children with obstructive sleep apnoea (Kelly et al., 2012), tramadol has been identified as a potentially suitable alternative for children with mild to moderate pain (Marzuillo et al., 2014). Tramadol is a weak opioid analgesic which also inhibits the reuptake of norepinephrine and serotonin, giving it anti-neuropathic qualities (ANZCA&FPM, 2020) and enhancing its analgesic action (Dale and Haylett, 2009). Tramadol is a medium potency analgesic that demonstrates similar efficacy to NSAIDs and one-tenth the potency of morphine (APAGBI, 2012). It has a lower incidence of constipation and pruritus, but it is not clear if it causes less respiratory depression in children than other opioids, and nausea and vomiting are its most common side effects (ANZCA&FPM, 2020). There is a lack of evidence for its use in infants (Anderson and Palmer, 2006).

Morphine

Morphine is the opioid of first choice in children due to its efficacy, familiarity in clinical practice and affordability (McGrath et al., 2014). Morphine is metabolised to morphine-6-glucuronide (which has analgesic activity) and morphine-3-glucuronide (which does not). Both are excreted via the renal system (McGrath et al., 2014). The ability of the child to clear morphine is an important factor to consider when administering opioids. Immature renal function and reduced metabolism in neonates causes reduced clearance and increased half-life of morphine and neonates require lower doses compared with older children (APAGBI, 2012). Similarly, children with impaired renal or liver function may require reduced opioid doses to prevent accumulation of morphine metabolites (McGrath et al., 2014). Common side effects of opioids and associated nursing care are presented in Table 3.9.

Table 3.9 Common side effects of opioids and associated nursing care

Side effect	Comments	Nursing care
Respiratory depression	Key concern in the patient receiving opioids Increased risk: • In infancy, especially for premature child (due to hepatic immaturity and decreased morphine clearance) • Obesity or underweight • Respiratory comorbidities or obstructive sleep apnoea (Chidambaran et al., 2014)	Close monitoring of: • Level of consciousness • Physiological signs, including respiratory rate and oxygen saturation Ready access to (and co-prescription of) opioid-antagonist naloxone, for use in the event of respiratory depression (McQueen et al., 2012) particularly if patient receiving intravenous administration Use of multimodal analgesia regime to minimise opioid requirements (McGrath et al., 2014)
Nausea and vomiting	Opioids may stimulate the chemoreceptor trigger zone, or inhibit gut motility (Neal, 2016)	Antiemetic therapy such as a 5-HT3 receptor antagonist (e.g., ondansetron) known to be effective (McGrath et al., 2014)
Pruritus (itching)	Release of histamines from mast cells may occur following the administration of morphine (Dale and Haylett, 2009)	Antihistamines are a common choice for managing morphine-related itching; however, their sedative properties should be considered when administered alongside opioids (McGrath et al., 2014)

SEE ALSO
CHAPTER 4

ACTIVITY 3.4: REFLECTIVE PRACTICE

Taking into account the information above, how would you plan the postoperative pain management for children of the following ages?

- Baby aged 2 weeks
- Child aged 7 years

ACTIVITY 3.5: REFLECTIVE PRACTICE

- Based on your experiences in clinical placement to date, how well do you think current practices adhere to the WHO (2012) two-step strategy?
- How might you adapt your practice to optimise evidence-based nursing?

NON-PHARMACOLOGICAL MANAGEMENT OF PAIN

Cognitive strategies

Cognitive strategies can be employed to reduce pain during procedures, including methods that alter the child's perception of pain by reducing brain activity in areas associated with pain processing (McGrath et al., 2014). These are summarised in Table 3.10.

Table 3.10 Cognitive strategies for managing procedural pain

Procedure	Comments	Evidence
Distraction	The child's ability to fully focus their attention on the painful experience is decreased by drawing their attention towards a distractor, thus decreasing their anxiety and pain (Koller and Goldman, 2012)	Strategies most frequently employed are: cartoons, non-procedural talk, and music-distraction (DeMore and Cohen, 2005). More recently, handheld electronic devices used as preparatory and distraction tools have become available (Miller et al., 2016)
Hypnosis	Suggestion by the hypnotherapist, which aims to change the child's perceptions, emotions, or behavioural response to a subjective experience (Richardson et al., 2006)	Changes in cerebral blood flow are higher during a hypnotic state and it is thought that hypnosis may modulate areas of the brain activated by painful stimuli (Wood and Bioy, 2008)
Deep breathing	Deep breathing or asking a child to blow up a balloon. Although the medical status of a child with respiratory difficulties should be assessed before employing this intervention (Birnie et al., 2018)	A response to danger or threat may trigger an autonomic nervous system 'fight or flight' response. Making the out-breath longer than the in-breath promotes a parasympathetic nervous system 'rest and relax' state that can have an anti-anxiety effect which may help relieve physical pain and emotional distress (Deadman, 2018). There is evidence supporting the use of breathing interventions for reducing needle-related procedural pain and distress, although the quality of evidence is low and further research is required (Birnie et al., 2018)

(Continued)

Table 3.10 (Continued)

Procedure	Comments	Evidence
Guided imagery	Redirecting attention from an anxiety-provoking medically evoked (external) painful stimuli, to an internal (imagery) focus (McGrath et al., 2014). The child is 'guided' by the health professional to explore the sights, smells and sounds of the imaginary experience thus engaging them more fully in the distraction (King, 2010)	Reduction in behavioural signs of pain in adolescents using relaxation and guided imagery during venepuncture (Forsner et al., 2014)
Virtual reality (VR)	Involves computer-generated three-dimensional environment which stimulates the auditory and visual senses (Koller and Goldman, 2012)	VR has proven benefits in reducing pain, anxiety, and duration of procedures in burns patients (Scapin et al., 2018). VR is more beneficial than passive distraction (video games) in reducing simulated pain (holding hand in cold water). Most beneficial in adolescents aged 11–14 years (Malloy and Milling, 2010)

Physical strategies

Physical strategies may reduce pain during painful procedures in neonates and are described in Table 3.11.

Table 3.11 Physical strategies for managing procedural pain in neonates

Strategy	Comments	Evidence
Non-nutritive sucking (NNS)	The use of a dummy to induce sucking (Twycross et al., 2014)	Effective in reducing pain in full-term neonate (but not preterm or older infants) immediately following a painful procedure (Pillai Riddell et al., 2015)
Sweet tasting solutions	The oral administration of sweet-tasting solutions (e.g. sucrose at concentrations greater than 20%) appear to have an analgesic effect during intramuscular injections and venipuncture, which may be enhanced if combined with techniques such as swaddling or NNS (ANZCA&FPM, 2020)	The safety and efficacy of repeated doses has not been tested (Stevens et al., 2013.) There is insufficient evidence to recommend sweet-tasting solutions for needle-related procedures in older children and further evidence is required for its use in children between 1 and 4 years of age (McGrath et al., 2014)
Swaddling	Swaddling is gently wrapping the infant in a blanket to contain their arms and legs (Twycross et al., 2014)	There is low-quality evidence supporting the efficacy of swaddling and facilitated tucking in reducing pain immediately following procedures in preterm infants and neonates (Pillai Riddell et al., 2015)
Facilitated tucking (also called 'containment')	Firm but gentle containment of an infant's head and lower limbs (with legs flexed) using the hands of the caregiver (Pillai Riddell et al., 2015)	
Breastfeeding	Breastfeeding an infant prior to, and until completion of, the painful procedure (Harrison et al., 2016)	Reduces pain in post-neonatal infants undergoing immunisation, reducing pain scores and duration of cry. More evidence is required to evaluate its efficacy during venepuncture or on hospitalised infants (Harrison et al., 2016)

CASE STUDY 3.2: KAREN

Karen has brought her 1-year-old child George to the community health centre for his vaccinations. George has been very distressed during previous vaccinations and Karen is anxious to know what can be done to limit any pain and anxiety George may experience. Taking into account the information above, how would you plan the procedural pain management for children of the following ages?

- Baby aged 2 weeks
- Child aged 8 years
- Adolescent aged 13 years

ACTIVITY 3.6: REFLECTIVE PRACTICE

- Based on your experiences in clinical placement to date, how consistently do you think non-pharmacological management of procedural pain is employed?
- How might you adapt your practice to ensure you are utilising evidence-based non-pharmacological strategies?

CHAPTER SUMMARY

- Unrelieved pain may potentially have several short- and longer-term consequences so it is important to ensure children's pain is assessed and managed effectively
- There are several validated pain assessment tools for children of all ages. The appropriate tool should be selected and used to assess (and reassess) children's pain
- There are three types of analgesic drugs used with children. If used together they have a synergistic effect
- Non-pharmacological strategies can be used to reduce pain during painful procedures

BUILD YOUR BIBLIOGRAPHY

Books

- Twycross, A., Dowden, S.J. and Stinson, J. (eds) (2014) *Pain Management in Children: A Clinical Guide for Nurses and Healthcare Professionals*, 2nd edn. Oxford: Wiley-Blackwell.
- Stevens, B.J., Hathway, G and Zempsky, W. T. (eds) (2021) *Oxford Textbook of Paediatric Pain*, 2nd edn. Oxford: Oxford University Press.

FURTHER READING

Journal articles

FURTHER
READING:
ONLINE
JOURNAL
ARTICLES

- Twycross, A., Williams, A., Bolland, R. and Sunderland, R. (2015) 'Parents' attitudes towards children's pain and analgesic drugs'. *Journal of Child Health Care*, 19: 402-11.
- Twycross, A., Parker, R., Williams, A. and Gibson, F. (2015) 'Cancer-related pain and pain management: sources, prevalence and the experiences of children and parents'. *Journal of Paediatric Oncology Nursing*, 32: 369-84.

Weblinks

FURTHER
READING
WEBLINKS

- WellChild et al., *My Child Is in Pain* https://mychildisinpain.org.uk/
- Australian Government, Department of Health, *FLACC Pain Scale* www.health.gov.au/internet/publications/publishing.nsf/Content/triageqrq~triageqrq~pain~triageqrq-FLACC
- RCN Guidelines on Acute Pain in Children www.rcn.org.uk/professional-development/publications/pub-003542

REFERENCES

Andersen, R.D., Langius-Eklöfb, A., Nakstadc, B., Bernkleve, T. and Jylli L. (2017) 'The measurement properties of pediatric observational pain scales: a systematic review of reviews'. *International Journal of Nursing Studies, 73*: 93–101.

Anderson, B.J. (2008) Review article: 'Paracetamol (acetaminophen): mechanisms of action'. *Pediatric Anesthesia, 18*: 915–21.

Anderson, B.J. and Palmer G.M. (2006) 'Recent developments in the pharmacological management of pain in children'. *Current Opinion in Anaesthesiology, 19*: 285–92.

Association of Paediatric Anaesthetists of Great Britain and Ireland (APA) (2012) 'Good practice in postoperative and procedural pain management, 2nd edition'. *Pediatric Anesthesia, 22*: 1–79.

Australian and New Zealand College of Anaesthetists and Faculty of Pain Medicine (ANZCA&FPM) (2020) *Acute Pain Management: Scientific Evidence*, 5th edn. Melbourne: Australian and New Zealand College of Anaesthetists.

Birnie, K.A., Noel, M., Chambers, C.T., Uma, L.S. and Parker, J.A. (2018) 'Psychological interventions for needle-related procedural pain and distress in children and adolescents (Review)'. *Cochrane Database of Systematic Reviews*, Issue 10. Art. No.: CD005179.

Castarlenas, E., Jensen, M.P., von Baeyer. C.L. and Miro, J. (2017) 'Psychometric properties of the numerical rating scale to assess self-reported pain intensity in children and adolescents: a systematic review'. *Clinical Journal of Pain, 33*: 376–83.

Chidambaran, V., Olbrecht, V., Hossain, M., Sadhasivam, S., Rose, J. and Meyer, M.J. (2014) 'Risk predictors of opioid-induced critical respiratory events in children: naloxone use as a quality measure of opioid safety'. *Pain Medicine, 15*: 2139–49.

Dale, M.M. and Haylett, D.G. (2009) *Pharmacology Condensed*. Edinburgh: Churchill Livingstone.

Deadman, P (2018) 'The transformative power of deep, slow breathing'. *Journal of Chinese Medicine, 116*: 56–62.

DeMore, M. and Cohen, L.L. (2005) 'Distraction for pediatric immunization pain: a critical review'. *Journal of Clinical Psychology in Medical Settings, 12*: 281–91.

Eccleston, C., Fisher, E., Howard, R.F., Slater, R., Forgeron, P., Palermo, T.M., Birnie, K.A., Anderson, B.J., Chambers, C.T., Crombez, G., Ljungman, G., Jordan, I., Jordan, Z., Roberts, C., Schechter, N., Sieberg. C.B., Tibboel, D., Walker, S., Wilkinson, D. and Wood, C. (2020) 'Delivering transformative action in paediatric pain: a *Lancet Child & Adolescent Health Commission'. The Lancet Child & Adolescent Health*, 5 (1).

Electronic Medicines Compendium (2022) Summary of Product Characteristics: Paracetamol Tablets 500mg (POM). Available at: www.medicines.org.uk/emc/product/5916/smpc#PHARMACOLOGICAL_PROPS (accessed 4 April 2022).

Forsner, M., Norström, F., Nordyke, K., Ivarsson, A. and Lindh, V. (2014) 'Relaxation and guided imagery used with 12-year-olds during venipuncture in a school-based screening study'. *Journal of Child Health Care*, 18: 241–52.

Grunau, R.E. (2020) 'Personal perspectives. Infant pain: a multidisciplinary journey'. *Paediatric and Neonatal Pain*, 2: 50–7.

Harrison, D., Reszel, J., Bueno, M., Sampson, M., Shah, V.S., Taddio, A., Larocque, C. and Turner, L. (2016) 'Breastfeeding for procedural pain in infants beyond the neonatal period'. *Cochrane Database of Systematic Reviews*, Issue 10. Art NO. CD011248.

Hicks, C.L., von Baeyer, C.L., Spafford, P.A., van Korlaar, I. and Goodenough, B. (2001) 'The faces pain scale – revised: toward a common metric in pediatric pain measurement'. *Pain*, 93: 173–83.

Hockenberry, M.J., Wilson, D. and Winkelstein, M.L. (2005) *Wong's Essentials of Pediatric Nursing*, 7th edn. St Louis, MO: Mosby.

International Association for the Study of Pain (IASP) (2015) *Declaration of Montréal – Declaration that Access to Pain Management Is a Fundamental Human Right*. Available at: www.iasp-pain.org/DeclarationofMontreal?navItemNumber=582 (accessed 16 June 2017).

Johnson, P. (2013) 'Fever and neutropenia in the pediatric oncology patient'. *Journal of Pediatric Health Care*, 27: 66–70.

Kelly, L.E., Rieder, M., van den Anker, J., Malkin, B., Ross, C., Neely, M.N., Carleton, B., Hayden, M.R., Madadi, P. and Koren, G. (2012) 'More codeine fatalities after tonsillectomy in North American children'. *Pediatrics*, 129: e1343–47.

King, K. (2010) 'A review of the effects of guided imagery on cancer patients with pain'. *Complementary Health Practice Review*, 15 (2): 98–107.

Koller, D. and Goldman, R.D. (2012) 'Distraction techniques for children undergoing procedures: a critical review of pediatric research'. *Journal of Pediatric Nursing*, 27: 652–81.

Lauridsen, M.H., Kristensen, A.D., Hjortdal, V.E., Jensen, T.S. and Nikolajsen, L. (2014) 'Chronic pain in children after cardiac surgery via sternotomy'. *Cardiology in the Young*, 24: 893–9.

Malloy, K.M. and Milling, L.S. (2010) 'The effectiveness of virtual reality distraction for pain reduction: a systematic review'. *Clinical Psychology Review*, 30: 1011–18.

Malviya, S., Vopel-Lewis, T., Burke, C., Merkel, S. and Tait, A.R. (2006) 'The revised FLACC observational pain tool: improved reliability and validity for pain assessment in children with cognitive impairment'. *Pediatric Anesthesia*, 16: 258–65

Marzuillo, P., Calligaris, L. and Barbi, E. (2014) 'Tramadol can selectively manage moderate pain in children following European advice limiting codeine use'. *Acta Pædiatrica*, 103: 1110–16.

Maurice, S.C., O'Donnell, J.J. and Beattie, T.F. (2002) 'Emergency analgesia in the paediatric population: Part II Pharmacological methods of pain relief'. *Emergency Medicine Journal*, 19: 101–5.

McGrath, P.J., Stevens, B., Walker, S.M. and Zempsky, W.T. (eds) (2014) *Oxford Textbook of Paediatric Pain*. Oxford: Oxford University Press.

McQueen, S., Bruce, E.A. and Gibson, F. (2012) *The Great Ormond Street Hospital Manual of Children's Practices*. Chichester: Wiley-Blackwell.

Medicines and Healthcare products Regulatory Agency (2013) MHRA confirms codeine not to be used in children under 12 years old. Available at: http://webarchive.nationalarchives.gov.uk/20141205150130/www.mhra.gov.uk/home/groups/comms-po/documents/news/con287049.pdf (accessed 10 May 2017).

Merkel, S.I., Shayevitz, J.R., Voepel-Lewis, T. and Malviya, S. (1997) 'The FLACC: a behavioral scale for scoring postoperative pain in young children'. *Pediatric Nursing, 23*: 293–7.

Miller, K., Tan, X., Hobson, A.D., Khan, A., Ziviani, J., O'Brien, E., Barua, K., McBride, C.A., Kimble, R.M. (2016) 'A prospective randomized controlled trial of nonpharmacological pain management during intravenous cannulation in a pediatric emergency department'. *Pediatr Emerg Care. 32* (7): 444-51.

Neal, M.J. (2016) *Medical Pharmacology at a Glance*, 8th edn. Chichester: Wiley–Blackwell.

Neubert, A., Verhamme, K., Murray, M.L., Picelli, G., Hsiaa, Y., Sen, F.E., Giaquinto, C., Ceci, A., Sturkenboomb, M., Wonga, I.C.K. and on behalf of the TEDDY Network of Excellence (2010) 'The prescribing of analgesics and non-steroidal anti-inflammatory drugs in paediatric primary care in the UK, Italy and the Netherlands'. *Pharmacological Research, 62*: 243–8.

Nilsson, S., Finnstrom, B. and Kokinsky, E. (2008) 'The FLACC behavioral scale for procedural pain assessment in children aged 5–16 years'. *Pediatric Anesthesia, 18*: 767–74.

Pillai Riddell, R.R., Racine, N.M., Gennis, H.G., Turcotte, K., Uman, L.S., Horton, R.E., Ahola Kohut, S., Hillgrove Stuart, J., Stevens, B. and Lisi, D.M. (2015) 'Non-pharmacological management of infant and young child procedural pain'. *Cochrane Database of Systematic Reviews*, Issue 12, Art. No.: CD006275.

Polkki, T., Pietila, A.-M. and Vehvilainen, K. (2003) 'Hospitalized children's descriptions of their experiences with postsurgical pain relieving methods'. *International Journal of Nursing Studies, 40*: 33–44.

Prins, S.A., Van Dijk, M., Van Leeuwen, P., Searle, S., Anderson, B.J., Tibboel, D. and Mathot, R. (2008) 'Pharmacokinetics and analgesic effects of intravenous propacetamol vs rectal paracetamol in children after major craniofacial surgery'. *Pediatric Anesthesia, 18*: 582–92.

Raphael, J., Ahmedzai, S., Hester, J., Urch, C., Barrie, J., Williams, J., Farqhuar-Smith, P., Fallon, M., Hoskin, P., Robb, K. et al. (2010) 'Cancer pain: part 1: pathophysiology; oncological, pharmacological, and psychological treatments: a perspective from the British Pain Society endorsed by the UK Association of Palliative Medicine and the Royal College of General Practitioners'. *Pain Medicine, 11*(5):742–64.

Richardson, J., Smith, J.E., McCall, G. and Pilkington, K. (2006) 'Hypnosis for procedure-related pain and distress in pediatric cancer patients: a systematic review of effectiveness and methodology related to hypnosis interventions'. *Journal of Pain and Symptom Management, 31*: 70–84.

Royal College of Nursing (RCN) (2015) *Pain Knowledge and Skills Framework for the Nursing Team*. London: RCN.

Royal College of Nursing (RCN) (2009) *The Recognition and Assessment of Acute Pain in Children – Recommendations: Revised*. London: RCN.

Scapin, S., Echevarría-Guanilo, M.E., Boeira Fuculo Junior, P.R., Gonçalves, N., Kuerten Rocha, P. and Coimbra, R. (2018) 'Virtual Reality in the treatment of burn patients: a systematic review'. *Burns, 44*: 1403–16.

Stevens, B., Johnston, C., Petryshen, P. and Taddio, A. (1996) 'Premature infant pain profile: development and initial validation'. *Clinical Journal of Pain, 12*: 13–22.

Stevens, B., Johnston, C., Taddio, A., Gibbins, S. and Yamada, J. (2010) 'The premature infant pain profile: evaluation 13 years after development'. *Clinical Journal of Pain, 26*: 813–30.

Stevens, B., Yamada, J., Lee, G.Y. and Ohlsson, A. (2013) 'Sucrose for analgesia in newborn infants undergoing painful procedures'. *Cochrane Database of Systematic Reviews*. Issue 1, Art. No.: CD001069.

Stinson, J., Yamada, J., Kavanagh, T., Gill, N. and Stevens, B. (2006) 'Systematic review of the psychometric properties and feasibility of self-report pain measures for use in clinical trials in children and adolescents'. *Pain, 125*: 143–57.

Taddio, A., Katz, J., Ilersich, A.L. and Koren, G. (1997) 'Effect of neonatal circumcision on pain response during subsequent routine vaccination'. *The Lancet, 349* (1): 599-603.

Tomlinson, D., von Baeyer, C.L., Stinson, J.N. and Sung, L. (2010) 'A systematic review of faces scales for the self-report of pain intensity in children'. *Pediatrics*, *126* (5): e1168–98.

Twycross, A., Dowden, S.J. and Stinson, J. (eds) (2014) *Pain Management in Children: A Clinical Guide for Nurses and Healthcare Professionals*, 2nd edn. Oxford: Wiley-Blackwell.

van der Westhuizen, F.Y., Kuo, P.W. and Holder, K. (2011) 'Randomised controlled trial comparing oral and intravenous paracetamol (acetaminophen) plasma levels when given as preoperative analgesia'. *Anaesthetic Intensive Care*, *39*: 242–6.

Wong, D. and Baker, C. (1988) 'Pain in children: a comparison of assessment scales'. *Pediatric Nursing*, *14*: 9–17.

Wood, C. and Bioy, A. (2008) 'Hypnosis and pain in children'. *Journal of Pain and Symptom Management*, *35*: 437–46.

World Health Organization (WHO) (2012) *Persisting Pain in Children Package: WHO Guidelines on the Pharmacological Treatment of Persisting Pain in Children with Medical Illnesses*. Geneva: World Health Organization.

MEDICATION: MANAGEMENT, ADMINISTRATION AND COMPLIANCE/ CONCORDANCE

4

MARY BRADY AND LINDA MOORE

THIS CHAPTER COVERS

- Issues involved in administration of medication to children
- Legislation underpinning medication administration
- Errors and adverse reactions in medication administration
- Parental role in medication administration
- Drug calculation

"Giving medicines is a large part of a nurse's role and can seem really daunting at first. As long as you take each step at a time, follow the six R's and adhere to NMC rules, you will soon grow in confidence. There are always lots of resources available, such as the BNFc, local guidelines and your practice assessor/ practice supervisor, if you get stuck. Even qualified staff need to use these."

Carol, children's nurse

INTRODUCTION

As indicated in the quote above, drug administration is a fundamental part of the role of the children's nurse and this chapter will help to guide you towards achieving the knowledge and skills to competently address this aspect of practice within the remits of the Nursing and Midwifery Council in *The Code: Professional Standards of Practice and Behaviour for Nurses, Midwives and Nursing Associates* (NMC, 2018). The Royal Pharmaceutical Society (RPS) collaborated with the Royal College of Nursing (RCN) to provide guidance for the administration of medicines in healthcare settings (RPS, 2019), which is an additional useful resource to this chapter. As a nursing student you will be observing your practice assessors/practice supervisors and other staff administer medication. You will also participate in drug calculations and some medication administration according to your student status; however, it is not until you are a registered nurse that you may administer medication with another children's nurse. Additionally, to administer intravenous medication, further training is required once a period of preceptorship has been undertaken. This training will have been commenced in your pre-registration nurse education programme and completed post registration.

This chapter will guide you, as a nursing student, towards the safe administration of all medication to children and young people. Current issues will be explored, so that you will have a useful overview of the knowledge required to be a safe practitioner. Current legislation will underpin the guidance regarding the ordering, storage and administration of drugs.

ACTIVITY 4.1: CRITICAL THINKING

Consider your own anxieties about drug administration to children.

ISSUES INVOLVED IN THE ADMINISTRATION OF MEDICATION TO CHILDREN

Medication routes used with children

Medication can be administered to children in similar ways as those used with adults; however, the nurse must be aware of the child's physical age and abilities, in addition to their cognitive ability. For instance, babies and younger children would not be able to swallow tablets. Children may refuse medication because of its taste or smell, or fear such as if needle phobic. In each case, the prescriber would need to ensure that the route of administration took these into account in their decision-making. The prescriber may be a doctor or a nurse with prescribing qualifications. However, the parents and child may be consulted by the prescriber regarding their recommendation to ascertain what is clinically suitable and appropriate for the child.

The use of 'unlicensed' and 'off label' prescribing and administration

It is not uncommon in children's nursing for 'unlicensed' or 'off label' drugs to be given to children and young people requiring specialised treatment, so it is important that the prescriber can justify the drug use and the nurse understands the rationale. Prior to this the senior Trust pharmacist would have expressed their approval. The use of unlicensed drugs can sometimes evoke ethical dilemmas and could potentially be dissonant to NMC guidance (NMC, 2018). Moreover, the nurse has a duty to advocate for the patient and escalate any concerns to senior staff as detailed in the Trust's 'Raising concerns' policy.

The National Institute for Health and Care Excellence (NICE) aims to provide national guidance and advice based on robust evidence. Evidence summaries (ESUOMs) are developed to guide practitioners in their decision-making regarding the use of unlicensed and 'off label' medication. These medications are only used when there is no other licensed medication available, and a significant number of people require treatment. However, it is worth noting that even though an ESUOM has been developed, NICE guidance may not yet have been developed, since NICE reviews all the evidence and practical implications prior to implementing guidance.

Concordance versus compliance in medication management

The words 'compliance' and 'concordance' are sometimes used interchangeably in medication management, but each has a distinct meaning and their use will depend on the overall attitudes of the child and their family towards health and the perceived severity of the illness (Blair, 2011; Ogden, 2022).

Compliance tends to infer obedience to instructions, whereas concordance shows an appreciation that people make their own decisions about taking medicines and have the right to decline them once informed of the benefits and risks. Thus, concordance with medication is a more fitting aim for partnership working with children and their families, since as children's nurses we aim to develop a therapeutic relationship with the unique child and their family or carers, providing care that is suitable for the individual. Working in partnership with the child and their family is an underpinning philosophy of children's nursing, where good communication and an appreciation of the diversity of family life is fundamental (Smith and Coleman, 2010). As a result of their qualitative research study into children's pain management, Vasey et al. (2019) urged that nurses must support parental involvement as they try to advocate and negotiate for appropriate care for their child.

Indeed as an advocate, nurses should be instrumental in providing up-to-date relevant information to empower the child and family to make decisions. Their approach can influence child and parental concordance with medication, so it is important that the nurse has the knowledge and skills not just to administer the medication correctly, but also to teach the parents/carers.

It is worth remembering that even when not formally teaching, the nurse is role modelling good practice that will be copied by others.

CASE STUDY 4.1: JOANNA

Joanna is 16 years old and has cystic fibrosis. Recently she has had an increasing number of hospital admissions for 2 weeks of intravenous antibiotics and intensive physiotherapy. Over the past 6 months she has been prescribed high-calorie supplemental drinks between meals. Prior to this she was rarely in hospital and had managed to keep a stable weight gain appropriate to her height on the 25th centile. You have built up a good rapport with her and she reveals that this is all a waste of time; she would prefer to die than continue with a lifetime of taking drugs. She craves to be normal like her friends.

- Why is she saying this?
- What can the children's nurse do to help her manage her life and treatment schedule?

In adolescence, the experience of illness and especially chronic life-limiting conditions may have a negative effect on development and can also interfere with the young person's need for autonomy and a positive self-image within their peer group. Risk-taking behaviour is another aspect of this stage in development where boundaries are tested as the young person moves towards making more autonomous decisions regarding the management of their condition. Young people are often capable of making complex decisions, but under stress their level of maturity may reduce to that of a younger child (Blair, 2011). This has increased relevance when the condition is chronic (such as with diabetes, sickle cell anaemia and cystic fibrosis) and the young person wants to be able to enjoy similar spontaneity as their peer group.

ACTIVITY 4.2: CRITICAL THINKING

For many young people acne is part of their adolescent years, challenging their ability to conform to a body image norm. Various medical treatments exist that can reduce the severity of the acne. However, they often require the medication to be given over a long period and at regular intervals.

- Why is body image important to this age group?
- What medication could be given?
- What are the side effects of such medication?
- How could the practice nurse, school nurse or children's nurse support the young person to be compliant with their medication?
- What other advice could be given?

Covert administration of medication

There may be times when, for a variety of reasons, a child refuses to take medication. This situation must be discussed with the child to explore their reasons and understanding of the rationale for the medication. If the healthcare professionals feel that the medication is in the best interests of the child, administration may then be disguised. This could mean that the medication is put into food to ensure the child takes it; however, crushing tablets to disguise in food may make the drug ineffective or unlicensed. Some tablets may be designed for slow release and by crushing, may lead to toxic blood levels and an overdose. Similarly, mixing some drugs with foods or drink may make them ineffective. Therefore, the covert administration of medication is not a decision solely made by one person but by all the healthcare professionals involved with the child and family.

——— SAFEGUARDING STOP POINT ———

It is not unknown for parents to administer medication to their children to initiate fabricated fictitious illnesses. In such instances, the registered nurse (RN) must adhere to safeguarding policies, alerting the appropriate staff and providing clear documentation.

LEGISLATION UNDERPINNING MEDICATION ADMINISTRATION

The safe administration of medication is governed by specific legislation and the professional expectations of the Nursing and Midwifery Council (NMC, 2018).

The Medicines Act 1968 established a Medicines Commission to ensure the implementation of the Act and to advise government ministers. It also set out the regulatory controls for the manufacture and distribution of all medication. The Act was further amended in 2005 by the Medicines and Healthcare products Regulatory Agency (MHRA) and serves to advise government ministers and local authorities about medicines and to also investigate and collect information should adverse reactions occur.

Drugs are categorised under three headings:

- Those that do not require a prescription and can be sold in, for example, supermarkets under a General Sales List (GSL)
- Those that can only be sold under the supervision of a pharmacist but do not require a prescription (P)
- Those that are prescription only medicines (POMs)

In the hospital environment, it is usual that two RNs check all drugs prior to administering to the child (please refer to your local policy). Medication is not left unattended; instead, it is given directly to the child, thereby preventing the drug from not being administered or being taken by another child. Often parents may be present and may want to assist. It is important that they understand how to administer the drug appropriately and are aware of any potential hazards if medication is left unattended or there is a delay in administration. Any equipment used such as oral syringes, medication spoons or pots must be disposed of safely as per Trust policy.

Occasionally medication is given via injection using needles and syringes that must be disposed of after use promptly and safely in appropriate sharps receptacles as per Trust policy (RCN, 2013).

General storage of medication

In compliance with the Medicines Act 1968, all medicines are stored in locked cupboards within a hospital ward. Some medication, such as antibiotics and insulin, are sensitive to ambient temperature, so oral antibiotics are often supplied to wards in powder form to be dissolved in water for administration later. The pharmacist, or on occasions ward nurses, will dissolve the powder in the appropriate amount of sterile water. The solution then needs to be stored in a fridge. Where oral antibiotics are prescribed for use within the home, advice needs to be given to the family regarding safe storage and ensuring that the medicine is out of the reach of children and away from foods where there may be a cross-contamination risk.

Safe storage of other medication within a child's home is also important and the nurse may have to provide guidance for the family regarding safe storage that is practical and manageable within their home. For instance, not all medicines are supplied in childproof containers, such as those supplied in blister packs; so, families need to store medication in cupboards (ideally lockable) that are out of reach of young children and at temperatures that comply with medication guidance. Prior to discharge from hospital, it is also important to watch medication being administered by the carer/parent, since sometimes incorrect techniques may be being used (for example, inhaler technique), which will render the medication less effective.

Frequently children require medication whilst at school, so the school needs to ensure that the medication is stored safely and appropriately, but accessible at all times (for example, bronchodilators for an asthmatic child). On some occasions the child may need to carry their medication with them, so the parents should liaise closely with the school to facilitate this whilst also being aware of any potential hazards to other pupils. The school nurse may be able to assist in the decision-making process.

CASE STUDY 4.2: PHOEBE

You are on placement with a health visitor and have accompanied her on a new birth visit. Mandy gave birth to Joshua 12 days ago and already has a 3-year-old daughter called Phoebe. Phoebe has an ear infection and has been prescribed amoxicillin. Whilst in the house you notice that Mandy has left a packet of paracetamol and a bottle of amoxicillin on the work surface in the kitchen.

- Why might this have happened?
- What should you as a children's nurse do?
- What advice should be given to Mandy?

Controlled drugs

The Misuse of Drugs Act 1971 controls the import, production, supply and possession of drugs. Controlled drugs are regulated under this Act since they have the potential to be harmful. These drugs have been further subdivided into three classes:

- Class A: diamorphine, cocaine, methadone
- Class B: codeine, amphetamines
- Class C: diazepam, anabolic steroids

Depending on their practice area, children's nurses can be involved in administering controlled drugs such as diamorphine, codeine, methadone and diazepam.

Nurses who are in charge of wards or areas where controlled drugs are administered to children and young people are responsible for the storage, ordering and administration of such drugs. Due to their potential for addiction, the storage of controlled drugs (CDs) is governed by various legislation; specifically, the Misuse of Drugs (Safe Custody) Regulations (1971, 2001 and 2007).

In hospital, the nurse in charge of the ward has responsibility for the possession, safe custody and issue of CDs. At times this might be delegated to another RN, but the nurse in charge remains responsible.

Storage of controlled drugs

CDs must be stored within a locked cabinet that is ideally made of steel fixed to a wall or the floor within another cupboard that is also lockable. The wall should be of 'suitable thickness'. The number of CDs stored within an area or ward must be kept to a minimum, whilst also being appropriate for the potential needs of the children/young people being cared for in that area/ward.

The stock levels of CDs are checked daily by two registered nurses (RNs) on most wards and prior to the preparation for administration to a child or young person. The RNs who check the drugs must document that the amount present is in accordance with the ward controlled drug record book.

When stock levels are low a requisition is completed from an ordering book with triplicate pages and sent to pharmacy. When new CDs are issued, they must be carried to the area in a lockable container and immediately checked into the CD cupboard by two RNs and the CD record book updated.

CASE STUDY 4.3: EMMANUEL

Your patient, Emmanuel, has been receiving a continuous infusion of morphine via an infusion pump as Patient Controlled Analgesia. The syringe is nearly empty, so you have asked your practice assessor for a new syringe. Together with another RN your practice assessor prepares to draw up another syringe. On checking the CD register, there appears to be fewer morphine ampoules present than on the register.

- What should happen next?
- What may have happened to create this situation?

Administration of controlled drugs to a child/young person

When a child requires a controlled drug (CD), two RNs check that the prescription is appropriate and that the existing stock level correlates with the record book. The correct amount of the drug is then prepared and administered to the correct child and any unused CD is recorded as wastage in the record book. Throughout the procedure, the two RNs work together to ensure that the administration and documentation adhere to current standards.

ERRORS AND ADVERSE REACTIONS IN MEDICATION ADMINISTRATION

Medication errors do happen and are an ongoing major clinical challenge in both hospital and community settings. They can result in significant morbidity and mortality for patients (General Medical Council, 2012; Quinn, 2022). Using research findings, the phenomena will be explored and interventions that may reduce the incidence of errors and adverse reactions will be suggested whilst also emphasising the need for continued vigilance by all staff.

The Medicines and Healthcare Products Regulatory Agency (MHRA) promotes the efficacy and safety of medicines and medical devices. Adverse incidents that occur in practice are reported to the MHRA via a yellow card system. This information can then be cascaded back to clinical areas as alerts to avoid further similar incidents. It is important that any adverse reaction that occurs in children is reported to the MHRA, especially since children are not usually involved in medical trials of drugs due to the ethical aspects of obtaining consent, so some of the drugs given to children will not have been licensed for their use. Furthermore, we know that children differ physiologically from adults, for example in the maturity of their organs, and therefore may react differently to medication.

Any miscalculation of the drug dose when prescribing or when administering is a potential hazard, thus numerical ability is an important requirement for all nurses. As a student your numerical ability will be tested frequently and as a registered nurse many Trusts impose mandatory annual testing to minimise the risk to patients.

WHAT'S THE EVIDENCE?

A study by Elliott et al. (2021) estimated that 327 million drug errors occur annually in England in both in-patient and community settings across all ages. These resulted in prolonged hospital stays or admissions from community settings and 0.038% resulted in death where the adverse drug error was a cause or contributory factor. Elliott et al. (2018) noted that the errors were due to administration (54%), prescribing (21%) and dispensing (16%). Furthermore, their findings were similar to earlier studies in the United States of America. However, they concluded that further study was required to develop a deeper understanding of the impact.

Furthermore, Stolic et al.'s (2022) systematic review that addressed errors involving student nurses in practice, found that numerical error was often an issue as well as knowledge about drugs and general confusion about the 'Rights' of medication (see Table 4.1). This re-emphasises the importance of accurate numeracy skills for nurses.

Drug errors are taken seriously; they have an impact on the child, young person, their family or carers as well as the NHS and the nurses(s) involved. Nurses who are negligent in their medication management and have harmed patients as a result are cautioned or disciplined, and they and/or their employers will be required to take remedial action. Organisations have a responsibility to create a culture of openness where errors are reported, and to minimise and manage future risk. To reduce the incidence of error, nurses should always check that the dose correlates with guidance from the British National Formulary for Children (BNFc). This is available in hard copy as well as an online application and mobile app.

As an advocate for children, it is imperative that the nurse is aware of correct drug dosages and checks the BNFc when unsure. Any errors in prescribing can be avoided if the nurse contacts the prescriber requesting that the appropriate amendments are made, using the BNFc to support this request. Thus, drug errors such as those mentioned above are taken seriously given the risk to the patients entrusted to the nurse's care. Ultimately, nurses who are negligent in their medication management must answer to their employer/professional body.

The children's nurse should remember the Rights of medication administration to reduce the potential for error in this important aspect of care (Table 4.1). Since it is nurses who administer the medication in most instances, they must also ensure that they have the knowledge and skills to prepare the drug appropriately. For instance, some oral drugs need to be dissolved in water. When preparing and administering intravenous medication, the agreed Trust policy and manufacturer's guidance must be adhered to regarding adding diluents and calculating the amount of liquid to be given, considering displacement volumes that arise when the diluent is added to the dried preparation. In addition, some intravenous drugs need to be infused slowly whilst others can be given safely as boluses. The intravenous administration of medication requires additional knowledge and skills and is normally undertaken once the newly qualified nurse has become established in that role. It is never undertaken by a nursing student. In short, all student and registered nurses must be aware of their own sphere of competence and always work within that sphere whilst seeking the knowledge to advance their abilities.

Table 4.1 Six 'Rights' of medication administration

Six Rights	Details
Right drug	Full generic name and strength
Right dose	Without abbreviations

(Continued)

Table 4.1 (Continued)

Six Rights	Details
Right route	Without abbreviations
Right time	Start, finish dates and frequency
Right patient	Full name of child or young person Age and/or date of birth For hospital patients: • Hospital number • Hospital and ward names
Right documentation completed	Child's weight in kilograms Allergies recorded Prescriber's signature Nurse(s) who administered the drug signature(s)

Adapted from: Blair, 2011, p.141

PARENTAL ROLE IN MEDICATION ADMINISTRATION

It is worth remembering that most illnesses that a child will suffer are treated at home by parents and carers. As a children's nurse, your advice and guidance may be required regarding the safe and appropriate administration and storage of medication – for instance, ensuring that medication is taken as prescribed but at realistic times that work in conjunction with family life to maximise compliance (indicated by parent voice below).

"As the parent of a child who requires administration of multiple medications every day at different times, I find the process very difficult and I am only human and have forgotten one or two on many occasions. As a family we have now set alarms for each dose and put up a visual reminder for my daughter in her room so if she goes to bed and we have forgotten her inhaler she remembers when she sees the poster and we can administer. When you're a working family, juggling medications can be harder as school can be reluctant to administer medications. It can feel like a full-time job just ensuring she takes everything at the right time. The GP has been very supportive, and we now do electronic repeat prescriptions which go straight to the pharmacy saving time and I can request these online which is very helpful. The pharmacy has also delivered when they needed to order in medications to save us a return trip. Overall, we find the support from healthcare professionals excellent; it's the day-to-day management that can feel like a struggle."

Debbie, parent

Safe storage within the child's home is important and the general storage advice given earlier should be adhered to. It is also important to watch medication being administered by the carer/parent since sometimes incorrect techniques may be being used (inhaler technique) which will render the medication less effective.

DRUG CALCULATION

Doses required for children frequently require understanding of the formulation of the drug and calculation of the amount required as prescribed. This is sometimes due to the drug being designed for adult use or because the drug is available in a liquid form in a volume requiring calculation. The formula used for calculating the correct volume is:

$$\frac{\text{The amount Needed multiplied by the volume you Have}}{\text{The Stock amount available}}$$

You may find this mnemonic useful: $\dfrac{\text{NH}}{\text{S}}$

Thus, if a child needed 50 milligrammes of ibuprofen and a bottle containing 100 milligrammes in 5 millilitres was available, the calculation would be:

$$\frac{50}{100} \times 5 = \frac{250}{100} = 2.5\,\text{millilitres}$$

Another example is a child needs 100 milligrammes of flucloxacillin. There is a bottle of 125 milligrammes in 5 millilitres available, the calculation is:

$$\frac{100}{125} \times 5 = \frac{500}{125} = 4\,\text{millilitres}$$

It is also worth considering the size of the child in relation to their age in order to make a 'rough' estimate prior to calculating the volume to be given, so that logic is used as well as accurate calculation.

CHAPTER SUMMARY

- As a nursing student you will help to administer medication to children and young people
- There is an expectation that this will be done competently and with adherence to current legislation. Thus, as a student, it is important that you witness and participate in best practice
- Drug knowledge of the medication administered in your practice area and numerical competence are absolute requirements for nurses
- In the event of any error, the nurse must be honest, promptly reporting the error to senior staff and efforts made to minimise its recurrence

BUILD YOUR BIBLIOGRAPHY

Books

- Blair, K. (2011) *Medicines Management in Children's Nursing*. London: Sage.

  Structured around the NMC Essential Skills Clusters for medicines management, this book covers legal aspects, drugs calculations, administration, storage, record keeping, introductory pharmacology, patient communication and contextual issues in medication.
- McFadden, R. (2019) *Introducing Pharmacology for Nursing and Healthcare*, 3rd edn. Abingdon: Routledge.

FURTHER
READING

This book addresses the related physiology and pathophysiology necessary to develop an understanding of how commonly used drugs work.

- Starkings, S. and Krause, L. (2015) *Passing Calculation Tests for Nursing Students*, 3rd edn. London: Sage.

This book provides drug and fluid calculations that will help build your confidence with this skill.

Journal articles

FURTHER
READING:
ONLINE
JOURNAL
ARTICLES

- Vasey, J., Smith, J., Kirshbaun, M.N. and Chirema, K. (2019) 'Tokensism or true partnership: parental involvement in a child's acute pain management'. *Journal of Clinical Nursing*, 28: 1491–505.

This paper described a small qualitative study to explore the reality of involving parents and other family members in pain management of children. The findings revealed that although nurses wanted to involve parents, they did not always follow this through in practice.

- Roberts, R.M., Albert, A.P., Johnson, D.D. and Hicks, L.A. (2015) 'Can improving knowledge of antibiotic-associated adverse drug events reduce parent and patient demand for antibiotics?' *Health Services Research and Managerial Epidemiology*, 1–5. Available at: http://journals.sage-pub.com/doi/pdf/10.1177/2333392814568345.

Some people believe that antibiotics are harmless, so this qualitative study was undertaken to assess the knowledge of adult patients and mothers of young patients. The findings revealed that nearly all mothers were aware that there were possible side effects with medications (including antibiotics); however, adult patients did not acknowledge this to the same extent.

- Marc, C., Vrignaud, B., Levieux, K., Robine, A., Gras Le Guen, C. and Launay, E. (2016) 'Inappropriate prescription of antibiotics in pediatric practice: analysis of the prescriptions in primary care'. *Journal of Child Health Care*, 20 (4): 530–6.

This paper addressed the inappropriate prescription of antibiotics in primary care and highlighted that GPs lacked the time to fully explain to parents why their child's infection did not warrant antibiotics and instead prescribed antibiotics that parents believed were required.

- Twycross, A.M., Williams, A.M., Bolland, R.E. and Sutherland, R. (2015) 'Parental attitudes to children's pain and analgesic drugs in the United Kingdom'. *Journal of Child Health Care*, 19 (3): 402–11.

This study explored parental attitudes towards analgesic administration to their child, highlighting that parents sometimes misread the amount of pain experienced by their child and their subsequent need for analgesia. Since many children will be discharged home after day surgery, this has relevance for parental advice prior to discharge so that the child's pain level is adequately managed.

Weblinks

FURTHER
READING:
WEBLINKS

- BNFC, *BNF Online* www.bnf.org/products/bnf-online The formulary is regularly updated providing information about drugs that may be given to children, their use, dosage, contraindications and side effects.
- Medicines and Healthcare products Regulatory Agency www.gov.uk/government/organisations/medicines-and-healthcare-products-regulatory-agency A regularly updated resource regarding medication, devices and all aspects of drug safety.
- NICE, *Medicines management – children* www.nice.org.uk/guidance/ng5

REFERENCES

Blair, K. (2011) *Medicines Management in Children's Nursing*. Exeter: Learning Matters.

Elliot, R.A., Camacho, I., Jankovic, I.D., Sculpher, M.J. and Faria, R. (2021) 'Economic analysis of the prevalence and clinical and economic burden of medication error in England'. *British Medical Journal Quality and Safety*, 30: 96–105.

General Medical Council (2012) *Investigating the Prevalence and Causes of Prescribing Errors in General Practice*. The PRACtICe Study. Available at: www.gmc-uk.org/about/what-we-do-and-why/data-and-research/research-and-insight-archive/investigating-the-prevalence-and-causes-of-prescribing-errors-in-general-practice (accessed: 15 November 2020).

Nursing and Midwifery Council (NMC) (2018) *The Code: Professional Standards of Practice and Behaviour for Nurses, Midwives and Nursing Associates*. London: NMC. Available at: www.nmc.org.uk/standards/code/.

Ogden, J. (2022 'Health psychology', in J. Naidoo and J. Wills (eds), *Health Studies: An Introduction*, 3rd edn. London: Palgrave Macmillan Education.

Quinn, H. (2022) 'Medication errors in children's care: what nurses need to know'. *Nursing Children and Young People*, 34 (4): 8–9.

Royal College of Nursing (RCN) (2013) *Sharps Safety: RCN Guidance to Support the Implementation of The Health and Safety* (Sharp Instruments in Healthcare Regulations). London: RCN.

Royal Pharmaceutical Society (2019) *Professional Guidance on the Administration of Medicines in Healthcare*. Available at: www.rpharms.com/Portals/0/RPS%20document%20library/Open%20access/Professional%20standards/SSHM%20and%20Admin/Admin%20of%20Meds%20prof%20guidance.pdf?ver=2019-01-23-145026-567 (accessed: 15 November 2020).

Smith, L. and Coleman, V. (2010) *Child and Family-centred Healthcare: Concept, Theory and Practice*, 2nd edn. Basingstoke: Palgrave Macmillan.

Stolic, S., Ng, L., Southern, J. and Sheridan, G. (2020) 'Medication errors by nursing students on clinical practice: an integrative review'. *Journal of Nurse Education*, 112: 1–9.

Vasey, J., Smith, J., Kirshbaun, M.N. and Chirema, K. (2019) 'Tokensism or true partnership: parental involvement in a child's acute pain management'. *Journal of Clinical Nursing*, 28: 1491–505.

INTERPROFESSIONAL WORKING

5

GEORGINA GREEN

THIS CHAPTER COVERS

- Core elements of interprofessional working (IPW)
- Benefits and challenges of IPW
- Current IPW practices across the UK
- Health and social care integration
- IPW and transition

> "Alone we can do so little. Together we can do so much."
>
> **Helen Keller**

INTRODUCTION

As children's nurses we have a unique and privileged position working with children, young people and their families; however, we cannot do this in isolation. An interprofessional working (IPW) approach is not just about other services you may refer to, it is how you collaborate with other professionals. It is a vital approach to ensure that we meet the complex, holistic needs of children and young people. This chapter will encourage you to explore the role of the children's nurse within IPW, focusing on communication and collaboration. The benefits and challenges of IPW across the UK will also be discussed along with the future of IPW within children's services.

ACTIVITY 5.1: REFLECTIVE PRACTICE

- Reflect on what 'collaboration' means to you.
- What disciplines can you think of that children's nurses may collaborate with?

CORE ELEMENTS OF INTERPROFESSIONAL WORKING

"Inter-agency professional working has helped achieve positive outcomes for the families I work with in many ways. Firstly, using a universal, child-centred framework provides a consistent assessment across many disciplines. In addition, it facilitates clear communication with common, understood professional language. This enables the sharing of information readily between professionals which facilitates timely identification of needs, appropriate referrals, and addressing any concerns promptly thus enabling positive outcomes for families."

Karen, Health Visitor

Karen has highlighted the importance of adopting a consistent assessment and the sharing of information to provide positive family-centred care. IPW happens when professionals work together to plan care to meet a common goal (Barr and Dowding, 2019; Delves-Yates, 2022). You may find that IPW, multidisciplinary and interdisciplinary are used interchangeably in practice. Multidisciplinary refers to individual involvement from other members of the health team and has largely been replaced by interprofessional/interdisciplinary as this approach is much more collaborative and beneficial for children and their families. For example, multidisciplinary may mean the children's nurse refers a child for specific input from another professional. The two professionals will be working together but they will each have very specific tasks to carry out and little collaboration (Day, 2018). Pullon et al. (2016) describe IPW as an 'active partnership' between professionals. Remembering that in IPW where two or more professionals are working together alongside the child, young person and family the aim is to achieve the best possible collaborative care decisions (Arnold and Underman Boggs, 2018). The United Nations Convention on the Rights of the Child (1989) established the right for children and young people to be listened to and for their opinions to be at the heart of any decision-making. This is also covered in Chapter 1, Involving children, young people and families in care.

SEE ALSO CHAPTER 1

The World Health Organization (WHO) defines interprofessional collaboration as 'Collaborative practice happens when multiple health workers from different professional backgrounds work together with patients, families, carers and communities to deliver the highest quality of care across settings' (WHO, 2010).

There are some IPW practices within children's services that are underpinned by legislation and policies. There are a number of high-profile safeguarding cases that have led to recommendations for national practice. Sadly, reviews from cases such as Victoria Climbié, Peter Connolly and Daniel Pelka all highlight the need for improved interprofessional collaboration, information-sharing processes, integrated training and improved communication (Laming, 2003, 2009). Despite the recommendations from these reviews we still see the same criticisms in serious case reviews and services failing children and young people. The statutory document *Working Together to Safeguard Children* (HM Government, 2018) has seen a number of revisions due to a number of public inquiries and has been updated following the Children Act 2004 which placed a duty on all agencies to work together to safeguard children. The 2018 statutory guidance focuses on early help and identifies three key agencies: Health, Police and Local Authority to ensure a local multi-agency response (HM Government, 2018). This topic is also covered in Chapter 9, Safeguarding children and young people.

SEE ALSO
CHAPTER 9

A review by the NSPCC and the Social Care Institute for Excellence (SCIE) in 2016 found that problems with interprofessional communication was still a common theme in serious case reviews. The NSPCC (2019) recommends the following principles when working as part of an interprofessional team:

- Improve communication – use clear language and don't use jargon. Have a common purpose and if possible shared records.
- Teamwork – understand everyone's roles and promote a collaborative culture.
- Consistency – parents should receive the same information from each professional.
- Build trusting, working relationships – respect and listen to each other. Be accountable, discuss and explore differences in opinions.
- Ensure appropriate resource allocation.

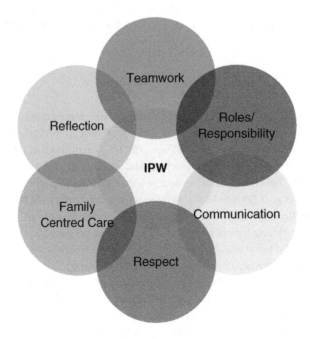

Figure 5.1   Model of IPW (adapted from Thistlethwaite and Moran, 2010)

Good record-keeping skills are essential to interprofessional working. Records should provide the reader with a summary of what has been done, what needs to be done, when does it need to be done, why it needs to be done and the outcome of any work already completed (Nursing and Midwifery Council (NMC), 2018). Care should be taken to avoid professional jargon as we know this is a common barrier to clear communication.

ACTIVITY 5.2: REFLECTIVE PRACTICE

- Look at the table set out below that highlights 10 competencies for interprofessional collaboration (Nancarrow et al., 2013).
- Reflect on a time in practice when you have been part of an IPW team. Which competencies did you observe that worked well?

1.	Identifies a leader who establishes a clear direction and vision for the team, while listening and providing support and supervision to the team members.
2.	Incorporates a set of values that clearly provide direction for the team's service provision; these values should be visible and consistently portrayed.
3.	Demonstrates a team culture and interdisciplinary atmosphere of trust where contributions are valued and consensus is fostered.
4.	Ensures appropriate processes and infrastructures are in place to uphold the vision of the service (for example, referral criteria, communications infrastructure).
5.	Provides quality patient-focused services with documented outcomes; utilizes feedback to improve the quality of care.
6.	Utilizes communication strategies that promote intra-team communication, collaborative decision-making and effective team processes.
7.	Provides sufficient team staffing to integrate an appropriate mix of skills, competencies, and personalities to meet the needs of patients and enhance smooth functioning.
8.	Facilitates recruitment of staff who demonstrate interdisciplinary competencies including team functioning, collaborative leadership, communication, and sufficient professional knowledge and experience.
9.	Promotes role interdependence while respecting individual roles and autonomy.
10.	Facilitates personal development through appropriate training, rewards, recognition, and opportunities for career development.

In the new NMC (2018) Future Nurse standards, nurses are expected to understand and apply the principles of IPW including the underpinning health and social policies that inform IPW practice (Platform 7.1, 7.2). Alongside this there are also standards around leading and managing interdisciplinary teams (Platform 5, Leading and managing nursing care and working in teams). The NMC places particular emphasis on the understanding of roles and responsibilities of all members of the interdisciplinary team.

The Centre for the Advancement of Interprofessional Education (CAIPE) defines Interprofessional Education (IPE) as 'Occasions when two or more professions learn with, from and about each other to improve collaboration and the quality of care' (CAIPE, 2016). IPE is seen by many as a positive step to ensuring that newly qualified staff understand roles within IPW and encourages students from differing professional disciplines to work together. As we have previously discussed, serious case reviews and reviews such as the review of maternity services at Shrewsbury and Telford Hospital NHS Trust continue to highlight a lack of communication and conflicting agency agendas as a factor in poor outcomes for children and their families (Ockenden, 2022).

IPE promotes collaborative practice and, if embedded successfully within undergraduate programmes, can enable professionals to build on active listening skills and the ability to make collaborative decisions (Wilkinson, 2022). IPE does, however, have to be a worthwhile experience and not one that focuses on multidisciplinary teams.

As students find through attending IPW workshops, they can gain an understanding of roles, a respect for differences in professional values, communicate with different philosophies and learn to negotiates differences through IPE (Ford and Gray, 2021). CAIPE highlight IPE as a way to improve collaboration and safe patient care whilst promoting professional respect, equality and instilling inter-professional values ensuring the identity of each profession is sustained (CAIPE, 2011). It is also an opportunity to introduce students to Group Theory concepts, such as those of Tuckman (1965). An understanding of how teams form can help students understand why there is often conflict within new teams and how to move forward through this (Day, 2018). Tuckman (1965) identified five stages of team development, as seen in Figures 5.2 and 5.3.

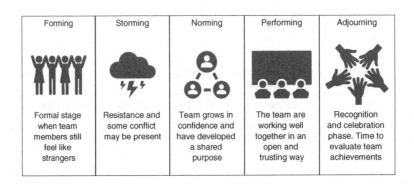

Figure 5.2 Five stages of team development

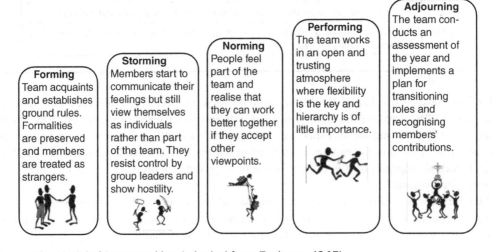

Figure 5.3 Model of team working (adapted from Tuckman, 1965)

BENEFITS AND CHALLENGES OF IPW

> "When I was unwell and in school CAMHS, school nurses and education support worked together, communicated and supported me. Children's mental health nurses made plans for within the school setting for certain situations and supported education to carry out these plans when and where needed. Overall, all professionals that were involved within my care worked together to support me, keep me safe and give me the best chance to have the best future possible! If it wasn't for these professionals working together I believe I wouldn't be doing as good as I am today!"
>
> **Elise, young person**

Elise has highlighted the importance of professionals working together and how truly life-changing this was for her. As children's nurses we are, quite rightly, very proud of our identity and our role in supporting children, young people and their families. As we have already discussed, we cannot do this in isolation.

There are, however, challenges when working with other professions. There are individual differences in education, experiences and values, along with organisational differences that can sometimes present barriers. Schot et al. (2019) identify that barriers such as separate IT systems, distinct professional domains and overlapping of roles can cause challenges for IPW.

> "Sometimes although IPW has many benefits no one wants to take on the lead role because it is seen as involving a lot of work. Everyone is busy but it often falls back to health to take on the lead. Sometimes I feel that we lose sight of the needs of the child and family and need to remember that we are all there for the common goal of ensuring they receive the best care and outcomes possible."
>
> **Jenna, community children's nurse**

Jenna highlights some of the challenges faced when working in an IPW team. There can be professional tensions as she mentions around workload/resource allocation and a lack of understanding around responsibilities.

Grant and Goodman (2019) identify a number of barriers that can occur as teams develop, including gender, differing professional education, differing lines of management, differing cultures and different values, all of which can impact the success of IPW.

The benefits and challenges of IPW can be summarised as follows:

Benefits of IPW

- Improved outcomes for children and young people
- Improved quality of care

- Sharing of expertise
- Children, young people and families central to decision-making
- Professional development

Challenges of IPW

- Resource allocation
- Organisational structure
- IT systems
- Overlapping of roles
- Professional tension

To overcome challenges there are a number of suggestions made for professionals within IPW. Key themes to overcome barriers identified from evidence include bridging gaps, negotiating roles, collaboration and organisational support (Schot et al., 2019). Barr and Dowding (2019) recommend that the benefits of IPW will be enhanced by embedding mutual support, friendship, regular feedback and the sharing of knowledge.

ACTIVITY 5.3: CRITICAL THINKING

Watch this video: 'Partnership working in child protection'
https://youtube/EtkcOLnIRPE

- What problems does the video highlight around IPW?
- What are the benefits of IPW ?

CURRENT IPW PRACTICES ACROSS THE UK

"As a School Nurse working remotely in Scotland I would not be able to fulfil my roles and responsibilities without the collaboration between other professionals and services. Because we have to travel such long distances (sometimes using boats!) I rely on education partners, social work, GP staff and midwives to keep me up to date with any concerns and changes. One of the most important skills I have learnt along the way is to respect and value the contribution that other professionals can make to ensure we provide the best care possible for children, young people and their families."

Kate, school nurse

There are numerous services involved in the care of children, young people and their families. Services vary across the UK but they all have common themes, chiefly that no one works in isolation.

Scotland

The Getting It Right for Every Child (GIRFEC) principles have been used in practice since 2006 and embedded in the Children and Young Peoples (Scotland) Act (Scottish Government, 2014). The GIRFEC approach focuses on the health and wellbeing of children and provides a framework for consistent assessment across all agencies. The GIRFEC National Practice Model combines wellbeing indicators with the 'my world triangle' assessment to ensure a shared understanding and common language for all children's services. The role of the lead professional is pivotal within this process to coordinate support required within a multi-agency child's plan. The lead professional will be a practitioner who has the appropriate skills and experience, remembering that in IPW two or more professionals are working together alongside the child, young person and family to achieve the best collaborative care decisions (Scottish Government, 2022).

All children and young people in Scotland are entitled to a Named Person, which will either be from Health (0–5) or Education (5–18). The Named Person acts as a clear point of contact and signposter for appropriate support. The role of lead professional is not to be confused with the Named Person, although in certain circumstances they may be the same. As a children's nurse you may undertake the named person role as a health visitor or as lead professional, for example as a community children's nurse.

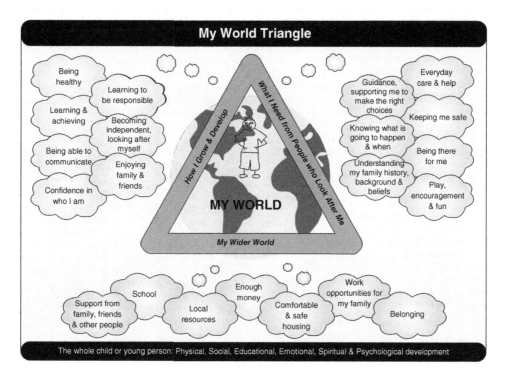

Figure 5.4 GIRFEC – My World Triangle (Scottish Government, 2018)

Northern Ireland

Northern Ireland has a network of over 29 Family Support Hubs which provide early intervention services across all children and young people. Understanding the Needs of Children in Northern Ireland (UNOCINI) is a multidisciplinary tool which aims to identify needs at an early stage. It is a framework adopted by all services involved in the care of children and young people to standard-ise and streamline assessment planning and the implementation of child and family processes to improve communication.

A key aim of the UNOCINI approach is to communicate needs of children and young people clearly and concisely to all professionals (Department of Health, Northern Ireland, 2011). A review of the UNOCINI began in February 2022.

England

The 'Early Help' model has now replaced the Common Assessment Framework. Early Help is a single, holistic assessment around the whole family which enables early assessment. It uses the 'signs of safety' approach which, as with the Scottish GIRFEC model, is a strengths-based approach to early intervention (HM Government, 2022). One of the main aims of Early Help is to improve multi-agency working through a coordinated approach. Once an Early Help Assessment has been completed a Team Around the Family (TAF) meeting will take place. The TAF approach brings together professionals from a number of different agencies including teachers, social workers, GPs, youth workers and nurses.

A TAF will coordinate an IPW plan, identifying a lead professional who will be the key contact. Alongside the TAF each local authority will have a threshold of need, which enables a consistent assessment that is understood by all professionals. It promotes effective communication, information sharing and engagement across all agencies. An example is shown in Figure 5.5.

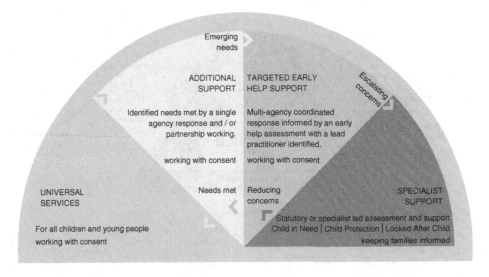

Figure 5.5 Example of a threshold of need framework (Hull City Council, 2022)

Wales

Wales has introduced the Families First programme which is administered by each local authority. Again, this model promotes multi-agency working to ensure a joined-up approach focusing on early intervention and prevention. Adopting a strengths-based approach as we have seen in other areas of the UK, Wales also utilises the Team Around the Family (TAF) following an initial child and family (CAF) assessment referral (Welsh Government, 2017).

A key worker will be identified through the TAF to coordinate services and ensure regular meetings take place to promote collaboration. As with the other UK nations, assessments will be based on a threshold of need framework.

Although each of the four nations have their own approaches we can identify key themes. Early intervention models have been adopted across the UK to promote a shared understanding and improve information sharing across the agencies (Selwyn, 2022). Children, young people and their families are at the centre of the assessment process. The success of all these practice models lies with staff understanding their roles along with robust information-sharing practices. Whether a key worker or lead professional is appointed they must be supported by all members of the IPW team to ensure the best outcomes for children and young people.

HEALTH AND SOCIAL CARE INTEGRATION - FUTURE OF IPW

The National Health Service Long Term Plan (2019) aims to improve care by bringing professionals together. There are a number of key measures to improve children and young people's health outcomes, and to facilitate the implementation of these the Children and Young People's Transformation Programme has been established [review the plans at www.rcpch.ac.uk/resources/nhs-long-term-plan-summary-child-health-proposals]. The NHS Long Term Plan set out to improve healthcare through greater collaboration through primary care networks, integrated care systems and the sustainability transformation partnerships.

Following the NHS Long Term Plan, the Health and Care Bill (2022) has now been passed in England and sees the implementation of 42 Integrated Care Systems (ICS). The aim of the ICS through integrating NHS services, local authority, support agencies and the third care sector is to ultimately improve collaboration to improve population health and reduce health inequalities (Department of Health and Social Care, 2022). As part of the ICS, the Integrated Care Boards have now replaced the Clinical Commissioning Groups and will be responsible for partnership planning to improve health in their local areas for children, young people and their families.

We know that the COVID-19 pandemic demonstrated the value of local authorities, NHS and third sector working together to provide joined-up care and support better outcomes for children and young people. The ICS will build on this and seek to embed collaboration at an organisational and statutory level (Department of Health and Social Care, 2022).

The UK Government has also announced plans for 'Start for Life' hubs across England (Department of Health and Social Care, 2021). These interprofessional services will support families and children in the first 1001 critical days of a child's life. Services working together within these hubs will include local authorities, the NHS, public health, social work, education, housing and third sector agencies. It is hoped that the family hub will provide a seamless service where services such as midwifery, health visiting, mental health support, parenting courses and infant feeding advice could all be accessed. There are a number of early implementation sites and emerging evidence of positive impact has been seen. The 'Start for Life' hubs appear to build on the previous success of Sure Start centres, which were established in 1999 but developed into the children centres we now see in some areas.

SEE ALSO
CHAPTER 11

WHAT'S THE EVIDENCE?

Review the 'Start for Life' policy: www.gov.uk/government/publications/the-best-start-for-life-a-vision-for-the-1001-critical-days

- Why are the first 1001 days critical in a child's life? How can services work together to improve outcomes?

Within Scotland the Getting It Right for Every Child (GIRFEC) framework is currently under review and still provides the guidance for all children's services. As part of the Children and Young People (Scotland) Act 2014 Community Planning Partnerships have been established in 2020 and there is a requirement that local collaborative planning takes place across integrated children's services. Each local authority must have a children's service plan in place (Scottish Government, 2020a).

Scotland has also published the NHS Recovery Plan 2021–2026, which has a number of objectives underpinned by greater joined up working and efficient allocation of resources. The integration authorities in Scotland are responsible for joint implementation and delivering services within local areas (Scottish Government, 2020b).

Wales has now established Regional Partnership Boards following the Social Services and Wellbeing (Wales) Act 2014 which will implement the National Models of Integrated Care (Department of Health and Social Care Wales, 2021).This follows the publication of 'A Healthier Wales – 10 year plan' (Department of Health and Social Care Wales, 2019) and places a statutory duty on health, social care, housing, education and the third sector to work together to improve population health and wellbeing.

In Northern Ireland a new Integrated Care System is under development to replace the Integrated Partnerships. Like the other UK nations, this will build on collaboration and integration to address the wider determinants of health through a population health approach (Health and Social Care Board, 2022). Northern Ireland also has a positive project 'no more silos' which aims to improve access to urgent and emergency care services across primary and secondary care. A main aim of this project is to break down professional boundaries (Department of Health, Northern Ireland, 2020).

ACTIVITY 5.4: CRITICAL THINKING

Connecting Care for Children (CC4C) Model

- View this video: https://youtube/GE6jStGLvJM
- Read the case study at: www.england.nhs.uk/integratedcare/resources/case-studies/child-health-hubs-see-patients-closer-to-home-and-reduce-unnecessary-hospital-trips/
- How has this model benefited children and young people?

IPW AND TEAM WORKING IN TRANSITION

Within children's services there are a number of key transition periods. Starting primary school, secondary school and the transition to adult services are significant changes in a child/young person's life. For children and young people who have complex needs, interprofessional working is essential to ensure a successful experience and positive outcomes for them. For young people transitioning to adult services the Care Quality Commission (2014) highlighted the use of health passports, a transition plan and improved engagement between services as crucial to ensuring a successful transition. The National Institute for Health and Care Excellence (NICE) (2016) transition guidance also reinforces the importance of a named worker, young person as equal partner in transition planning, and ensuring health and social care work together collaboratively. In a review of how babies, children and young people experience healthcare, NICE (2021) found that children and young people do not like having to repeat healthcare history on multiple occasions and find good communication between professionals is really helpful.

CASE STUDY 5.1: GEORGE

George is almost 3 and was born with Patau's syndrome. He has been diagnosed with developmental delay and complex physical disabilities. George is non-verbal, non-mobile, has limited vision and epilepsy. As George lives in Scotland he has a named health visitor who has, alongside a number of other professionals and his parents, developed a Child's Plan. Each professional has contributed to the assessment and an action plan to meet his needs has been agreed. As George will be starting nursery soon education staff have been invited to a Child Plan meeting to review the current plans and start the transition process for nursery. George has a number of needs that education staff will need to plan for, including a feeding tube, mobility issues, personal care, epilepsy management including medication and communication difficulties. The health visitor has also made a referral to the local social work disability team to complete a self-directed assessment to explore available funding for further family support.

- What do you think the challenges will be for George once he starts school?
- Which professionals do you think will be involved in George's Child Plan?
- Looking back at the 'My World Triangle' (Figure 5.4), what do you think George needs from the people who look after him?

Go further: Look up Patau's syndrome.

SPECIAL EDUCATIONAL NEEDS AND DISABILITY (SEND)

Effective, coordinated interprofessional and interdisciplinary working in relation to transition for children and young people with special educational needs is essential to achieve the best possible outcomes.

The Children and Families Act 2014 and the subsequent SEND code of practice (Department of Health and Social Care, 2014) set out key principles for IPW. One key recommendation was that children, young people and their families should play a central part in making decisions about the way in which their needs could best be met. There was also strong emphasis on education, health and social care services working closely together to meet children and young people's needs, rather than as separate entities. The Care Quality Commission (CQC) found that robust and consistent joined up cross-agency working can have a profoundly positive impact on the lives of children and young people (CQC, 2022). The Children's Commissioner for England in 'Beyond the labels' (2022) also emphasises the importance of working in partnership with children and their families in a shared vision to ensure they achieve their goals.

The Children and Families Act 2014 states that CCGs, NHS Trusts and NHS Foundation Trusts must inform the appropriate local authority if they identify a child under compulsory school age as having, or probably having, special educational need or a disability. A unique and key leadership role within child health services is that of the Designated Clinical Officer for SEND. This role ensures that health services are fully embedded within the local authority process (Council for Disabled Children, 2019).

SEE ALSO CHAPTER 34

The following case study demonstrates how one element of the SEND reforms (Duty to Notify) was implemented within a local area with a focus on the importance of interprofessional working.

CASE STUDY 5.2: ELLI BORRILL, SPECIALIST COMMUNITY PUBLIC HEALTH NURSE

I was employed as the Designated Clinical Officer (DCO) for a large city in the North of England. One of my key priorities was to formalise the work previously undertaken to implement the Notification Process and roll it out across all health services within the local area. I re-established and chaired the SEND Health steering group, inviting senior representation from across health, social care and education. This group was able to sign up to and agree a process by which any health professional could inform the appropriate local authority if they identified a child under compulsory school age as having, or probably having, SEN or a disability. The most challenging element to getting this process up and running was in communicating the need for it in a way that demonstrated to front-line practitioners that it would really make a difference to children and families in the longer term. It was my role not only to provide leadership, education and information to my fellow colleagues regarding the importance of our statutory responsibilities, but also to foster a mutual respect of professional boundaries and roles that had been historically challenging. Simply getting to know my colleagues on a more personal level and building relationships was very important to me. This way we could get to grips with any barriers to progress, fully understand what they were and how we could overcome them together as a team rather than a group of individuals from different organisations with different priorities. Having the privilege of working with children with complex needs for over 20 years I also felt and tried to convey a shared passion and vision for our children that could result in significant changes to local SEND services. Often, we are asked to undertake interventions that seem overly driven by paperwork and seem a low priority in the face of high workloads and competing demands. The transition for children between health services and educational provision is highly complex and can involve multiple professionals from many different agencies all with different priorities. Keeping the focus on the child and family was a crucial aspect of getting this process up and running. The partnership between education, health and social care is stronger and there is greater collective ambition for children and young people with SEND in our local area.

- What examples of effective collaboration can you identify from this case study?

CHAPTER SUMMARY

- It is clear that the COVID-19 pandemic has had far-reaching implications for child services across all of health and social care. We have seen rapid responses to very challenging times and this has perhaps promoted IPW in very positive ways
- Future research exploring IPW and of the pandemic may help to shape positive improvements and inform and improve interprofessional working practices
- As children's nurses we never work in isolation. Holistic, effective, safe and family-centred care is achieved when we collaborate effectively with other professions
- Successful IPW is achieved through effective communication
- Children, young people and their families are at the heart of IPW and key partners in its success

---
BUILD YOUR BIBLIOGRAPHY

Books

- Day, J (2018) *Interprofessional Working: An Essential Guide for Health and Social Care Professionals*, 2nd edn. Andover: Cengage Learning.

  This book explores further underpinning theoretical and practical knowledge, skills and understanding to work effectively as a member of an interprofessional team.
- Goodman, B. and Clemow, R. (2010) *Nursing and Collaborative Practice: A Guide to Interprofessional Learning and Working.* London: Sage.

  Explores effective collaboration further.

FURTHER READING

Journal articles

- Hood, R., Gillespie, J. and Davies, J. (2016) 'A conceptual review of interprofessional expertise in child safeguarding'. *Journal of Interprofessional Care*, 30 (4): 493-8.

  This article reviews interprofessional working within a safeguarding context.
- Darling, J., Bamidis, P., Burberry, J. and Rudolf, M. (2020) 'The First Thousand Days: early, integrated and evidence-based approaches to improving child health: coming to a population near you?' *Archives of Disease in Childhood*, 105: 837-41.

  This article explores the first 1001 days further and the importance of integrated services within this.

FURTHER READING ONLINE JOURNAL ARTICLES

Weblinks

- Interprofessional Collaboration - complete this e-learning module:
- https://health.ubc.ca/collaborative-health-education/tbc-run

- Healthy Child Programme - complete the module Communication and Interprofessional working:
- https://portal.e-lfh.org.uk/myElearning/Index?HierarchyId=0_97_97&programmeId=97

- Early Help - North Yorkshire Early Help Strategy - review the video:
- www.youtube.com/watch?v=DaDz5eocKPs

FURTHER READING: WEBLINKS

REFERENCES

Arnold, E.C. and Underman Boggs, K. (2018) *Interpersonal Relationships: Professional Communication Skills for Nurses*, 7th edn. Professional [eBook]. Saunders/Elsevier.

Barr, J. and Dowding, L. (2019) *Leadership in Health Care*, 4th edn. London: Sage.

Care Quality Commission (CQC) (2014) *From the Pond into the Sea: Children's Transition to Adult Health Services*. Newcastle upon Tyne: CQC.

Care Quality Commission (CQC)/ OFSTED (2022) *Joint Inspections of Local Area SEND Provision*. Available at: www.gov.uk/government/publications/local-area-send-inspections-information-for-families/joint-inspections-of-local-area-send-provision (accessed 6 July 2022).

Centre for the Advancement of Interprofessional Education (CAIPE) (2011) *Principles of Interprofessional Education*. Available at: www.caipe.org/resources/publications/barr-low-2011-principles-interprofessional-education (accessed 5 May 2022).

Centre for the Advancement of Interprofessional Education (CAIPE) (2016) *Statement of Purpose*. Available at: www.caipe.org/resource/CAIPE-Statement-of-Purpose-2016.pdf (accessed 5 May 2022).

Children and Families Act 2014. Available at: www.legislation.gov.uk/ukpga/2014/6/contents/enacted (accessed 1 June 2022).

Children and Young People (Scotland) Act 2014. Available awww.legislation.gov.uk/asp/2014/8/contents/enacted (accessed 7 July 2022).

Children's Commissioner for England (2022) A SEND system which works for every child, every time. Beyond the Labels. Available at: www.childrenscommissioner.gov.uk/wp-content/uploads/2022/11/cc-beyond-the-labels-a-send-system-which-works-for-every-child-every-time.pdf (accessed 1 December 2022).

Council for Disabled Children (2019) *Designated Medical/Clinical Officer Handbook*, rev. edn. London: National Children's Bureau.

Day, J. (2018) *Interprofessional Working: An Essential Guide for Health and Social Care Professionals*, 2nd edn. Andover: Cengage Learning.

Delves-Yates, C. (ed.) (2022) *Essentials of Nursing Practice*, 3rd edn. London: Sage.

Department of Health, Northern Ireland (2011) *Understanding the Needs of Children in Northern Ireland*. Available at: www.health-ni.gov.uk/publications/understanding-needs-children-northern-ireland-unocini-guidance (accessed 1 June 2022).

Department of Health, Northern Ireland (2020) *Covid 19 – Urgent and Emergency Care Action Plan*. Available at: www.health-ni.gov.uk/NoMoreSilos (accessed 2 July 2022).

Department of Health and Social Care (2014) *SEND Code of Practice*: 0–25 years. Available at: www.gov.uk/government/publications/send-code-of-practice-0-to-25 (accessed 3 July 2022).

Department of Health and Social Care (2021) *The Best Start for Life – A Vision for the first 1001 Critical Days*. Available at: www.gov.uk/government/publications/the-best-start-for-life-a-vision-for-the-1001-critical-days (accessed 6 June 2022).

Department of Health and Social Care (2022) Health and Care Bill. Available at: www.legislation.gov.uk/ukpga/2022/31/contents/enacted (accessed 6 July 2022).

Department of Health and Social Care (Wales) (2019) *A Healthier Wales – Long Term Plan for Health and Social Care*. Available at: https://gov.wales/healthier-wales-long-term-plan-health-and-social-care (accessed 6 July 2022).

Department of Health and Social Care (Wales) (2021) *Regional Partnership Boards*. Available at: https://gov.wales/regional-partnership-boards-rpbs (accessed 5 July 2022).

Ford, J. and Gray, R. (2021) *Interprofessional Education Handbook for Educators and Practitioners incorporating Integrated Care and Values-Based Practice*. Available at: www.caipe.org/resources/caipe-publications (accessed 1 June 2022).

Grant, R. and Goodman, B. (2019) *Communication & Interpersonal Skills in Nursing*, 4th edn. London: Sage.

Health and Social Care Board (2022) *Integrated Care System Northern Ireland*. Available at: https://hscboard.hscni.net/icsni/ (accessed 29 June 2022).

HM Government (2018) *Working Together to Safeguard Children: A Guide to Inter-agency Working to Safeguard and Promote the Welfare of Children*. London: DfE. Available at: www.gov.uk/government/publications/working-together-to-safeguard-children–2 (accessed 16 May 2022).

HM Government (2022) *Supporting Families: Early Help System Guide*. London: DfE. Available at: www.gov.uk/government/publications/supporting-families-early-help-system-guide (accessed 5 July 2022).

Hull City Council (2022) *Threshold of Need*. Available at: www.hull.gov.uk/sites/hull/files/media/thresh_needs_0.pdf (accessed 1 July 2022).

Laming, Lord (2003) *The Victoria Climbié Inquiry*. CM5730. Norwich: TSO. Available at: http://dera.ioe.ac.uk/6086/2/climbiereport.pdf (accessed 7 June 2023).

Laming, Lord (2009) *The Protection of Children in England – A Progress Report*. Available at: www.gov.uk/government/publications/the-protection-of-children-in-england-a-progress-report (accessed 6 July 2022).

Nancarrow, S.A., Booth, A., Ariss, S. et al. (2013) 'Ten principles of good interdisciplinary team work'. *Human Resources for Health*, 11: 19. doi.org/10.1186/1478-4491-11-19.

National Health Service (2019) *The National Health Service Long Term Plan*. Available at: www.longtermplan.nhs.uk/wp-content/uploads/2019/08/nhs-long-term-plan-version-1.2.pdf (accessed 1 July 2022).

National Institute for Health and Care Excellence (NICE) (2016) Transition from children's to adults' services for young people using health or social care. NICE guideline [NG43]. Available at: www.nice.org.uk/guidance/ng43 (accessed 6 July 2022).

National Institute for Health and Care Excellence (NICE) (2021) Babies, children and young people's experience of health care. NICE guideline [NG204]. Available at: www.nice.org.uk/guidance/ng204 (accessed 7 July 2022).

NSPCC (2019) Interagency Working. Available at https://learning.nspcc.org.uk/child-protection-system/multi-agency-working-child-protection#heading-top (accessed 15 June 2022).

NSPCC/SCIE (2016) *Learning into Practice: Inter-Professional Communication and Decision Making – Practice Issues Identified in 38 Serious Case Reviews*. London: NSPCC/SCIE.

Nursing and Midwifery Council (2018) *Future Standard: Proficiencies for Nurses*. Available at: www.nmc.org.uk/standards/standards-for-nurses/standards-of-proficiency-for-registered-nurses/ (accessed 1 July 2022).

Ockenden, D. (2022) Final report of the Ockenden review. Findings, conclusions and essential actions from the independent review of maternity services at the Shrewsbury and Telford Hospital NHS Trust. Available at: www.gov.uk/government/publications/final-report-of-the-ockenden-review (accessed 2 July 2022).

Pullon, S., Morgan, S., McDonald, L. and McKinlay Gray, B. (2016) 'Observation of interprofessional collaboration in primarycare practice: a multiple case study'. *Journal of Interprofessional Care*, 30 (6): 787–94

Schot, E., Tummers, L. and Noordegraaf, M. (2019) 'Working on working together. A systematic review on how healthcare professionals contribute to interprofessional collaboration'. *Journal of Interprofessional Care*, 34 (3): 332–342.

Scottish Government (2014) *Getting It Right for Every Child*. Available at: www.gov.scot/policies/girfec/ (accessed 1 July 2022).

Scottish Government (2020a) *Children's Service Planning*. Available at: www.gov.scot/publications/children-young-people-scotland-act-2014-statutory-guidance-part-3-childrens-services-planning-second-edition-2020/ (accessed 5 July 2022).

Scottish Government (2020b) *Statutory Guidance for Integration Authorities*. Available at: www.gov.scot/publications/statutory-guidance-directions-integration-authorities-health-boards-local-authorities/ (accessed 6 July 2022).

Scottish Government (2022) *Getting It Right for Every Child (GIRFEC) Practice Guidance 3 – The Role of the Lead Professional*. Available at: www.gov.scot/publications/getting-right-child-girfec-practice-guidance-3-role-lead-professional/pages/1/ (accessed 14 February 2023).

Selwyn, R. (2022) 'Early help for children and families'. *Paediatrics and Child Health*, 32 (3): 81–87.

Social Services and Well Being Act (Wales) 2014. Available at: www.legislation.gov.uk/anaw/2014/4/contents (accessed 6 July 2022).

Thistlethwaite, J. and Moran, M. (2010) 'Learning outcomes for interprofessional education (IPE): literature review and synthesis'. *Journal of Interprofessional Care*, 24 (5): 503–513.

Tuckman, B.W. (1965) 'Developmental sequence in small groups'. *Psychological Bulletin*, 63 (6): 384–399.

United Nations Convention on the Rights of the Child (1989) (UNCRC) 'Your rights under the UNCRC'. United Nations Children's Fund (UNICEF) Youth Voice. Available at: www.unicef.org.uk/youthvoice/pdfs/uncrc.pdf (accessed 1 July 2022).

Welsh Government (2017) *Families First Guidance*. Available at: https://gov.wales/families-first-guidance-local-authorities (accessed 1 June 2022).

Wilkinson, E. (2022) 'Why medicine must catch up on interprofessional education for a safer NHS'. *British Medical Journal*, 377.doi: https://doi.org/10.1136/bmj.o1547.

World Health Organization (2010) *Framework for Action on Interprofessional Education and Collaborative Practice*. Geneva: WHO.

ORGANISATION AND SETTINGS FOR CARE OF CHILDREN AND YOUNG PEOPLE

6

JANE HUGHES, AMANDA KELLY, TRACEY JONES AND ORLA McALINDEN

THIS CHAPTER COVERS

- History of the nursing process
- Assessment strategies in a range of settings
- Nursing skills and patient assessment
- Identifying and planning care needs
- Implementing and evaluating care plans
- Developing technology in the organisation of care

> "Children are cared for in diverse settings and consideration of the impact, tensions and challenges is an essential component of caring for children and families."
>
> **Carter et al., 2014, p.97**

INTRODUCTION

As nursing professionals it is important to be aware of the way in which we give nursing care to our patients or clients and, in particular, to children, young people and their parents and carers. As highlighted in the opening quotation, children and young people (CYP) are cared for in a variety of settings. In this chapter we will consider assessment, planning care, implementing and evaluating care, and the handover and referral of care. In all these we will look at how we organise and deliver care and why we do this in the way we do.

In community settings, organisation and delivery of care may focus much more on who provides the services – health, social care, or education – and key strategies for promoting and protecting health. In acute clinical environments, assessment of risk and prevention of harm may be a significant issue and focus for care delivery. As the Code (Nursing and Midwifery Council, 2018a) directs us, also as part of clinical governance, we must be seen to practise effectively and deliver safe care, although as part of reducing costs from litigation, Clinical Negligence Schemes for Trusts (CNST) require clear risk assessment and management systems as part of the scheme (NHS Litigation Authority, 2016).

ACTIVITY 6.1: REFLECTIVE PRACTICE

Consider your current area of practice. What systems or frameworks govern the way that you work and why?

HISTORY OF THE NURSING PROCESS

In the past, nurses had a number of ways to deliver care (Carter et al., 2014). Some of this was dictated by doctors, although Florence Nightingale and early nurse leaders might have argued otherwise. Some was based on tradition and the need to prevent infection and promote cleanliness. While these systems were not based on evidence and holistic patient-centred care, they had a purpose in that things were not forgotten or missed and were systematic in their approach; they reflected nursing theory of the time. McFarlane (1986) argued, however, that there had been a need to change this approach.

From 1967 the 'nursing process' became known through the work of Yura and Walsh (1967). The nursing process represented a systematic approach that demonstrated a holistic basis for care and asked nurses to see the care process in a cyclical manner based on the patient's needs. This process still underpins many of the systems that we use today. This was also the basis for the development of individualised care plans.

Nursing models

Nursing models are theoretical frameworks devised to support the assessment and delivery of nursing care; defined as 'abstract frameworks, linking facts and phenomena, that assist nurses to plan nursing care, investigate problems related to clinical practice, and study the outcomes of nursing actions and intervention' (McFerran, 2008). Another way of understanding this is the idea that models represent what nursing is, a picture or representation of nursing (Pearson et al., 1996).

Nursing models were originally developed in the 1960s and were mainly North American in origin. Murphy et al. (2010) describe how a range of influences brought about their development. Technological advances in medicine and a need to recognise the profession of nursing led to early nurse theorists' wish to demonstrate the unique body of knowledge specific to nursing, hence the development of dedicated nursing models. In an attempt to define nursing, most theorists appeared to reflect on one of our earliest influences, Florence Nightingale, and her focus on health and the environment (Nightingale, 1859).

From the 1970s, and more so in the 1980s, there was a proliferation of UK-based texts demonstrating an interpretation of the initial models and their application to UK settings (Aggleton and Chalmers, 1986; Kershaw and Salvage, 1986; Walsh, 1991).

In defining the concept of a nursing model, most authors at the time described key concepts or aspects that a nursing model would incorporate. These included:

- The person – receiving nursing care
- The environment – and surroundings where the person is situated
- Health – the illness or wellness state
- Nursing actions (Kershaw and Salvage, 1986; Fawcett, 1995)

Each nursing model depends on the setting or underlying philosophy and reflects nursing from a different perspective, such as psychological or sociological principles. Nurses were encouraged to seek out the most appropriate model of nursing to their setting and patients (Walsh, 1991).

The dominance of the medical model of care based on illness-focused assessment and treatment was to some degree the political driver for nurses to develop their own framework for nursing towards a more patient-focused model which reflected what nurses actually do. However, it could be argued that the most popular models, such as Roper et al. (1985), do reflect a systems-based approach but more closely focused on the needs of human beings. Known as the activities of daily living, these are:

- Maintaining a safe environment
- Communicating
- Breathing
- Eating and drinking
- Eliminating
- Personal cleansing and dressing
- Controlling body temperature
- Mobilising
- Working and playing
- Expressing sexuality
- Sleeping
- Dying

In acute care settings in both adult and children's settings, these activities are frequently reflected in nursing documentation today.

So, it is clear that in different environments and client groups, patient/clients require their care to be organised to reflect their needs, hence the development of models or philosophies to reflect this.

ACTIVITY 6.2: REFLECTIVE PRACTICE

Thinking about your current or most recent practice placement, what nursing model or underlying principles underpin how nursing care is delivered? If you could identify one model of choice, why might this be important to your clients?

Ann Casey developed the 'Casey Partnership model' in 1988 to represent how we work with children and families as children's and young people's nurses. Casey utilised five paradigms (a typical example or pattern of something, or a model): child, health, environment, family, nurse. Casey also demonstrated the interaction between child, family and nurse.

SEE ALSO CHAPTER 2

The principles of the model are that it demonstrates mutual respect for the child and family; it recognises the age continuum, recognises care at home and in hospital, and involves negotiation and sharing/a partnership approach. Although the model has not been further developed, the principle underlies much of how children's nursing care is delivered, and to this end it could be argued that the principle of 'family-centred care' is also a model for children's nursing practice (Smith et al., 2002; Shields et al., 2006).

Smith et al. (2002) outlined the evolving concept of family-centred care in their now key text *Family-Centred Care*. Coleman reflects that changing society and policy together to reflect the wider family is such that family-centred care is a cornerstone of children's nursing practice. Their model/concept demonstrates a continuum of involvement of families, partnership with nurses to parent-led care agreed following negotiation with the parent and child. Congruent with developing knowledge and a changing approach to children and their families, the second edition of this text is entitled *Child and Family-Centred Healthcare* (Smith and Coleman, 2010; Queensland Government, 2021).

There has been some debate around the validity of family-centred care in clinical practice (Shields et al., 2008) and recently 'child-centred nursing' has been promoted as a more appropriate term to promote the idea that children are at the centre of our thinking as active participants in their care (Carter and Ford, 2013; Carter et al., 2014; Smith, 2017; Al Motlaq et al., 2019, 2021; Carter et al., 2021). So, it could be argued that 'child-centred care' is the most preferred current model for nursing practice (Al Motlaq et al., 2019).

ASSESSMENT STRATEGIES IN A RANGE OF SETTINGS

Assessment is the foundation for the provision of patient-focused care. It is key when planning the correct care process and it is integral to effective patient and family-centred care planning. Assessment is about gathering information about a patient in order to identify their needs.

Assessment usually occurs following the initial referral of care. This referral may be from a variety of sources (see below). Assessment is an essential skill that all nurses must have in order to make subsequent decisions and decide on the next step of care. This might be at delivery for resuscitation of a preterm infant to the admission of a 15-year-old who has consumed excessive amounts of alcohol.

Nursing assessment, is vital for planning safe care and a structured framework is essential. This is not a new concept but one that has evolved over time as nursing assessment tools have been developed. Nursing assessment is not deemed an easy process to complete and therefore the use of assessment tools has become an integral part of the process. These will be discussed later. An important aspect of a nurse's role in all areas where children are cared for is the ability to undertake a systematic assessment which is reliable and valid.

SCENARIO 6.1: JAKE

Jake is a 4-year-old brought by his parents directly to the emergency department with wheezing. Jake has had no previous medical input or assessment. Consider the same child 2 hours later being admitted to a children's ward from the emergency department.

- You are the admitting nurse: how would the assessment process differ to that completed by the emergency department nurse? See the definitions below to help with this.

Assessment on admission requires a comprehensive nursing assessment, including patient history, general appearance, physical examination and vital signs completed at the time of admission.

The child in the above scenario, when admitted to the emergency department, would have required a complete assessment including a full history from the parents.

Assessment, when taking over patient care on a shift, differs slightly. It requires a concise nursing assessment completed at the commencement of each shift, or if the patient's condition changes at any other time during your shift. If you were the nurse taking over the care of the child in the above scenario the information received from the thorough assessment in the emergency department would reduce the need for a full assessment on the ward. You should prioritise vital signs to ensure that the condition has not changed during the time between admission and transfer to the ward. Your focus will include ensuring that the child is safe and comfortable.

A focused assessment includes a detailed nursing assessment of specific body system(s) relating to the presenting problem or current concern(s) of the patient (Royal Children's Hospital Melbourne, 2015; RCPCH, 2023).

A child who has received no medical input would require a more urgent assessment to alleviate any immediate concerns. This assessment may not take the same approach as that by staff working on the acute ward admitting a child who has received previous care either by the emergency department staff or by the team in theatre. There should be a structured approach. However, the priority may differ from that of immediate safety to pain control or emotional and family support.

The baseline observation and recording of clinical data forms the foundation of the process, irrelevant of the order that it takes. Accurately recording significant data such as the child's blood pressure, temperature, respiratory rate and oxygen saturations can not only form a baseline foundation to measure against but can escalate care and avoid deterioration. It is often the nurse who will have initial contact with the child and family when they enter a healthcare environment. It is the information obtained by the nursing assessment, therefore, that can direct the care provision. The respiratory rate has been identified as one of the most important clinical signs observed, especially in children, and one that can direct care to alleviate life-threatening symptoms, which has however been omitted in the past (Breakell, 2004; Watson, 2006; NICE, 2022; RCPCH, 2023).

SCENARIO 6.2: JAKOB

You are taking over care of a 2-day-old baby named Jakob on a children's ward. Jakob was admitted the previous day with respiratory distress. Following a clinical assessment and some oxygen therapy the child is now deemed ready for discharge. All monitoring has therefore ceased.

During your shift assessment you acknowledge that the infant now has a raised respiratory rate and subcostal recession.

- Why would this cause you concern?
- And what other assessments might you now consider?
- What would your next action be?

Children's conditions can change rapidly and the skills of assessment to recognise these changes are fundamental to the nursing role. The reliable identification of changes in a child's condition can alleviate further deterioration or even prevent admission to intensive care areas. It has been recognised that deterioration of critically ill patients has usually been present prior to collapse (NICE, 2022). However, the NICE 2022 guidelines came in for some criticism as '*not being reliable*' (Clark et al., 2022). This again flags up the importance of using only tools which are 'reliable and valid'.

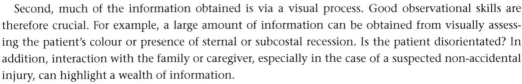

ACTIVITY 6.3: REFLECTIVE PRACTICE

Consider the assessment of a child with whom you have been recently involved during a placement.

- Did you utilise all of your senses when carrying out this assessment? Discuss how you did this.
- Which sense was your most useful tool?
- Discuss and define what is meant when we speak of the 'reliability' and 'validity' of a tool. Why is this important?

NURSING SKILLS AND PATIENT ASSESSMENT

Nurses require a set of key skills to be effective in the process of patient assessment. First, they require an understanding of human physiology across the lifespan (Peate, 2021). In order to highlight deviations from the normal it is vital to have the ability to recognise the normal. It is important to have an understanding of why the respiratory rate in a child who has an underlying respiratory condition may be vital in the speed of escalation required. Nursing assessment of the child often requires additional skills and knowledge in addition to anatomy and physiology. The relationship between age, development and communication ability is particularly significant and it is therefore important for the nurse to have a clear understanding of developmental milestones as these may offer additional assessment information.

SEE ALSO
CHAPTER 2

Second, much of the information obtained is via a visual process. Good observational skills are therefore crucial. For example, a large amount of information can be obtained from visually assessing the patient's colour or presence of sternal or subcostal recession. Is the patient disorientated? In addition, interaction with the family or caregiver, especially in the case of a suspected non-accidental injury, can highlight a wealth of information.

SEE ALSO
CHAPTER 9

One of the most fundamental aspects of nursing assessment and a priority area is communication. Unlike adult patient care, where a large proportion of information is gathered directly from the patient, children's nurses work with an array of age groups some of which may not be able to communicate effectively. This is where an ability to adapt your skills is important. An understanding of child development will enable you to adapt your communication skills in order to engage effectively and gather the correct information needed for an appropriate plan of care or referral. Consider two types of questioning and how they might affect the response. Open-ended questions are more likely to elicit more detailed information. This might lead to a more probing approach to questioning should a need be perceived. Lambert et al. (2011) suggest that in practice health professionals position children as either passive bystanders or active participants in the communication process, which is a consideration when reflecting on your skills during the assessment process. This is relected in later literature about the meaning and practice of family-centred care (Smith at al., 2017; Al Motlaq et al., 2019, 2021b; Neill et al., 2021; Queensland Government, 2021).

One of the most effective tools you can use are listening skills. The information divulged can be vital for the nursing assessment to establish the key areas of concern, both for the patient and the family.

The use of assessment tools

Assessment tools are what offer the mechanism to gather a score or referral algorithm. Whatever tool you use it must be current and reliable and valid, approved for use for the intended care group. Because of the nature of the scoring system, all early warning systems utilise the benefits of technology in some way to aid with scoring saturation, heart rate monitoring, etc. Watson (2006) suggests that nurses have in the past been required to record but not necessarily interpret clinical observations. This, however, is not the case in many clinical areas where nurses are at the first point of patient contact and are often the gatekeepers to specific medical input. Competency is therefore paramount to safe assessment. Many acute areas now work with a triage system. Being able to interpret clinical information to direct clinical care is a skill which is required by all nurses carrying out assessment and is part of the required competencies by NMC for the 'Future Nurse' programme (2018b).

SBAR (Situation, Background, Assessment, Recommendation)

Many children's observation and assessment units utilise an SBAR tool (NHS Institute, 2013). This enables the handover of care from the GP in the community to the acute paediatric area. The SBAR enables nursing coordinators not only to prepare for the child's arrival but to anticipate what has already been assessed prior to arrival. This involves communicating what treatment has already been commenced. There has been an increase in the need for nurses to assess and refer patients correctly in order to increase efficiency of care. The areas where children are cared for are constantly evolving in order to be more clinically effective and efficient. This has resulted in more responsibility being placed upon nursing assessment. Remember, no tool is foolproof, it is only as good as the user.

PEWS (Paediatric Early Warning Score)

In many acute areas, the use of a PEWS is a common early warning tool. Early warning tools highlight clinical deterioration based on physiological parameters. Early warning tools were first used in adult nursing but have been adapted to suit paediatric patients (children and young people population). Although no early warning score for the use of children has been *universally* validated, many areas have adopted such a tool and these will be developed over time. Using the most current tool is essential.

The PEWS enables clinical teams to recognise patients who are deteriorating and act accordingly. This tool can be adapted according to the patient group. It must, however, have the key areas of physiological assessment embedded, which in turn indicate a clear need for referral or escalation. Alongside the scoring tool there needs to be a recommendation flow chart, which allows the nurse to act upon the score obtained. This action may relate to an increase in clinical observations, or in more serious situations an urgent referral to the medical teams. The sequence of a clinical assessment may require some adaptation according to the age or needs of the child. Assessment often leads to referral to other professionals. There has been some comment in recent years that this tool should include reference to parental opinion, as the parents tend to know their well child best and can spot early any subtle signs of deterioration in their child (Salama et al., 2021).

IDENTIFYING AND PLANNING CARE NEEDS

Following the underpinning approach reflected in *The Nursing Process* (Yura and Walsh, 1967) and in other developments of this cyclical process (see Figure 6.1), the second and third stages focus on the identification and planning of care needs. This follows earlier assessment of the child and family as discussed in the previous section.

Planning care needs will depend on the setting and client group, and this context may mean that different language is used to reflect the process. Early versions of the nursing process used the term 'problem' or 'patient problem', 'patient need', or 'nursing diagnosis', often in North American settings

(NANDA, 2008). There is also consideration of the cause and nature of the problem – an anatomical or physiological malfunction or the inability of the person to adapt their behaviour to the situation they find themselves in. Problems or needs may be physical, social, psychological and/or spiritual, and their identification may depend on the focus of that assessment, the practitioner and the client.

Planning care can and does also take into account potential problems or assessment of risk, such as the risks of an anaesthetic or operation, or the risks to physical or mental health of certain behaviours. However, it could be argued that potential problems are not necessarily the child or family's problem, but pertain to the nurse's role in minimising risk.

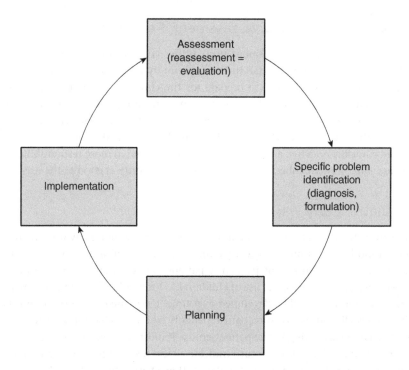

Figure 6.1 The nursing process

ACTIVITY 6.4: REFLECTIVE PRACTICE

In your practice setting, when you have identified patient needs and are planning 'goals', to what degree are these goals those of the child and family or the nurse? Consider the earlier discussion in the section on nursing models about the debate around child-centred care/family-centred care.

The focus on holistic and individualised patient care from the development of the nursing process implies that needs and goals should be patient-centred and should be negotiated with the child and family (Aggleton and Chalmers, 1986). In current policy it is an expectation that clients and carers are involved in all aspects of planning and that practitioners should have this philosophy at the heart of what we do (NMC, 2018a). This principle has existed for many years in policy and guidance around caring for children.

Once problems and goals have been identified it is important to consider priorities in the care of children and their families. The nurse should be able to clearly articulate and document priorities in care, communicate effectively with the child and family, and encourage and support negotiation of care planning (NMC, 2018a and 2018b).

Problems and goals may be further prioritised by considering level of need, risk and availability of resources For example, for the child who is admitted to the emergency department following a head injury and is currently unconscious, although there are also safeguarding issues the child's immediate physical health would take priority and the level of risk of further harm would be reduced if the child were admitted to hospital. The availability of access to resources such as the multidisciplinary team out of hours might be reduced at certain times, hence the need for the nurse to make competent judgements based on knowledge and experience; team working is essential (NMC, 2018a and 2018b).

It is recommended that goals are **SMART** – specific, measurable, achievable/agreed, realistic and time limited – which may be appropriate in some settings more than others. However, the introduction of time parameters could serve as the impetus for evaluation and reassessment of the original goal.

SCENARIO 6.3: SARAH

Sarah is 10 years old and has a diagnosis of cystic fibrosis. She was admitted to an acute medical children's ward. The hospital policy is that all medication must be administered by the nursing team. A delay in this administration caused the mother to verbalise her distress and frustration at not being given the authority to administer medication that she gives daily at home.

- How could this situation have been better managed?
- Is this a time-critical drug?
- Should an 'incident form' (I R 1 or Datix) be completed?

Care planning in different settings may be adapted further by the use of documentation and other systems which in some cases allow standardisation of care plans. In the case of operative procedures, many Trusts utilise integrated care pathways.

An integrated care pathway (ICP) is a multidisciplinary outline of anticipated care, within an appropriate timeframe, to help a patient with a specific condition or set of symptoms move progressively through a clinical experience to positive outcomes. Integrated care pathways are usually agreed within an organisation and are usually child-specific. Variation from the pathway can be indicated to show individual patient need. They may also minimise risk where key actions are necessary.

Many acute clinical areas also use standardised care plans that can be adapted to the individual patient, which may be more time-efficient. Emergency departments also incorporate clinical guidance by developing condition-related algorithms or decision trees in order to standardise treatment in fast-paced environments.

"I have used ICPs and standardised care plans whilst in practice. I found that standardised care plans and pathways are a helpful tool for students who have little experience or knowledge in how to care for children with particular illnesses as they outline the care and procedures nurses need to deliver in each circumstance. I found as a student, it is a useful guide to follow which I can use to plan and implement care for the child."

Natalie, 3rd-year children's nursing student now a RN (Child)

In community settings where the focus of care is on the wider family, parenting and/or areas of other need, documents such as the Common Assessment Framework (CAF) are frequently used to identify significant areas of need to support the child in his or her environment (see the section on referrals below). The assessment of a child and family using a CAF requires the involvement of the child/family, assessing professional and any other professionals who are subsequently required to meet any identified needs of the child and/or family. There have been criticisms from professionals (head teachers, school nurses, health visitors) that the CAF is not very friendly to the whole family and has been too focused on assessing and meeting the needs of the child. And so the move to the use of 'Early Help Assessments' (EHAs) in places like Manchester in the north-west of England (Manchester City Council, 2015), support the 'Think Family' approach and emphasises that any kind of early intervention assessment should be based on a conversation with the families about their needs and what they would like to get out of their involvement with agencies.

——————— SAFEGUARDING STOP POINT ———————

If a child is subject to a Child Protection Plan, there is a statutory requirement for all agencies to meet as a core group with the child and parents/carers to review the plans at regular intervals as set out at the initial child protection conference. The care plans of looked after children are reviewed within 28 days of the child coming into care, then at 6-monthly intervals whilst the child remains looked after. Health professionals are seen as active partners in the planning process for young people subject of CPPs and care orders and they can request additional meetings if plans are not fulfilling the needs of the child or additional risk factors are identified.

Once care is identified and care plans are agreed practitioners are required (NMC, 2018a and 2018b) to communicate plans with the child and family but also the multidisciplinary team (HM Government, 2015b). Please make yourself familiar with local arrangements for safeguarding procedures in your own area.

A number of formats and approaches may be used in different settings; this may depend on priority, risk and availability of resources as before. However, some form of written/permanent communication would normally be required to support a verbal handover via face to face or telephone, etc. The standard of documentation would be required to be in keeping with minimal Nursing and Midwifery Council guidance (NMC, 2018a) and Trust Caldicott Guardian principles for information governance (HSCIC, 2015b).

IMPLEMENTING AND EVALUATING CARE PLANS

Following on from the previous section, as care is planned and goals are agreed it is important as practitioners that we also consider the nature of the care and how it is delivered.

The NMC (2018a and 2018b) direct nurses to ensure that care is safe and effective and that practitioners should maintain skills and knowledge for effective practice. We should also be confident that the care we implement is based on the best evidence; research and development has helped practitioners by the development of guidance, such as NICE, SIGN, clinical nursing procedures and Trust guidelines for practice. Be sure to always use the most current versions. Some of the care we give is not necessarily based on empirical research. McKenna et al. (2000) explore this argument in some detail and the central arguments still stand. As nurses, using our clinical judgement in addition to the available evidence is key to the recognition of professional practice (NMC, 2018).

Care that is planned may not necessarily be delivered by the person who instigated the care plan; it may be handed over or delegated to another person. The NMC (2018) is very clear about the need to work cooperatively and maintain communication with others (this is explored further in the referral section of this chapter). In addition, care that is delegated should be within the competence of the person it is delegated to and the practitioner should ensure that care meets the required standard (NMC, 2018).

A registered nurse can delegate to a student a task such as recording vital signs, but the member of staff must be sure the nursing student is able to do this appropriately as well as report back on it.

Where care is delivered will also have an influence on how it is delivered. In acute settings, there is not only local and national guidance but frequently a variety of other personnel whom practitioners can draw on for help and advice should the situation require this. In community settings, practitioners often work alone and the opportunity to seek advice and support is not so easily available. Hence, those working in community settings need to draw on a greater level of knowledge and experience in order to work independently.

Working in families' homes also brings about other considerations, in respect of the family's own environment and their family time (Neill and Coyne, 2018).

Recording and documenting care given is also pertinent (NMC, 2021). Legal challenges have highlighted cases where care was apparently given but not documented, and decisions were given in favour of the patient where the legal point in law 'not recorded not done' was used in support of this.

The final stage of evaluation provides the end/beginning point of the cycle to allow reassessment of the situation and to assess whether the nursing intervention has been effective. Setting goals or timescales for reassessment or reassessing care on a recognised schedule allows clear pathways to evaluate and align care more closely with patient need. However, as previously discussed, the practitioner should have skills to evaluate the care and outcome with the child and family and redefine the next stage of care or decide to discharge the child from the current setting. Unfortunately, this is not always the case (see Amy's scenario).

SEE ALSO
CHAPTER 7

SCENARIO 6.4: AMY

Amy is 15 years old and is being placed in foster care following child protection concerns and ongoing health issues. As a result of this move Amy has changed schools. Due to a delay in the transfer of health records the school nurse at Amy's new school has no information regarding the previous child protection concerns and therefore fails to make relevant preparations for her arrival in the school. This resulted in Amy being placed in a vulnerable situation and health needs continuing to be unmet.

- Reflect on how this situation could be avoided.

Referrals

In the community care of children where there are child protection concerns, documented evaluations of care are paramount to effective transfer of care.

The referral process often involves the transfer of clinical responsibility from one health professional to another professional. A referral is often not a simple process but a highly complex interaction involving multiple stakeholders influenced by a wide range of factors. Not all referrals are alike and research studies have put forward several typologies for distinguishing between the different types:

- Establishing diagnosis
- Treatment or operation
- Specified test/investigation
- Advice on management

- Specialist to take over management
- Reassurance/second opinion
- Reassurance for the patient and/or their family
- Other reasons

It is important to note that referrals can be emergency, routine and elective and as such will determine the differing referral processes.

SMART referrals in a technologically advancing healthcare environment are paramount if we want children to receive optimum healthcare that will enable them to improve their life chances.

Both commissioners and providers of healthcare need to be abreast of the health predictors affecting children today so that health organisations can employ effective strategies, systems and structures to meet the demands of increasingly complex issues ranging from acute and community care needing specialist intervention to safeguarding some of the most vulnerable groups in society. Prevention of harm is paramount whether by act or omission (NMC, 2018a and 2018b).

Historically, children's health services were hosted and managed by different organisations and access to these services was often by a number of independent referral routes, differing in terms of entry, urgency criteria, who is eligible to refer and working to different geographical boundaries. Poor communication and coordination between services often led to duplication of work or confusion about who was responsible for meeting which particular part of a child and family's needs. Transition of care across organisations and interfaces is a high-risk area and should be carefully managed and planned (NHS England, 2018).

The initial Health and Social Care Act 2012 introduced a new ideology for health and social care services, modernising service delivery, developing new ways of working and providing integrated care. As a result, the strong focus on integration of primary, community, acute, specialist healthcare and social care should mean that services are more unified and organised around the needs of children and their families.

The multifaceted needs of children and families today mean referrers need referral pathways that readily navigate health systems so there is no delay or duplication and identify the most appropriate service. Single points of entry or single points of care (SPE, SPOC) systems and referral management schemes (RMS) aim to simplify and streamline access to children's health services, thus addressing issues of equity of access and coordination highlighted in *Improving Children and Young People's Health Outcomes: A System Wide Response* (Department of Health, 2013a).

Many different referral pathways exist and local commissioning and resources differ from area to area and country to country depending on the needs of the local population.

Where children and young people are referred to the hospital, ambulatory assessment units (AAU) provide rapid access to care without hospital admission and, if admission is necessary, discharge patients home as soon as possible. Many conditions can be effectively managed at home with advice and support from specialist nurses and allied health professionals, so if necessary, following discharge from hospital or clinic, referrals need to be directed to appropriate services such as diabetes or asthma nurse specialists, health visitors and school nurses. These services can then work in collaboration with the multi-agency team and through ongoing reassessment and evaluation, identify if referrals to other services are required, such as counselling or health weight management.

Local areas should also have good working relationships with third party and charitable organisations, and referrals can then be progressed for children who may need additional support around issues that can have health impacts. These can include services that help young people who may go missing from home or are at risk of child sexual exploitation, which can have an impact on emotional, sexual and physical wellbeing.

The National Institute for Health and Care Excellence (NICE) also provides standards that guide health professionals in decision-making when progressing referrals for specific conditions. This too aims to improve early diagnosis and access to the most effective treatments. NICE guidelines are evidence-based, and set out clear patient referral criteria and timeframes. Children have needs that are different from adults, and research does not define what a good quality referral entails but recognises it is multidimensional. If practitioners assessing these needs want to drive forward quality improvements, they need to consider the following for any referral they complete (NICE, 2016; Royal College of Nursing, 2022):

- Necessity: Are patients referred as and when necessary?
- Timeliness: Is this done without avoidable delay?

- Destination: Are patients referred to the most appropriate destination first time?
- Process: Is the process of referral a high-quality one, in the following respects:
- Does the referral contain the necessary information in an accessible format?
- Are children and families offered a choice of time and location, and are they supported in making this decision?
- Can the referrer, patient and specialist form a shared understanding of the purpose and expectations of the referral?
- Is pre-referral management adequate?

School nurses, health visitors and community nurses are well positioned to work with their multi-agency partners such as education and social care to utilise the Early Help Assessment (EHA) framework for assessing the needs of children and families. The framework allows them to identify what support is needed and, therefore, lead on progressing referrals to the appropriate services without duplication. By working with a child- and family-centred approach and consulting with other agencies they can streamline professional involvement.

The framework allows practitioners to identify where needs lie and to make a clinical judgement on the impact to the child's health using the levels of need descriptors.

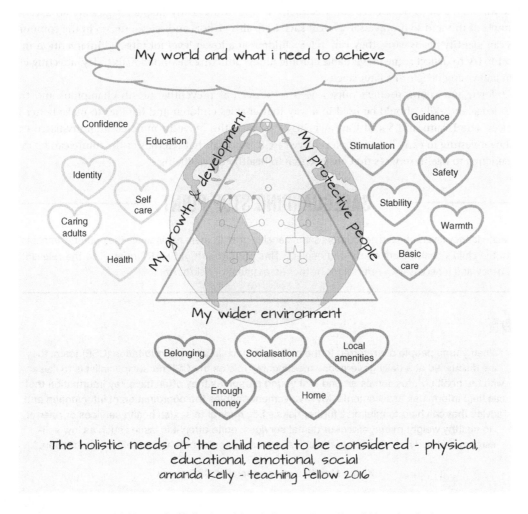

Figure 6.2 My world (Amanda Kelly, teaching fellow, University of Manchester)

WHAT'S THE EVIDENCE?

Most families will at some point face an issue that requires a level of support, whether related to health, employment, poverty or other social problems. As an example, it is estimated that around 20-30% of children and young people will have additional needs at some point in their lives – some for a limited period, and others for longer. The human costs of reaching crisis point before services intervene and the financial costs of providing acute-level services are significantly higher than those associated with earlier interventions, leading to the logical conclusion that providing support at an earlier stage will save money over the longer term and improve individuals' quality of life (Rallings and Payne, 2016, p.5).

Referral to treatment (RTT) within an ever-changing and technologically advancing health service is beset with potential obstacles in an effort to navigate children and families not only to the correct service but within the maximum waiting time in order to meet equality and consistency targets, and patient satisfaction and experience.

Children don't often need to be 'treated' per se; but they do need expert guidance from universal and specialist services in order to help them make healthier choices with a desired outcome so that they will not need to be referred for 'treatment' in the future. Early help strategies are an excellent example of this and so if universal services such as health visitors and school nurses in the communities can identify needs early, they can 'refer' children at a lower level for targeted intervention in an effort to try to deflect some preventable chronic illness afflicting the individuals today, affecting children and young people at a later stage.

Children and young people's nurses need to be seen as preventive health champions and their knowledge and skills should be used in a way that enables children and families to make better life choices. The Health and Social Care Act 2012 activated the move to more community-based care, and by investing in early help and preventive care it is hoped that referrals of the future can be more streamlined to health services that are essential to health and wellbeing.

SAFEGUARDING STOP POINT

Multi-agency levels of need descriptors should enable practitioners to evidence the potential impacts to the child's health from abuse and neglect. This will facilitate a SMART referral to the relevant agency and if necessary a referral for further assessment of risk/harm.

"When young people are referred to the multiagency child sexual exploitation (CSE) team, they are discussed at a daily governance meeting. My role as the CSE nurse specialist is to liaise with the health professionals around that young person as they often have key information that can help inform risk assessments. My involvement enables the coordination of intervention and advice that can help to minimise further risks – i.e., referral to sexual health services or referral to healthy weight management or dental services; quite often it is issues such as low self-esteem and body confidence that can leave young people more vulnerable to exploitation."

Kathy March, senior specialist CSE nurse

DEVELOPING TECHNOLOGY IN THE ORGANISATION OF CARE

The development of a range of technology over the last 30 years has changed the way that we deliver care in a number of ways, and as technologies continue to develop, nurses need to be aware of the potential benefits to care for children and their families and considerations for professional practice.

As nurses we are generally very familiar with some of the developments of monitoring equipment and day-to-day equipment that we use. It can be difficult to consider how we would be able to function without what we now consider to be basic items of equipment, such as the bed that is adjustable in height and position, moving and handling equipment, and the increase in availability of monitoring systems for taking vital signs – even the electronic thermometer. Consider using a mercury thermometer with a wriggling child. Another example would be the use of pulse oximeters – some of you will not remember a time when this invaluable piece of equipment was not available. While the benefits are clear for preventing injury, reducing risk and promoting comfort for the child, as professionals we should be mindful of the appropriate use of technology for the correct purpose, the need for training and the importance of maintenance of equipment. Some would argue that overuse of technology can lead to an overreliance on monitoring readings and a loss of key skills in assessment.

The availability of equipment that is now more portable can have a direct and positive impact on the care of children in community and home settings (such as monitoring equipment, adaptations for the home, feeding devices and other technology). Children can be cared for at home and avoid hospital admissions where community nurses, GPs and families have access to such technology and innovation.

'eHealth' is defined by the Royal College of Nursing as a 'means of promoting, empowering and facilitating health and wellbeing with individuals, families and communities and enhancing professional practice through the use of information management and information and communication technologies' (RCN, 2012). This can include telephone consultations, telephone or text health advice and management, submission of patient health information, remote consultation between patient and doctor – telemedicine, Internet-based social networks and support groups. Increases in communication technology mean that consultations can occur in real time, but remotely – invaluable in certain clinical situations.

ACTIVITY 6.5: CRITICAL THINKING

Are you using any of the above aspects of eHealth with children and their families? What benefits do you see for children and their families?

Future developments projected by NHS England (2015) for funding across a range of NHS Trusts include:

- Digitally enabled observation management
- Mobile access to digital care records across the community
- Digital capture of clinical data at point of care
- Safer clinical interventions
- Real-time digital nursing dashboards
- Smart workforce deployment

- Remote face-to-face interaction
- Digital images for nursing care

There are a number of considerations and potential drawbacks outlined in RCN guidance (2012). These include access issues, patient and staff attitudes, support for alternative language and sensory restrictions, and overuse of services.

As nurses we are both professionally and legally required to account for our actions, which involves keeping a record of assessments, conversations, care given and referrals made. We are guided by the NMC Code (2018a), 'Keep clear and accurate records relevant to your practice'.

The updated guidance includes six key aspects:

- Completing records at the time
- Identifying risks and the steps taken to deal with them
- Accurate record-keeping and reporting if someone else has not done so
- Attributing records to yourself with the date and time, and no jargon or speculation
- Keeping records secure and confidential
- Treating all data and research findings appropriately

NHS Trusts are required to audit the documentation of their employees on a regular basis as a part of clinical governance requirements. Trusts also have responsibilities following the Caldicott Review in 1997 to appoint a Caldicott Guardian (HSCIC, 2015a) who is responsible for information governance. This involves training for all employees, safe and secure systems for all records to ensure confidentiality but also appropriate access to those who need information. The move to electronic data and records brings new challenges for the NHS in developing information systems that are compatible and robust for the 21st century, particularly where health and social care professionals need to communicate and share information.

As highlighted earlier in this chapter, sharing information is key to joined-up working in healthcare practice, in particular in safeguarding information (Department of Health, 2013b; HM Government, 2015). It is also indicated a number of times in the NMC Code (2018a) in relation to working cooperatively. Considering the range of settings in which children are cared for it is understandable that there may be difficulties in accessing and sharing information, between nurses and other professions.

Community nurses may have paper-based records which they need to carry with them during visits and need to store safely between visits. In some services the records are kept in the patient's home or a duplicate version is kept with the child at home. Increasingly though, school and community nurses are using electronic records, although these systems are not always compatible. In community settings eHealth developments may include the use of specific apps and websites which support children and families with particular conditions.

In acute areas many Trusts are now 'paperless', which includes electronic records, recording of vital signs on computer systems and medicines administration supported by technology. Thus, it is important to recognise these are not without their limitations, such as problems with access, availability of resources, the need for training, systems, individual error and breaches of data protection.

A final consideration with regard to documentation and technology is that patients have a legal right to access to their records under the Freedom of Information Act 2000. This is also supported by the Code (NMC, 2018a). As nurses we should consider how we can support children and their families in accessing their records and being partners in their care. New developments in technology may help or hinder their access to information.

CHAPTER SUMMARY

- Different environments and client groups require their care to be organised to reflect the needs of individual children and young people
- Assessment is the foundation of care delivery and is an ongoing process which should be carried out collaboratively
- When planning care and setting goals it is important to recognise the context and the need to work with children and families to ensure that care is delivered and evaluated in a collaborate manner
- Looking forward, nurses need to recognise developments in technology and eHealth and utilise the benefits for children and families while being mindful of potential problems
- All interventions, plans and policies should have the child at the centre of consideration

BUILD YOUR BIBLIOGRAPHY

Books

- Queensland Government (2021) *Child and Family Centred Care: evidence based principles for the care of critically unwell children.* Brisbane: State of Queensland (Queensland Health). E-version available at: www.childrens.health.qld.gov.au/wp-content/uploads/PDF/qcycn/child-and-family-centred-care-principles-paper.pdf.

FURTHER READING

Journal articles

- Stafford, V., Hutchby, I., Karim, K. and O'Reilly, M. (2016) '"Why are you here?" Seeking children's accounts of their presentation to Child and Adolescent Mental Health Service (CAMHS)'. *Clinical Child Psychology and Psychiatry*, 21 (1): 3-18.

  This article explores, on referral to a Child and Adolescent Mental Health Service (CAMHS), the naturally occurring first assessments to discover the beliefs that children hold regarding their reasons for attendance and the implications this has for the trajectory of the appointment and later engagement with interventions.

FURTHER READING: ONLINE JOURNAL ARTICLES

- Tointon, K. and Hunt, J.A. (2016) 'How holistic nursing can enhance the quality of life of children with cystic fibrosis'. *Nursing Children and Young People*, 28 (8): 22-5.

  This article draws on a case study to demonstrate a holistic approach to providing care in both home and hospital settings for a 15-year-old girl with cystic fibrosis.

Weblinks

- NHS England, *NHS Digital Technology: Harnessing the Information Revolution* www.england.nhs.uk/digitaltechnology This NHS-supported website highlights developments in digital technology across the NHS.
- Nursing and Midwifery Council (NMC) (2018) *The Code for Nurses, Midwives and Nursing Associates* www.nmc.org.uk/standards/code The NMC website offers support and guidance for nurses, employers and the public around standards and expectations of all nurses. There are a number of publications, including *The Code* and information about hearings.

FURTHER READING: WEBLINKS

- Don't Forget the Bubbles www.dontforgetthebubbles.com This is a dedicated website to make us all better at caring for children and young people. New videos are posted each Thursday on a wide variety of clinical topics.

REFERENCES

Aggleton, P. and Chalmers, H. (1986) *Nursing Models and the Nursing Process*. London: Macmillan.

Al Motlaq, M., Carter, B., Nell, S., Kristensson–Halstrom, I., Foster, M., Coyne, I., Arabiat, D., Darbyshire, P., Feeng, V.D. and Shields, L. (2019) 'Towards developing consensus on family centred care: an international descriptive study and discussion'. *Journal of Child Health Care*, 23 (3): 458–67.

Al Motlaq, M., Neill, S., Foster, M.J., Coyne, I., Houghton, D., Angelhoff, C., Rising-Holstrom, M. and Majamanda, M. (2021) 'Position statement of the International Network for Child and Family Centred Care: Child and family centred care during the pandemic'. *Journal of Pediatric Nursing*, 61: 140–3.

Breakell, A. (2004) 'The Respi-check oxygen mask'. *British Journal of Resuscitation*, 3 (2): 21.

Casey, A. (1988) 'The partnership model with child and family'. *Senior Nurse*, 4: 8–9.

Carter, B. and Ford, K. (2013) 'Researching children's health experiences: the place for participatory, child centred, arts-based approaches'. *Research in Nursing and Health*, 36 (1): 95–107.

Carter, B., Bray, L., Dickinson, A., Edwards, M. and Ford, K. (2014) *Child Centred Nursing: Promoting Critical Thinking*. London: Sage.

Carter, B., Foster, M., Al Motlaq, M., Neill, S., O Sullivan, T., Majamanda, M., Lim Abdullah, K., Hallstrom, I., Quaye, A., English, C., Viskers, A., Coyne, I., Adama. E. and Morelius, E. (2021) Seeing lockdown through the eyes of children from around the world: Reflecting on a children's artwork project. Nursing praxis in Aoetaroa NZ https://research.edgehill.ac.uk/en/publications/seeing-lockdown-through-the-eyes-of-children-from-around-the-worl last accessed 5/7/2023

Clark, A., Cannings-John, R., Blyth, M., Hay, A.D., Butler, C. and Hughes, K. (2022) 'Accuracy of the NICE traffic light system in children presenting to general practice; a retrospective cohort study'. *British Journal of General Practice*, 72 (719): e398–e404.

Department of Health (2013a) *Improving Children and Young People's Health Outcomes: A System Wide Response*. London: DH.

Department of Health (2013b) *Information: To Share or Not to Share? The Information Governance Review*. London: DH.

Fawcett, J. (1995) *Analysis and Evaluation of Conceptual Models of Nursing*. Philadephia, PA: F.A. Davis.

HSCIC (Health and Social Care Information Centre) (2015a) *Caldicott Guardians*. Available at: http://systems.hscic.gov.uk/infogov/caldicott. [The HSCIC is now called NHS Digital.]

HSCIC (Health and Social Care Information Centre) (2015b) *Information Governance Toolkit*. Available at: www.igt.hscic.gov.uk/Caldicott2.aspx?tk=423455759240822&cb=cd0a4b06-5736-4743-bd01-8f18dd41b04d&lnv=18&clnav=YES (accessed 9 December 2015). [The HSCIC is now called NHS Digital.]

HM Government (2015) *Information Sharing: Advice for Practitioners Providing Safeguarding Services to Children, Young People, Parents and Carers*. London: DfE.

Holmes, L. and McDermid, S. (2014) 'The Common Assessment Framework: the impact of the lead professional on families and professionals as part of a continuum of care in England'. *Child and Family Social Work*. DOI: 10.1111/cfs.12174.

Kershaw, B. and Salvage, J. (1986) *Models for Nursing*. Chichester: Wiley.

Lambert, V., Glacken, M. and McCarron, M. (2011) 'Communication between children and health professionals in a child hospital setting: a child transitional communication model'. *Journal of Advanced Nursing*, 67 (3): 569–82.

Manchester City Council (2015) *Multi-Agency Levels of Need and Response Framework: April 2015. Delivering Effective Support for Children, Young People and Families.* Available at: www.manchester.gov.uk/download/downloads/id/21076/multi_agency_need_and_reponse_framework

McFarlane, J. (1986) 'The Value of Models for care' and 'Looking to the Future' in B. Kershaw and J. Salvage (eds) *Models for Nursing.* Chichester: Wiley.

McFerran, T. (2008) *Oxford Dictionary of Nursing*, 5th edn. Oxford: Oxford University Press.

McKenna, H., Cutclife, J. and McKenna, P. (2000) 'Evidence based practice: demolishing some myths'. *Nusing Standard*, 14 (16): 39–42.

Murphy, F., Williams, A. and Pridmore, J. (2010) 'Nursing models and contemporary nursing 1: their development, uses and limitations'. *Nursing Times*, 106: 23.

Neill, S. and Coyne, S. (2018) 'The role of felt or enacted criticism in parents' decison making in differing contexts and communities: towards a formal grounded theory'. *Journal of Family Nursing*, 23 (3): 443–69.

Neill, S., Roland, D., Carter, B., Rishes, L., Bayes, N., Hughes, J., Bray, L., Palmer-Hill, S., Carrol E.D., O'Donnell, J. and Pandey, P. (2021) 'Learning from pre-hospital journeys: uncertain illness trajectories for young children with serious infection illness.' Available at: https://pearl.plymouth.ac.uk/handle/10026.1/17298 (accessed 7 June 2023).

NANDA (North American Nursing Diagnosis Association) (2008) 'Appendix C 2007–2008 NANDA-approved nursing diagnoses'. Available at: http://wps.prenhall.com/wps/media/objects/3918/4012970/NursingTools/koz74686_AppC.pdf (accessed 9 December 2015).

NHS England (2015) *Digital Transformation.* Available at www.england.nhs.uk/digitaltechnology (accessed 9 December 2015).

NHS England (2018) Supporting young people through transition into adult care services. The Atlas of Shared Learning. 27 November 2018. Available at:www.england.nhs.uk/atlas_case_study/supporting-young-people-through-transition-into-adult-care-services/ (accessed 17 March 2023).

NHS Institute for Innovation and Improvement (NHSIII) (2013) SBAR – *Situation Background Assessment Recommendation.* Available at: www.institute.nhs.uk/safer_care/safer_care/situation_background_assessment_recommendation.html (accessed 21 December 2015).

NHS Litigation Authority (2016) *Clinical Claims.* Available at: www.nhsla.com/Claims/Pages/Clinical.aspx (accessed 20 June 2017).

NICE (National Institute for Health and Care Excellence) (2016) *Transitions from children's services to adults' services for young people using health or social care service.* NICE guideline [NG43]. Available at: www.nice.org.uk (accessed 17 March 2023).

NICE (National Institute for Health and Care Excellence) (2022) Traffic light system for identifying risk of serious illness in under 5s. [NG143] Trafffic light tool. Available at: www.nice.org.uk/guidance/ng143/resources/support-for-education-and-learning-educational-resource-traffic-light-table-pdf-6960664333 (accessed 17 March 2023).

Nightingale, F. (1859) *Notes on Nursing What It Is and What It Is Not.* Pall Mall: Harrison (original edition).

Nursing and Midwifery Council (NMC) (2018a) *The Code: Professional Standards of Practice and Behaviour for Nurses, Midwives and Nursing Associates.* London: NMC. Available at: www.nmc.org.uk/standards/code/.

Nursing and Midwifery Council (NMC) (2018b) *Future Nurse: Standards of Proficiency for Registered Nurses.* London: NMC.

Nursing and Midwifery Council (NMC) (2021) Keep records of all evidence and decisions. Available at: www.nmc.org.uk/employer-resource/local-investigation/guiding-principles/record-evidence-decisions/ (accessed 17 March 2023).

Pearson, A., Vaughan, B. and Fitzgerald, M. (1996) *Models for Nursing Practice*. Oxford: Butterworth Heinmann.

Peate, I. (2021) *Fundamentals of Children and Young People's Anatomy and Physiology*, 2nd edn. London: Wiley–Blackwell.

Queensland Government (2021) *Child and Family Centred Care: evidence based principles for the care of critically unwell children*. Brisbane: State of Queensland (Queensland Health).

Rallings, J. and Payne, L. (2016) *The Case for Early Support*. London: Barnardo's. Available at: www.barnardos.org.uk/case-for-early-support-2016.pdf (accessed 30 August 2017).

RCPCH (Royal College of Paediatrics and Child Health) (2023) Spotting the Sick Child. www.rcpch.ac.uk/resources/spotting-sick-child-online-learning (accessed 17 March 2023).

Roper, N., Logan, W.W. and Tierney, A. (1985) *The Elements of Nursing*. Edinburgh: Churchill Livingstone.

Royal Children's Hospital Melbourne (2015) *Clinical Guidelines (Nursing)*. Available at: www.rch.org.au/rchcpg/hospital_clinical_guideline_index/Nursing_Assessment (accessed 21 December 2015).

Royal College of Nursing (2012) *Using Technology to Complement Nursing Practice: An RCN Guide for Healthcare Practitioners*. London: RCN.

Salama, M., Emms, K., Hemlesly, A., Amber, O., Higgs, J., Valler-Jones. T. and Duncan, H. (2021) '1412 Incorporating parental concern as an integral escalation entity on a paediatric early warning system'. *Archives of Disease in Childhood*, 106: Issue Suppl 1.

Shields, L., Pratt, J. and Hunter, J. (2006) 'Family centred care: a review of qualitative studies'. *Journal of Clinical Nursing*, 15 (10): 1317–23.

Shields, L., Pratt, J., Davis, L. and Hunter, J. (2008) 'Family-centred care for children in hospital (review)'. *The Cochrane Foundation*, 3.

Smith, J., Shields, L., Neill, S. and Darbyshire, P. (2017) 'Losing the child's voice and "the captive mother": an inevitable legacy of family centred care?' *Evidence Based Nursing*, 20 (3): 67–9.

Smith, L. and Coleman, V. (2010) *Child and Family-centred Healthcare: Concept, Theory and Practice*, 2nd edn. Basingstoke: Palgrave Macmillan.

Smith, L., Coleman, V. and Bradshaw, M. (2002) *Family-centred Care*: Concept, Theory and Practice. Basingstoke: Palgrave.

Walsh, M. (1991) *Models in Clinical Nursing*. London: Bailliere Tindall.

Watson, D. (2006) 'The impact of accurate patient assessment on quality of care'. *Nursing Times*, 102 (6): 34–7.

Yura, H. and Walsh, M.B. (1967) *The Nursing Process: Assessing, Planning, Implementing, Evaluating*. Norwalk, CT: Appleton-Century-Crofts.

COMMUNITY CARE AND CARE IN NON-HOSPITAL SETTINGS FOR CHILDREN AND YOUNG PEOPLE

7

GARETH JONES, SARAH JONES, ORLA McALINDEN AND JACQUI SCRACE

THIS CHAPTER COVERS

- An introduction and current guidance on providing community care to babies, children and young people under the age of 18, in various community settings
- Gives a brief overview of the antecedents of community care for children and young people in the UK from 1950s
- Gives an exemplar of how to maximise efficient, effective evidence-based care in contemporary community nursing care provision for children and families

> "
> "To see a child at home with their family is something I will never forget. I felt honoured to provide nursing care in the home as the child felt far more relaxed and comfortable than in a hospital ward. It also meant they didn't have to attend either a hospital or outpatients department and could have their nursing treatment at home and even at school!"
>
> **Nursing student's voice**
> "

INTRODUCTION

The provision of clinical care to children and young people is no longer confined to a hospital setting as nursing care can be provided in a variety of community settings (nurseries, special schools, short break providers). It is not a new concept. Children and their families can find it easier to receive appropriate clinical interventions in the community setting, as it ensures that care delivery is less disruptive to family life and eases the pressures on the acute/hospital settings. There are many different groups of professionals that provide care in the community to children and young people, which includes public health nurses (health visitors, school nurses) and clinical nurse specialists. For the purpose of this chapter it will focus on Community Children Nursing.

Current guidance and vision

Latest (2021) guidelines from NICE recommend ensuring children and young people are 'fully informed about their health so that they are empowered to take an active role in their healthcare'. With that in mind Community Children's Nurses (CCNs) are highly skilled and educated autonomous practitioners working to ensure that children remain as close to their home as possible and still have their healthcare needs met.

"Younger patients have historically been seen as more 'passive' recipients of healthcare than adults, but supporting them to truly understand their condition and treatment can help them to feel more confident engaging with healthcare staff. This is the first guideline we have published that specifically addresses the experience of [patients] aged under 18. We hope that it will provide healthcare staff with clear advice on how to engage effectively with younger [patients] … we are very pleased that this guideline has been developed with input from children and young people."

Paul Chrisp, Director Centre for NICE Guidelines, 2021

The overarching principles of the 2021 NICE guidelines for care are identified as:

- Safeguarding
- Disabilities
- Competence
- Age and developmentally appropriate care
- Changes in need and preference
- Digital access

With appropriate attention to cultural sensitivity, shared decision-making, consent, privacy and confidentiality in the assessment, planning, implementation, delivery and evaluation of care interventions. Advocacy and support as well as self advocacy and independent advocacy are all identified as quality indicators of improving the healthcare experience (NICE, 2021).

The design of CCN services is important to engage and deliver appropriate services to the child, young person and family, wherever they may be in the community, and refers to looked-after, refugee, disability and end of life care. Collecting feedback to evaluate care is essential to the development of appropriate services from all service users, including those from under-represented groups (minority ethnic groups, disadvantaged groups, LBGT+ as well as those who choose not to use the services). For these reasons co-production of provision is important (NHS England, 2022).

Co-production may be defined as 'working in partnership by sharing power between people who draw on care and support, carers, families and citizens'. An example of this can be seen in SCIE (2022).

Developments in CCN can be seen in changing healthcare legislation. The Health and Care Act 2022, with the advent of the new Integrated Care Boards (ICB) and Integrated Care Systems (ICS), has given CCN teams the impetus to strive to improve services further and innovate nursing practice and delivery in the community. The latter has never been more pertinent than during the COVID-19 pandemic to ensure children remained at home and avoided hospital admissions wherever possible.

The Queen's Nursing Institute, Public Health England and Department of Health (2018) describe the CCN role as: 'Highly complex and requires skills in negotiating, coaching, teaching and supporting the families and carers of babies, children and young people whilst collaborating with a range of other agencies and services.' This highlights the need for education, practice, leadership and excellence as well as the ability for CCNs to work both autonomously as well as with others as required. This is in contrast to historical care of children in the community.

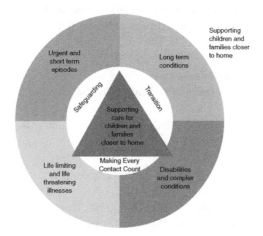

Figure 7.1 Maximising the role of CCN teams service contribution to high-quality, compassionate and excellent health and wellbeing outcomes for children cared for in community setting

www.england.nhs.uk/6cs/wp-content/uploads/sites/25/2015/11/ccn-visual.pdf)

HISTORY OF COMMUNITY CHILDREN'S NURSING (CCN) SERVICES

Community Children's Nursing (CCN) services first began emerging during the latter years of the 19th century. The first CCN team was formed in Rotherham in 1949. This was around the same time that District Nursing and Health Visiting services were becoming established (Whiting, 2000).

This service in Rotherham was introduced to address the concerns of a high rate of infant deaths which was thought to have occurred due to poor infection control leading to cross-infections in hospital. Referrals to this service were made by the local General Practitioner (GP). Four advantages of this service were described by Gillet (1954). These were:

- The child remaining at home in familiar surroundings is less likely to fret
- The danger of cross-infection is lessened
- The mother is encouraged to help in the nursing of the child and the health teaching to parents and relatives done in these cases is considerable
- The call on hospital beds for sick children has been reduced

Similar advantages were identified for the domiciliary Nursing Service for infants and children in Birmingham and the St Mary's Paediatric Home Care project in Paddington, London, both of which were also established in 1954 (Whiting, 2000). Whilst CCN services have continued to develop since 1954, arguably these advantages remain the same.

The care of the sick child has moved steadily from being almost exclusively the responsibility of a hospital setting towards various community settings (Sidey and Wilddas, 2005; Chilton and Bain, 2017). The development of CCN teams was identified by the Department of Health (England) as significantly contributing to, whilst supporting, the safe delivery of care to children and young people (CYP) and their families closer to home (Royal College of Nursing (RCN), 2020).

CCN services have since established themselves as an important part of interdisciplinary and multi-agency teams aiming to provide a high-quality, safe and effective care to CYP in the community (RCN, 2020). Children have a recognised specific health needs spectrum and practitioners need to understand how a healthy child develops towards adulthood to minimise the impact of illness (Queen's Nursing Institute ..., 2018).

In 2011 the Department of Health in England described four identified groups (below) to ensure that the needs of ill and disabled children are met. The DH described CCN services as the 'bedrock of the care pathway' for these groups of CYP (Department of Health (DH), 2011):

- Children with acute and short-term conditions
- Children with long-term conditions
- Children with disabilities and complex conditions including those requiring continuing care and neonates
- Children with life-limiting, life-threatening illnesses, including those requiring palliative and end-of-life care

These children can move between the groups as above and require staff with the skills to meet the needs of these children and young people (DH, 2011).

The Queens Nursing Institute (QNI ..., 2018), recognises that a CCN team provide a vital service to CYP with complex and often long-term illness and disability, delivering care to some of the most vulnerable CYP. The QNI acknowledges that CCNs will not only provide the clinical care but also recognises the role CCNs play in providing the emotional support to families and carers in addition to meeting the child's physical needs and promote their health outcomes.

CRITICAL THINKING STOP POINT

Working in a family's home or other community settings, you may often work autonomously. There may be times when you will need to escalate clinical concerns – how would you go about doing this?

There is a clear policy shift to community-based integrated health and social care in all UK countries and an enhanced focus on admission avoidance, early discharge and greater support for families and others caring for CYP with complex needs in the home or community setting. CCN services play a major role in preparing young people for adulthood and supporting them through the transition process. This is in line with the newly formed Integrated Care Boards, previously known as Clinical Commissioning Groups (CCGs).

Currently, few CCN services are able to meet *all* the needs of all ill and disabled CYP that fall into the categories (above) as there are different models of CCN provision across the United Kingdom (DH, 2011). Ideally there would be a working consensus as to models of care and how they are delivered and evaluated, with an aim for parity of reach and involvement in accordance with the United Nations Convention on the Rights of the Child (United Nations, 1989).

Models of Community Children's Nursing

There is no nationally defined 'best' model of Community Children's Nursing (CCN) care delivery as there is for District Nursing and Public Health Nursing, so this has led to CCN services evolving in response to the local geographical population need, through the development of service specifications. This allows the CCN role to be very flexible and without boundaries and the CCN offer can vary greatly across the regions (RCN, 2020).

There is also very limited recent research on the models of CCN delivery although the main aim of a CCN service remains the same as Eaton (2001) describes, which is to reduce the length of a hospital admission and ideally to avoid a hospital admission altogether, and to provide a service that is of a high quality and cost-effective.

CCN services are usually either based in a hospital setting or in the community. In 2001, Eaton described the 6 models of service delivery:

Model 1 – Hospital outreach or a generalist CCN service

Model 2 – Hospital outreach or specialist

Model 3 – Community-based team

Model 4 – Hospital at home (virtual ward)

Model 5 – District Nursing service

Model 6 – Ambulatory or assessment unit

These models still appear to be relevant, although may have evolved, such as hospital at home, which is now defined as a virtual ward although the concepts remain the same. Some teams across the United Kingdom will incorporate several of the above models of delivery, for example an outreach service and a hospital at home service.

Each of the CCN models will have its own advantages, but the most important factor is that services are designed to focus on the needs of the children, young people and their families and are integrated at the point of service delivery (NICE, 2021).

CRITICAL THINKING STOP POINT

There is an ever-increasing pressure for hospital/acute beds. What would you need to consider from a community perspective regarding

- Admission avoidance?
- Safe and timely discharge from hospital into the community?

And

- How can hospital and community nursing services influence change to ensure the child is kept as close to home as possible?

Please see this link for additional information www.england.nhs.uk/6cs/wp-content/uploads/sites/25/2015/11/ccn-visual.pd

Despite a variety of documents (DH, 2011; NHS England, 2019) that support and highlight the need for a CCN role, there remains at times a lack of clarity in what a CCN team should provide. Models and guidance such as these and the NICE (2021) guideline can signpost the essential components expected from a CCN service for babies, children and young people.

Whatever model or aspiration is used, it should not stifle opportunity for innovative development of services that can be responsive to the ongoing, often changing needs of the local population, the evolving healthcare system and advances in medical technology and treatment options. The global COVID-19 pandemic is a good example where CCN services had to rapidly review and adapt their model of delivery to achieve the balance of continuing to support the most complex and vulnerable CYP and their families, and also manage the risks to this group. This led to changing communication methods with virtual consultations, reviews, updates, training/teaching sessions undertaken virtually along with multidisciplinary meetings.

Whilst face-to-face visits and communications are considered preferable and clinical tasks will still need to be performed, digitalisation and improved technology has expedited CCN teams to explore ways of working into their service delivery. This can give children and young people alternative options to choose how they would like services to be delivered and models to be developed in future. It should be remembered also that children and young people are already 'digital natives' (those who are familiar with digital technology because they have grown up with it) and in many cases are ahead in this respect of those who plan, deliver and evaluate services.

CASE STUDY 7.1: COVID-19 SYSTEM RESPONSE – A COMMUNITY PERSPECTIVE

During the COVID-19 pandemic it was essential that children and young people were kept safe at home and avoided being admitted to hospital. Many children living in the community with complex health needs have significant vulnerabilities of their immune system. A systems response for community settings was required to integrate hospital and community care for CYP.

A systems response is when organisations from statutory services and the voluntary sector all work together as one 'system' to support the child and family. In one area of the Southwest the CCN team, palliative care team, hospital team, hospice, Clinical Commissioning Group (now an Integrated Care Board) and short break teams worked together to ensure that the needs of children were coordinated and supported at a system level (four CCG/local authority areas).

This is a summary of this work.

The challenges

- Depletion of usual workforce
- Increased pressures on hospital services
- PPE and equipment supply issues

What was in place that could be built on

- IT connectivity and regular meetings (thrice weekly at start of the pandemic)
- Enhanced collaborative working and track record of flexibility and adaptability

Shared goals

- Support end-of-life/symptom management needs / Those CYP that meet Children's Continuing Care criteria (ensure care package stability)
- Hospital avoidance (where appropriate)
- Support for families where family resilience impacted by CYP being out of school and/or care package impacted by COVID-related staffing issues

Outputs

- Triaged and co-developed shared caseload across system of CYP with complex and palliative and end-of-life care (PEoLC) needs across four Integrated Care System (ICS) areas
- Identified CYP that must have care needs met (those who met Children's Continuing Care criteria or end of life)
- Ensured that 100% of shift coverage for those requiring packages of care was met. Not one CYP on this shared caseload was admitted to hospital during lockdown 1
- Letter from local MP was sent to the system response praising the work undertaken by the team involved

Together for Short Lives (2020) predict that the number of CYP being diagnosed and living with a complex condition is likely to rise by 11% by 2030, so CCN teams will need to ensure that they are planning for the future and have the capacity to meet this increasing demand. This is particularly challenging in the current climate where the recruitment and retention is greatly stretching the resources of CCN teams. Children living longer with complex needs and the development of technology available to children at home is exciting and very positive; however, it is all adding to the CCN's increased workload. These challenges that CCN teams face further demonstrates that services are going to need to continue to look at innovative, efficient, resilient and sustainable ways of working which suit the needs of those in receipt of the service (United Nations, 1989).

CRITICAL THINKING STOP POINT

CCNs often work alone – how would you ensure your safety in working out in the community?

CASE STUDY 7.2: MIA

What makes a 'good' visit? Sometimes it is not possible to carry out a 'standard' home visit.

Carol is a CCN who is due to visit Mia, aged 10, and her mum at home in an urban housing development in order to assess and attend to her wound following minor surgery. The appointment is in winter, at the weekend and the housing development is well known to be a place where there is often civil unrest, drug dealing and vehicle hijacking; previously several CCNs have been approached to see if they are carrying drugs in their nursing kit.

Mia's mother on the phone has said that the wound on Mia's leg is healing well, giving no pain and that all is well, except that there may be some 'trouble on the estate this evening'. In this situation, consider various options of what to do next.

The future of Children's Community Nursing

The pivotal role of CCN is now increasingly becoming recognised at national level. To reflect this, the recruitment and retention of nurses into the community is one of the Chief Nursing Officer for England's priorities (NHS, 2019).

Investment in the strategic development of community nursing services is described as essential to achieve the ambitions of the NHS Long Term Plan (Bedford, 2022; Clennell, 2022). The move to Integrated Care Systems (ICS) provides a real opportunity for community nurses everywhere to raise the profile of the incredibly valuable and highly skilled work that they do to support this transformation agenda. There is now a statutory requirement for greater integration of health and care services, improving population health and reducing inequalities, supporting productivity and sustainability of services, to help the NHS to support social and economic growth. The future success of community nursing should build on its existing strengths and requires the involvement of people at every level, from the public to politicians, from system leaders and educators, and across the diverse family of community nurses who make up the workforce (Clennell, 2022).

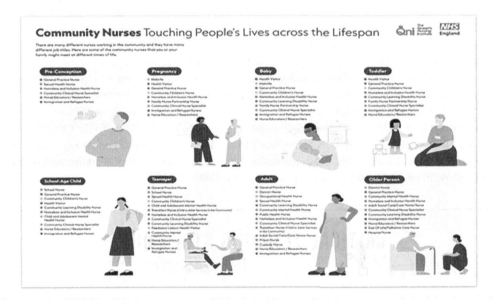

Figure 7.2 Community nurses touching people's lives across the lifespan

HEALTH INEQUALITIES AND POPULATION MANAGEMENT

Data consistently show that poverty and inequality impact a child's whole life, affecting their education, housing and social environment and in turn affecting their health outcomes. The Royal College of Paediatrics and Child Health (RCPCH, 2020) note that action to reduce health inequalities must start before birth and be followed through the life of the child. The importance of investing in the early years is key to preventing ill health later in life; however, this requires a whole system approach with collaboration across a range of stakeholders, including community and hospital settings, local authorities and the third sector (Marmot et al., 2020).

SEE ALSO
CHAPTER 11

Population Health Management (PHM) focuses on the wider determinants of health, recognising that only 20% of a person's health outcomes are attributed to the ability to access good-quality healthcare. It is a partnership approach across the different sectors, of which all have a role to play in addressing the interdependent issues that affect people's health and wellbeing. This approach is pivotal to the way ICSs will work together to improve the health of their local populations. It enables health and care services to be tailored to the needs of local people, reducing duplication and workload pressures (NHS England, n.d.).

Core20PLUS5 (NHS, 2022) is a national NHS England approach to support the reduction of health inequalities at both national and system level. The approach, which originally focused on adults, has been adapted for children and young people and defines a target population cohort, alongside an additional '5' focus clinical areas requiring accelerated improvement.

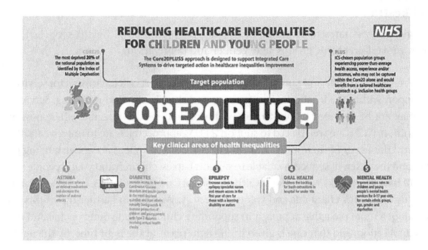

Figure 7.3 Reducing healthcare inequalities for children and young people

Core20 focuses on the most deprived 20% of the national population as identified by the national Index of Multiple Deprivation (IMD).

PLUS population groups include ethnic minority communities; inclusion health groups; people with a learning disability and autistic people; coastal communities with pockets of deprivation hidden amongst relative affluence; people with multi-morbidities; and protected characteristic groups; amongst others. Specific consideration should be taken for the inclusion of young carers, looked after children/care leavers and those in contact with the justice system.

Inclusion health groups include people experiencing homelessness, drug and alcohol dependence, vulnerable migrants, Gypsy, Roma and Traveller communities, sex workers, people in contact with the justice system, victims of modern slavery and other socially excluded groups (NHS, 2022).

The final part sets out five clinical areas of focus. The five areas of focus are part of wider actions for Integrated Care Board and Integrated Care Partnerships to achieve system change and improve care for children and young people. Governance for these five focus areas sits with national programmes; national and regional teams coordinate local systems to achieve aims.

1. **Asthma**
   - Address over-reliance on reliever medications; and
   - Decrease the number of asthma attacks.

2. **Diabetes**
   - Increase access to real-time continuous glucose monitors and insulin pumps across the most deprived quintiles and from ethnic minority backgrounds; and
   - Increase proportion of those with Type 2 diabetes receiving recommended NICE care processes.

3. **Epilepsy**
   - Increase access to epilepsy specialist nurses and ensure access in the first year of care for those with a learning disability or autism.

4. **Oral health**
   - Tooth extractions due to decay for children admitted as inpatients in hospital, aged 10 years and under to decrease.

5. **Mental health**
   - Improve access rates to children and young people's mental health services for 0–17-year-olds, for certain ethnic groups, age, gender and deprivation.

Infants, children, young people and families should have equitable access to cross-sector services, resources, advice and support within the local community to support their health and wellbeing. Services within the community may not be provided by health services but should seek to integrate where possible (RCPCH, 2020). By definition, CCNs are well placed to support a PHM approach to care to improve health outcomes. They understand the needs of their individual patient caseloads as well as an understanding of their local communities and the different services available to support babies, children and young people and their families. CCNs will have good links with other health and social care professionals, both locally and across the wider system, including the charitable and voluntary sectors. Working in partnership in this way, empowers CCNs to adopt a more proactive approach in supporting children and young people and their families, ensuring less duplication, and that care is given in the right place, at the right time, by the right person.

PERSONALISED OUTCOME MEASURES FOR CHILD- AND FAMILY-CENTRED CARE

The NHS Long Term Plan (2019) set out the vison that personalised care will become business as usual across the health and care system.

> "Personalised Care will benefit up to 2.5 million people by 2024, giving them the same choice and control over their mental and physical health that they have come to expect in every other aspect of their life. A one-size-fits-all health and care system cannot meet the increasing complexity of people's needs and expectations."
>
> **NHS England, Personalised care (accessed 2022)**

Personalised care for CYP should give rise to identification of their individual strengths and needs.

There are several approaches by which CCNs can ensure this takes place. First and foremost, a holistic nursing assessment needs to be undertaken, this will then identify needs. The concept of child-centred care encourages healthcare professionals to place the child and their interests at the centre of thinking.

One example where CCNs can support children is by working to promote personal health budgets. It is often the role of a CCN to identify individual needs. Personal health budgets can improve people's quality of life and their experience of care as there should be more choices about how their healthcare needs are met.

A personal health budget is an option that could currently apply to children in receipt of Children's Continuing Care (Department of Health, 2016).

The role of the CCN should provide a holistic, child-centred approach to care to allow a focus on pursuit of normal childhood activities (Coombes, 2022).

As Leonard (2020) states, care and support plans are written jointly with the family to identify their individual priorities. This plan is used to determine a budget and allows people to purchase services and equipment to meet their self-defined health outcomes. Forder (2012), as part of an independent evaluation of personal health budgets, suggested they give rise to cost-effectiveness, reduced inpatient care, and led to significant improvement in the care-related quality of life and wellbeing. With ever-increasing pressure on hospital services, enabling bespoke packages of care around the child and family can keep children at home and, where possible, avoid hospital admissions. Furthermore, child-centred care must be directed by children's views on their priorities to develop improved accessibility, coordination and availability of health services to meet their individual needs.

Given the wide range of services involved in community settings are far reaching, from social care, education and a wide range of voluntary sector services (i.e., respite or hospice care), the role of nurses in the community should use and develop specific health outcomes for CYP to help identify care needs.

Allard (2014) suggests that for children with neurodisability, using a framework to determine health outcomes can identify CYP priorities such as communication methods, mobility, pain, self-care, interpersonal relationships improving wellbeing and gaining independence for future aspirations into transitioning into adult life. Communication was regarded as highly important because it was fundamental to making choices, decision-making, independence and social interaction in the wider community context (Allard, 2014).

Nursing in community settings must ensure close working relationships to identify individual need with the aim to improve health outcomes, ensure improved coordination of the wide range of services that can support our children, young people and families.

Responding to the needs of children and young people

Integrated Care Boards commission Community Services (and in the case of Public Health Nursing, local authorities). Community Services involve a wide variety of the multiprofessional teams (i.e., CCNs, Public Health Nurses, Clinical Nurse Specialist (CNSs), paediatrics and allied health professionals). These services should have clear core offers and pathways and the focus on such services should have meaningful person-centred outcomes for individuals and carers, valuing impact, rather than individual contacts or tasks (Evans, 2015).

Integrated Care Boards and in turn Community Services should focus on person-centred outcome measures as this method can lead to streamlining the delivery of patient care (Evans, 2015). The King's Fund (Foot et al., 2014) also suggests that community nursing needs to move away from task- and contact-based care to person-centred outcome-based care.

Community Services and nurses specifically are in prime position to start developing outcome-based nursing for community services. As part of the commissioner-provider contracts, Foot et al. (2014) suggest that providers need to evidence their impact using outcome measures. These measures might include: patient care outcomes – dying in the preferred place of care; quality outcomes – experience of care; clinical performance outcomes – i.e. wound care.

The Royal College of Nursing (2019) suggest that outcomes may be identified as part of a clinical nursing pathway to demonstrate a staged approach to achieving patient-centred outcomes. There are many ways to record Patient Reported Outcome Measures (PROMs); these can evidence the impact of healthcare on a patient's health and support the patient's perspective. PROMs can be generic as measured in a quality of life tool, e.g. EuroQo or EQ-5D, or specifically more patient-centred, such as a specific health outcome, for example pain (Royal College of Nursing, 2010).

In summary, personalised approaches that are commissioned through Integrated Care Boards should give rise to improving individualised outcomes for CYP and their families. There are a variety of ways to undertake this, and community nursing services can support this delivery for improved coordinated and targeted care.

CASE STUDY 7.3: TRANSITION – A PARENT AND CHILD PERSPECTIVE

Martin is 16 and has been with his CCN team for 5 years due to his health needs around asthma. He has had a very good relationship with his nurse and is aware that soon he will need to transfer to adult services. He is not looking forward to this at all and has expressed some anxiety to Zara, his current CCN. His mother, Martha, also has concerns mainly around continuity of care, starting a new relationship with the nurses and building up trust in the new service.

• What should be happening for Martha and for Martin in relation to their fears and expectations around transition to adult services?

SAFEGUARDING STOP POINT

What would be the role of a community children's nurse in terms of safeguarding children and young people with special educational needs and/or disability?

WHAT'S THE EVIDENCE?

The Children and Families Act 2014 requires education, health and social care agencies to work together more closely than they have in the past. This Act promoted integrated practices in identification and assessment of needs and integrated planning to meet their needs.

It also includes joint commissioning of services for children and young people with SEND and their families.

To support a more integrated approach to assessment and care planning for those with the most complex needs, the Act replaced the former statutory assessment process and Statements of SEN, and the former post-16 Learning Difficulty Assessments with the integrated Education, Health and

Care (EHC) needs assessment and Education, Health and Care Plan (EHC Plan). This brings together practitioners from different agencies to contribute to a single assessment of needs and a single plan.

It is imperative where there is an identified nursing need that a nursing needs assessment and input into an EHC Plan is developed with the child and young person.

The Act also enforces increased personalisation of services and introduced personal budgets to give families with an EHC Plan more control over how the funding available to meet their child's needs is spent.

The Act also introduced a requirement for every local authority to publish a 'Local Offer' website of information about services for those aged 0–25 with SEND and their families. This site must also provide a forum for families to give feedback and influence local service developments.

The CCN role has been to have awareness of this Act, especially in relation to their contribution for EHC Plans and transitioning young people to adult healthcare services.

CHAPTER SUMMARY

- The importance and understanding the complexities of nursing children and their families in the community setting from an historical and contemporary perspective
- Current NHS strategies
- Overview of some models of care in CCN services
- Brief overview of the role of the CCN in population health management
- Ensuring the child, young person and family are seen as individuals whose rights to efficient, effective community care should be recognised as part of contemporary multi-agency working
- The importance of transitional care from child to adult services

REFERENCES

Allard, A., Fellowes, A., Shilling, V. et al. (2014) 'Key health outcomes for children and young people with neurodisability: qualitative research with young people and parents'. *BMJ Open*, 2014;4:e004611. Doi: 10.1136/bmjopen-2013-004611.

Bedford, R. (2022) 'Raising the profile of children's community nursing'. *Journal of Community Nursing*, 36 (3): 66–7.

Children and Families Act 2014. Available at: legislation.gov.uk (accessed 2 September 2022).

Chilton, S. and Bain, H. (2017) *A Textbook of Community Nursing*, 2nd edn. London: Routledge.

Clennell, J. (2022) 'Developing the national community nursing plan'. *British Journal of Community Nursing*, 27 (3): 105.

Coombes, L., Braybrook, D., Roach, A. et al. (2022) 'Achieving child-centred care for children and young people with life-limiting and life-threatening conditions—a qualitative interview study'. *European Journal of Pediatrics*, 181, 3739–52.

Department of Health (2011) *NHS at Home: Community Children's Nursing Services*. London: DH.

Department of Health (2016) *National Framework for Children and Young People's Continuing Care*. London: DH.

Eaton, N. (2001) 'Models of community children's nursing'. *Paediatric Nursing*, 13 (1): 32–6.

Evans, K. (2015) Framework for Commissioning Community Nursing. London: NHS England. Available at: www.england.nhs.uk/wp-content/uploads/2015/10/Framework-for-commissioning-community-nursing.pdf (accessed 25 February 2023).

Foot, C., Sonola, K., Bennett, L., Fitzsimons, B., Raleigh, V. and Gregory, S. (2014) *Managing Quality in Community Health Care Services*. London: The King's Fund.

Forder, J., Jones, K., Glendinning, C. et al. (2012) Evaluation of the personal health budget pilot programme. Discussion Paper 2840_2. www.phbe.org.uk.

Gillett, J.A. (1954) 'Children's Nursing unit'. *British Medical Journal*, 1 (4863): 684–5.

Leonard, H. (2020) 'Children with complex health needs personal health budgets'. *Archives of Disease in Childhood*, 105 (3): 211–13.

Marmot, M., Allen, J., Boyce, T., Goldblatt, P. and Morrison, J. (2020) *Health Equity in England: The Marmot review 10 years on*. London: Institute of Health Equity. Available at: www. instituteofhealthequity.org/resources-reports/marmot-review-10-years-on/the-marmot-review-10-years-on-full-report.pdf (accessed 9 January 2023).

NHS (2019) NHS Long Term Plan. Available at: www.longtermplan.nhs.uk/ (accessed 26 February 2023).

NHS England (2022) Core20PLUS – An approach to reducing health inequalities for children and young people. Available at: www.england.nhs.uk/long-read/core20plus5-infographic-children-and-young-people/ (accessed 23 February 2023).

NHS England (n.d.) Personalised care. Available at: www.england.nhs.uk/personalisedcare/ (accessed 2 September 2022).

NHS England (n.d.) Population Health and the Population Health Management Programme. www. england.nhs.uk/integratedcare/what-is-integrated-care/phm/ (accessed 7 June 2023).

NICE (National Institute for Health and Care Excellence) (2021) Babies', children and young people's experience of healthcare. NICE guideline [NG204]. Available at: nice.org.uk/guidance/NG204 (accessed 22 February 2023).

Queen's Nursing Institute, Public Health England and Department of Health (2018) 'Maximising the role of Community Children's Nursing teams' [Online resource]. Available at: www.england.nhs. uk/6cs/wp-content/uploads/sites/25/2015/11/ccn-visual.pdf (9 June 2023).

Royal College of Nursing (2010) *PROMS: Patient Reported Outcome Measures. The Role, Use and Impact of PROMs on Nursing in the English NHS* (Policy Briefing). London: RCN.

Royal College of Nursing (2020) *Futureproofing Community Children's Nursing* [RCN Guidance]. Available at: www.rcn.org.uk/professional-development/publications/pub-007844 (accessed 9 June 2023).

RCPCH (Royal College of Paedicatrics and Child Health) (2020) *State of Child Health in the UK*. Available at: https://stateofchildhealth.rcpch.ac.uk/ (accessed 23 February 2023).

SCIE (Social Care Institute for Excellence) (2022) Coproduction: what it is and how to do it. Available at: www.scie.org.uk/co-production/what-how#:~:text=Co%2Dproduction%20is%20not%20 just,any%20project%20that%20affects%20them. (accessed 23 February 2023).

Sidey, A. and Widdas, D. (2005) *Textbook of Community Children's Nursing*, 2nd edn. London: Elsevier.

Together for Short Lives (2020) Research shows a significant rise in the number of children with life-limiting conditions. Available at: www.togetherforshortlives.org.uk/new-research-reveals-a-significant-rise-in-the-number-of-children-with-life-limiting-conditions/ (accessed 23 February 2023).

United Nations (1989) *Convention on the Rights of the Child (UNCRC)*. Available at: www.unicef.org.uk/ what-we-do/un-convention-child-rights (accessed 9 June 2023).

Whiting, M. (2000) '1888–1988: 100 years of community children's nursing', in J. Muir and A. Sidey (eds), *Textbook of Community Children's Nursing*. London: Ballière Tindall.

LAW AND POLICY FOR CHILDREN AND YOUNG PEOPLE'S NURSING

8

ORIGNALLY WRITTEN BY MARC CORNOCK AND ORLA McALINDEN, REVISED BY MARC CORNOCK

THIS CHAPTER COVERS

- Policy, procedure and law – what are the differences?
- How law can interact with and affect care delivery for children and young people in all settings
- Clinical scenarios and identification of key principles of care for the child
- Expert guided discussion around the professional and lawful care of children and families and their varying health and social care needs

> "The end of law is not to abolish or restrain, but to preserve and enlarge freedom. For in all the states of created beings capable of law, where there is no law, there is no freedom."
>
> **John Locke, 1690**

INTRODUCTION

The opening quotation demonstrates succinctly what the law seeks to do in the context of nursing and healthcare – to enable and facilitate the provision of nursing care, to preserve what is good and restrict what is wrong. In the case of children and young people's nursing this may be seen to be enshrined in the UN Convention on the Rights of the Child (United Nations, 1989). These rights are applicable in health and social care and are relevant to the aspiring children's nurse.

The practice of nursing children in the 21st century is a complex and multifaceted set of skilled and interlinked evidence-based interventions. The contemporary children's nurse in the health and social care setting is expected to be fit for the practice of the art and science of nursing, fit for the purpose of meeting the needs of children in all health and social care settings and, last but not least, fit for the award of an academic as well as professional qualification. In a nutshell, that is what you are doing on your current academic and professional programme. If you are reading this you are most likely in year 2 or 3 of your university programme, either at undergraduate level or at continuing education/ postgraduate level.

Why do you need to understand the material in this chapter, as it relates to care in children's nursing? As a registered nurse, you will be expected to be responsible, accountable and liable for the care you assess, plan, deliver and evaluate. It is not simply about knowing the rationale or evidence base for actions; rather it is a working awareness of the often complex interactions between people, health, society, culture and organisations. This chapter provides you with the opportunity to explore these areas and gain an understanding of them now as a nursing student, in preparation for your role as a registered nurse.

Please have a look at *The Code: Professional Standards of Practice and Behaviour for Nurses, Midwives and Nursing Associates* (Nursing and Midwifery Council (NMC), 2018). Remember that these are periodically updated and you should check that you are reading the current edition. You can do this by accessing the NMC website.

SEE ALSO
CHAPTER 1

Children's nurses are required to safeguard the interests of children at all times, practise in a non-discriminatory manner and remain vigilant to the legal and ethical aspects of their practice. A challenging aspect of working with children is navigating the interplay of decision-making with policy, law and procedure in dealings with children, families and the multidisciplinary team (McAlinden, 2012). Interpreting and applying codes and policies and upholding the law can be a major juggling act. By year 2 most students are mastering their clinical skills fairly well, and their attention turns to the complexities of delivering 'whole care' and not just 'the bits' that involve a clinical (psychomotor) skill. This involves the policies, procedures, codes and laws associated with delivering safe and effective multidisciplinary health and social care.

> "Legislation in children's nursing is everywhere and conveyed within the NMC Code, which sets out professional standards and is underpinned by the law. As a student, you will constantly refer back to the Code and reflect on your practice. The law is important to me because having heard about cases in university and viewed bad practice reports online, I want to ensure that I practise responsibly within legal frameworks."
>
> **Thomas, 2nd-year children's nursing student**

Although having to manage the various aspects of children's care – including clinical care, relationships with children and their families, decision-making, and the interplay of polices, law and ethics – all at the same time can be terrifying, it is a vital and important skill to master. You are not alone in your apprehension about being able to achieve this skill. Practice does make perfect, and your practice assessor and your university lecturer will help you progress towards achievement of this skill. So too will listening to the views and wishes of children and their families. A reassuring technique is to ask yourself, 'Am I acting in my patient's best interests using the best available evidence and within my sphere of competence?' If you can answer yes, then you should be practising effectively.

ACTIVITY 8.1: CRITICAL THINKING

Although mastering complex skills can appear daunting at first, think back to when you first started to learn to drive. At the beginning you were probably solely 'task focused' and unable to 'look, mirror, signal, manoeuvre and read the road' all at the same time as dealing with the mechanics of actually 'driving' the car. With practice and increasing confidence you started to master the integration of the tasks, skills and knowledge – then one day you found yourself doing it with increasing ease. If you are not a driver you can probably think of other examples yourself where you had to master both cognitive and practical skills at the same time and suddenly found that they became second nature to you without you really noticing that you had mastered them.

- Reflect on recent experience in your practice where you have realised that you are completing care fairly effortlessly when previously you were worried about that same aspect of care. At what point did you realise you could complete this aspect of care without too much concern? How does this make you feel now about that aspect of care?

POLICY, PROCEDURE AND LAW - WHAT ARE THE DIFFERENCES?

Please read the *Oxford English Dictionary* definitions of these terms in Table 8.1.

Table 8.1 Definitions of policy, procedure and law

Policy	Procedure	Law
A course of action proposed or agreed by an organisation or individual	A correct, official or usual way of doing something	A rule or system of rules, usually made by a particular government or community, that orders the way a society behaves and which may be enforced by penalties

Source: Adapted from Oxford English Dictionary

Nursing is governed by specific legislation from country to country, for example in the UK this is The Nursing and Midwifery Order 2001.

ACTIVITY 8.2: CRITICAL THINKING

Access The Nursing and Midwifery Order 2001 in the UK, or the relevant law for your country. Read and note the requirements in law of (1) a registered nurse and (2) nursing as a professional body.

HOW LAW CAN INTERACT WITH AND AFFECT CARE DELIVERY FOR CHILDREN AND YOUNG PEOPLE IN ALL SETTINGS

'Ethics and law are an important aspect of healthcare practice because they provide the foundation upon which practice can develop' (Cornock, 2021, p.5). Further, it can be said that 'ethics and law work together for the benefit of society. Ethics outline the shared values and the law enforces these values' (Cornock, 2021, p.22). However, it is the law which has a more direct effect upon healthcare practice through its ability to enforce its principles.

The law which governs nursing is overarching of all care interventions and the standard set in law is the minimum standard that must be achieved by all those working in health and social care. Interestingly, the professions all tend to set their professional expectations in excess of the legal standing in their codes of professional conduct. This is to make clear their emphasis on protection of the public, which is the key aspect of the professional regulator bodies such as the NMC.

It is helpful to remember that the law sets out the minimum expected standards whilst the Code sets out the best possible standards expected (McAlinden, 2012). Together these concepts can be thought of in the following way:

Law + Code = intention is to protect the public

For nurses in the UK, the NMC Code is an example in point. The NMC Code sets the standard that all registered nurses have to meet. It is the NMC Code that provides protection to the public. For nurses in other countries you should become familiar with the legislation and nursing codes and standards of your own particular jurisdiction.

The NMC Code (2018) uses a 'principles'-based approach to the care of patients and clients; it also indicates how the law both intertwines with and informs healthcare practices. The NMC Code is a lengthy professional guidance and directive on how nurses must protect those in their care and is a combination of 'positive rules' (binding) and 'normative' rules (what a person should do). This reflects the reality and complexity of contemporary health and social care delivery.

"A lot of emphasis is put on the NMC Code in university and on placement, which really highlights how much it underpins my practice, now as a student and when I qualify as a registered nurse. I do find the NMC Code very easy to read and relate to. It is well laid out in sections, making it easy to refer to, which I often do, particularly in university work."

Amber, 3rd-year children's nursing student

"I have found the NMC Code and standards very helpful in my learning as a children's nursing student, particularly with linking my theory into practice and references for assignments. It is available online, easy to understand and I like to keep updated with any revisions. I think it is important to keep referring back to the Code in everything you do as a nursing student because it has derived from the law and when working with children and their families we want to practise legally as competent practitioners."

Thomas, 2nd-year children's nursing student

Duty of care and duty of candour

Two important legal principles in healthcare practice are the duty of care a nurse has to those they care for and the duty of candour that applies if something untoward occurs.

Duty of care

The legal duty of care relates to the legal obligations that one person has towards another. In the healthcare setting the legal duty of care is related to ethical and professional duties. The legal duty of care for nurses requires that nurses provide care to all those whom they have a responsibility for and that the patients and clients of the nurse receive the care to a particular standard and do not come to any harm as a result of the nurse's actions or omissions (Cornock, 2017).

Duty of candour

This is not a new concept as it is concerned with openness and honesty in dealing with patients and their families. However, more recently, following events at Mid Staffordshire and subsequently serious care failings at Morecambe Bay (Kirkip, 2015), much more attention has been on what happens when failings in care occur. This led to consideration of how failings should be addressed and when. As a result, the concept of a legal duty of candour was proposed. The Francis Report (2013) proposed a shift from the existing contractual duty of care to advise patients and their families of failings in care (required by employers) to a statutory (required by law) obligation on all organisations, providers and individuals.

There are two types of duty of candour. The first is owed by an organsation to those it treats, this is what is referred to when speaking of the 'duty of candour'. The second is that owed by healthcare professionals to their patients and clients, either individually or jointly; this is generally referred to as the 'professional duty of candour'.

The professional duty of candour requirements are to:

- Make sure the healthcare professional acts in an open and transparent way with relevant persons in relation to care and treatment provided to people who use services in carrying on a regulated activity
- Tell the relevant person in person as soon as reasonably practicable after becoming aware that a notifiable safety incident has occurred, and provide support to them in relation to the incident, including when giving the notification
- Provide an account of the incident which, to the best of the health service body's knowledge, is true of all the facts the body knows about the incident as at the date of the notification
- Advise the relevant person what further enquiries the provider believes are appropriate
- Offer an apology
- Follow this up by giving the same information in writing, and providing an update on the enquiries
- Keep a written record of all communication with the relevant person (NMC and GMC, 2015)

CLINICAL SCENARIOS AND IDENTIFICATION OF KEY PRINCIPLES OF CARE FOR THE CHILD

ACTIVITY 8.3: REFLECTIVE PRACTICE

For all relevant reports and legislation (specific to your country) visit the appropriate websites and make a note of pertinent material to your practice:

(Continued)

- England:www.gov.uk/government/organisations/department of health
- Northern Ireland:www.health-ni.gov.uk
- Scotland:www.scotland.gov.uk
- Wales:http://gov.wales
- Republic of Ireland:www.gov.ie
- Irish Health Reports: www.hiqa.ie/
- World Health Organization: www.who.org
- United Nations Convention on the Rights of the Child: www.unicef.org/child-rights-convention

WHAT'S THE EVIDENCE?

Francis, R. (2013) The Report of the Mid Staffordshire NHS Foundation Trust Public Inquiry.

Access the Francis Report and take time to read it as this has particular resonance for all nursing practice. List six of the key recommendations from this report.

EXPERT GUIDED DISCUSSION AROUND THE PROFESSIONAL AND LAWFUL CARE OF CHILDREN AND FAMILIES AND THEIR VARYING HEALTH AND CARE NEEDS

SCENARIO 8.1: SOPHIE

Sophie, a 2nd-year nursing student, is new to the Day Surgery Unit.

She has been asked to admit a 5-year-old boy called Felix who needs dental extractions and is on the afternoon list for surgery. Her mentor is nearby and has instructed Sophie to start the admission and call for assistance with anything that she is not sure about.

Sophie introduces herself to Felix and his grandmother who has accompanied him. She takes Felix's vital signs and notes the time he last ate or drank. She records this along with his preferences and demographic details and asks both Felix and his granny if they understand why he is there.

Granny signals covertly to Sophie and takes her aside. She says that Felix doesn't know about the dental extractions; they have told him he's going for a nice sleep and when he's asleep the nurse will clean his teeth and make them all shiny and white. Sophie is not sure that this is the best way to deal with Felix but she says nothing at this point. Sophie watches as the surgeon asks granny for her signature on the hospital consent form. Sophie is not very happy about this either but is reluctant to speak up and tell the surgeon that she is the grandmother and not the mother – surely he would know? She is also not sure about telling her mentor that Felix has no idea why he's there.

- What would you do in Sophie's situation?

Compare your answers with the following discussion.

It is tempting to begin our discussion by considering whether Sophie has done anything wrong. However, a more useful starting point may be to consider the respective roles of all concerned in this scenario:

- Felix is going to have some teeth removed
- Felix's grandmother is supporting him
- Sophie has been instructed to start Felix's admission
- Sophie's practice assessor has to ensure that Felix is safely admitted to the Day Surgery Unit
- The surgeon is responsible for ensuring that Felix has his dental extractions safely

There is a complex interplay of legal responsibility, Trust policies and professional accountability in this scenario, as well as legal considerations regarding the operation itself. It may therefore be easiest to go through the scenario step by step to ensure that we have covered all these.

Sophie's practice assessor instructing her to start the admission is the first point we need to consider. Sophie's practice assessor is accountable for Felix's admission. He has delegated the starting of this to Sophie but this does not remove his accountability. Whilst tasks can be delegated, it is not possible to delegate accountability for that task (Cornock, 2014). Therefore, overall accountability for Felix's admission remains with Sophie's practice assessor. This means that he has to check that Felix's admission has been undertaken correctly.

Sophie has responsibility for starting Felix's admission. As this has been delegated by her practice assessor, she is not accountable to the NMC for this as she is not on the NMC register. However, she is liable for her actions in law and has to perform her role to the necessary standard as required by law (Cornock, 2017). This standard is known as the 'Bolam test' (because it arose out of the *Bolam* v. *Friern Hospital Management Committee* [1957] court case) and means that Sophie must perform her role in the same way as another 2nd-year nursing student. Sophie must also adhere to any Trust policy regarding the admission of a child to the hospital and the Day Surgery Unit.

Sophie is then informed by Felix's granny that Felix does not know about the surgery but believes he is having his teeth cleaned. Sophie seems unsure whether this is the best way to deal with Felix. She is right to be concerned. All healthcare is a partnership with the patient. Felix's treatment will not end when his teeth are extracted; he will need aftercare, including pain relief and the need to rinse his mouth. He will also need to go for a check-up to ensure that everything has healed correctly. If Felix wakes up in pain and not knowing what has happened, he may be unwilling to have any further assessment or treatment for his mouth and may also be mistrustful of hospitals, nurses and doctors. On the other hand, if a child-centred care approach is taken and everything is explained to him, he will understand what is happening and why and this may be a more positive experience for him. (For further discussion on child-centred care, see Carter et al., 2014.)

At this point, Sophie's concern would seem to be that expected of a 2nd-year nursing student.

The next point to concern us is obtaining consent. The surgeon is liable and accountable for ensuring that valid consent is obtained for Felix's operation. As a 5-year-old, Felix is not legally competent to provide his own consent. A child is able to provide their own consent if they can demonstrate to the relevant healthcare professional that they are Gillick competent (Cornock and Montgomery, 2014). This means that the child (a minor) can demonstrate they have the necessary emotional and intellectual maturity to understand the nature of the proposed procedure, as well as any possible side effects, along with the risks and possible complications, and also the risk associated with not having the treatment. The term 'Gillick competent' arises from the Gillick case (*Gillick* v. *West Norfolk and Wisbech AHA* [1985]).

As Felix cannot consent for himself, the law says that for a child, someone with parental responsibility can provide valid consent. Sophie notes that Felix's granny signs the consent form. However, it is not automatic that the grandmother has parental responsibility for Felix. Parental responsibility normally rests with the parents of a child, unless this has been changed, such as via a court order, to the contrary – for example, adoption of the child or a residence order (Cornock, 2015). It is the surgeon's responsibility to ensure that the correct person signs the consent form. However, Sophie watches this being done and has not informed the surgeon that he has been talking with Felix's granny. It may be that Felix's granny has parental responsibility for him, but Sophie has not checked this and so does not know either way.

At this point Sophie is aware that Felix does not know why he is at the Day Surgery Unit and also that it was Felix's granny who signed the consent form. We must remember that she is responsible for starting Felix's admission as it was delegated to her.

The nursing student–practice assessor relationship is based on trust and communication. If either of these is absent then the relationship will not work. Furthermore, Sophie was told by her practice assessor to ask for assistance if she is unsure of anything. Let's also not forget that Sophie is responsible for her own actions and has to meet the required standard in undertaking these.

So what should Sophie do? We need to consider what another 2nd-year nursing student would do in Sophie's situation. This is the application of the 'Bolam test' discussed above. We do not need to consider the best 2nd-year student, just the average one. We would expect that a 2nd-year student unsure of something would seek the assistance of their practice assessor.

Therefore, to fulfil her responsibility to the required standard, Sophie needs to discuss the situation with her practice assessor who will become aware of Felix's lack of knowledge about his operation and be able to check whether Felix's granny has parental responsibility for him or not. The practice assessor can then decide how best to proceed regarding Felix's understanding of why he is at the Day Surgery Unit, and also inform the surgeon, if necessary, regarding consent.

We should note that Sophie's legal responsibility can be satisfied by Sophie informing her practice assessor of the relevant facts. This is not an onerous duty on Sophie. As stated above, it should be part of her relationship with her practice assessor. She needs to ensure that her practice assessor is aware of the facts before Felix undergoes his treatment. If she doesn't then she may be said to have fallen below the required standard.

If Sophie did not inform her practice assessor of the relevant facts, her practice assessor would still be expected to discuss Felix's admission with Sophie as part of their accountability in delegating the admission to Sophie. At this stage it would be hoped that the relevant facts would come to light and for the practice assessor to act on them as discussed above. In this situation Sophie would have breached her duty, but no harm would have occurred as her practice assessor would have established the facts and acted accordingly.

If Sophie does not discuss the situation with her practice assessor, and her practice assessor does not check with Sophie regarding Felix's admission, both Sophie and her practice assessor would have failed in their respective responsibility and accountability regarding Felix's operation.

SCENARIO 8.2: MICHAEL

Nursing student Michael loves his placement with the community children's nurse (CCN) and the health visitors; this could well be an area he would like to work in after he registers with the NMC, though it is so very different from working in an acute area. This morning he and the CCN are planning on visiting Petra, a 9-year-old at home, to check and renew a wound dressing. On arrival there is no answer for quite a while, then finally Petra opens the door. Her mum is at work, she says. When undertaking the dressing, Michael and the CCN note that Petra has a lot of fresh bruising on her arms and goes silent when asked how these bruises happened. Michael wonders how this incident and suspicions relating to safeguarding children will be managed by the CCN.

- What do you think the CCN should do regarding Petra's situation?

Compare your answers with the following discussion.

There are two issues that we need to examine in this scenario. The first is that a 9-year-old child appears to have been left alone in the house. The second is that the child has unexplained bruising on her arms, both potential safeguarding points. Let's take the issue of an unsupervised minor at home first. Michael and the CCN need to make sure that Petra is indeed alone and that there is no-one else in the house before taking any action. It could be that there is someone else in the house, perhaps another adult asleep, or that Petra's mum has gone to the shops for some food and is not at work. From a legal perspective we need to note that there is no specific age at which a child becomes old enough to be left alone on their own, or any minimum age. Rather, each child needs to be judged on their own maturity to be left alone at home. However, the National Society for the Prevention of Cruelty to Children (NSPCC) has published guidance on leaving a child at home which has links to the law on leaving children alone in England and Wales, Scotland and Northern Ireland, and this suggests that most children under 12 would not be considered mature enough to be left at home for any considerable period of time (NSPCC, 2021).

Whilst the law has no specific age limit when a child can be left alone, it does make it an offence to leave a child alone if they are placed at risk, and the relevant person can be prosecuted for neglect. Therefore, if Petra has indeed been left alone for the whole time that her mother is at work, this could be seen to be an issue. The CCN would need to assess if, in her opinion, Petra is mature enough to look after herself or is at risk. We will come back to what she should do if she considers that Petra is at risk after discussing the issue of Petra's bruising. Michael and the CCN note that there is a lot of bruising on Petra's arms and that these bruises are fresh. Again, caution needs to be applied and further investigation of the bruising undertaken. The CCN should gently question Petra further to try to ascertain how the bruising occurred. The reason for this is that it is possible that Petra is an active young girl who suffers knocks and bruising in her playing. On the other hand, it could be that the bruising has been deliberately inflicted by someone else and that Petra is at further risk of being abused. The CCN has to try to determine which of these two causes is the more likely. If the CCN believes that Petra's bruising may be caused as a result of neglect or abuse she has to take action. Likewise, if she believes that Petra is at risk by being left alone she has to take action. The CCN may take the view that there are two areas of concern and this is reason to act further. It isn't necessary to be absolutely certain in these cases; suspicions or concerns should be raised so that they can be investigated by the relevant authorities. All the action that the CCN now takes has to be in Petra's best interests in order to protect and safeguard her.

All organisations that come into contact with children are required to have safeguarding policies and procedures for child protection in place. The CCN should contact her manager or the person who is responsible in her organisation for child protection issues and explain the situation, what she has found and what her concerns are. This also needs to be documented in the child's notes.

The manager or responsible person then needs to make contact with the appropriate authorities. In this instance it may be a social worker in the child protection team who is able to arrange for Petra to be either removed to a place of safety or for someone to protect Petra by staying with her. The CCN and Michael would need to stay with Petra until someone else is able to come to the house and take responsibility for Petra's safety. A key aspect of managing this situation for the CCN is communication and scrupulous record-keeping. The CCN needs to make sure that she has recorded all the relevant facts, including why her suspicions were raised, the actions she took and the names of the individuals she contacted as well as any subsequent action. It is possible that the police may be involved in this case and action taken against Petra's mother for neglect. If this does occur, Michael and the CCN may be asked to provide statements to the police regarding their involvement and actions.

SEE ALSO
CHAPTER 9

"Safeguarding children is a key role of a children's nurse as often they are the first to see signs of abuse and neglect. In university we focus a lot on child protection and when I go on placement it becomes obvious why we do have so much emphasis on safeguarding. As a 1st-year children's nurse student I was horrified when I realised the number of safeguarding issues that were unfolding in a hospital so close to my hometown. Now, as a 3rd-year student, I have seen many cases where children have been brought into hospital with injuries that are thought to be non-accidental and have found it very interesting working with the entire multidisciplinary team to come to conclusions about what has happened to the children and seeing social workers and other agencies becoming involved. Many of the cases are heart-breaking but it is comforting to know that as nurses, we are protecting the child and ensuring the best future for them."

Amber, 3rd-year children's nursing student

SCENARIO 8.3: KATHY

Whilst on lunch break in the coffee bar in the foyer, Kathy, a nursing student, has her friends enthralled as she tells them all about her morning's experiences in the A&E Department. You wouldn't believe it, she says, as she tells them all about the young person who came in with an overdose, the 13-year-old who turned out to be pregnant and the road traffic collision caused by the local school bus driver. The coffee shop is used by everyone, not just nursing staff. Some visitors are listening.

- Do you think that Kathy has done anything wrong?

Compare your answers with the following discussion.

Kathy has a duty of care to all her patients; even as a nursing student this duty exists. Part of this duty is to respect the patient's right to confidence. The right to confidence is known as confidentiality and is a fundamental principle of healthcare, encompassing law, ethics and professional regulatory principles.

To maintain a patient's confidentiality means to protect information that is obtained about or from the patient in the course of your professional practice. If you do not maintain patient confidentiality then you will have failed in your duty of care to that patient, unless there are public interest reasons to disclose the information, such as to prevent or detect serious crime or where the information needs to be disclosed to protect the patient or another person from serious harm.

So, has Kathy breached any of her patients' confidentiality?

She is in a public area discussing patients with her friends; it doesn't matter if Kathy's friends are nurses or not. The only time you should discuss patient information is when the other individual needs the information in order to care for that patient.

However, has she passed on any patient details? From the information we have it does not appear as if Kathy is actually naming her patients when she is discussing them with her friends. Does this mean that she is maintaining her patients' confidentiality?

No, Kathy may breach confidentiality even if she does not pass on the patient's name. It all depends upon the information Kathy is disclosing to her friends. If one of the visitors listening in to Kathy's conversation is able to identify one of their neighbours from the information that Kathy is sharing, such as how they were dressed and some identifiable feature such as a mole in a particular place on their face, or their job (such as school bus driver), Kathy will have breached her duty of confidentiality to those patients.

Even if Kathy does not provide identifiable features in her discussion with her friends, the question to be asked is why she is discussing her patients with her friends in a public place. Whilst this may not be breaching any law, it is unethical in that it shows a lack of respect for her patients.

So, has Kathy done anything wrong? Yes, she has. At best she has shown a lack of respect for her patients. At worst she has breached their confidentiality and the duty of care she owes to them.

"Confidentiality can be a complex issue, particularly with changing family dynamics. I find confidentiality is even more complex in children's nursing than it is in other areas of nursing as it can be difficult to know who you should and should not share information with. I have been involved with the care of an adolescent during my training who didn't want his parents to know about his health issue and this was a difficult situation to manage."

Amber, 3rd-year children's nursing student

Working with children is both a privilege and a challenge. This book is primarily intended for those who are studying towards their registration in this area, although it is equally applicable to the registered children's nurse and those wanting an insight into the work of children's nurses.

Working with children requires awareness and promotion of the principles of empowerment, protection of rights and respect for children and their families. Indeed, the primary role of the children's nurse is to put the children first at all times.

Nurses working with children need to understand the legal underpinning of their work, such as their duty of care to children. Through the use of specifically selected practice-focused case studies and expert commentary, this chapter has explored legislation and policy applicable to the children's nurse, such as duty of care, duty of candour, communication, accountability, consent, safeguarding and confidentiality.

Attaining registration as a children's nurse is an immense achievement but it is not the end of the journey, just the beginning of the next stage. Remaining fit to practise is the responsibility of all nurses and is a requirement of the NMC as well as a societal expectation. It is what we demonstrate in the Revalidation process (NMC, 2019). It requires that all nurses demonstrate the required knowledge, skill and respect for those in their care.

SEE ALSO CHAPTER 1,2 AND 5

By working through this chapter you will have had the opportunity to critically reflect, explore and discuss the implications of delivering contemporary child-centred nursing care as part of a multidisciplinary and multi-agency endeavour.

CHAPTER SUMMARY

- Law + Code = the intention is always to protect the public. Each registered nurse should follow policies, procedures and the law in their individual as well as multiprofessional and multidisciplinary practice

- You have gained awareness of the relevance of duty of care and duty of candour
- As a children's nurse you should regularly refresh your knowledge of the Code, and general and local policies and procedures for each area in which you work
- As a children's nurse you should refresh your knowledge of child protection legislation and policy at frequent intervals
- As a children's nurse you should deliver child-centred and relevant associated care and put the child first
- You should always ask your mentor or seniors if unsure – do not hesitate to seek advice. Even senior nurses seek advice and check their understanding as this is a hallmark of being a professional

BUILD YOUR BIBLIOGRAPHY

Books

FURTHER
READING

- Carter, B., Bray, L., Dickinson, A., Edwards, M. and Ford, K. (2014) *Child-Centred Nursing. Promoting Critical Thinking*. London: Sage.

  This book is an excellent resource for those wishing to better understand the imperatives under-pinning contemporary child-centred nursing care.
- Cornock, M. (2021) *Key Questions in Healthcare Law and Ethics*. London: Sage.

  This book provides a reader-friendly discussion of ethical and legal issues in relation to health-care practice.
- Smith, L. and Coleman, V. (2009) *Child and Family-centred Healthcare: Concept, Theory and Practice*. Basingstoke: Palgrave Macmillan.

  This book provides a clear focus on child-centred care in interprofessional and multidisciplinary settings as well as in community care.
- Watson, G. and Rodwell, S. (2014) *Safeguarding and Protecting Children, Young People and Families: A Guide for Nurses and Midwives*. London: Sage.

  This book offers a clear explanation of the ways in which children's nurses can safeguard their patients and considers many of the challenges that a children's nurse may encounter.

Journal articles

FURTHER
READING:
ONLINE
JOURNAL
ARTICLES

- Cornock, M. (2010) 'Hannah Jones, consent and the child in action: a legal commentary'. *Paediatric Nursing*, 22 (2): 14-20.

  This article explains consent relating to the child, in an accessible manner and using a real-life clinical case as the focus for contemporary discussion.
- Gilmore, S. and Herring, J. (2011) '"No" is the hardest word: consent and children's autonomy'. *Child and Family Law Quarterly*, 23 (1): 3-25.

  This article explores the difficulties associated with legal definitions of consent in children's care.
- McFarlane, A. (2011) 'Mental capacity: one standard for all ages'. *Family Law*, 41 (5): 479-85.

  This article looks at mental capacity and what it means for issues of consent.

Weblinks

- Children Act 1989 www.legislation.gov.uk/ukpga/1989/41/contents An example of key legislation which you should explore in more depth is the Children Act 1989 (or the equivalent in other countries). This sets out the legal expectations and requirements around the protection and welfare of children.
- UNICEF, United Nations Convention on the Rights of the Childs www.unicef.org.uk/what-we-do/un-convention-child-rights The UNCRC is important reading for the children's nurse.
- NSPCC, *Child Protection in the UK and Safeguarding Deaf and Disabled Children* https://learning.nspcc.org.uk/safeguarding-child-protection https://learning.nspcc.org.uk/safeguarding-child-protection/deaf-and-disabled-children Useful resources on child protection in England, Northern Ireland, Scotland and Wales.

FURTHER
READING:
WEBLINKS

REFERENCES

Bolam v. Friern Hospital Management Committee [1957] 2 All ER 118.

Carter, B., Bray, L., Dickinson, A., Edwards, M. and Ford, K. (2014) *Child-centred Nursing: Promoting Critical Thinking*. London: Sage.

Cornock, M. (2014) 'Legal principles of responsibility and accountability in professional healthcare'. *Orthopaedic and Trauma Times*, (23): 16–18.

Cornock, M. (2015) 'The child and consent'. *Orthopaedic and Trauma Times*, (27): 13–15.

Cornock, M. (2017) 'Clinical negligence'. *Orthopaedic and Trauma Times*, (32): 10–13.

Cornock, M. (2021) *Key Questions in Healthcare Law and Ethics*. London: Sage.

Cornock, M. and Montgomery, H. (2014) 'Children's rights since Margaret Thatcher', in S. Wagg and J. Pilcher (eds), *Thatcher's Grandchildren*. Basingstoke: Palgrave.

Francis, R. (2013) *The Report of the Mid Staffordshire NHS Foundation Trust Public Inquiry*. London: The Stationery Office.

Gillick v. West Norfolk and Wisbech AHA [1985] 1 All ER 533.

HM Government (2018) *Working Together to Safeguard Children: A Guide to Inter-agency Working to Safeguard and Promote the Welfare of Children*. London: DfE. Available at: www.gov.uk/government/publications/working-together-to-safeguard-children--2 (accessed 1 February 2021).

Kirkip, B. (2015) *The Report of the Morecambe Bay Investigation: An Independent Investigation into the Management, Delivery and Outcomes of Care Provided by Maternity and Neonatal Services at the University Hospitals of Morecambe Bay NHS Foundation Trust from January 2004 to June 2013*. London: TSO.

Locke, J. (1690) *Second Treatise of Civil Government*. Available at: www.constitution.org/jl/2ndtreat.htm (accessed 5 April 2017).

McAlinden, O. (2012) 'Ethical and legal implications when planning care for children and young people', in D. Corkin, S. Clarke and L. Liggett (eds), *Care Planning in Children and Young People's Nursing*. Chichester: Wiley–Blackwell.

NSPCC (National Society for the Prevention of Cruelty to Children) (2021) Staying home alone. Available at: www.nspcc.org.uk/keeping-children-safe/in-the-home/home-alone/ (accessed 1 February 2021).

Nursing and Midwifery Council (NMC) and General Medical Council (GMC) (2015) *Openness and Honesty When Things Go Wrong. The Professional Duty of Candour*. Available at: www.gmc-uk.org/guidance/ethical_guidance/27233.asp (accessed 8 May 2017).

Nursing and Midwifery Council (NMC) (2018) *The Code: Professional Standards of Practice and Behaviour for Nurses Midwives and Nursing Associates*. London: NMC. Available at: www.nmc.org.uk/standards/code/ (accessed 1 February 2021).

Nursing and Midwifery Council (NMC) (2019) Revalidation. Available at: http://revalidation.nmc.org.uk/ (accessed 1 February 2021).

Oxford English Dictionary (2017) Available at: www.oed.com (accessed 5 April 2017).

United Nations (1989) *United Nations Convention on the Rights of the Child (UNCRC)*. Available at: www.unicef.org.uk/what-we-do/un-convention-child-rights (accessed 6 June 2023).

SAFEGUARDING CHILDREN AND YOUNG PEOPLE

9

CAMERON COX AND ZOE CLARK

THIS CHAPTER COVERS

- An overview of safeguarding children, young people and families
- Multi-agency working within safeguarding
- Multi-agency safeguarding models
- An exploration of the issues and concerns linked to contemporary issues

> "I was so confused but knew what he was doing was wrong. I wanted it to stop but part of me was afraid to speak out because I didn't want to get him into trouble."
>
> **Lee, child, NSPCC**

INTRODUCTION

Safeguarding children and young people is everyone's business and will form an essential part of the role of a qualified nurse. However, safeguarding remains the responsibility of any individual in contact with children and their families, including nursing students. Safeguarding is far more than simply knowing the risk factors and being on alert; it is understanding what risks are posed to children in today's society, it is understanding that families are vulnerable, and with this come complications with development of children and safety. This chapter aims to give you an understanding of how agencies work together to safeguard children and how to seek support from these agencies. Overall, safeguarding is a combination of knowledge including policies, research and sometimes simple 'gut instinct'. Building on the opening quote, the take-home message from this chapter is that if you have any concerns about a child or family, always raise this with someone senior, always do something and never do nothing.

AN OVERVIEW OF SAFEGUARDING CHILDREN, YOUNG PEOPLE AND FAMILIES

'Safeguarding children' and 'child protection' are terms commonly interlinked and it is clear within the guidance (RCN, 2019) that everybody who comes into contact with children has a responsibility to safeguard their welfare and ensure they are protected from harm. Nursing students are often drawn to this profession as they have a wish to help children.

> "I got into children's nursing because I am compassionate and focused on the quality of care I feel I could give to patients in the future."
>
> **Laura, 2nd-year children's nursing student**

In recent years there has also been a movement away from children being placed on a child protection register to children having a Child Protection Plan (CPP), suggesting a more positive action to the families involved, **provided it is in the best interests of the child** (London Safeguarding Children Board (LSCB), 2022).

In the *Working Together to Safeguard Children* guidance (HM Government, 2018), safeguarding and promoting the welfare of children is defined as:

- Protecting children from maltreatment
- Preventing impairment of children's health or development
- Ensuring that children are growing up in circumstances consistent with the provision of safe and effective care
- Taking action to enable all children to have the best life chances

Child protection is identified as a part of safeguarding and promoting welfare for children. However, it is focused more on the activity undertaken to protect specific children who are either suffering or are likely to suffer significant harm (HM Government, 2018). Section 47 of the Children Act 1989 provides local authorities with a duty to make enquiries into whether action is required to be taken to protect a child who is believed to be suffering or likely to suffer significant harm (LSCB, 2022). So, how do we define harm?

Harm is more commonly referred to as abuse within the framework of safeguarding children. Somebody may abuse or neglect a child by inflicting harm, or by failing to act to prevent harm. Children may be abused in a family or in an institutional or community setting by those known to them or by others (e.g., via the Internet, social media). They may be abused by an adult or adults, or another child or children.

This can be further broken down into four main categories of abuse which children may need protecting from in relation to safeguarding children (HM Government, 2018; Welsh Government, 2019; Scottish Government, 2021; Safeguarding Board for Northern Ireland, 2022)

1. **Physical abuse**: A form of abuse which may involve hitting, shaking, throwing, poisoning, burning, or scalding, drowning, suffocating or otherwise causing physical harm to a child. Physical harm may also be caused when a parent or carer fabricates the symptoms of, or deliberately induces, illness in a child (known as fabricated illness).

2. **Emotional abuse**: The persistent emotional maltreatment of a child such as to cause severe and persistent adverse effects on the child's emotional development. It may involve conveying to a child that they are worthless or unloved, inadequate, or valued only insofar as they meet the needs of another person. It may include not giving the child opportunities to express their views, deliberately silencing them or 'making fun' of what they say or how they communicate. It may feature age or developmentally inappropriate expectations being imposed on children. These may include interactions that are beyond a child's developmental capability, as well as overprotection and limitation of exploration and learning, or preventing the child participating in normal social interaction. It may involve seeing or hearing the ill-treatment of another. It may involve serious bullying (including cyberbullying), causing children frequently to feel frightened or in danger, or the exploitation or corruption of children. Some level of emotional abuse is involved in all types of maltreatment of a child, though it may occur alone.

3. **Sexual abuse**: Involves forcing or enticing a child or young person to take part in sexual activities, not necessarily involving a high level of violence, whether or not the child is aware of what is happening. The activities may involve physical contact, including assault by penetration (for example, rape or oral sex) or non-penetrative acts such as masturbation, kissing, rubbing and touching outside of clothing. They may also include non-contact activities, such as involving children in looking at, or in the production of, sexual images, watching sexual activities, encouraging children to behave in sexually inappropriate ways, or grooming a child in preparation for abuse (including via the Internet). Sexual abuse is not solely perpetrated by adult males. Women can also commit acts of sexual abuse, as can other children.

4. **Neglect**: The persistent failure to meet a child's basic physical and/or psychological needs, likely to result in the serious impairment of the child's health or development. Neglect may occur during pregnancy as a result of maternal substance abuse. Once a child is born, neglect may involve a parent or carer failing to:

   - Provide adequate food, clothing and shelter (including exclusion from home or abandonment)
   - Protect a child from physical and emotional harm or danger
   - Ensure adequate supervision (including the use of inadequate caregivers)
   - Ensure access to appropriate medical care or treatment. It may also include neglect of, or unresponsiveness to, a child's basic emotional needs

CASE STUDY 9.1: FRAN

Fran (age 30) is a mother of two children: Katlin (14) and Oisin (4 months). The family lives in a two-bedroom flat. Adam (34), the father of Oisin, works as a security guard. He works night shifts and often comes back to the flat to sleep during the day. Fran is unemployed and does not like leaving the house.

Katlin is in Year 10 of the local high school. She was born prematurely at 32 weeks and has mild learning difficulties. She has an education and healthcare plan to support her to stay in mainstream education. However, she is often reported by teachers to be disengaged, tired and withdrawn in class. She does not have a big circle of friends and teachers have noted she is often isolated. Katlin has type 1 diabetes and was diagnosed aged 4 years. She has been having repeated admissions to hospital for poorly controlled blood sugar levels and is not compliant with her insulin regime.

Oisin is a small baby whose weight at his postnatal check was measured on the 0.4th centile. He has not been taken to any further postnatal appointments. Fran called an ambulance for Oisin 2 weeks ago as he was 'floppy' and 'not himself'. Oisin was admitted to the ward from Accident and Emergency due to malnutrition and dehydration. Fran is keen to get him discharged as she wants to be back at home. However, the nurses on the ward have concerns about Fran's capacity to care for Oisin.

- What are the safeguarding concerns?
- What categories of abuse are relevant to this case study?

MULTI-AGENCY WORKING WITHIN SAFEGUARDING

A wide range of health professionals including nurses, GP, health visitors, school nurses, midwives, child and adolescent mental health, drug and alcohol services and emergency care services have a critical role in safeguarding children and young people under 18 years (HM Government, 2018).

Multi-agency teams have been introduced to improve safeguarding approaches through better information sharing as well as high-quality and timely safeguarding approaches (HM Government, 2018). These structures of joint assessment were developed in response to child protection inquires (Laming, 2003; Munro, 2011), where there had been a tragic failure in services (Davis and Smith, 2012).

When safeguarding children, multi-agency working is paramount. Achieving successful joint working (while safeguarding children) requires professionals to communicate effectively and recognise each other's areas of expertise (Jahans-Baynton and Grealish, 2022).

Working Together to Safeguard Children (HM Government, 2018) and *National Guidance for Child Protection in Scotland* (Scottish Government, 2014) provides statutory guidance for multi-agency professionals to safeguard and promote the welfare of children (Welsh Government, 2019; Safeguarding Board for Northern Ireland, 2022). The guidance is for local agencies such as health, education, housing and police, who have a duty under section 11 of the Children Act 2004, to ensure the safeguarding needs and welfare of children are considered when carrying out their work.

Working Together to Safeguard Children (HM Government, 2018) also guides local safeguarding children boards (LSCBs) and local authorities to work together to safeguard children locally to provide evidence-based services to address their needs.

The following are examples of nurses that have a crucial role in multi-agency arrangements to safeguard children:

- School nurses
- Health visitors
- Community children's nurses

- Specialist safeguarding midwives
- Safeguarding nurse leads and/or advisors
- Looked after children's nurses: looked after child is a term defined in law under the Children Act 1989 and refers to a child or young person who is cared for by the local authority for a period of more than 24 hours (RCN, 2022)
- Accident and Emergency liaison nurses/health visitors)

SEE ALSO
CHAPTER 5

ACTIVITY 9.1: REFLECTIVE PRACTICE

Take a moment to consider the nurse's role when working as part of multi-agency teams associated with safeguarding the health and wellbeing of children. The next section will discuss these models and their implications.

MULTI-AGENCY SAFEGUARDING MODELS

Multi-agency safeguarding hub (MASH)

There are several multi-agency safeguarding models and the most common is the Multi-Agency Safeguarding Hub (MASH). In some local authorities MASH teams are in place to screen child safeguarding referrals (LSCB, 2022). The Home Office (2014) underlines the aims of MASH: to improve safeguarding for children and young people through better information sharing and timely safeguarding responses. It is largely based on three common principles (see Figure 9.1) that enable effective communication across agencies and improved service delivery (Home Office, 2014). The MASH comprises five core elements (Table 9.1):

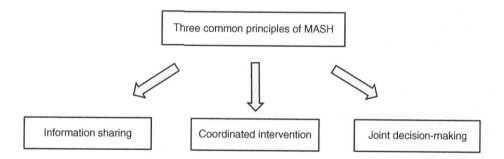

Figure 9.1 MASH

Synthesised from Home Office, 2014 and London Safeguarding Children Board, 2022

ACTIVITY 9.2: CRITICAL THINKING

Take some time to investigate your local area to establish what multi-agency models are used to safeguard children. You can find out more about these in the next section.

Table 9.1 A MASH team comprises five core elements

	Core element	Procedure
1	Acts as a single point of entry	The aim is for all concerns, no matter what the level, to be routed through the MASH to enable a single route and decision-making process
2	Information-sharing	A team of professionals from core agencies deliver an integrated service that will research, interpret and determine what information is proportionate and relevant to share (see Activity 9.3)
3	Confidentiality	MASH activity takes place in a confidential environment due to the sensitive nature of the information provided. The information is viewed by those who actually need to see it. It is disclosed on a strictly need-to-know basis
4	An agreed process for analysing and assessing risk	This enables the MASH to identify potential risks and have the opportunity to further address the risks through coordinated interventions
5	Early intervention	A process to identify victims, perpetrators and emerging harm through research and analysis. Early identification of these individuals and families enables services to intervene and prevent the need for more intensive interventions at a later stage

Synthesised from: The Home Office, 2014 and London Safeguarding Children Board, 2022

Multi-agency risk assessment conference

Multi-agency risk assessment conferencing (MARAC) is a local meeting that usually takes place monthly with a primary focus on the safety of high-risk victims of domestic abuse (10% of local cases) (LSCB, 2022).

The main purpose of a MARAC is to:

- Reduce the risk of serious harm or even death of victims
- Share information to enhance the health, safety and wellbeing of the adult victim and children
- Decide whether the alleged perpetrator poses a significant risk to either individuals and/or the general community
- Jointly construct and implement a risk management plan that provides professional support to all those at risk and reduce harm (LSCB, 2022).

Agencies that should always be invited to a MARAC are:

- Police
- Children's social care (local authority)
- Probation services
- Health services
- Education (local authority)
- Other agencies such as the women's safety unit, youth offending teams, community mental health nurse, but it usually depends on whether they have specific involvement with the victims (LSCB, 2022)

Collaborative working is essential in safeguarding practice as discussed here by a health visitor:

"Through collaborative working with healthcare professionals and single fathers I enabled my local NHS Trust to identify the need for a local resource specifically for single fathers, one which is available to health professionals to refer to within health promotion and its application to practice."

Shaun Lewis, children's nurse

Multi-agency sexual exploitation meeting (MASE)

Child sexual exploitation (CSE) can involve children and young people being subject to a number of exploitative situations that render them vulnerable to the risk of sexual exploitation. Commonly, the children do not see themselves as victims of sexual exploitation. Consequently, professionals, including nursing students, from all agencies should be alert to the possibility of sexual exploitation in children and report it to the appropriate child safeguarding professionals (LSCB, 2022).

Sexual exploitation leaves a lasting imprint on children, and they will often have long-term mental health concerns and/or physical illness following a period of exploitation. All children are at risk of sexual exploitation, both boys and girls and from all backgrounds and cultures. However, some risk factors have been identified to highlight children at an increased risk of sexual exploitation. These include children who have a history of running away/going missing from home, are in foster care, have special needs, are migrant children, are asylum seekers, are disengaged from education, are involved in use of drugs and alcohol or in gangs.

The overall aim for the perpetrator of sexual exploitation is to induce a power imbalance between themselves and the child. This can be in the form of threatening behaviour, violence and forced entrapment. However, encouraging sexual acts through the use of gifts, money and support may also be used. The perpetrator will form what the child feels is a safe nurturing relationship where they are spoilt with gifts and affection in return for sexual acts with them or any other person the perpetrator suggests. Often this relationship begins this way – for example, with online grooming where the child is persuaded to share sexual pictures of themselves online in return for gifts and praise. This can quickly turn, and the child is then threatened into sending more and more images due to the threat of the other images being shared online, for example on social media (DfE, 2017; Welsh Government, 2019; Scottish Government, 2021).

WHAT'S THE EVIDENCE?

The Child Exploitation and Online Protection Centre (CEOP, 2011) published a thematic assessment to increase understanding of child sexual exploitation. The aim of this research was to raise awareness and knowledge to enhance prevention by understanding patterns of offenders, and the victimisation and vulnerability of children to sexual exploitation.

Highlight the main findings from this evidence.

MASH teams (as mentioned earlier) play a vital role in identifying those at risk of CSE through the warning signs seen within referral notifications. MASH remains the first point of contact for any individual or professional who has concerns about a child or young person they feel is at risk of CSE.

Another team associated with CSE is MASE, which works in line with local safeguarding policy and procedures but unlike MASH it is not an established route for first-time referrals of CSE. Also, MASE do not work with individual cases; the prime aim is to provide a framework for regular information sharing and action planning to tackle CSE. The aim is for professionals to identify themes, patterns and trends in relation to CSE – for example, the identification of serial perpetrators, gang involvement, locations and premises associated with CSE – to discuss and address the risks and how to facilitate support that will remove the young person from the threat. (LSCB, 2022). No agency should delay taking action whilst waiting for a discussion at the next meeting (LSCB, 2022). Each MASE should discuss and focus on all agencies working together:

- To ensure everything is being done to protect the victims and disrupt and prosecute offenders
- To ensure relevant information is being recorded on specific systems to provide appropriate agencies with access to that information
- To coordinate actions with children's social care and other processes such as MARAC and MASH when required (LSCB, 2022)

Membership of MASE is statutory for some agencies and others are encouraged to attend. It is essential they do if they have relevant information for the meeting.

Statutory agencies

- Police
- Children's social care
- Health
- Education
- Agencies that are contracted by the local authority to support victims of CSE
- Youth offending services

ACTIVITY 9.3: REFLECTIVE PRACTICE

Take some time to reflect on why information sharing is so important in safeguarding. You will find out more on this in the following section.

In recent years there have been several serious case reviews that have highlighted that poor information sharing has contributed to the death or serious injury of a child or children. Organisations such as health services and local authorities should have arrangements in place which set out clear guidance around the principles of information sharing (HM Government, 2018).

The LSCB (2022), for example, bases their information-sharing principles for domestic abuse on the following:

- Professionals receiving information about domestic violence should explain that priority will be given to ensuring the safety of the mother/victim and child/ren
- If there are concerns about risk and/or significant harm to a child then it is every professional's duty to protect the child
- Professionals also have a duty to protect the mother/victim and should do so under the Crime and Disorder Act 1998. This allows accountable local authorities to share information where a crime has been committed or is going to be committed

The case study below involving Amisha helps you to further explore issues inherent in information sharing.

CASE STUDY 9.2: AMISHA

Amisha was a 19-year-old woman who had a troubled upbringing. She was first made homeless at the age of 13 and had 'sofa surfed' from then onwards. She was in and out of education and had contact with the local IAPT (Improving Access to Psychological Therapies) team for most of her adolescence. Amisha was known by two different general practitioners and she was constantly struggling to fight addiction to both alcohol and drugs. During this time she had a referral to a consultant psychiatrist to make a full mental health assessment to meet her needs. Housing was providing input to assist in her finding accommodation in privately rented accommodation. At this point Amisha attended the GP to state that she was pregnant. She also saw the drug rehabilitation team and the psychiatrist in the same week. She disclosed her housing and financial difficulties to all professionals. However, she stated that she was not taking drugs or drinking as she was happy to be pregnant. Amisha was allocated a midwife and the midwife received no history on Amisha and relied only on what was told to her.

During the later stages of her pregnancy the specialist midwife for supporting vulnerable mothers documented that a referral may be needed. However, this was never carried out. A baby was born to Amisha but died aged 2 days. At post-mortem, unlicensed and unprescribed drugs were found in her system. These drugs most likely passed through the placenta or breastmilk (Wonnacott, 2013).

Consider the above case study:

- What are some of the lessons learnt from this case study?
- What does the literature say in relation to information sharing?

AN EXPLORATION OF CONCERNS LINKED TO CONTEMPORARY ISSUES

As students, it is essential for you to have an overview of contemporary safeguarding issues which include female genital mutilation and trafficking.

Female genital mutilation

Female genital mutilation (FGM) is the practice of mutilation of the outer parts of the female genitals. FGM is illegal in the UK and it is also illegal to remove a girl from the UK to another country to perform FGM (DH, 2020). Overall, there are approximately 180,000 women and children at risk of FGM in England and Wales. However, the true figures are estimated to be much higher due to the hidden nature of FGM (European Union, 2013). Estimates suggest that 20,000 girls are at risk of FGM in the UK and 66,000 women living in the UK have experienced FGM (WHO, 2017). In the period from January to March 2022, 1685 women and girls had an attendance with a healthcare professional and FGM was identified (NHS Choices, 2022). There are four types of FGM (see Table 9.2). Currently, FGM is mainly performed on females under the age of 15 and before puberty. However, FGM may be performed on adolescents between the ages of 15–19 years. UNICEF (2022) estimates that in some countries (e.g., Kenya and Tanzania) the numbers of adolescents undergoing FGM are falling dramatically in comparison to 30 years ago. Global efforts have impacted in a positive way on the rates of FGM; however, sustaining these achievements remains challenging (UNICEF, 2022).

FGM has many health effects for women, varying from short-term initial effects through to longer-term effects (see Table 9.3), including depression and anxiety.

To learn more about FGM, watch this video: www.youtube.com/watch?v=HN1mulqwv5g.

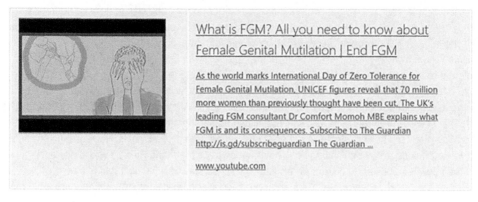

Figure 9.2 What is FGM?

www.youtube.com/watch?v=HN1mulqwv5g

Table 9.2 Different types of FGM (WHO, 2022)

Classification	Description
Type 1	Clitoridectomy: partial or total removal of the clitoris (a small, sensitive and erectile part of the female genitals) and, in very rare cases, only the prepuce (the fold of skin surrounding the clitoris)
Type 2	Excision: partial or total removal of the clitoris and the labia minora, with or without excision of the labia majora (the labia are 'the lips' that surround the vagina)
Type 3	Infibulation: narrowing of the vaginal opening through the creation of a covering seal. The seal is formed by cutting and repositioning the inner, or outer, labia, with or without removal of the clitoris
Type 4	All other harmful procedures to the female genitalia for non-medical purposes – e.g., pricking, piercing, incising, scraping and cauterising the genital area

Table 9.3 Overall effects of FGM (NHS Choices, 2014)

Short-term effects	Long-term effects
Infection	Persistent urine infections
Difficulty or inability to urinate	Abnormal periods
Damage to urethra and/or bowel	Kidney impairment and possible kidney failure resulting from difficulty or inability to pass urine
Risk of contracting HIV/hepatitis B and hepatits C	Psychological damage, including low libido, depression and anxiety (see below)
Shock/blood loss	The need for later surgery to open the lower vagina for sexual intercourse and childbirth
Pain	Complications in pregnancy and newborn deaths
	Pain from the formation of scar tissue
	Damage to the reproductive system, including infertility
	Pain during sex and lack of pleasurable sensation

Trafficking

Another essential contemporary safeguarding issue for consideration is the trafficking of humans, including children. Human trafficking is the movement of human beings into and out of countries including the UK. Human trafficking can affect women, men and children of all ages. However, for the purpose of this chapter the focus will be on children.

Children are trafficked through the use of force, coercion, abuse or any other form of deception with the sole purpose of exploitation. This exploitation comes in many forms and is not solely linked to sexual exploitation, as often is the misconception. Trafficking of children may be for labouring in big industries producing mass-produced goods through to domestic duties within a home environment. Children may also be trafficked to be forced into criminal activity including street crimes such as stealing and forced begging. Organ harvesting and forced marriage are also reasons to traffic children out of the UK (NSPCC, 2014).

Due to the difficulties in identifying these children it is hard to give exact figures to highlight the extent of the problem. However, the United Nations International Children's Emergency Fund (UNICEF) currently estimates that 10 children are trafficked every week out of the UK (National Crime Agency, 2017).

The following are Potential 'Red Flags' to keep a look out for in practice that a child is at risk of trafficking:

- CYP inappropriately dressed for age, time of day or weather
- Unkempt appearance or presence of unusually expensive items
- Unusual behaviour including marked wariness, agitation, aggression, belligerence, sexualized manner, fear, timidity or submission
- CYP appears unusually tired, sallow or sleep deprived
- May be with an accompanying person who appears controlling or who insists on speaking for the child and may appear particularly 'charming'
- Healthcare attendance related to alcohol, illegal substances, inappropriate medication use, self-harm, or suicidality
- Delayed presentation with advanced or severely complicated health needs (including child or adolescent pregnancy/abortion) that would have been readily supported or resolved if help had been received at an early stage
- CYP homeless or unsure of home address, current location or contact numbers of responsible adults
- CYP is not registered with a general practitioner or school
- CYP has no or limited local language skills
- CYP asking for help and safety (verbally or non-verbally)
- Carer requesting help due to child's behaviour deterioration, missing episodes, drug use

(Royal College of Paediatrics and Child Health, 2022)

Importantly, a strong correlation between adverse childhood experiences and trafficking was identified by Middleton et al. (2022), who state that children who experience physical abuse, emotional abuse, domestic abuse and sexual abuse are 70% more likely to be a victim of trafficking. Children who have been trafficked are exposed to high levels of violence and physical abuse, and sexual exploitation which may include forced sexual acts and rape. Controlling behaviour of the responsible adult is a sign that the child has been trafficked; this may include withdrawing the right to education, confiscation of passports and neglect in general of the child.

Trafficking of children is a very serious issue of rising concern for professionals in the UK who work closely with this group. The difficulty often faced by professionals is that these children may not be aware that they have been trafficked, especially if they have come from a country outside of the European Union into the UK. These children will be fearful of the UK authorities and may lack understanding around what abuse and exploitation are. They may not disclose information, even during a visit from a health professional for example. Children trafficked out of the UK are often taken quickly and without much prior warning or signs and therefore are a difficult group to identify and protect (NSPCC, 2014).

You may have contact in your career with a child who has been the victim of trafficking. In this instance, trust your professional instinct and do not raise concerns with the adult accompanying the child. Seek support from a more experienced member of the team and attempt to assess the child without the adult present. However, consider factors such as language barriers and, if needed, make use of interpreter services. Remember that the child may be fearful of divulging information. Ensure they understand that they are safe and can talk to you. However, when responding, do not make promises you can't keep and be open about the next steps. Allow the child time to open up and never let cultural factors stand in the way of making an overall assessment (NSPCC, 2014).

Safeguarding children is everyone's responsibility and a fundamental part of children's nursing practice. In today's ever-changing society it is essential to know what constitutes child abuse and how it can be addressed and prevented. Appropriate training allows professionals to recognise signs of child abuse or early indicators of concern, provide support, share information and carry out approved assessments. Joint working between agencies requires professionals to communicate effectively and respect each other's area of expertise.

CHAPTER SUMMARY

- Safeguarding children and young people is everyone's business and will form an essential part in the role of the qualified nurse. In addition, it remains the responsibility of any individual in contact with children and their families including nursing students
- Child protection is part of safeguarding and promoting the welfare of children, but the main focus is to protect specific children who are suffering or likely to suffer significant harm
- Within the framework of safeguarding children, harm is often referred to as abuse. The four main categories of abuse which children may need protecting from are physical, sexual, emotional and neglect. Understanding the definitions of child abuse is an essential aspect of safeguarding children and young people
- Multi-agency working is paramount in safeguarding practice. There are several models, the most common being the MASH and others such as MARAC and MASE, which are directed at more specific areas of safeguarding children and young people
- It is essential to pursue help and advice if you are concerned a child has suffered or is at risk of suffering abuse

BUILD YOUR BIBLIOGRAPHY

Books

FURTHER
READING

- Cleaver, H., Cawson, P., Gorin, S. and Walker, S. (2009) *Safeguarding Children: A Shared Responsibility*. Chichester: Wiley-Blackwell.

    This book covers key areas in the principles and processes of safeguarding children, including an excellent chapter (Chapter 1) on the effectiveness of multi-agency working.

- Corby, B., Shemmings, D. and Wilkins, D. (2012) *Child Abuse: An Evidence Base for Confident Practice*, 4th edn. Maidenhead: Open University Press.

  This book raises students' awareness of child abuse. See Chapter 4 on defining child abuse.
- Dimond, B. (2015) *Legal Aspects of Nursing*, 7th edn. Harlow: Pearson Education.

  The chapter on children and young people provides an overview of legal aspects associated with child protection in healthcare.
- Megele, C. (2017) *Safeguarding Children and Young People Online: A Guide for Practitioners.* Bristol: Policy Press.

  This book presents an overview on e-safety and online risks to children and young people.
- Powell, C. (2015) *Safeguarding and Child Protection for Nurses, Midwives and Health Visitors: A Practical Guide*, 2nd edn. Maidenhead: Open University Press.

  An excellent book with an informative chapter that uses case studies to highlight importance of prevention and early help when safeguarding children and young people. See Chapter 2 on prevention and early help.

Journal articles

- Featherstone, B., Morris, K., Daniel, B., Bywaters, P., Brady, G., Bunting, L., Mason, W. and Mirza, N. (2019) 'Poverty, inequality, child abuse and neglect: changing the conversation across the UK in child protection?', *Children and Youth Services Review*, 97 (February): 127-33.
- Gonzalez-Izquierdo, A., Ward, A., Smith, P., Walford, J., Ioannou, Y. and Gilbert, R. (2014) 'Notifications for child safeguarding from an acute hospital in response to presentations to healthcare by parents'. *Child: Care, Health and Development*, 41 (2): 186-93.

  An interesting study into notifying children's social care services of safeguarding concerns when parents present at acute hospitals with drug, alcohol, mental issues and violence.
- Jahans-Baynton, K. and Grealish, A. (2022) 'Safeguarding communications between multi-agency professionals when working with children and young people: a qualitative study'. *Journal of Child and Adolescent Physciaric Nursing*, 35 (2): 171-8.

  A study exploring safeguarding communications between multi-agency professionals who work with children and young people.

FURTHER READING: ONLINE JOURNAL ARTICLES

SEE ALSO CHAPTER 8

Weblinks

- London Safeguarding Children Board - www.londonscb.gov.uk An excellent resource for London Child Protection Procedures and Practice Guidance.

FURTHER READING: WEBLINKS

REFERENCES

Child Exploitation and Online Protection Centre (CEOP) (2011) *Out of Mind, Out of Sight: Making Every Child Matter … Everywhere*. Executive Summary. Available at: https://childhub.org/en/child-protection-online-library/out-mind-out-sight (accessed 4 July 2022).

Davis, J.M. and Smith, M. (2012) *Working in Multi-Professional Contexts: A Practical Guide for Professionals in Children's Services*. London: Sage.

Department for Education (DfE) (2017) *Child Sexual Exploitation: Definition and a guide for practitioners, local leaders and decision-makers working to protect children from child sexual exploitation*. London: DfE. Available at: www.gov.uk/government/publications/child-sexual-exploitation-definition-and-guide-for-practitioners (accessed 6 July 2022).

Department of Health (DH) (2020) *Multiagency statutory guidance on female genital mutilation*. Available at: www.gov.uk/government/publications/multi-agency-statutory-guidance-on-female-genital-mutilation (accessed 30 June 2022).

European Union (2013) *Communication from the Commission to the European Union and Croatia*. Available at: http://eige.europa.eu/rdc/eige-publications/female-genital-mutilation-european-union-report (accessed 5 July 2023).

Gov.Uk Female Genital Mutilation: Help and Advice. Available at: www.gov.uk/female-genital-mutilation-help-advice (accessed 5 July 2023).

HM Government (2018) *Working Together to Safeguard Children: A Guide to Inter-agency Working to Safeguard and Promote the Welfare of Children*. London: DfE. Available at: www.gov.uk/government/publications/working-together-to-safeguard-children–2 (accessed 16 May 2022).

Home Office (2014) *Multi Agency Working and Information Sharing Project Final Report*. Available at: https://assets.publishing.service.gov.uk/government/uploads/system/uploads/attachment_data/file/338875/MASH.pdf (accessed 4 July 2022).

Jahans-Baynton, K. and Grealish, A. (2022) 'Safeguarding communications between multiagency professionals when working with children and young people: a qualitative study'. *Journal of Child and Adolescent Psychiatric Nursing*, 35 (2): https://doi.org/10.1111/jcap.12363.

Laming, Lord (2003) *The Victoria Climbié Inquiry*. Cm 5730. Norwich: TSO. Available at: http://dera.ioe.ac.uk/6086/2/climbiereport.pdf (accessed 7 June 2023).

London Safeguarding Children Board (2017) *London MASH Project: The Five Core Elements*. Available at: www.londonscb.gov.uk/wp-content/uploads/2016/04/1.-Five-CORE-ELEMENTS-Final-1.pdf (accessed 29 June 2022).

London Safeguarding Children Board (2021) *The London Child Sexual Exploitation Operating Protocol*, 2nd edn. Available at: https://cscp.org.uk/wp-content/uploads/2021/03/The-London-Child-Exploitation-Operating-Protocol-2021-MPS.pdf (accessed 30 June 2022).

London Safeguarding Children Procedures and Practice Guidance. Updated: 31st March 2023. Available at: /www.londonsafeguardingchildrenprocedures.co.uk (accessed 5 July 2023).

Middleton, J., Edwards, E., Roe-Sepowitz, D., Inman, E., Frey, L.M. and Gattis, M.N. (2022) 'Adverse childhood experiences (ACEs) and homelessness: a critical examination of the association between specific ACEs and sex trafficking among homeless youth in Kentuckiana'. *Journal of Human Trafficking*, doi: 10.1080/23322705.2021.2020061.

Munro, E. (2011) *The Munro Review of Child Protection: Final Report: A Child-centred System*. London: DfE. Available at: www.gov.uk/government/uploads/system/uploads/attachment_data/file/175391/Munro-Review.pdf (accessed 8 May 2017).

National Crime Agency (2017) *National Referral Mechanism Statistics: End of Year Summary 2016*. Available at: www.antislaverycommissioner.co.uk/media/1133/2016-nrm-end-of-year-summary.pdf (accessed 29 August 2017).

NHS Choices (2022) *Female Genital Mutilation*. Available at: www.nhs.uk/Conditions/female-genital-mutilation/Pages/Introduction.aspx (accessed 30 June 2022).

NSPCC (National Society for Prevention of Cruelty to Children) (2014) *Stop Child Trafficking in Its Tracks: Advice for Health Visitors*. London: NSPCC.

Royal College of Nursing (RCN) (2019) *Safeguarding Children and Young People: Roles and Competences for Health Care Staff: Intercollegiate Document*, 4th edn. London: RCN. Available at: www.rcn.org.uk/professional-development/publications/pub-007366 DCFS.

Royal College of Nursing (RCN) (2022) *Looked after Children*. Available at: www.rcn.org.uk/clinical-topics/children-and-young-people/looked-after-children (accessed 30 June 2022).

Royal College of Paediatrics and Child Health (RCPCH) (2022) *Guidance: Child Modern Slavery and Human Trafficking.* Available at: www.rcpch.ac.uk/sites/default/files/2022-05/Child%20 Modern%20Slavery%20and%20Human%20Trafficking%20guidance.pdf (accessed 27 May 2022).

Safeguarding Board for Northern Ireland (2022) *Role of SBNI.* Available at: www.safeguardingni.org/ (accessed 17 July 2022).

Scottish Government (2021) *National Guidance for Child Protection in Scotland 2021.* Available at: www. gov.scot/publications/national-guidance-child-protection-scotland-2021/documents/ (accessed 30th June 2022).

UNICEF (2022) Female genital mutilation. Available at: hwww.unicef.org/protection/female-genital-mutilation (accessed 30 June 2022).

Welsh Government (2019) *Wales Safeguarding Procedures.* Available at: www.safeguarding.wales/index. html (accessed 30 June 2022).

Welsh Government (2021) *Safeguarding Children from Child Sexual Exploitation.* Available at: https:// gov.wales/safeguarding-children-child-sexual-exploitation-0 (accessed 30 June 2022).

Wonnacott, J. (2013) *On Baby Z: Serious Case Review.* Available at: www.westsussexscb.org.uk/ wp-content/uploads/Isle-of-Wight-Baby-Z.pdf (accessed 6 July 2022).

World Health Organization (WHO) (2017) Female genital mutilation. Fact Sheet. Available at: www. who.int/news-room/fact-sheets/detail/female-genital-mutilation (accessed 30 June 2022).

PART 2 CHILD AND INFANT WELLBEING AND DEVELOPMENT

GENETICS AND EPIGENETICS: EFFECTS ON CHILDREN AND YOUNG PEOPLE

10

GILL LANGMACK AND ELISABETH O'BRIEN

THIS CHAPTER COVERS

- The concepts of genetics, genomics and epigenetics
- The variation in inheritance
- The concept of risk
- The essential ethical and legal implications of genomics

"My advice to nursing students would be to look at all families with a genetic eye and don't be afraid to ask the family the difficult questions. Are there specific health problems running through a family? Understand that sometimes bad news can be good news for families, which is not something you expect as a nurse."

Marjie, genetic nurse counsellor

INTRODUCTION

Before starting this chapter you should know how genes pass from grandparents to parents and to children. You should understand chromosomes, genes and cell division/replication and the terms 'autosomal dominant' and 'recessive inheritance', 'monogenic' and 'mitochondrial inheritance'.

REQUIRED KNOWLEDGE

It would helpful to have an understanding of genetics and epigenetics before you start this chapter. Please read Boore et al. (2021), Chapter 3: 'Genetic and epigenetic control of biological systems'.

Using case studies, this chapter aims to explore the basis of genetics and epigenetics through the changes that are seen when the child inherits their parents' genome. This chapter can only form an introduction but should help you start to link the child's genetic make-up to their ongoing condition. For example, it is already well known that some people respond to medications, including analgesia, differently if their genes provide the instructions to make the cytochrome P450 enzyme. The diagnosis and treatment of many conditions – for example, some types of leukaemia, asthma and solid tumours – is increasingly dependent on accurate information about an individual's genome.

The opening quotation from a genetic counsellor, Marjie, identifies the need for all nurses to consider the role of genetics in that everyone's health status and risk of developing diseases may be based on a genetic variation. She also indicates that there is a national move to include diagnostic testing within care pathways, which may occur before referral to genetic counselling services.

It is now known that all diseases lie on a spectrum from being 100% caused by genetic factors to being completely determined by the environment. During your nursing career, you will come across families and their children with symptoms, conditions and underlying syndromes that are unfamiliar to you. An understanding of the underlying principles of genetics and epigenetics can be very helpful.

The increasing complexity of genetics and genomics has resulted in the gradual development of competencies for preregistration nurse. Competencies have developed through work by Kirk, Tonkin and Skirton (2011, 2014), the HEE/National Genetics and Genomics Education Centre (2013) and Biosciences in Nurse Education (BINE) (2016). This results in the need for all nurses to 'demonstrate knowledge of ... genomics' (s2.2) applying this within 'full and accurate person-centred nursing assessments' (s3.2) to plan nursing care (Nursing and Midwifery Council, 2018). In summary, these competencies include:

- Demonstrating core knowledge and understanding of how genetics and genomics underpins effective nursing practice.
- Explaining how changes occurring within the genome influence both health and disease processes.
- An ability to recognise clinical indicators suggesting individuals need referral to genetic services.
- Providing sensitive, supportive, evidence-based information at the time of diagnosis, as ongoing support through periods of uncertainty, and facilitate referral to local genetic services when appropriate.
- Advocating for, and individualising support in respect of differing cultures, religious beliefs and the child's age and developmental stage. This may include being aware of conditions which may mimic non-accidental injury or abuse, such as osteogenesis imperfecta or conditions that result in failure to thrive.
- Working in partnership as a trusted and informed partner with the family, to deal with feelings of anger, guilt or blame as parents acknowledge their own genetic contribution to the child's situation or as they consider prenatal diagnosis in a future pregnancy. This may include working with the child growing up with the genetic condition, such as muscular dystrophy or cystic fibrosis, as they may be probing increasingly for information about condition, its prognosis and effect on their life plans.

ACTIVITY 10.1: REFLECTIVE PRACTICE

Children's nurses and health visitors work across a range of settings, at primary, secondary and tertiary levels of care. Think about situations in an acute or community setting when issues to do with genetics have arisen.

Look at Figure 10.1 to remind you of the typical areas you may have seen on practice placement. Consider to what extent you and your practice supervisor/assessor were able to assess the family's genetics.

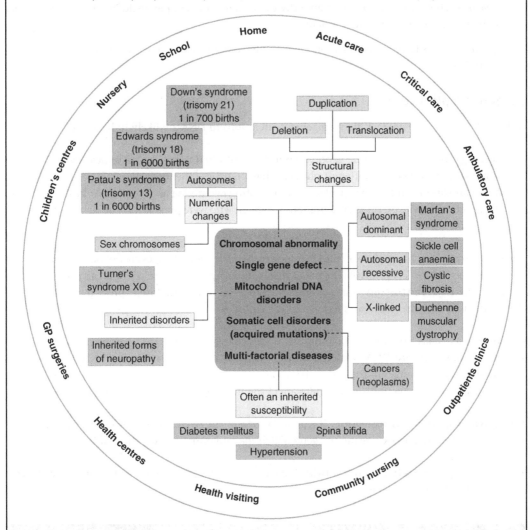

Figure 10.1 Genetic changes that can occur and the typical places where knowledge of genetics can be helpful

THE CONCEPTS OF GENETICS, GENOMICS AND EPIGENETICS

With significant advances in computing speeds and molecular techniques, our knowledge of human genetics has developed rapidly since the beginning of the Human Genome Project (HGP) in 1990. At first, the goal was to sequence the genes and produce a map of the human genome. When the full sequence of the human genome was mapped in 2003, there was an astonishing discovery that only about 1–2% of the bases code for proteins. The total number of identified genes that code for proteins is approximately 30,000. This means that the role of 98% of human deoxyribonucleic acid (DNA) is not known.

Genetics: This is the study of how genes are inherited from one generation to the next, and how the DNA provides the building blocks for the body's phenotype (the person's appearance). Genes can be switched 'on' or 'off' by various external factors, but also through ribonucleic acid (RNA) which is coded by 'junk' DNA.

Genomics: This is the study of all of an individual's genes, or genome, including how they interact with other genes and the environment.

Epigenetics: This term refers to factors that influence the way our genes are expressed in the cells of our body.

Epigenetic alterations

If the following criteria are met, then epigenetic alterations in DNA are likely to have occurred.

1. Two organisms have the same genotype but different phenotypes, e.g., identical twins have the same DNA (genotype) but different physical characteristics (phenotype).
2. An organism continues to be affected by an initiating event long after that event has passed, e.g., the effects of famine on the grandchildren of women who were pregnant at the time of the famine (Stein and Susser, 1975).

Epigenetic marks can change the way the DNA message is read. These changes are not permanent and can alter over time (Sharma et al., 2010). The major mechanisms by which these changes can occur include:

Stem cell differentiation: Some processes change the way genes are expressed which changes the instructions for cells and tissues to form in the embryo.

- *Methylation*: adds a methyl group to the DNA. This changes how the DNA is transcribed into RNA
- *Histone modifications:* DNA is packed around proteins known as histones. The tightness of the packing causes changes in the gene expression
- *RNA changes:* tiny micro-RNA molecules affect the messenger RNA which makes enzymes

De-activating an X chromosome: If a gene on one of the X chromosomes is deactivated, it prevents both chromosomes expressing the gene which may potentially affect the child.

- **Phenotype in Twins:** Identical twins have the same DNA and genotype but different physical characteristics (phenotype)

WHAT'S THE EVIDENCE?

Increasingly, it is being identified that susceptibility to illness in adulthood has a basis in genetics and pre-natal/infant/child health which result in adverse childhood events (ACEs).

For example, mental illness appears to have epigenetic mechanisms that stem from maternal and prenatal stressors (DeSocio, 2018). Bale (2014) identifies a three-hit model underpinning mental illness. Within this model the hits include:

Genetic predisposition - this is borne out by the familial tendency for offspring to develop mental illness

Prenatal insult - potentially, through exposure to maternal stress, anxiety or depression within pregnancy

Life stress - following birth, environmental stressors may precipitate symptoms of mental illness

Stress on the foetus can increase the risk of prematurity, potentially altering, and therefore increasing, the risk for epigenetic changes in physical illnesses in addition to mental illness, such as cardiovascular disease, and insulin resistance in adulthood (Arabin and Baschat, 2017). Current research into prenatal and infant factors include exploring the foetal stress response and DNA methylation changes (Moore et al., 2022; Wigley et al., 2022) as the foetus adapts to changes in the intrauterine environment.

THE VARIATION IN INHERITANCE

If a diagnosis is made that may have an underlying genetic cause, the question needs to be asked if there are others in the family who have a similar problem. A pedigree shows relationships between family members and indicates which individuals have certain genetic pathogenic variants, traits, and diseases within a family as well as vital status. A pedigree can be used to determine disease inheritance patterns within a family.

Identifying the family pedigree

When starting to develop a family pedigree, a family may immediately discuss a set of illnesses in one part of the family, but it is important to be specific and systematic to explore the links between family members. This needs to include the biological relationships, not the social relationships – for example, step-siblings do not have the same genetics as they are not biologically related. Family members can also be 'hidden' or 'forgotten' within families, particularly when looking at the grandparent generation, aunts, uncles and cousins.

The types of questions (British Society for Genetic Medicine (BSGM), 2021) need to include:

- Major medical, physical or mental health problems
- Anyone requiring hospital admission
- Serious illnesses or operations
- Age when the condition was diagnosed
- Cause of death and age at death – this should include stillborn infants
- Conditions or illnesses which seem to run on either side of the family

It is traditional to look at three or four generations in the family. The resulting family pedigree can help to define the risks of the condition in others in the family. Whilst it would not usually be ethical to ask about the health of others in a family, where the questions are asked for a medical purpose, as in this situation, the questions are acceptable (Royal College of Physicians, Royal College of Pathologists and British Society for Human Genetics, 2011).

Drawing the pedigree

A standard set of symbols is used to draw a family pedigree (Bennett et al., 1995; Genomics Education Programme, 2021) (Figure 10.2).

When taking a history, it is essential to record the date of birth, age at death and relevant medical information. This includes symptoms or diagnosis and the age of occurrence in addition to documenting who gave the information, who drew the pedigree and the completion date.

The following case study should help you to develop an understanding of the complexity of assessing inheritance. Use Dwayne's family pedigree to develop your understanding of how a pedigree is constructed from the family history.

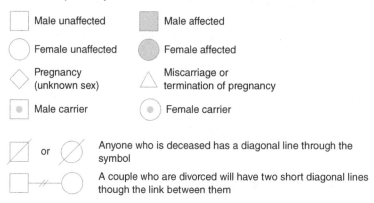

Figure 10.2   Symbols used in drawing a pedigree

CASE STUDY 10.1: DWAYNE

Dwayne is a 3-year-old who has had intermittent symptoms of feeling tired and lethargic with a racing heartbeat for the last 2 months. Following investigations, the doctors diagnose a conduction problem in how his heart beats, known as 'short Q-T syndrome'. His mum remembers an old discussion that a cousin of hers had a sudden heart attack as a child.

A family pedigree is developed to explore the pattern of inheritance as Dwayne's condition has a genetic basis (Figure 10.3). The risk can then be determined for his parents having other children and within the wider family.

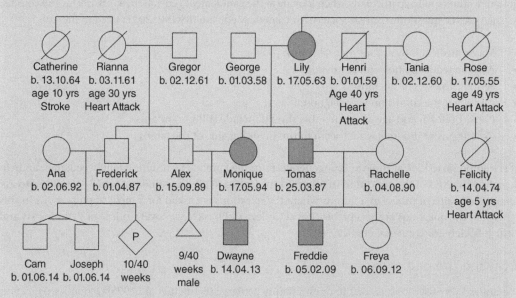

Figure 10.3   Dwayne's pedigree, showing the members of his family who have the cardiac conduction problem

- Identify which members of Dwayne's family are affected by short Q-T syndrome.
- How would you describe the pattern of inheritance seen in Dwayne's pedigree?

Although you may not have done this in practice, mapping a pedigree is a useful skill that enhances a thorough family history.

ACTIVITY 10.2: REFLECTIVE PRACTICE

Using the symbols in Figure 10.2, draw your own family pedigree. Try putting in three generations. Can you add in a fourth generation?

THE CONCEPT OF RISK

If a chromosomal abnormality or a single gene mutation exists, then it is possible to estimate the potential risk of a further child having the abnormality. Where one child has a condition, it does not mean the next child will not get the illness, the probability will remain the same. Predicting the potential risk of a subsequent child having a genetic condition is difficult and the family is currently offered the opportunity to be referred to a regional genetics centre to be seen by a specialist team.

Autosomal dominant patterns have an equal number of males and females affected, with each affected child having at least one affected parent, but two affected parents may have an unaffected child (see Case study 10.1: Dwayne).

Autosomal recessive patterns are often seen where unaffected parents have an affected child, for example where a child has single gene mutation that causes cystic fibrosis.

Case study X-linked patterns show more males are affected and there are no male-to-male transmissions. An example of this would be Fragile X inheritance.

Genetic risk

Estimating the genetic risk can be undertaken by developing a tree diagram and/or a Punnett square and assessing the probability of subsequent children having inherited the affected gene (Genomics Education Programme, 2021). Both diagrams are used (see Figure 10.4); however, the Punnett square is more easily understood .

The chance of having a subsequent child with a specific trait is seen in the tables and probability analysis in Figure 10.4.

Where both parents are carriers for a child who has cystic fibrosis (see Case study) the probability of having another child with cystic fibrosis (rr = 1 in 4 chance) would be worked out as follows:

(Child 1) 0.25 × (Child 2) 0.25 = 0.0625 or 6.25%

The probability of this child's parents having two further children who do not have cystic fibrosis – so having a genotype of either RR (1 in 4 chance) or Rr (1 in 2 chance) would be:

(Child 1) (0.25 + 0.5) × (Child 2) (0.25 + 0.5) = 0.75 x 0.75 = 0.5625 or 56.25%

The probability calculations become even more complex where one parent has no family history or where there are epigenetic influences. Assessing a family's understanding of risk is an integral part

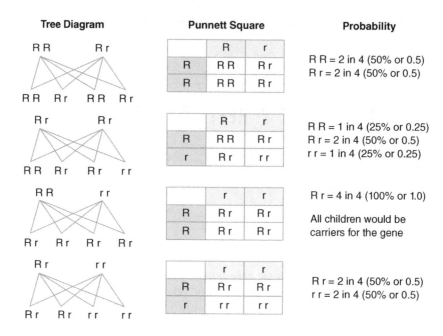

Figure 10.4 Patterns of inheritance showing dominant (R) and recessive (r) traits

of genetic counselling – for example, some people will think that a 1 in 4 chance of inheritability is greater than a 25% risk when in fact they are equal.

THE ESSENTIAL ETHICAL AND LEGAL IMPLICATIONS OF GENOMICS

Genetics is at the cutting edge of science, and therefore at the forefront of ethics and law. When planning, assessing and delivering children's care nurses should be aware of the legal, ethical and moral implications of procedures and tests and their potential consequences. This is particularly relevant to today's students as genetics testing is increasingly taking place outside mainstream genetics services.

The four fundamental principles of medical ethics developed by Beauchamp and Childress (2019) have a wide consensus. These principles of autonomy, beneficence, non-maleficence and justice might seem theoretical at first glance but have implications for practice, research and policy.

Issues to consider for health professionals

There are many methods for diagnosing genetic disorders and abnormalities in the first two trimesters of pregnancy, including non-invasive testing. Prenatal diagnosis and offers of termination raise difficult questions for the individuals concerned and wider questions about the way society cares for and values those with disability.

Justice is a concept that emphasises fairness and equality. Patients in similar situations should be treated similarly, and in a broader sense, benefits and costs should be fairly distributed across a population. There is general agreement in the UK that sex selection for social preferences or family balancing is not justified as grounds for termination.

Health staff should consider the principle of *beneficence*, or acting in the child's best interests. As a general rule, the benefit should outweigh the harm and testing is best left until the child is old enough to consent, unless there are health implications which mean that treatment should begin earlier.

Testing children younger than 12 years of age is not generally justified unless there is a clear benefit. For example, if an adult has familial adenomatous polyps (FAP) then close family members will be offered screening from 12 years of age as, if any children have the altered gene, it is likely the bowel polyps, some of which may lead to cancer, will appear before the age of 20.

The principle of *non-maleficence* (or the principle of not doing harm) should be remembered. There are many issues relating to a genetic disease that a family may wish to keep private or to share. There is the difficulty of sharing results between regional genetics services when many family members are seen. Confidentiality would only be breached under extreme circumstances.

The principles underpinning genetic counselling are that it is non-directive and aims to ensure that decision-making is informed choice. Families should be given full information including the risks, limitations, outcomes and implications of genetic testing and the option of not participating. The consequences of each course of action should be explored. For families to have *autonomy* they should be empowered when decisions need to be made. This means they need accessible information but should feel free to opt out of genetic testing at any stage.

ACTIVITY 10.3: CRITICAL THINKING

On a recent insight visit, you encountered the following situations where health professionals need to consider the balance between the conflicts that inevitably arise in practice. Based on the issues you have just read about, what are the ethical, legal and societal questions that arise for each case?

- *Prenatal diagnosis:* Sunil and Lucy are expecting a second baby and have asked to know the sex of the foetus with a view to termination if it is a boy. Their first child has a condition they know is more common in boys. Overall, the risk of having another child with the same condition is 5% (1 in 20).
- *Children and predictive testing:* Daniel and Isha have requested testing to see if their child has inherited an adult onset autosomal dominant condition that they have just found out runs in the family.
- *Implications for individuals, immediate and extended family:* Sam is a 14-year-old boy who comes to clinic with his father after a referral from Sam's GP. Sam's dad wants him to have genetic testing for type 1 osteogenesis imperfecta but Sam is reluctant. Sam has an older sister who is due to get married and wants to start a family before her career takes her overseas.

To find out more about ethical principles, please read the chapter by Northway and Beech (2022, second edition).

In complex cases the practical considerations of care management are not straightforward and there may be competing claims to ethical principles. In some cases the advice of the hospital ethics committee can be sought.

An example of this can be heard on the radio programme *Inside the Ethics Committee* (BBC, 2016), which discusses the ethics of sharing genetic information. Is the duty of care to the patient, or also to the wider family? How do staff balance the right to privacy with the wider family's right to information that could save their lives? This examines a real-life complex dilemma facing a woman who discovers her father has Huntington's disease. Should she get tested and what does this mean for her young son?

Both Avery (2022), and Griffith and Dowie (2019) provide excellent resources for those looking to further explore contemporary legal and ethical issues in healthcare.

As Marjie indicates at the very beginning of this chapter, understanding the nature of the way health problems run through succeeding generations in a family pedigree can provide the child and their family with the information they require to make informed decisions about care and future pregnancies.

SEE ALSO
CHAPTER 8

FROM GENETICS TO GENOMICS - FUTURE DIRECTIONS

Whereas genetics focuses on the 2% of our DNA which is in our genes, genomics looks at the gene and all the DNA in between. In the future, sequencing the genome could help with:

- Diagnosis and personalising medicine via clinical diagnostic testing, whole genome sequencing and tailored therapies, e.g., diagnosing sub types of chronic lymphocytic leukaemia.
- Predicting the chance of developing the disease later in life, e.g., targeted screening programmes such as an expansion of the newborn blood spot test.
- Helping with decisions about treatment options: Cancer is primarily an acquired disease of the genome. Genetic variations and rearrangements all contribute to the make-up of the disease, meaning genomic-led diagnosis is critical to understanding cancer better.

According to a recent report from Genome UK (HM Government, 2021, p.1), 'The strength of our genomics science base, our leading life sciences industry, and public sector funding has allowed us to truly lead the world in sequencing the COVID-19 virus.' This critical data, involving early sequencing, has informed the pandemic response across the world and highlighted the importance of genomics to the public.

Emerging evidence also shows how an individual's genome can affect their immune response to COVID-19 (Pairo-Castineira et al., 2021). One criticism is that the largest data sets analysed arise from studies on European cohorts. This decreases the potential transferability across different populations, although this issue is correctly acknowledged and highlighted in the report as a limitation.

The advances in technology also highlight ethical questions that concern healthcare professionals and the general public: those of informed consent, issues of confidentiality, sample ownership, test regulation, genetic discrimination and incidental findings.

──────────────── **CHAPTER SUMMARY** ────────────────

- Knowledge of human genetics has developed rapidly since the beginning of the Human Genome Project (HGP) in 1990
- Understanding the nature of the way health problems run through succeeding generations via a family pedigree can provide the child and their family with information
- Genetics is at the cutting edge of science, and therefore at the forefront of ethical and legal controversies

BUILD YOUR BIBLIOGRAPHY

You can find references to useful books, book chapters and weblinks throughout the chapter.

Journal articles

- House, S.H. (2013) 'Transgenerational healing: educating children in genesis of healthy children, with focus on nutrition, emotion, and epigenetic effects on brain development'. *Nutrition and Health*, 22 (1): 9-45.

  This article provides an overview of epigenetic changes illustrated using historical events to show the differences between genetic inheritance and epipgenetic influences focusing on nutrition and brain development.

- Letourneau, N., Giesbrecht, G.F., Bernier, F.P. and Joschko, J. (2014) 'How do interactions between early caregiving environment and genes influence health and behavior?' *Biological Research for Nursing*, 16 (1): 83-94.

  This article explores the effects of stress on gene expression in relation to attachment and behaviour in childhood.

- Wigley, M.I.L.C., Mascheroni, E., Bonichini, S. et al. (2022) 'Epigenetic protection: maternal touch and DNA-methylation in early life'. *Current Opinion in Behavioral Sciences*, 43: 111-17.

  This article focuses on the role of maternal touch in protecting the epigenetic changes and promoting mental and physical health throughout life

FURTHER READING: ONLINE JOURNAL ARTICLES

REFERENCES

Arabin, B. and Baschat, A.A. (2017) 'Pregnancy: an underutilized window of opportunity to improve long-term maternal and infant health-an appeal for continuous family care and interdisciplinary communication'. *Frontiers in Pediatrics*, 5: 69.

Avery, G. (2022) 'Law', Chapter Six in C. Delves-Yates and F. Everett (eds), *Essentials of Nursing Practice*, 3rd edn. London: Sage.

Bale, T.L. (2014) 'Lifetime stress experience: transgenerational epigenetics and germ cell programming'. *Dialogues in Clinical Neurosciences*, 16(3): 297–305.

BBC (2016) 'Sharing genetic information'. (Inside the Ethics Committee: Series 12). Available at: www.bbc.co.uk/sounds/play/b07nrxd4 (accessed 13 December 2021).

Beauchamp, T.L. and Childress, J.F. (2019) *Principles of Biomedical Ethics*, 8th edn. Oxford: Oxford University Press.

Bennett, R.L., Steinhaus, K.A., Uhrich, S.B., O'Sullivan, C.K., Resta, R.G., Lochner-Doyle, D., Markel, D.S., Vincent, C. and Hamanishi, J. (1995) 'Recommendations for standardized human pedigree nomenclature'. *American Journal of Human Genetics*, 56 (3): 745–52.

Biosciences in Nurse Education (BiNE) (2016) *Quality Assurance Framework for Biosciences Education in Nursing: Learning Outcomes for Biosciences in Preregistration Nursing Programmes*. Available at: https://s3.eu-west-2.amazonaws.com/assets.creode.advancehe-document-manager/documents/hea/private/bine_biosciences_qa_framework_b-qaf_july_16_1568037218.pdf (accessed 5 July 2023).

Boore, J. (2021) 'Genetic and epigenetic control of biological systems', in Boore, J., Cook, N. and Shepherd, A. (eds), *Essentials of Anatomy and Physiology for Nursing Practice*. London: Sage.

British Society for Genetic Medicine (2021) *Taking and Recording a Family History*. Available at: www.bsgm.org.uk/healthcare-professionals/taking-and-recording-a-family-history/ (accessed 13 December 2021).

DeSocio, J.E. (2018) 'Epigenetics, maternal prenatal psychosocial stress, and infant mental health'. *Archives of Psychiatric Nursing*, 32 (6): 901–6.

Griffith, R.B. and Dowie, I. (2019) *Dimond's Legal Aspects of Nursing: A Definitive Guide to Law for Nurses*, 8th edn. Harlow: Pearson Education.

Genomics Education Programme (2021) Taking and drawing a family history. Available at: www.genomicseducation.hee.nhs.uk/taking-and-drawing-a-family-history/#resources (accessed 14 December 2021).

HM Government (2021) Genome UK: 2021 to 2022 implementation plan. Available at: www.gov.uk/government/publications/genome-uk-2021-to-2022-implementation-plan (accessed 14 December 2021).

Kirk, M., Tonkin, E. and Skirton, H. (2011) *Fit for Practice in the Genetics Era: A Revised Competence Based Framework with Learning Outcomes and Practice Indicators. A Guide for Nurse Education and Training*. Available at: http://genomics.research.southwales.ac.uk/media/files/documents/2013-09-05/ffpgge-nursing-learning-outcomes.pdf (accessed 14 December 2021).

Kirk, M., Tonkin, E. and Skirton, H. (2014) 'An iterative consensus-building approach to revising a genetics/genomics competency framework for nurse education in the UK'. *Journal of Advanced Nursing*, 70 (2): 405–20.

Moore, S.R., Merrill, S.M., Sekhon, B. et al. (2022) 'Infant DNA methylation: an early indicator of intergenerational trauma?' *Early Human Development*, 164: 105–19.

Northway, R. and Beech, I. (2022) 'Ethics', in C. Delves-Yates and F. Everett (eds.), *Essentials of Nursing Practice*, 3rd edn. London: Sage.

Nursing and Midwifery Council (NMC) (2018) *Future Nurse: Standards of Proficiency for Registered Nurses*. London: NMC.

Pairo-Castineira, E., Clohisey, S., Klaric, L. et al. (2021) 'Genetic mechanisms of critical illness in COVID-19'. *Nature*, 591: 92–98.

Royal College of Physicians, Royal College of Pathologists and British Society for Human Genetics (2011) *Consent and Confidentiality in Clinical Genetic Practice: Guidance on Genetic Testing and Sharing Genetic Information*, 2nd edn. Report of the Joint Committee on Medical Genetics. London: Royal College of Physicians and Royal College of Pathologists.

Sharma, S., Kelly, T.K. and Jones, P.A. (2010) 'Epigenetics in cancer'. *Carcinogenesis*, 31 (1): 27–36.

Stein, Z. and Susser, M. (1975) 'The Dutch famine, 1944–1945, and the reproductive process. I. Effects on six indices at birth'. *Pediatric Research*, 9: 70–6.

Wigley, M.I.L.C., Mascheroni, E., Bonichini, S. et al. (2022) 'Epigenetic protection: maternal touch and DNA-methylation in early life'. *Current Opinion in Behavioral Sciences*, 43: 111–17.

INFANT MENTAL WELLBEING AND HEALTH OR 'HOW TO GROW A HEALTHY ADULT'

ORLA McALINDEN

11

THIS CHAPTER COVERS

- What is meant by infant mental health (IMH) and why is it so important?
- Strategies to improve infant mental health
- Which strategies work and how do we know this?

> "But the hearts of small children are delicate organs. A cruel beginning in this world can twist them into curious shapes. The heart of a hurt child can shrink so that forever afterward it is hard and pitted as the seed of a peach. Or again, the heart of such a child may fester and swell until it is a misery to carry within the body, easily chafed and hurt by the most ordinary things."
>
> Carson McCullers, 1951, 'The Ballad of the Sad Café

INTRODUCTION

The concept of infant mental health (IMH) is not new. In the 1930s Sigmund Freud began examining the impact of child mental development on the later life of the adult, and this scrutiny continued with a string of interested theorists throughout the 20th century. It is now a newly resurgent topic of interest to multidisciplinary teams and a global effort of enquiry, practice and research. This is led in some part by recent advances in science and genetics, in particular the earliest stages of a child's life, before they have been born.

Whilst the science and psychological theory may be complex, the topic is an important one for you to engage with as it has a direct impact on the services that are currently offered and being developed to support wellbeing from early life onward. The quotation at the start of this chapter, for instance, aptly summarises the importance of the influences on the 'hearts of small children', and it is an important role as a children's nurse to tend to the psychological mental and physical wellbeing of your CYP charges. This may be in early-years care, or as a nurse caring for the school age or older child right into the adolescent and early years of adulthood. By association, it also means considering the welfare of the parent and family as well (RCN, 2021).

Today's society has many children in need of the essential universal health services, as well as children with very particular needs (e.g., complex physical and intellectual needs, learning disability, looked after children, children leaving care, children in the custody and youth justice system, child and adolescent mental health tiers, refugees and those who are displaced and exploited for varying complex reasons). The children's nurse of today and tomorrow needs to understand what interventions are needed, why, and the robustness of the evidence underpinning them (Dubicka, 2021; UNICEF, 2021).

Research (Barlow and Svanberg, 2009; O'Donnell et al., 2009) clearly shows that what happens in the womb and early years can affect the development of a child into adulthood and beyond. This is why the topic is so important to all health and social care professionals: the best start in life is needed for a good finishing chance – this is part of what a 'good outcome' looks like for children.

SEE ALSO
CHAPTER 10,
11, 13 AND 14

This chapter will first explore definitions of infant mental wellbeing and health as a touchstone for measuring the success of identified interventions, and explore why it is so important, giving a summary of seminal and recent scientific and psychological research. It will then look at how services and interventions address emotional and mental wellbeing for all, not just those at risk, how the services are developing and the evidence behind them. Finally, it will examine one of the main recent developments in the UK and USA – the Family Nurse Partnership (FNP).

SEE ALSO
CHAPTER 35

WHAT DO WE MEAN BY INFANT MENTAL HEALTH AND WHY IS IT SO IMPORTANT?

Infant mental health (IMH) and why it matters

IMH is the capacity to:

- form close relationships;
- recognise and express emotions; and
- explore and learn about their environment

Babies are wired for connection! During pregnancy and infancy, it is obvious how physically reliant babies are on their parents and caregivers. They are also socially and emotionally connected to us in so many fascinating ways. The way we interact with babies and infants literally shapes their brain development. This occurs particularly during pregnancy, and continues up to the age of 3 years, when our brains are growing at the fastest rate. We now know that 'mirror neurons' in the brain mean that how we act and interact with our children explains their 'copy-cat' behaviours. It all sounds like a huge responsibility but in fact, it's the small, day-to-day interactions with babies and infants that make the greatest difference (Nath et al., 2018; McAliskey and Meehan, 2020; Children's Society, 2022).

There are varying definitions and some criticism that the above timeframes start too early and end too soon. Barlow and Svanberg (2009) prefer broad timeframes which include the important pre- and perinatal periods. They and others (O'Donnell et al., 2009; Ball et al., 2012; Svanberg and Barlow, 2013) place great importance on the role of the placenta in the early influences on the developing foetus and strongly support the idea that early intervention should start ideally in the pre-conceptual and antenatal/perinatal periods if an improvement in children's life and health chances is sought. The 'First 1001 Days Movement' works with the 'Conception to Age Two All-Party Parliamentary Group' to raise awareness of the importance of the earliest years of life. The importance of perinatal mental health is equally important as many mothers feel unable to ask for help and often the signs of impaired wellbeing and altered mental health go undetected. According to Ralph and Clarke (2019), 'The impact of poor maternal mental health can be devastating, not only for the woman herself but also for her baby and other children, her partner and wider family. Perinatal depression, anxiety and psychosis also carry a staggering long-term cost to society for each annual cohort of births in the UK.' NHS England (2018) https://www.england.nhs.uk/publication/the-perinatal-mental-health-care-pathways/ have developed perinatal mental health care pathways which along with a growing awareness of IMH present another prong towards raising awareness and early prevention and detection of issues. This is also clearly a human rights issues (Children Act 1989; UNCRC, 1989; Human Rights Act 1998; Lundy, 2007, 2019).

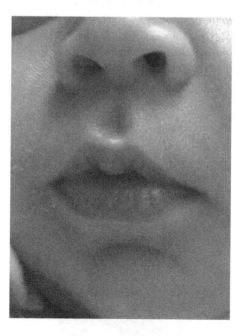

Figure 11.1 Baby face

There is now much more research and enquiry into these periods, which is enhanced by the increased contemporary scientific and research technology capability available. There is also growing recognition that IMH is influenced both by parenting and the environment, which includes the placenta as an 'environment' with a hitherto under-recognised role (O'Donnell et al., 2009; Knight et al., 2018; NHS England, 2018).

There is greater will to provide a good start in life for infants and children, one which will optimise their life chances and improve their resilience to multiple adverse childhood events (ACEs); in other words, help them cope better with life and family stresses and go on to be a young adult who is better equipped to deal with negative life events. This includes consideration of the effects of the COVID-19 pandemic and the emerging data on the negative effects of the pandemic on the mental and emotional wellbeing of children and young people (Crawford and Crawford, 2021; Dubicka, 2021). Safeguarding practices for children and young people have had to significantly adapt in response to COVID-19. In November 2020, there was a 12% fall in referrals to children's services, suggesting there is a growing number of unidentified vulnerable children due to COVID-19 lockdown restrictions. 'The pandemic has exacerbated several existing challenges for safeguarding services, including an increase in mental health issues and a rise in online abuse. As lockdown measures are relaxed or lifted, new cross-sector approaches will be needed to identify and respond to unreported cases of abuse and protect vulnerable children and young people' (Working in Partnership to Safeguard Children & Young People Conference, 2021; Children's Society, 2022).

SEE ALSO
CHAPTER 10

SEE ALSO
CHAPTER 37

Emotional wellbeing

Emotional wellbeing is important for all children. It should not be left until problems with emotional, psychological and mental health surface in later years and is an excellent reason why knowledge of this area should be reflected in all health, social care and education interventions. For an example, see the children's strategy for your country by visiting the appropriate government website.

There is strong evidence to support preventing mental and emotional ill health rather than trying to deal with the negative outcomes in later years. Remember that as a children's nurse you have a social, ethical/professional and employment imperative to do the best for your children and their families.

Recent developments in psychology indicate a shift in orientation from a deficit (the skills you do not have) to a strengths perspective (the skills you do have). This is known as 'positive psychology' and aims to promote adaptation and recovery to a stage where there is a limited dysfunction of life experiences, giving a better quality of life for the individual.

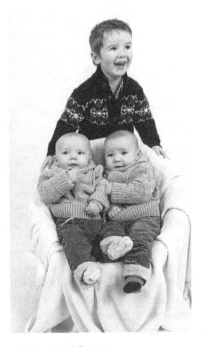

Figure 11.2   Darragh with twins Cathal and Conor

It is generally becoming better recognised in the literature that what happens in early childhood will shape the later stages of childhood and adulthood (Minnis et al., 2007; Barlow and Svanberg, 2009; Ball et al., 2012), and there is growing awareness of the potential for shaping positive outcomes in the emerging areas of epigenetics and neurobiology (Barlow and Svanberg, 2009; Svanberg and Barlow, 2013). These biogenetic elements appear to shape infant and children's future development and adjustments in life.

This understanding of good IMH is crucial because the message is clear that early intervention is important in order to ensure that infants and children have the best possible start in life. This also involves multiprofessional learning and working, at all levels and across agencies, skills which a children's nurse should be both familiar with, and competent in demonstrating (RCN, 2021).

Infant Mental Health Awareness Week runs annually every June. It provides an opportunity for everyone working in the sector to raise awareness of the importance of babies' social and emotional development. The goal of each IMHAW theme is to encourage everyone working in children and young people's mental health policies, strategies and services to think about and include babies. 'Children and young people's mental health should refer to the mental health of all children from 0–18 and beyond, but too often it is focussed on older children. It is recognised that there is a '"baby blindspot" made worse by the effects of covid' (Institute of Health Visiting 2023 and Parent–Infant Foundation 2021). This report also highlights how services have not returned to normal and that this will severely impact future global generations.

This has major implications for parenting and shaping of global health and social policy and for strategies for teaching and educating parents, families and communities as well as current and future students of health and social care (Wakelyn, 2019).

All children's and mental health nurses should be particularly well placed to influence positive parenting and promote emotional wellbeing in infants and children in order to stabilise and promote the foundations of resilience.

SEE ALSO
CHAPTER 10

SEE ALSO
CHAPTERS 2
AND 5

SEE ALSO
CHAPTER 9

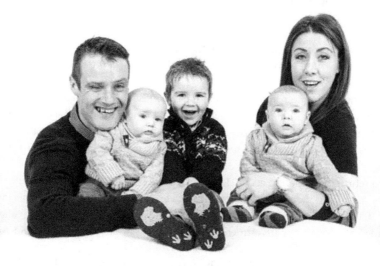

Figure 11.3 Peter and Deirdre and their children

It is also true that adult nurses, and indeed anyone who comes into contact with infants, children and families, can make an impact on the future development of that individual. This development is also inextricably linked with the issue of safeguarding.

STRATEGIES TO IMPROVE INFANT MENTAL HEALTH

Public health strategies from all four UK countries, the Republic of Ireland and further afield recognise the importance of the findings discussed above, as well as the role of the nurse (in all four fields of practice) in enhancing the path from the prenatal period, through to childbirth and early years and on towards adolescence and adulthood.

There have been numerous initiatives and programmes designed to support the improvement of infant mental health. They include:

- Infant massage techniques
- Brazelton Neonatal Behavioural Assessment Scale
- First Steps Parenting Programme
- Family Partnership Model of intervention and support
- The Parental Couple in Parenting
- PEEP Model – Learning together
- Early screening and intervention re. secure attachment
- Black and Ethnic Minorities (BEM)
- Mellow Babies
- Mellow Bumps
- Solihull Approach
- Solihull Plus
- Ounce of Prevention
- Working with mothers who have mental health needs
- Parenting with support for parents who have learning difficulties
- Breastfeeding initiatives and WHO 'Baby Friendly' policies
- Developing infant-centred services
- Sure Start programmes from 2000 onwards
- Child and family centres

There are also many US programmes, including the Abecedarian Project, High Scope/Perry Preschool, Chicago Child–Parent Centers, Early Head Start, HomeVisiting, and the Doula Program (theounce.org) amongst others.

These interventions cannot effectively work alone but must be part of a broader drive and focus on research education practice and policy in order to succeed. There needs to be ongoing consistent evidence to show that the gains will be worth the initial early investment. This is particularly important in times of global austerity when there must be compelling evidence to show that investment works (the 'invest-to-save' principle).

The expected return (gain) period on IMH investment is estimated to be in the region of seven years of no return, or actual loss, before any material gains can be seen in monetary terms (Marmot, 2010; Munro, 2011; Tickell 2011; Wakelyn and Katz, 2020). This means that IMH is particularly vulnerable to underfunding or inconsistent investment unless a strong approach is taken and followed by all countries.

Approaches and interventions should ideally mean seamless access for all families. This includes midwives, health visitors, GPs and children's centres, and services should engage with families as soon as possible, not waiting for dysfunction or a crisis to occur. Ideally the approach should be during or before pregnancy. All contact that parents have with services before and after the birth of their child provides a unique opportunity to work with them at the stage which is an essential precursor to the healthy development of our children.

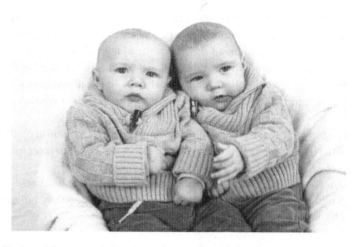

Figure 11.4   Cathal and Conor

SEE ALSO
CHAPTER 2
AND 14

WHICH STRATEGIES WORK AND HOW DO WE KNOW THIS?

Central to any decision about introducing new policy or strategy is the question 'What works and what evidence is there?' In recent times this has been gaining more interest and importance as governments and policy-makers aim to raise the topic higher on the health, social care and justice agenda (Dubicka, 2021).

The Child Psychotherapy Trust document *An Infant Mental Health Service* (2012) and the Ounce of Prevention website are good starting places for an overview of the experiences of the early years and the importance of evidence informing early years intervention.

The UK Cross-Party Manifesto called 'The 1001 Critical Days' (Leadsom et al., 2014; Department of Health and Social Care, 2021a, 2021b), the first of its kind, stressed that the approach should be one of agency rather than passive engagement and in the foreword states:

> as our understanding of the science of development improves, it becomes clearer and clearer how the events that happen to children and babies lead to the structural changes that have life-long ramifications ...

> ... we know too that not intervening now will affect not just this generation of children and young people but also the next. Those who suffer multiple adverse childhood events achieve less educationally, earn less, and are less healthy, making it more likely that the cycle of harm is perpetuated into the following generation ...

Leadsom et al. (2014) set out key areas for attention as:

- The importance of the foundation years: All children should be able to enjoy their childhood, in a supportive and nurturing environment, and be protected from harm. The United Nations Convention on the Rights of the Child (1989) also sets the precedent here to make clear that children's needs are a right and not an afterthought.
- Parents and families at the heart of services: There has often been insufficient focus on the central role of families in children's earliest years, which has meant that mothers and fathers have not always received enough, or sufficiently timely, advice and support. Recognition and inclusion of fathers as parenting partners and positive role models is another goal (RCM, 2014; Widarsson et al., 2015).

- Focusing on child development and intervening early: The 'Healthy Child Programme' can be fully and consistently implemented. This programme, from pregnancy to age five, is the overarching framework for NHS foundation years provision for all children, with additional early help for vulnerable families needing support using tools such as those at the National Child and Maternal Health Network.
- Skilled professionals: There has not been a sufficiently coherent framework to date for professional development and progression, highlighting the critical importance of continuing to improve the skills and qualification levels of workforces.
- A strong relationship with the sector: Children's centres in the community will be developed to provide access to a range of integrated universal and targeted services to meet locally defined need.

In 2021, there was a further call for the UK government to have a more co-ordinated access to help and services under plans to improve children's health in England including family hubs and the digitilisation of the 'Red Book':

> Infant mental health is about more than babies. It's about improving our whole lives and striving for better outcomes that have a profound effect from cradle to grave. (Department of Social Care, 2021a)

Evidence for interventions

Good quality evidence which underpins practice is a key concern, especially in times of austerity. It is required for ethical, professional, accountable practice and justification for the spending of public money. It is also a key election driver and can be used to influence health and social care policy at each term of government (Wilson et al., 2022).

There is a wide range of early years interventions employed UK-wide in order to improve and empower parenting capability and bolster infant mental health practices. The evidence is not readily available for some, and for others the evidence suggests that there may be ways of better managing interventions, either because of cost or because of outcome.

Other research over the years suggests that early intervention can work well (Center on the Developing Child, n.d.; Svanberg and Barlow, 2013; Galloway, 2014; Wakelyn, 2019; Heckman, 2000; Wakelyn and Katz, 2020).

All services aimed at family and parenting support must be non-stigmatising, empowering, have a participatory and strengths-based orientation, be accessible to all and must be underpinned by a child-rights approach, and be readily accessible (Lundy 2007, 2019).

Moulin et al. (2014) conducted research into parenting and providing a secure attachment for children, and this work yields some interesting evidence. The report clearly identifies how secure attachment can also narrow the 'school readiness' gap and improve children's life chances. This study suggests that more support from health visitors, children's centres and local authorities in helping parents bond with young children could play a role in narrowing the education gap. The report also found that securely attached children are more resilient to poverty, family instability, parental stress and depression. For example, boys growing up in poverty are two and a half times less likely to display behaviour problems at school if they formed secure attachments with parents in their early years.

In cases where mothers have poor bonds with their babies, research suggests their children are also more likely to be obese as they enter adolescence. Parents who were insecurely attached themselves, who are living in poverty or who have poor mental health find it hardest to provide sensitive parenting and bond with their babies.

Secure attachment develops through sensitive and responsive parenting in the first years of life and parenting plays a causal role in attachment: an improvement in parental sensitivity is necessary for an improvement in attachment security.

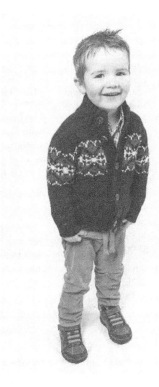

Figure 11.5   Darragh aged two-and-a-half years

WHAT'S THE EVIDENCE?

In the research discussed above, Moulin et al. (2014, pp.22-7) looked at several programmes (summarised below) promoting parenting, attachment and socio-emotional development for under-3s, identifying each model's elements:

- Evaluation
- Benefits to child and family
- Approximate cost of the intervention

Table 11.1   Baby bonds

Family Nurse Partnership	Intense one-to-one home-visiting Relationship building with first-time teenage mothers	Randomised control trial (Memphis, USA) with low-income, first-time, young mothers	FNP children had better emotional development at age 4, amongst other positive, lasting gains	£3,000 per family, per year
	Nurses	15-year follow up		
	From early pregnancy to age 2	Trialled in the UK and elsewhere		

(Continued)

Table 11.1   (Continued)

Circle of Security	Parent education, therapy and peer support in small groups of 5-7 Therapists Weekly 75-minute sessions over 20 weeks	Pre-test/post-test, 65 parents recruited through Head Start and Early Head Start Federal programmes for low-income families in the USA	The number of children securely attached rose from 20% to 54% after treatment. Number with highest risk (disorganised) attachment fell from 60% to 25%	£1,200 for training per head
Minding the Baby	Home-visiting supports reflective parenting Specialist social workers and nurses working together From the third trimester of pregnancy weekly until age 1, fortnightly until age 2	A randomised control trial (RCT) in Connecticut, USA is a work in progress An independent RCT in the UK with 320 first-time mothers under 25 began in spring 2014	RCTs still underway Early US findings show improved reflective functioning and more secure attachment	Not yet available
Child-Parent Psychotherapy	Child-Parent Psychotherapy and Parenting Educational therapists Sessions over 10 to 12 months	RCT with high-risk families in New York State, USA	At age 2, 61% formed a secure attachment, compared to 2% of the control in the control group of standard community services	£1,900 a head for training
Incredible Years	Social-learning model using video, role-play, peer support Masters-level group leaders and parenting practitioners 8-10 sessions for babies under 1 and toddlers 1-3	Parent Training for 4-8 year olds has undergone multiple randomised control trials in the USA	Benefits for other programmes include improved positive affect, emotional regulation and behaviour	£850 for the programme materials
Parents Early Education Partnership (PEEP)	Home-visiting and group sessions, based on reflective functioning for first-time parents Level-3 qualified parenting practitioners One prenatal home visit, 3 group sessions and 4 postnatal group sessions	An evaluation by Warwick Medical School began in 2014 It is a controlled realist evaluation with 25 families and 25 in the control	The aim is to impact on secure attachment through increased parental reflective functioning	£450 to train a practitioner; £450 per family for 8 sessions

| Oxford Parent Infant Project (OXPIP) | One-to-one support, video-feedback

Therapists

Average of 10 sessions, from conception to age 2 | Small, internal pre-test, post-test evaluation in Oxford, UK | The proportion of infants who were rated 'adapted' or 'well adapted' rose from 3% to 29% after the intervention | £800 per family on average

£4,000 a head for training |

Adapted with permission from Moulin, S., Waldfogel, J. and Washbrook, E. (2014) *Baby Bonds: Parenting, Attachment and a Secure Base for Children*. London, UK: The Sutton Trust

This study by Moulin concludes that:

1. Early interventions can work with all, especially with very high-risk or troubled families with children under 3 years of age.
2. Early interventions can promote secure attachment and development, especially when skilled practitioners support parents.
3. For both national and local policy-makers, this would represent a sound preventative investment.

ACTIVITY 11.1: CRITICAL THINKING

- Consider what you know so far about attachment and write a definition in your own words. Read the report by Moulin et al. (2014) and consider their definition of attachment. Does this match or exceed your own definition?
- Which political parties have a consistent track record of promoting infant and child welfare?
- What specific services to promote infant and child welfare are there in your area or country? (Refer to your local jurisdiction websites)

A rapid health review (PHE, 2015) provided compelling evidence updates in relation to key areas affecting IMH, including: parental mental health; smoking; alcohol/drug misuse; intimate partner violence; preparation and support for childbirth and the transition to parenthood; attachment; parenting support; unintentional injury in the home; safety from abuse and neglect; nutrition and obesity prevention; and speech, language and communication. The Children and Young People's Mental Health Taskforce has produced key reports (Department of Health (DH), 2015; Department of Health and Social Care, 2021b), which recognise that:

> Our childhood has a profound effect on our adult lives. Many mental health conditions in adulthood show their first signs in childhood and, if left untreated, can develop into conditions which need regular care. (DH, 2015 p.5)

The Family Nurse Partnership (FNP)

The FNP programme was originally developed in the USA by Professor David Olds (Olds et al., 1986, 2010). It is an intensive 'nurse' home visiting programme designed to improve the health, wellbeing and self-sufficiency of first-time parents and their children. FNP visits start early in pregnancy and continue until the child reaches 24 months. The specially trained nurse home-visitor's attention is focused on the social, emotional and economic context of the client's life, and activities are based on understanding human interactions.

At the time of writing, the FNP is widely used in the UK and is led by the Family Nurse Partnership National Unit which heads the national delivery of the FNP programme and supports local organisations with implementation as commissioned by the Department of Health, which holds the licence in England. The National Unit also works closely with NHS England to assure the quality of local programme delivery and to support preparation in new areas. Their role includes:

- Providing strategic direction and working with national partners
- Overseeing research and development
- Providing the Family Nurse Partnership learning programme for family nurses and supervisors
- Providing clinical guidance to supervisors and family nurses
- Advising on programme set-up in local areas and sub-licensing organisations to provide the programme
- Supporting local and national quality improvement and providing technical advice and guidance to local areas
- Leading adaptations to the programme so it remains relevant to the UK social context and developing knowledge
- Developing related models and products that support children's development in pregnancy and the early years

The FNP programme has been evaluated mostly positively to date (Ball et al., 2012), with further reviews and evaluations expected from both UK and US data as the programme is further refined and developed.

The pivotal element of the home visits and one of the distinguishing characteristics of the Nurse Family Partnership (NFP) model, as it is known in the USA, is building a therapeutic relationship between the nurse and the client. The aim is to build and empower clients' skills, confidence and hope in a manner that values the clients' ability to determine their own futures. The programme in England has been renamed the Family Nurse Partnership to better reflect the UK method of working but practitioners also made a collective decision to call themselves family nurses (FNs) to distinguish their role from previous posts such as health visitor or community health nurse. It remains essentially the same as the original US Nurse Family Partnership (NFP). It is an evidence-based, manualised, preventive intervention and according to FNP this is one of the main reasons that it was selected rather than any alternative UK interventions with weak or no evidence (Ball et al., 2012).

Evidence for the FNP programme is of higher quality than many other early intervention programmes and it is commonly named when examples of programmes with good evidence for success are sought (Ball et al., 2012). Whether this evidence-based US intervention can be applied in a different cultural and institutional context has been considered. It is also relevant that some 'competing' interventions developed within the UK context may feel that their programmes are as effective, but have not as yet been able to conduct the necessary randomised trials with long-term follow-up that the NFP/FNP has achieved to date.

Initial UK results in the Ball et al. (2012) study showed that the parents involved liked FNP in comparison with other services, particularly the different way they were perceived by FNP staff, not judged and undermined but supported and strengthened. Most participants found the programme better than they had expected, particularly some of the young men interviewed as they felt more involved as 'fathers to be'. These appear to be significant measures of the success of the FNP in the UK, with research and evaluation data still being collected. Importantly, the role of the FNP family nurse is seen as a separate, specialist role, different from that of a health visitor or community nurse. You can read more about FNP as well as more recent outcomes at The Family Nurse Partnership (fnp.nhs.uk).

Two of the three theories upon which FNP is based – attachment theory (Bowlby, 1969) and ecological systems theory (Bronfenbrenner, 1979) – are widely understood and used to plan interventions and guide interactions.

SCENARIO 11.1: BERNEICE AND ZARA

Berneice was pregnant at 17 and her boyfriend did not stay with her. Berneice felt abandoned and afraid. She knew she could not rely on her mother, also a single parent, as Berneice's own upbringing had been chaotic and complicated, with several episodes of social work involvement due to concerns about Berneice's growth and development. Her boyfriend had been her only constant companion for the previous year, and now he had abandoned her. Berneice lived at home with her mother. Initially she was not at all sure about the FNP nurse and was reluctant to engage but with time and patience she grew in confidence over her pregnancy, had a successful birth of Zara, and was supported by her mother. Over the first months and years Berneice developed her communication skills, insight and awareness of her own strengths and limitations. She worked hard with her FNP nurse to maximise her strengths and practical parenting skills, and her mother seemed to benefit from the support also. Gradually, Berneice was able to start to think about her future with Zara and started a part-time animal welfare course at the local college. The college had a crèche which helped with childcare and enabled Berneice to concentrate on her studies.

- Make notes on Berneice's story and critically reflect on the main negative and positive issues in her story.
- Critically reflect upon whether it is a children's nurse's role to facilitate successful attachment bonding and development of parenting skills.
- Cross-reference your notes with:
  o the UN Convention on the Rights of the Child
  o the NMC Code (use the most current edition)
  o your own country's current children's welfare policy

ACTIVITY 11.2: CRITICAL THINKING

How good are our children's lives? What do they say?

Read and reflect upon the information given by children in the report from the Jacobs Foundation (2015) and the UNICEF report (2021), The State of the World's Children.

- Take some time out to reflect on the various elements of these studies.
- Make notes on where you might like to grow up if you had a choice, and why.
- Do these findings in any way surprise you?

The research and case studies above demonstrate some of the ways the relationship between the family nurse and the family can, with consent and motivation, be strengthened to increase capacity and improve outcomes for the child and family.

- Start a media or social media 'watch' to capture any coverage of campaigns or intervenions on the topic of IMH. This will help you focus on what is happening locally and nationally (e.g., Sure Start programmes, early years iniatiatives, Baby Friendly services, breast feeding friendly organisations and places, baby massage sessions, parenting skills – including for fathers).
- Shadow a public health nurse, health visitor or FNP nurse to enhance your understanding and evidence base. This will help you see very clearly the ways in which public health strategies and services can marry up. You can see policy in action and also see gaps in services. You can use this as reflection for revalidation or for lobbying for better local services. You can also gain valuable experience from role-modelling opportunities.
- Access websites for health and social care for your country and check what is available locally for children and maternity care services. You may also develop your literature search skills and knowledge of your locality. This information may prove very useful to you later in your practice.
- View the Association of Infant Mental Health UK's short clip video series on 'Getting to Know Your Baby' at Getting to Know Your baby Videos – AiMH.

The following section is a reflective exercise considering the negative effects of poor infant mental health or parenting.

ACTIVITY 11.3: CRITICAL THINKING

'In every nursery there are ghosts. They are the visitors from the unremembered pasts of the parents, the uninvited guests at the christening ... These intruders from the past have taken up residence in the nursery, claiming tradition and rights of ownership. They have been present at the christening for two or more generations. While no one has issued an invitation, the ghosts take up residence and conduct the rehearsal of the family tragedy from a tattered script ... The baby in these families is burdened by the oppressive past of his parents from the moment he enters the world. The parent, it seems, is condemned to repeat the tragedy of his own childhood with his own baby in terrible and exacting detail' (Fraiberg et al., 1975, pp.164-5).

- What do you feel when you read this representation of the intergenerational effects of disrupted attachment, bonding and parenting upon the child?
- What are your thoughts on the apparent inevitability of 'repeating the tragedy'? Is this only applicable in 'extreme' cases?
- Find out what the specific provision is in your local area for enhancing attachment, bonding and parenting skills in the early years of a child's life.

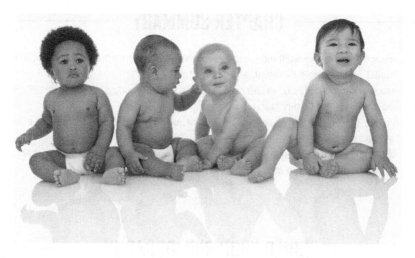

Figure 11.6 Baby group

Overall, the main focus of debate in recent years on health and social care has been biased towards an ageing population, with less regard evident for the outcomes for children (DH, 2015).

This appears to be a false economy and furthermore is a shocking indictment of how we as a group of nations view and value our youngest citizens.

This must change and is the basis for the ongoing professional argument for the introduction of a national child and young person's health strategy – this should include early as well as ongoing mental and emotional health action and outcomes fulfilment.

Building capacity, improving life chances and resilience to deal better with adverse situations and events and achieve better emotional and mental health is key to building a healthy adult. Finding the best strategies, through good quality research and evidence, and working in an effective interdisciplinary and interagency manner, in accordance with the wishes and needs of the child and family is the ongoing 'Holy Grail'. Our children and families need you to recognise and support them as part of your professional duty of care. One excellent free resource is the Watch Me Play! Manual (Wakelyn and Katz, 2020). This was first developed in First Step as an intervention to promote child-led play, to enhance relationships and create better understanding of different child strengths.

ACTIVITY 11.4

Visit the Watch Me Play! approach research page for information about the research background to Watch Me Play! and current research in the UK, Italy and Japan: https://tavistockandportman. nhs.uk/research-and-innovation/our-research/research-projects/watch-me-play-feasibility-study/ (accessed 22 February 2023).

CHAPTER SUMMARY

- Infant mental health and wellbeing is a resurgent and evidenced-based topic which can positively impact on the whole development of the child
- There are several examples of evidence-based theoretical models used in the UK. Perhaps the most well-known is the Family Nurse Partnership
- Ongoing and long-term follow up research is required to continue to test theories of 'what works' in the area of Infant mental health
- There should be an interdisciplinary approach involving statutory and voluntary services across care settings to promote and share good examples of IMH

BUILD YOUR BIBLIOGRAPHY

Books and Reports

FURTHER READING

- RCPCH (2016) Securing Better Health for Northern Ireland's Infants, Children and Young People: A vision for 2016. Available at: www.rcpch.ac.uk/system/files/protected/news/RCPCH%20 NI%20vision_Embargoed%2019Nov_0.pdf

This report from the Royal College of Paediatrics and Child Health (RCPCH) sets out the vision for Northern Ireland's children and families in terms of best practice aspirations.
- Leadsom, A., Field, F., Burstow, P. and Lucas, C. (2014) *The 1001 Critical Days: The Importance of the Conception to Age Two Period.* Available at: www.wavetrust.org/sites/default/files/ reports/1001%20Critical%20Days%20-%20The%20Importance%20of%20the%20 Conception%20to%20Age%20Two%20Period%20Refreshed_0.pdf (accessed 5/7/23).

This above publication was the first of its kind in UK where cross-party commitment to infant mental health is recommended.
- MBRRACE-UK. Saving Lives, Improving Mothers' Care Core Report – Lessons learned to inform maternity care from the UK and Ireland Confidential Enquiries into Maternal Deaths and Morbidity 2018-20. Oxford: National Perinatal Epidemiology Unit, University of Oxford 2022.

Report looking at direct cause of death in the year after pregnancy. This latest report indicates that mental ill health is an increasing cause of maternal death.
- Hogg, S. and Mayes, G. (2022) *Casting Long Shadows. The ongoing impact of Covid-19 pandemic on babies, their families and the services that support them.* Institute of Health Visiting with First 1001 Days Movement. Available at: https://parentinfantfoundation.org.uk/wp-content/ uploads/2022/11/F1001D-Casting-Long-Shadows-FINAL-NOV-22.pdf (accessed 10 June 2023).

Journal articles

FURTHER READING: ONLINE JOURNAL ARTICLES

- Mountain, G., Cahill, J. and Thorpe, H. (2017) 'Sensitivity and attention interventions in early childhood: A systematic review and meta analysis'. *Infant Behaviour and Development*, 46: 14–32.

This article looks at the effects on infant behaviour of parental input such as increased handling, cuddling, speaking to the infant and other nurturing interventions.
- De Pascalis, L., Kkeli, N., Chakrabarti, B. et al. (2017) 'Maternal gaze to the infant face: Effects of infant age and facial configuration during mother–infant engagement in the first nine weeks'. *Infant Behavior and Development*, 46: 91-9.

This article similarly looks at the matenal-child gaze and recognition of same by infant in the first few weeks of life.

- Newland, R., Parade, S., Dickstein, S. and Seifer, R. (2016) 'The association between maternal depression and sensitivity: Child-directed effects on parenting during infancy'. *Infant Behaviour and Development*, 45: 47–50.

This paper explores how maternal sensitivity in general and in particular towards the infant can be blunted during a period of maternal depression

Weblinks

FURTHER
READING:
WEBLINKS

- The Association for Infant Mental Health (AIMH) Association of Infant Mental Health UK's short clip video series on 'Getting to Know Your Baby': https://aimh.org.uk/getting-to-know-your-baby/ AIMH provides discussion, comment and resources on the topic as well as evidence-based reports and information on conferences.
- Family Nurse Partnership: http://fnp.nhs.uk The Family Nurse Partnership website sets out the evidence for the programmes and provides valuable resources and links for supporting infants and parents in the early years.
- Institute of Health Visiting (IHV): http://ihv.org.uk The IHV website contains many excellent resources and signposts to relevant materials relevant to early years wellbeing.
- NHS England, NHS Improvement, National Collaborating Centre for Mental Health: The Perinatal Mental Health Care Pathways (May 2018): www.england.nhs.uk/publication/theperinatal-mental-health-care-pathway
- Nursing and Midwifery Council (NMC) (2018) *Standards for Competence that Apply to Specific Fields of Nursing: Children's.* London: NMC: www.rcn.org.uk/Professional-Development/publications/pub-005942
- Nursing and Midwifery Council (NMC) Professional Duty of Candour Guidance: www.nmc.org.uk/standards/guidance/the-professional-duty-of-candour/read-the-professional-duty-of-candour
- Parent-Infant Foundation: https://parentinfantfoundation.org.uk/our-work/imhaw/
- Parent-Infant Foundation: The Vision, Mission and Consensus Statement (2021): https://parentinfantfoundation.org.uk/1001-days/
- Royal College of Nursing (RCN) (2017) *Standards for Assessing, Measuring and Monitoring Vital Signs in Infants, Children and Young People.* London. RCN Publications. Code 005 942: www.nmc.org.uk/globalassets/sitedocuments/standards/nmc-standards-for-competence-for-registered-nurses.pdf
- Royal College of Nursing (RCN) (2018) *Recordkeeping. The Facts.* London RCN Publications. Code 005 343: www.rcn.org.uk/Professional-Development/publications/rcn-record-keeping-uk-pub-011-016
- Watch Me Play! https://tavistockandportman.nhs.uk/research-and-innovation/our-research/research-projects/watch-me-play-feasibility-study/ Current research in the UK, Italy and Japan.
- Working in Partnership to Safeguard Children & Young People Conference Online (2021): https://childsafeguardingconf.co.uk/

REFERENCES

Ball, M., Barnes, J. and Meadows, P. (2012) *Issues Emerging from the First 10 Pilot Sites Implementing the Nurse–Family Partnership Home-visiting Programme in England.* London: DH.

Barlow, J. and Svanberg, P.O. (2009) *Keeping the Baby in Mind: Infant Mental Health in Practice.* London: Routledge.

Bowlby, J. (1969) *Attachment and Loss*. Vol. 1: Attachment. New York: Basic Books.

Bronfenbrenner, U. (1979) *The Ecology of Human Development*. Cambridge, MA: Harvard University Press.

Center on the Developing Child (n.d.) Available at: https://developingchild.harvard.edu/ (accessed 5/7/ 2023).

Child Psychotherapy Trust (2012) *An Infant Mental Health Service: The Importance of the Early Years and Evidence-based Practice*. London: CPT.

Children Act 1989. www.legislation.gov.uk/ukpga/1989/41/contents.

Children's Society (2022) The impact of COVID-19 on children and young people. Available at: www.childrenssociety.org.uk/sites/default/files/2021-01/the-impact-of-covid-19-on-children-and-young-people-briefing.pdf (accessed 5/7/2023).

Crawford, P. and Crawford, J. (2021) *Cabin Fever: Surviving Lockdown in the Coronavirus Pandemic* (Society Now series). Bingley: Emerald Publishing.

Department of Health (2015) *Future in Mind: Promoting, Protecting and Improving Our Children and Young People's Mental Health and Wellbeing*. London: Children and Young People's Mental Health Taskforce/DH.

Department of Health and Social Care (2021a) New focus on babies' and children's health as review launches. Available at: www.gov.uk/government/news/new-focus-on-babies-and-childrens-health-as-review-launches (accessed 14 February 2023).

Department of Health and Social Care (2021b) Policy Paper: The best start for life: a vision for the 1001 critical days. Available at: www.gov.uk/government/publications/the-best-start-for-life-a-vision-for-the-1001-critical-days (accessed 14 April 2021).

Dubicka, B. (2021) 'Editorial: Evidence, policy and practice – gold standard, good enough or doing it differently?' *Child and Adolescent Mental Health*, 26 (1): 1–2.

Fraiberg, S., Adelson, E. and Shapiro, V. (1975) 'Ghosts in the nursery. A psychoanalytic approach to the problems of impaired infant-mother relationships'. *Journal of the American Academy of Child & Adolescent Psychiatry*,14 (3): 387–421.

Galloway, S. (2014) *Infant Mental Health: The Scottish Context. NSPCC Scotland*. Available at: www.nspcc.org.uk/globalassets/documents/consultation-responses/nspcc-scotland-2012-briefing-infant-mental-health-policy-context.pdf (accessed 10 June 2023).

Gov.uk (2015) Healthy child programme: rapid review to update evidence. *Rapid review of the evidence base supporting the healthy child programme (HCP) 0 to 5 years*. Available at: www.gov.uk/government/publications/healthy-child-programme-rapid-review-to-update-evidence (accessed 5 July 2023).

Heckman, J.J. (2000) *Invest in the Very Young*. Chicago, IL: Ounce of Prevention Fund and University of Chicago Harris School of Public Policy Studies.

Human Rights Act 1998. www.legislation.gov.uk/ukpga/1998/42/contents

Institute of Reproductive and Developmental Biology at Imperial College London (n.d.) Begin before Birth. Available at: https://beginbeforebirth.org/the-science-epigenetics/ (accessed 5 July 2023).

Jacobs Foundation (2015) *Children's Views on Their Lives and Well-being in 15 countries: A Report on the Children's Worlds Survey, 2013–14*. York: Children's Worlds Project.

Knight, M., Bunch, K., Tuffnell, D. et al. (eds) on behalf of MBRRACE-UK. (2018) *Saving Lives, Improving Mothers' Care - Lessons learned to inform maternity care from the UK and Ireland Confidential Enquiries into Maternal Deaths and Morbidity 2014–16*. Oxford: National Perinatal Epidemiology Unit, University of Oxford.

Leadsom, A., Field, F., Burstow, P. and Lucas, C. (2014) *The 1001 Critical Days: The Importance of the Conception to Age Two Period*. Available at: www.wavetrust.org/sites/default/files/reports/1001%20

Critical%20Days%20-%20The%20Importance%20of%20the%20Conception%20to%20Age%20 Two%20Period%20Refreshed_0.pdf (accessed 16 May 2017).

Lundy, L. (2007) 'Voice is not enough: conceptualising Article 12 of the United Nations Convention on the Rights of the Child'. *British Educational Research Journal*, 33 (6): 927–42.

Lundy, L. (2019) *National Strategy on Children and Young People's Participation in Decision-Making*. Department of Children, Equality, Disability, Integration and Youth. Eire.

Marmot, M. (2010) *Fair Society, Healthy Lives: The Marmot Review: Strategic Review of Health Inequalities in England Post-2010*. London: Department for International Development.

McAliskey, D. and Meehan, M. (2020) 'What is infant mental health and why does it matter so much during COVID-19? Available at: www.publichealth.hscni.net/node/5161 (accessed 8 April 2021).

McCullers, C. (1951) *The Ballad of the Sad Café. Boston*. MA: Houghton Mifflin.

Minnis, H., Reekie, J., Young, D., O'Connor, T., Ronald, A., Grayand, A. and Plomin, R. (2007) 'Genetic, environmental and gender influences on attachment disorder behaviours'. *British Journal of Psychiatry*, 190: 490–5.

Moulin, S., Waldfogel, J. and Washbrook, E. (2014) *Baby Bonds: Parenting, Attachment and a Secure Base for Children*. London: The Sutton Trust.

Munro, E. (2011) *The Munro Review of Child Protection: Final Report – A Child-Centred System*. London: TSO.

Nath, S., Ryan, E.G., Trevillion, K. et al. (2018) 'Prevalence and identification of anxiety disorders in pregnancy: the diagnostic accuracy of the two-item Generalised Anxiety Disorder scale (GAD-2)'. *BMJ Open*, 2018; 8:e023766.

NHS England (2018) The Perinatal Mental Health Care Pathways. Available at: www.england.nhs.uk/ publication/the-perinatal-mental-health-care-pathways (accessed 5 July 2023).

O'Donnell, K., O'Connor, T.G. and Glover, V. (2009) 'Prenatal stress and neurodevelopment of the child: focus on the HPA axis and role of the placenta'. *Developmental Neuroscience*, 31 (4): 285–92.

Olds, D.L. (2006) 'The nurse–family partnership: an evidence-based preventive intervention'. *Infant Mental Health Journal*, 27: 5–25.

Olds, D.L., Henderson, C.R., Tatelbaum, R. and Chamberlin, R. (1986) 'Improving the delivery of prenatal care and outcomes of pregnancy: a randomized trial of nurse home visitation'. *Pediatrics*, 77, 16–28.

Olds, D.L., Kitzman, H.J., Cole, R.E. et al. (2010) 'Enduring effects of prenatal and infancy home visiting by nurses on maternal life course and government spending'. *Archives of Pediatric Adolescent Medicine*, 164 (5): 419–24.

Ralph, T. and Clarke, N. (2018) Clinical Review: Perinatal Mental Health. Available at: www. healthprofessionalacademy.co.uk/docs/default-source/resourcesdoc/house-resources/perinatal- mental-health-review.pdf?sfvrsn=267a4723_0&fbclid=IwAR0-8CxMNIv4lXsT7iIi5XhArqdlG6TvBk Gf4ZmWxqExQkWuZ-T4e-jddqI (accessed 8 February 2023).

Royal College of Midwives (RCM) (2014) *Making the Most of Fathers to Improve Maternal and Infant Health*. London: RCM.

Royal College of Nursing (RCN) (2021) *Children and Young People's Nursing: A Philosophy of Care*. London: RCN Publications. Code 009 433.

Svanberg, P.O. and Barlow, J. (2013) 'The effectiveness of training in the Parent–Infant Interaction Observation Scale for health visitors'. *Journal of Health Visiting*, 1 (3): 162–6.

Tickell, C. (2011) *The Early Years: Foundations for Life, Health and Learning. An Independent Report on the Early Years Foundation Stage to Her Majesty's Government*. London: DfE.

UNICEF (2021) The state of the world's children. Annual Report. Available at: www.unicef.org/ reports/state-worlds-children-2021 (accessed 10 June 2023).

United Nations (1989) United Nations Convention on the Rights of the Child (UNCRC). Available at: www.unicef.org.uk/what-we-do/un-convention-child-rights (accessed 6 June 2023).

Wakelyn, J. (2019) *Therapeutic Approaches with Babies and Young Children in Care: Observation and Attention*. London: Routledge.

Wakelyn, J. and Katz, A. (2020) *Watch Me Play! Manual for Parents*, Version 2. Tavistock and Portman NHS Foundation Trust, Gateway number: PUB20_64. Available at: https://tavistockandportman. nhs.uk/care-and-treatment/our-clinical-services/watch-me-play/.

Widarsson, W., Engström, G., Tydén, T., Lundberg, P. and Hammar, L.M. (2015) 'Paddling upstream': fathers' involvement during pregnancy as described by expectant fathers and mothers'. *Journal of Clinical Nursing*, 24 (7–8): 1059–68

Wilson, D.M, Underwood, L., Sungmin, K., Olukotun, M. and Errasti-Ibarrondo, B. (2022) 'How and why nurses became involved in politics or political action, and the outcomes or impacts of this involvement'. *Nursing Outlook*, 70(1): 55–63.

FACTORS INFLUENCING WELLBEING AND DEVELOPMENT IN CHILDREN AND YOUNG PEOPLE

12

MELANIE ROBBINS AND CILLA SANDERS

THIS CHAPTER COVERS

- What are health and wellbeing?
- Parenting capacity
- Family and environmental factors

> "Relationships are at the heart of children's well-being. When children talk about what is important in their lives, they highlight their need for love, support, respect, fairness, freedom and safety ... Children acknowledge that material items are important, but they see them as secondary to relationships."
>
> The Children's Society, 2022, www.childrenssociety.org.uk/sites/default/files/2022-09/GCR-2022-Full-Report.pdf (accessed 5 July 2023)

INTRODUCTION

It is acknowledged that children's development and wellbeing are influenced by many factors and that these begin before the child is born. Once the child is born, these factors can support or sabotage the child in meeting their full potential physically, emotionally and cognitively, and as the quote above acknowledges, children identify these aspects, somewhat surprisingly, as more important than material aspects. Your role as a children's nurse requires you to be aware of these factors so that you can assess, plan and implement a holistic approach to care, which can support or mitigate these factors and ensure that the child and family voice is heard at policy level.

Most of the documentation used in a clinical setting directs us towards assessing the physiological systems – for example, the cardiovascular system – before eventually assessing the child and family situation, and wider influences. However, the trend for shorter stays in acute care may limit the effectiveness of that holistic assessment. If you truly want to improve the health and wellbeing of children, an understanding of the wider influences needs to become a cornerstone of your care alongside assessment of physiological status.

WHAT ARE HEALTH AND WELLBEING?

Health is a complex issue and many authors have tried to define it. The World Health Organization's (WHO) seminal definition (1948) stated that 'Health is a complete state of physical, mental and social wellbeing not merely the absence of disease or infirmity'. This is considered an idealised view that few would recognise as being related to everyday life. The WHO developed their definition, stating that:

> a conception of health is the extent to which an individual or group is able, on the one hand, to realise aspirations and satisfy needs, and, on the other hand, to change or cope with the environment. Health is, therefore, seen as a resource for everyday life, not just the object of living. (WHO, 1986)

ACTIVITY 12.1: CRITICAL THINKING

Is it possible for the children below to achieve a state of health?

- A child with a congenital condition – for example, talipes
- A child who has learning disabilities
- A child who has a long-term condition – for example, type 1 diabetes

---

Develop your understanding of the factors that influence health by accessing the video on the Social Determinants of Health or read *Health Inequalities and the Social Determinants of Health* (RCN, 2012).

You need to consider how children may define health, which is closely linked to cognitive and emotional development and life experiences. This will enable you to provide care that incorporates the child's perspective. However, life experiences may accelerate their understanding of health and illness – for example, a young child with a life-threatening illness as a brief experience versus a child who has to manage a chronic life-limiting disease.

ACTIVITY 12.2: CRITICAL THINKING

Watch the video entitled *We asked London children – What does being healthy mean to you?* Make notes on what you think about the children's views and if they surprise you or not. Would these views be different in another country or part of the world?

A number of studies have linked a child's understanding of illness to Piaget's stages of development, but this approach has been criticised on the grounds that Piaget's stages underestimate a child's development and development is not always linear. It has been shown that a child's understanding of health is separate from illness. Myant and Williams's (2005) work shows that children can hold separate concepts of what it means to be healthy and what it means to be ill. They explored this in different age ranges and for different illnesses, those which are contagious (common cold, chicken pox) and those which are not (asthma). As the child grows, a more complex understanding develops which includes aspects of health-promoting behaviours – that is: eating well, wearing appropriate clothing against the cold – rather than just an absence of illness.

You can see that when establishing what health means, you need to consider the biological *and* the psychosocial and emotional influences.

WHAT'S THE EVIDENCE?

Our understanding of how children process information and develop their understating is evolving. Toyama (2016) extends the work of Myant and Williams (2005), demonstrating that even young children recognise that illness is not the result of a misdemeanour and that children actually obtain information from a wide source, including parents, teachers, television and other media sources. Katz et al. (2015) explore the use of the Internet in teenagers in assisting with homework, health information and development of self and found that parents are poor at assessing how frequently their children use this source for these activities. The Office for National Statistics (ONS) survey (2020) found that there were core concepts children raised that help form their perception of health and wellbeing. This includes feeling loved, positive supportive relationships, feeling safe and being able to express themselves without judgement. Children were aware of the impact of financial matters on the family, such as the ability to pay for basic needs, developing social inclusion and the effect of stress on mental health, but they also recognised money does not equal happiness (p.2).

- How can you use this information to aid a child's understanding of an illness? Think about how we explain signs, symptoms and disease processes to children.
- We should acknowledge that children are accessing online information but should we also take into account the quality of the information and assess the accuracy of their understanding?
- We need to ascertain what children understand about factors that can influence their family's health and wellbeing.

SCENARIO 12.1: SAMIRA

Samira is 7 years old and has suffered repeated urinary tract infections since she was 2. She takes prophylactic antibiotics and has regular scans to monitor renal functioning. Samira lives in privately

(Continued)

rented accommodation with her mum and brother, aged 3 years. Mum, Jamila, does not work at the moment and suffers with depression and anxiety and relies on child benefit and Jobseeker's Allowance to financially support the family.

Their house does not provide the best living conditions – the children share a bedroom, whilst Jamila sleeps in the lounge. The kitchen is basic; the fridge is old and only two rings on the cooker work. Samira hates the cold, damp bathroom and delays using the toilet. As a consequence, she occasionally wets herself.

Samira attends school, which she enjoys, but she has made few friends and one of her peers has called her smelly.

Jamila does her best to look after her children on her own but sometimes she wishes she could just stay in bed. She knows she needs to encourage Samira to empty her bladder regularly but her brother demands so much of her attention that Samira doesn't get a look in. Jamila feels guilty as she sometimes forgets to give Samira her medicine.

- What do you think Samira's definition of health would be?
- List the influences, both positive and negative, on Samira's health and wellbeing.
- Do you think Samira's definition of health would be the same as Jamila's?

These concepts have been summarised in *Working Together to Safeguard Children* (HM Government, 2018).

It is not by chance that a child's developmental needs, parenting capacity and family and environmental factors are portrayed as sides of a triangle. Each contributes uniquely to the hoped-for outcome, a healthy and well child. A child needs the fundamental aspects to be met: nutrition to grow physically and also to be stimulated and nurtured and educated, including learning how to get along with others so that they grow cognitively and emotionally. The environment they live in influences positively or negatively the carer's ability to provide these aspects but also the child's ability to utilise these to the fullest.

You now need to consider these aspects, reviewing the evidence and degree of influence in more depth.

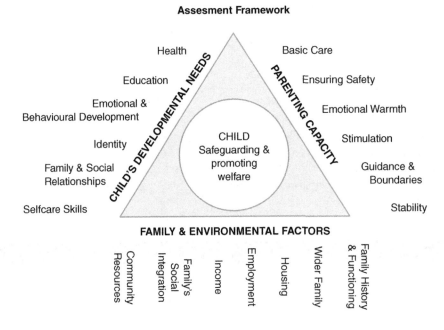

Figure 12.1 The Assessment Framework

HM Government, 2018, p.30. © Crown copyright

PARENTING CAPACITY

When exploring the effects of parenting on child health and illness, many studies review what happens when aspects of parenting capacity are absent or negative. We know that where parents provide warmth and love this mitigates, to some degree, other aspects such as poverty. However, even in the warmest of environments, poverty limits opportunity and life experiences, which can hinder the child's cognitive and emotional growth, impacting on their choice of career, earning capacity and so adversely affects subsequent generations. Genetic primacy has long held to be true that we are what we inherit, but there is now growing evidence that the environment also influences how those genes work. You will have explored the importance of genetics and the health of the mother before conception and during pregnancy in previous chapters. A key component of providing basic care is nutrition. There is a wealth of evidence that demonstrates that breastfeeding has many immediate and longer-lasting benefits for the child and mother.

SEE ALSO
CHAPTER 11
AND 14

SEE ALSO
CHAPTER 37

Basic care and nutrition

The UNICEF breastfeeding initiative (2013) summarised a number of studies which outline the benefits, which include:

SEE ALSO
CHAPTERS 10
AND 11

- Reduced risk of admission of the newborn for respiratory conditions and gastroenteritis
- A correlation between higher rates of breastfeeding prevalence and lower rates of inpatient admissions among infants under 1 year old for a number of conditions
- Evidence from America also suggests that babies who have not been breastfed have a higher risk of obesity, hypertension and type 2 diabetes
- UNICEF UK (2017) produced Breast Feeding Standards for health services to promote and sustain breastfeeding; these include standards for universities so that the future workforce is able to support breastfeeding, as the UK breastfeeding continuation rates (to 6 months) remain the lowest in the world.

Petherick (2010) suggests that the current debate between breast versus formula feeding is polarised, with both groups exaggerating their position that one is better than the other. However, the more we know about the micro-constituents of breast milk the more we realise formula cannot replicate breast milk. The Promotion of Breastfeeding Intervention Trial (PROBIT), a study conducted in Belarus, divided centres into those which:

- Delivered the WHO Baby-Friendly Hospital Initiative (BFHI) (where healthcare professionals received specific training and education in breastfeeding support)
- Offered normal care, which did not include any specific breastfeeding initiatives or support

They found differences in weight and reduction of illnesses in the PROBIT group up to the age of 1 year. Ongoing reviews found that by the age of 6, weight and height were similar but in the 'exclusively breastfed for 6 months' group, teachers rated the children's IQ scores as being higher. However, Martens (2012) suggests caution because the study groups did not include non-breastfed children, and that non-breastfed children or other influencing factors need to be considered. In Belarus it is normal for mothers to be with their children for the first three years of life, so other factors cannot be excluded. Nevertheless, the findings led to a change of policy for the WHO as it now advocates exclusive breastfeeding for the first 6 months of life and the continuation of breastfeeding, alongside solid foods, for 2 years (WHO, 2003). Indeed, understanding confounding issues is key when reviewing an issue such as breastfeeding, as women who breastfeed are more likely to be of a higher social group, better educated and have the income to enable them to take maternity leave. However, Iacovou and Sevilla-Sanz (2010, p.2) reviewed the evidence assessing the benefits of breastfeeding on the impact of cognitive development for children in England and concluded that in English, maths and science there is a statistical significance in improved scores which continues to the age of 14 and they suggest this effect grows over time.

Nutrition is important throughout life. We know we have an obesity problem in the Western World. Measuring child obesity is via Body Mass Index (BMI) but is more complicated as factors such as age, sex and ethnicity influence the assessment of whether BMI is too high or too low. In the UK, the UK 1990 population threshold used for population monitoring states that being above the 85th and 95th centiles indicates the person is overweight and obese, respectively (the UK 1990 clinical thresholds are 91st and 98th, indicating clinical intervention is needed) (SACN & RCPCH, 2012). A further complication is that data are collected differently across the UK making comparison difficult and this is compounded by the effect of the COVID-19 pandemic. However, all surveys show that obesity is on the rise, and the rate is higher in areas of deprivation.

Table 12.1   Percentage of children classified as obese in the UK

	Age 4-5		Primary 1 (aged around 5-6)	Age range - see within box		Gender differences
	Over-weight	Obese	Over- weight or obese	Over- weight	Obese	
England*	13.3	14.4%		10-11 years old 15.4%	10-11 years old 25.5%	Aged 4-5, more boys are overweight or obese compared to girls, 28.3% vs 27.2%. This increases significantly by ages 10-11 when the rates are 44.3% (boys) and 37% (girls). Rates were higher in the more deprived areas.
Wales**	14.7%	12.6%				In 4-5 age slightly more boys are overweight or obese compared to girls and those children living in the most deprived areas of Wales were twice as likely to be obese than in the least deprived.
Scotland+			29.5			Boys continue to have a slightly higher risk than girls, but those in the least deprived areas continue to be at risk of becoming overweight or obese.
Northern Ireland++				Age 2-15 years 16% were recorded as being overweight	Age 2 -15 years 11-15 18% were obese	The difference between boys and girls is smaller but boys continue to be more overweight (17% vs. 15%) and be obese (20% vs. 16%)

Adapted from House of Common Library Research briefing paper on Obesity Statistics 16 March 2022. Available at: https://researchbriefings.files.parliament.uk/documents/SN03336/SN03336.pdf (accessed 3 October 2022)

*National Child Measurement Programme England, 2020/21 school year. **The Child Measurement Programme for Wales 2018/19. +Public Health Scotland (2021) term the rates as 'risk of obesity' rather than obese. ++Health Survey Northern Ireland (Department of Health, 2020).

NHS Digital (2017) reviews the evidence on the effects of obesity in childhood and suggests that children are more likely to miss schooling and have other health-related illnesses such as asthma, type 2 diabetes, cardiovascular disease and muscular skeletal disease, and that whilst the evidence is not conclusive that obesity impacts on a child's self-esteem, adolescents who are obese are more at risk of low self-regard and impaired quality of life. PHE states clearly that an obese or overweight child is more likely to become an obese adult with all the potential health risks. Another influence that is explored later in this chapter is that of food insecurity and the quality of food available to the family.

Social interaction and emotional warmth

Social interaction and emotional warmth are also important factors in promoting a child's health development. This is a difficult area to research because we cannot deliberately put a child in an environment that does not meet their needs, therefore research tends to be at the extremes, where the child demonstrates clear anti-social behaviours, or where there is extreme deprivation or abuse. Much of the work exploring emotional warmth has been around attachment, attachment theory and the study of children where attachment has been adversely affected, such as mothers with postnatal depression (PND). However, this is a difficult area to study because of many interlinked themes, such as:

- Parenting styles (high or low warmth, consistent parenting approach)
- Poverty
- Availability and type of social support

The evidence is growing that a child's resilience against adversity is influenced by the quality of care giving (Julian et al., 2017) and that where care giving is poor quality it increases the risk of disorganised attachment and relationships (Humphreys et al., 2022). The Department of Health's characterisation of good parenting in DCSF (2010) is old but still relevant:

> Good parenting involves caring for children's basic needs, keeping them safe, showing them warmth and love, and providing the stimulation needed for their development and to help them achieve their potential, within a stable environment where they experience consistent guidance. (Department for Children, Schools and Families (DCSF), 2010, p.2)

These characteristics of good parenting are reflected in the Assessment Framework (HM Government, 2018) above.

A child needs stability and an environment demonstrating love and security to be able to grow, develop and take advantage of experiences offered to them. A child who lacks a secure attachment is less likely to be able to form secure and meaningful relationships in later life. They also need to feel secure to be able to explore their environment and to try new experiences, as exploration develops a child's imagination, their inquisitiveness and ability to assess and manage risks (McCluskey and Robbins, 2009). McManus and Poehlmann's (2011) study explored the effect of maternal postnatal depression (PND) on the cognitive development of pre-term infants and found that infants' cognitive development was influenced in those whose mothers showed PND symptoms. The presence of PND symptoms at 9 months post-birth was associated with lower cognitive functioning at 16 months of age. Their study supports other studies that socioeconomic factors and maternal social support can mitigate the effects of PND.

Resilience

The concept of resilience explores whether building resilience within the child and/or family, by providing them with strategies or resources, could help them manage adverse life events. However, resilience is recognised as difficult to define. Joslyn (2016) suggests that it could be described as either a group of positive characteristics that individuals display even if they have experienced negative situations earlier in their life, or a level of competence gained and utilised even in times of great stress. Factors which can help resilience develop or not, include:

- Being secure – a physical (safe environment) and emotional feeling of safety
- The ability to develop and sustain social relationships which involves being able to negotiate and demonstrate empathy with others
- A positive view of themselves, feeling they have worth and can contribute to society

Promoting effective parenting programmes (1)

Furlong and McGilloway (2014) reviewed a parenting programme of children aged 3–8 years where the child was demonstrating 'anti-social behaviour' (though not defined) and how long its effects could be seen in families. For 14 weeks the parents attended sessions where trained facilitators worked with them to develop positive child–parent relationships through actions such as:

- Play
- Positive reinforcement – for example, praise and rewards
- Ignoring negative behaviours
- Operating 'time out' strategies

In these ways they provided a consistent approach for the child. The families were followed up at 6, 12 and 18 months post-intervention. They found that 18 months after the intervention the majority of parents were still able to use the interventions with good effect. Interestingly, the parents also reported positive outcomes around self-efficacy and self-empathy. They viewed themselves more positively, recognising that they could bring about a change in their child's behaviour, sometimes seeking appropriate help to do so – for example, contacting the school when the issue involved a teacher. However, many of the families did report relapses lasting between 2 and 4 months, linked to families not continuing with the parenting practices at stressful times – for example, pressures of work or family, bereavement and other negative factors relating to school, neighbourhood or having an uncooperative partner. Parents who then re-implemented the positive parenting plan reported an improvement in the child's behaviour. This study has limitations, particularly because the study group was small and may not have been representative or generalisable to older children.

Promoting effective parenting programmes (2)

'Minding the Baby' is a study conducted by the NSPCC in three locations in Scotland and the north of England. It utilises work undertaken in the USA and is based on attachment theory, that fostering good attachments will provide for the emotional and cognitive development of the child through attachment-based interdisciplinary home visiting from health visitors and social workers. The study faced recruitment challenges which means there are limitations on the conclusions. Whilst there was evidence of improved child behaviour at 2 years of age and improved maternal mental health, there were no significant differences in mothers' mental health or increase in parental sensitivity (Longhi et al., 2019).

However, a study in America using the same 'Minding the Baby' programme found mothers in the study group were more likely to show improved level of reflective functioning (mothers' ability to understand the infant behaviour in terms of emotions and mental state), whilst the infants were more likely to demonstrate secure attachments and less likely to be disorganised (Slade et al., 2020), but again sample size was small.

You may want to visit Ainsworth's work on the four types of primary attachment, explored in 'The Strange Situation Procedure' (Ainsworth et al., 1978).

ACTIVITY 12.3: REFLECTIVE PRACTICE

Review the video *Saving Brains, A Grand Challenge*, which explores how all these factors affect brain development.
    How can you:

* Ensure you maintain stimulation for children in hospital?
* Encourage parents to engage in stimulating their child?

Gertler et al. (2014) followed up the Saving Brains study 20 years later and found, significantly, that the earnings of the children in the stimulation group and nutritional and stimulation group were 25% higher than the control group and that they had caught up with the children in the comparison group, that of well-fed children. The Saving Brains programme is a partnership of a number of organisations that support projects in low- and middle-income countries to improve the health of children focusing on the following three areas: health, nutrition, and enrichment and protection.

ACTIVITY 12.4: REFLECTIVE PRACTICE

Visit the Saving Brains website to investigate some of the funded studies: www.grandchallenges.ca/programs/saving-brains/.

SAFEGUARDING STOP POINT

A lack of parenting capacity must always be assessed by considering safeguarding issues. Neglect is a form of abuse whether it is by deliberately withholding basic needs, warmth and love or where circumstances, such as lack of finance or knowledge, make it difficult to provide for these needs. However, that does raise the question, 'Who is the abuser, parents or society?'

ACTIVITY 12.5: CRITICAL THINKING

Review Samira's story presented in Scenario 12.1. What are the positive and negative factors that are influencing Jamila's ability to parent Samira?

FAMILY AND ENVIRONMENTAL FACTORS

The discussion above focuses on the relationship between parents and children, and the capacity of parents to nurture and respond to their child's developmental needs. We must acknowledge that children (and indeed their parents) do not exist within a softly cushioned vacuum. The Assessment Framework (HM Government, 2018) urges us to consider the impact that family, environment and society can have on parents, and consequently their child's development and wellbeing.

Family functioning

The role of the family in promoting a child's development and wellbeing is an important one. Non-statutory guidance for local authorities on parenting and family support makes the point that 'what happens within the family has more impact on children's wellbeing and development than any other single factor' (DCSF, 2010, pp.16–17). 'It is argued that the fundamental promotive experiences gained from parental nurturing and protection have life-long benefits including health, growth and increased learning' (Britto et al., 2017). Extensive research demonstrates that the quality of relationships between parents can have a positive effect on parenting, and directly results in improved outcomes for children (Coleman and Glen, 2009; Harold and Leve, 2012; Britto et al., 2017). Coleman and Glenn (2009) found that parents who experienced a happy and loving relationship together, promoted mental and physical health for all members of the family. Parents are role models and in a loving home, children learn how to relate to others, share, be kind, say sorry and manage conflict (DCSF, 2010). Conversely, children experiencing high levels of parental conflict can have increased anxiety, depression and even hostility and criminality (Harold and Leve, 2012). Close relationships with other family members can help children cope with family stress. Being able to talk about their feelings and knowing they are loved can help children deal with stressful family situations, with the added benefit of building resilience; giving them strategies to deal with stressful situations in the future.

SAFEGUARDING STOP POINT

Conflict is frequently hidden from the outside world, even from the family. It has been estimated that 1.6 million women and 695,000 men between the ages of 16 and 74 years experienced domestic abuse in the year ending March 2018 (Office for National Statistics, 2018). Phraseology has changed in recent years – with domestic 'abuse' being the preferable term as it acknowledges all forms of abuse. Further reading to raise your awareness of the signs and symptoms of domestic abuse or intimate partner violence (IPV) is recommended.

When children are admitted to hospital, diagnosed with a health problem or are living with a chronic and complex health need, this can often lead to acute and ongoing psychological stress for parents and other family members. In our nursing assessment and care of children and their families, we need to consider how parents are coping with their child's illness and their additional health needs. This includes being aware of signs of parental conflict, domestic abuse and as a result children/young people being exposed to domestic abuse.

The wider family

Parents and their children are influenced by members of their wider family. In today's society, it can be difficult to define exactly who 'the wider family' are – for example, grandparents, aunts, uncles, step-parents, half-siblings, neighbours, childminders and babysitters can all be thought of as part of the wider family. Each person, with their own family history and upbringing, can subsequently have positive and negative influences on parenting style, and on the decisions parents make about their child's health and wellbeing.

ACTIVITY 12.6: REFLECTIVE PRACTICE

Reflect and discuss with a practice assessor/supervisor or peers what influences:

- A parent's decision to immunise their child.
- How a parent disciplines their child.
- A parent's attitude towards their teenagers drinking alcohol.

Each parent's personal family history, their upbringing and relationships in addition to external factors such as education, money, society and the media may override our attempts to provide parents with the knowledge and skills they require to meet their child's needs. But by developing our knowledge and skills in forming therapeutic relationships with families we can begin to work in partnership to promote a parent's understanding about child development and wellbeing.

Poverty in the UK

The choice to have children has financial implications; most parents hope they can provide for and meet the needs of their child. For some, this equates to buying designer nappies, £1000 travel systems and intellectually stimulating toys that claim to nurture the inner Einstein in their offspring. For many other parents, however, ensuring the basic needs of food, warmth and shelter can be a daily struggle. Rising food, fuel and housing costs, increasing since the COVID pandemic, have pushed more and more households into poverty (Hill and Webber, 2022).

There are numerous definitions of – and opinions about – the concept of poverty. Townsend provided a useful definition in the 1970s, which is still relevant today:

> Individuals, families and groups in the population can be said to be in poverty when they lack resources to obtain the type of diet, participate in the activities and have the living conditions and amenities which are customary, or at least widely encouraged and approved, in the societies in which they belong. (Townsend, 1979, p.31)

In the UK, the concept of 'relative poverty' is used. A household is in relative poverty (also called relative low income) if their income is below 60% of the median household income. Because the government is measuring quality of living rather than earning power, incomes are measured after taxes and benefits (Full Fact, 2019).

It is disconcerting that employment is not a guaranteed route out of poverty. The Department of Work and Pensions (DWP, 2021) states that 75% of children growing up in poverty live in a family where at least one person works. This is known as 'in-work poverty' (DWP, 2021). The period following the COVID pandemic created a lack of stability in work; increasing low paid work, increased childcare costs and reduced benefit payments have put particular families at higher risk. Furthermore, children living in lone-parent, Bangladeshi, Pakistani and Black families and those families where there are three or more children are at a greater risk of being poor.

Child poverty

Child poverty has risen from 27% in 2013–2014 to 31% in 2019–20 (Joseph Rowntree Foundation, 2022a,b). This equates to nearly 1 in 3 children in the UK being classed as poor. Poverty impacts upon every aspect of a child's life, not least access to food, warmth and shelter.

Providing food – food insecurity

It is claimed that 75% of those visiting Food Banks (Bramley et al., 2021) are from low-income families and are subject to food insecurity, defined as 'a lack of regular access to enough safe and nutritious food for normal growth and development and an active and healthy life' (Food and Agricultural Organization of the United Nations, 2022). COVID accentuated already difficult circumstances for parents. A loss of income and caps on benefits (Rae and Carruthers, 2022), together with the added responsibility of feeding their family for the duration of the lockdown, prompted an 84% increase in the number of food parcels distributed by the Trussell Trust (Bramley et al., 2021).

A review of 109 papers seeking to discover the impact of food insecurity on children (Aceves-Martins et al., 2018) found that they had:

- higher rates of asthma, dental caries and hospitalisations
- poor social wellbeing, including poor social skills, lower happiness scores and lower life satisfaction scores
- lower reading and maths scores and lower school attendance resulting in reduced educational outcomes.

ACTIVITY 12.7: CRITICAL THINKING

If families are reliant on Food Banks and have a lack of control in the type of food they have:

- How do families ensure their children have a nutritious diet; one that will help them grow and develop? A diet that includes protein and iron, five fruit and veg per day, wholegrain carbohydrates, calcium-rich foods and healthy fats (British Dietetic Society, 2021).
- Think about the specific nutritional needs of the following groups and how Food Banks may or may not sufficiently meet their needs:
  - a weaning baby
  - a maturing adolescent
  - a child with an acute illness
  - a complex or continuing health need – when the need for a nutritious diet is even more important.

Providing warmth - fuel poverty

Due to the current rise in fuel costs, once families have paid their utility bills many will find themselves in relative poverty. The director of the institute of Health Inequity, Sir Michael Marmot, highlighted this year that 'millions of children face a humanitarian crisis of fuel poverty' (Marmot et al., 2022). Children living in cold accommodation are:

- twice as likely to suffer from respiratory problems such as asthma and bronchitis (Marmot Review Team, 2011)
- more likely to have colds or the flu – which in young children can cause serious illness (Public Health England and Institute of Health Equity, 2014)
- more likely, as infants to suffer poor weight gain using more calories to keep warm
- likely to have poor quality of sleep, slower developmental progress and a higher level of hospital admissions in the first 3 years of life (Marmot Review, 2010).

ACTIVITY 12.8: CRITICAL THINKING

Be mindful that children and young people with complex care needs may have higher fuel costs. For example, a child who

- is dependent on a NIPPY ventilator
- is incontinent, they may need frequent washes/baths and there may be an increase in amount of laundry.

Providing shelter - poor housing

It has been long recognised that poor housing has a detrimental effect on health. The National Children's Bureau (2016) highlights that households with dependent children are more likely than those without to live in private or social rented accommodation. The Department for Levelling Up, Housing and Communities (2022) identifies that social rented flats and bedsits are amongst some of the poorest quality housing in the UK, exposing low-income families and children to a higher rate of negative health consequences.

The UK housing charity Shelter (2013) published a key report that highlighted the impact that poor housing can have on children's physical and mental health, education and opportunities in adulthood. Many researchers since have added support to these findings (Bilal, 2022). Overcrowded and poor housing can:

- Increase the spread of infection, increasing susceptibility to respiratory problems, tuberculosis and meningitis
- Increase symptoms such as coughing and wheezing, leading to poor sleep, and slow growth
- Increase the risk of accidents, leading to long-term morbidity and disability
- Result in low school attendance due to increased illness and infections, in turn leading to delays in cognitive developmental and communication skills.

In our assessment of where a child and family live, we should use our knowledge of the geographical area, areas of wealth or deprivation, the location of social housing and available local services and amenities.

Each local authority and Integrated Care Board (ICB) now has the responsibility of carrying out a Joint Strategic Needs Assessment. This involves an assessment of the current and future health and social care needs of the local community, including wider factors that impact on their community's health and wellbeing, and local assets that can help to improve services and reduce inequalities. This information is of value to both acute and community-based children's nurses, enabling accurate assessment of the issues that may affect a child and family, and providing insight into local services that may offer support.

"When visiting one mother and child it was obvious this mother knew exactly what this child needed to be safe, e.g., baby gates on the stairs and locked kitchen cupboards so the child couldn't access them. However, every time the health visitor attended the house the mother hadn't put these in place. It then became apparent she couldn't afford to purchase these items and therefore was provided with help from the local children centre who helped her get all the necessary safety equipment for her child.

On a hospital placement after this, I saw multiple children who attended hospital with preventable falls and consumption of liquids/tablets they should not have taken. I then saw the importance of good education to children and parents as well as contacting health visitors to continue with the support and also sign-posting parents to other agencies who could the help them keep their children safe."

Sarah-Louise, 3rd-year nursing student

To conclude, the factors influencing children's health and wellbeing fall under three distinct headings:

- Children's growth and development
- Parenting capacity
- Social and environmental factors

However, these headings mask the complexity of the issues. Whilst for ease of reading these have been separated within the chapter, in truth they are interlinked and interdependent. As a children's nurse you must understand how these can impact on a family and tailor your care and advice to ensure these factors are considered. You need to be aware of how social policy decisions and service provision may help or hinder a child and family's health and wellbeing.

CHAPTER SUMMARY

- There are various definitions of health which are complex and ever-changing
- There are many factors that affect parenting which can impact on the health and wellbeing of a child and family due to the complex interaction of social factors
- Identifying positive coping strategies and protective factors can influence the development of children and families
- Resilience is a concept that needs caution in applying to children and young people

BUILD YOUR BIBLIOGRAPHY

Books

FURTHER READING

- Green, L. (2016) *Understanding the Life Course: Sociological and Psychological Perspectives.* Cambridge: Polity Press.

  The book discusses traditional theories surrounding child development and offers insight into the social and psychological issues that can impact upon the life course.
- Joslyn, E. (2016) *Resilience in Childhood: Perspective, Promise and Practice.* London: Palgrave.
- Zanni, L. (2021) *Human Kind: Resilience.* Braeside, VIC: Five Mile Books.

  This book for children analyses the concept of resilience, a topic of scholarly interest for several decades. Part One introduces the concept. Part Two explores theory and research of the topic. Part Three considers the practical applications.
- Lundgaard, P. (2018) *Developing Resilience in Children and Young people: A Practical Guide.* London: Routledge.

  A discussion of the complexities and determinants of health and the need for nurses to understand and engage with health policy.

Journal articles

FURTHER READING: ONLINE JOURNAL ARTICLES

- Moore, C. (2019) 'Resilience theory: a summary of the research'. *Positive Psychology,* https://positivepsychology.com/resilience-theory/ (accessed 20 February 2023).

  This article summarises the development of risk and resilience theory to date and what it offers to our understanding of how families manage the complex nature of their lives.
- Gartland, D., Riggs, E., Muyeen, S. et al (2019) 'What factors are associated with resilient outcomes in children exposed to social adversity?' *BMJ Open,* 9 (4): 024870 (published online 11 April 2019).

  The article highlights many of the theories that seek to discover how the family unit works, factors affecting family functioning (including socio-economic inequalities), and how child health and development can be supported by the family.

Weblinks

FURTHER READING: WEBLINKS

- The Children's Society, *The Good Childhood Report* www.childrenssociety.org.uk/sites/default/files/TheGoodChildhoodReport2015.pdf Children identify what are important influences in their lives. We need to understand what key worries for the children in our care are, so we can ensure we tailor care packages that meet these needs.
- Centre on the Developing Child Resilience www.developingchild.harvard.edu
- Extend your knowledge on the effects of domestic abuse on children and families by reviewing some of the available government literature: HM Government (2021) *Tackling Violence Against Women and Girls: A guide to good practice communication.* www.gov.uk
- This factsheet outlines some of the areas you need to consider in your assessment of parenting capacity: www.nspcc.org.uk/globalassets/documents/information-service/factsheet-assessing-parenting-capacity.pd:
- Read the definitions of poverty: The Poverty Site, *Relative Poverty, Absolute Poverty and Social Exclusion* www.poverty.org.uk/summary/social%20exclusion.shtml
- Review some of the Saving Brains projects: www.grandchallenges.ca/programs/saving-brains/ www.grandchallenges.ca/programs/saving-brains/

REFERENCES

Aceves-Martins, M., Cruickshank, M., Fraser, C. and Brazzelli, M. (2018) *Child Food Insecurity: A Rapid Review*. Southampton (UK): NIHR Journals Library; 2018 Nov. PMID: 30475559. Available at: www.ncbi.nlm.nih.gov/books/NBK533784/ (accessed 26 October 2022).

Ainsworth, M.D.S., Blehar, M.C., Waters, E., and Wall, S. (1978) *Patterns of Attachment: a Psychological Study of the Strange Situation*. Hillsdale, NJ: Erlbaum.

Bilal, N. (2022) 'Does poor quality housing impact on child health? Evidence from the social housing sector in Avon, UK'. *Journal of Environmental Psychology*, 82: 1–10.

Bramley, G., Treanor, M., Sosenko, F. and Littlewood, M. (2021) *State of Hunger. Building the evidence on poverty, destitution and food insecurity in the UK: Year Two Main Report*. The Trussell Trust. Available at: www.trusselltrust.org/wp-content/uploads/sites/2/2021/05/State-of-Hunger-2021-Report-Final.pdf (accessed 24 October 2022).

British Dietetic Society (2021) Healthy Eating for Children: Food Fact Sheet. Available at: www.bda.uk.com/resource/healthy-eating-for-children.html (accessed 26 October 2022).

Britto, P.R., Lye, S.J., Proulx, K., Yousafzai, A.K., Matthews, S.G., Vaivada, T., Perez-Escamilla, R., Rao, N., Ip, P., Fernald, L.C.H., MacMillan, H., Hanson, M., Wachs, T.D., Yao, H., Yoshikawa, H., Cerezo, A., Leckman, J.F., Bhutta, Z.A. and the Early Childhood Development Interventions Review Group, for the Lancet Early Childhood Development Series Steering Committee (2017) 'Nurturing care: promoting early childhood development'. *Lancet* 389 (10064): 91–102.

Children's Society (2022) www.childrenssociety.org.uk/sites/default/files/2022-09/GCR-2022-Full-Report.pdf (accessed 5 July 2023).

Coleman, L. and Glenn, G. (2009) *When Couples Part: Understanding the Consequences for Adults and Children*. London: One Plus One.

Department for Children, Schools and Families (DCSF) (2010) *Parenting and Family Support: Guidance for Local Authorities in England*. London: DCSF.

Department of Health (2020) Health survey Northern Ireland: first results 2019/20. Available at: www.health-ni.gov.uk/publications/health-survey-northern-ireland-first-results-201920 (accessed 5 July 2023).

Department for Levelling Up, Housing and Communities and Clark, G. (2022) New standards for rented homes under consideration. [Press Release] Available at: www.gov.uk/government/news/new-standards-for-rented-homes-under-consideration (accessed 27 October 2022).

Department for Work and Pensions (2021) Households below average income: an analysis of the income distribution FYE 1995 to FYE 2020. Available at: www.gov.uk/government/statistics/households-below-average-income-for-financial-years-ending-1995-to-2020/households-below-average-income-an-analysis-of-the-income-distribution-fye-1995-to-fye-2020 (accessed 26 October 2022).

Food and Agricultural Organization of the United Nations (2022) Hunger and food insecurity. Available at: www.fao.org/hunger/en/ (accessed 24 October 2022).

Full Fact (2019) *Poverty in the UK: A Guide to the Facts and Figures*. Available at: https://fullfact.org/economy/poverty-uk-guide-facts-and-figures/ (accessed 24 October 2022).

Furlong M. and McGilloway, S. (2014) 'The longer term experiences of parent training: a qualitative analysis'. *Child Care, Health and Development*, 41 (5): 687–96.

Gertler, P., Heckman, J., Pinto, R., Zanolini, A., Vermeersch, C., Walker, S., Chang, S.M. and McGregor S.G. (2014) 'Labor market returns to an early childhood stimulation intervention in Jamaica'. *Science*, 344 (6187): 998–1001.

Harold, G.T and Leve, L.D. (2012) 'Parents as partners: How the parental relationship affects children's psychological development', in A. Balfour, M. Morgan and C. Vincent (eds), *How Couple*

Relationships Shape Our World: Clinical practice, research, and policy perspectives. London: Routledge (e-book 2019).

Hill, K. and Webber, R. (2022) *From Pandemic to Cost of Living Crisis: Low-Income Families in Challenging Times.* York: The Joseph Rowntree Foundation.

HM Government (2018) *Working Together to Safeguard Children: A Guide to Inter-agency Working to Safeguard and Promote the Welfare of Children.* London: DfE. Available at: https://assets.publishing.service.gov.uk/government/uploads/system/uploads/attachment_data/file/942454/Working_together_to_safeguard_children_inter_agency_guidance.pdf (accessed 27 September 2022).

Humphreys, K.L., King, L.S., Guyon-Harris, K.L. and Zeanah, C.H. (2022) 'Caregiver regulation: a modifiable target promoting resilience to early adverse experiences'. *Psychological Trauma: Theory, Research, Practice, and Policy*, 14(S1), S63–S71. Available at https://doi.org/10.1037/tra0001111 (accessed 3 October 2022).

Iacovou, M. and Sevilla-Sanz, A. (2010) *The Effect of Breastfeeding on Children's Cognitive Development.* Colchester: Institute for Social and Economic Research. Available at: www.iser.essex.ac.uk/research/publications/working-papers/iser/2010-40 (accessed 17 May 2017).

Joseph Rowntree Foundation (2022a) Overall UK Poverty Rates. Available at: www.jrf.org.uk/data/overall-uk-poverty-rates#:~:text=Child%20poverty%20continues%20to%20rise,of%20those%20in%20couple%20families (accessed 24 October 2022).

Joseph Rowntree Foundation (2022b) UK Poverty 2022: The essential guide to understanding poverty in the UK. Executive summary. Available at: www.jrf.org.uk/report/uk-poverty-2022 (accessed 27 October 2022).

Joslyn, E. (2016) *Resilience in Childhood: Perspective, Promise and Practice.* London: Palgrave.

Julian, M. M., Lawler, J. M. and Rosenblum, K.L. (2017) 'Caregiver-child relationships in early childhood: interventions to promote well-being and reduce risk for psychopathology'. *Current Behavioral Neuroscience Reports*, 4: 87–98. Available at: https://link.springer.com/article/10.1007/s40473-017-0110-0 (accessed 3 October 2022).

Katz, S., Lee, T. and Byrne, S. (2015) 'Predicting parent–child differences in perceptions of how children use the Internet for help with homework, identity development, and health information'. *Journal of Broadcasting and Electronic Media*, 59 (4): 574–602.

Longhi, E., Murray, L., Wellsted, D., Hunter, R., MacKenzie, K., Taylor-Colls, S., Fonagy, P. and Fearon, P. (2019) Minding the Baby (MTB) home-visiting programme for vulnerable young mothers: results of a randomised controlled trial in the UK. London: NSPCC. Available at https://psycnet.apa.org/doiLanding?doi=10.1037%2Ftra0001111 (accessed 3 October 2022).

Marmot, M., Sinha, I. and Lee, A. (2022) 'Millions of children face a "humanitarian crisis" of fuel poverty'. *British Medical Journal*, 378:o2129. Available at: www.bmj.com/content/378/bmj.o2129 (accessed 26 October 2022).

Marmot Review (2010) *Fair Society, Healthy Lives.* Available at: www.parliament.uk/globalassets/documents/fair-society-healthy-lives-full-report.pdf (accessed 26 October 2022).

Marmot Review Team (2011) *The Health Impacts of Cold Homes and Fuel Poverty.* Friends of the Earth and The Marmot Review Team. Available at: www.instituteofhealthequity.org/resources-reports/the-health-impacts-of-cold-homes-and-fuel-poverty

Martens, P.J. (2012) 'What do Kramer's Baby-Friendly Hospital Initiative PROBIT studies tell us? A review of a decade of research'. *Journal of Human Lactation*, 28 (3): 335–42.

McCluskey, H. and Robbins M. (2009) 'Safeguarding children', in A. Glasper, G. McEwing and J. Richardson (eds), *Foundation Studies for Caring.* Basingstoke: Palgrave Macmillan.

McManus, B.M. and Poehlmann, J. (2011) 'Maternal depression and perceived social support as predictors of cognitive function trajectories during the first 3 years of life for preterm infants in Wisconsin'. *Child: Care, Health and Development*, 38 (3): 425–34.

Myant, K.A. and Williams, J.M. (2005) 'Children's concepts of health and illness: understanding of contagious illnesses, non-contagious illnesses and injuries'. *Journal of Health Psychology*, 10 (6): 805–19.

National Children's Bureau (2016) Housing and the Health of Young Children. Policy and evidence briefing for the VCSE sector. London: NCB. Available at: www.ncb.org.uk/sites/default/files/uploads/files/Housing%2520and%2520the%2520Health%2520of%2520Young%2520Children.pdf (accessed 27 October 2022).

NHS Digital (2017) Health Survey for England 2017 Adult and child overweight and obesity. Available at: http://healthsurvey.hscic.gov.uk/media/78619/HSE17-Adult-Child-BMI-rep.pdf (accessed 5 July 2023).

Office for National Statistics (2018) Domestic abuse: Findings from the Crime Survey for England and Wales: year ending March 2018. Available at: https://backup.ons.gov.uk/wp-content/uploads/sites/3/2018/11/Domestic-abuse-findings-from-the-Crime-Survey-for-England-and-Wales-year-ending-March-2018.pdf (accessed 24 October 2022).

Office for National Statistics (2020) Children's views on well-being and what makes a happy life: UK 2020. Available at: www.ons.gov.uk/peoplepopulationandcommunity/wellbeing/articles/children sviewsonwellbeingandwhatmakesahappylifeuk2020/2020-10-02#main-points (accessed 3 October 2022).

Petherick, A. (2010) 'Development: mother's milk: a rich opportunity'. *Nature*, 468: S5–7.

Public Health England and Institute of Health Equity (2014) Local action on health inequalities: Fuel poverty and cold-home related health problems. UCL Institute of Health Equity. Available at: https://assets.publishing.service.gov.uk/government/uploads/system/uploads/attachment_data/file/355790/Briefing7_Fuel_poverty_health_inequalities.pdf (accessed 26 October 2022).

Public Health Scotland (2021) Primary 1 Body Mass Index (BMI) statistics. Scotland School year 2020 to 2021. Available at: https://publichealthscotland.scot/publications/primary-1-body-mass-index-bmi-statistics-scotland/primary-1-body-mass-index-bmi-statistics-scotland-school-year-2020-to-2021/ (accessed 3 October 2022).

Rae, M. and Carruthers, J. (2022) 'Childhood poverty is rising in the UK, but the government continue to ignore it'. *British Medical Journal*, 377:o872. www.bmj.com/content/377/bmj.o872. publication

Royal College of Nursing (RCN) (2012) *Health Inequalities and the Social Determinants of Health*. London: RCN.

SACN & RCPCH (Scientific Advisory Committee on Nutrition and the Royal College of Paediatrics and Child Health) (2012) Defining child underweight, overweight and obesity in the UK. Available at: https://assets.publishing.service.gov.uk/government/uploads/system/uploads/attachment_data/file/339411/SACN_RCPCH_defining_child_underweight__overweight_and_obesity_in_the_UK_2012.pdf (accessed 3 October 2022).

Shelter (2013) *Chance of a Lifetime: The impact of bad housing on children's lives*. Available at: https://assets.ctfassets.net/6sxvmndnpn0s/4LTXp3mya7IigRmNG8x9KK/6922b5a4c6ea756ea94da71ebdc001a5/Chance_of_a_Lifetime.pdf (accessed 24 October 2022).

Slade, A., Holland, M., Ordway, M., Carlson, E., Jeon, S., Close, N. et al. (2020) 'Minding the Baby®: Enhancing parental reflective functioning and infant attachment in an attachment-based, interdisciplinary home visiting program'. *Development and Psychopathology*, 32 (1): 123–37.

Townsend, P. (1979) *Poverty in the United Kingdom*. London: Allen Lane.

Toyama. N. (2016) 'Adults' explanations and children's understanding of contagious illnesses, non-contagious illnesses, and injuries'. *Early Child Development and Care*, 186 (4): 526–43.

UNICEF (2013) *The Evidence and Rationale for the UNICEF UK Baby Friendly Initiative Standards*. Available at: www.unicef.org.uk/wp-content/uploads/sites/2/2013/09/baby_friendly_evidence_rationale.pdf (accessed 17 May 2017).

UNICEF UK (2017) *Guide to the UNICEF UK Baby Friendly Initiative Standards*. Available at www.ons. gov.uk/peoplepopulationandcommunity/wellbeing/articles/childrensviewsonwellbeingandwhatm akesahappylifeuk2020/2020-10-02#main-points (accessed 3 October 2022).

World Health Organization (WHO) (1948) *Preamble to the Constitution of the World Health Organization as adopted by the International Health Conference*, New York, 19–22 June 1946.

World Health Organization (WHO) (1986) *The Ottawa Charter for Health Promotion*. First International Conference on Health Promotion, Ottawa, 21 November 1986. Available at: www.who.int/ healthpromotion/conferences/previous/ottawa/en (accessed 17 May 2017).

World Health Organization (WHO) (2003) *Global Strategy for Infant and Young Child Feeding*. Available at: www.who.int/nutrition/topics/global_strategy/en (accessed 17 May 2017).

UNIVERSAL SCREENING AND THE ROLE OF THE HEALTH VISITOR

13

MANDY BRIMBLE AND SARAH REDDINGTON-BOWES

THIS CHAPTER COVERS

- The role of the health visitor
- The value of universal screening and the evidence that underpins practice
- Universal screening programmes in the UK
- How screening activities are used to monitor development and promote health

"A popular perception is that health visitors drink cups of tea and weigh babies. That's certainly all I knew about the service."

Terry, 2nd-year children's nursing student

INTRODUCTION

Many children's nursing students undertake a health visitor placement, so understanding their role is important for improving your own practice and gaining an appreciation of the difference they make to children and families. The quotation above from a 2nd-year nursing student is typical, not only of nursing students but also the general public. Health visiting is so much more than this and is a highly skilled role. It is a role that adapts to ongoing situations. For example, during the lockdowns of the COVID-19 pandemic modes of contact such as telephone and video calling were used to deliver the health visiting services alongside the traditional home visiting model. This chapter will outline how health visitors carry out universal screening programmes in the UK, together with the evidence that underpins them. Case studies are used to bring practice to life and to highlight typical issues and interventions. Working in partnership with parents is essential for successful relationships which benefit the child and family.

SEE ALSO
CHAPTER 7

THE ROLE OF THE HEALTH VISITOR

The work of health visitors is embedded in public health and reflects its history, which began in 1862 when the Manchester and Salford Ladies Sanitary Reform Association decided to employ 'sanitary visitors' to offer practical help, advice and health education in people's homes (Adams, 2012). This primary focus on public health makes it unique among the caring professions (Malone et al., 2003 in Baldwin, 2012) and, in fact, the formal title of a health visitor is 'specialist community public health nurse' (SCPHN). The principles of health visiting underpin the work of the profession and are:

- The search for health needs
- The stimulation of an awareness of health needs
- The influence on policies affecting health
- The facilitation of health enhancing activities (Cowley and Frost, 2006, p.1)

The first two points mean that health visitors carry out assessments to determine the health needs of children and families and in some cases highlight that a need exists – some families may be unaware that they have a health need if their upbringing, culture or outlook normalises something which is detrimental to their health. The third principle applies to all nurses. However, health visitors are autonomous and closely linked to communities so they have first-hand, detailed knowledge of the needs of local populations. They have, therefore, a key role in responding to government consultation documents and may be involved in lobbying for change which promotes health. The final principle involves instigating activities which promote health – for example, baby massage classes which promote parent–child attachment, parenting groups and postnatal depression support groups. The principles of health visiting (Cowley and Frost, 2006) have been identified as being as relevant today as when they were first set out in the 1970s (Clark, 2020).

To qualify as a health visitor, registered nurses undertake an intensive and rigorously assessed year-long programme of academic study and practice placement (Nursing and Midwifery Council, 2022). They are knowledgeable in all aspects of child and maternal health and are skilled communicators with excellent interpersonal skills (Robinson, 2016). Their role requires tact and diplomacy whilst being assertive and upholding the primary principle of the Children Act 1989 – that is, the welfare of the child is paramount. Whilst health visiting practice is highly autonomous, health visitors are an integral part of the primary care multidisciplinary team, and partnership working with colleagues across health and social care is essential (Holland et al., 2022).

Health visiting is a universal service (offered to all). Universalistic services are effective in reaching those who do not identify their own needs or are reluctant/unable to take up services. This is especially important as these sections of the population are usually those in most need (Black, 1980). Most health visitors work with families who have children aged 0–5 years, although there are roles that cover specific conditions like diabetes and population groups such as travelling families. Health visitors often work with families for a long time, sometimes over a decade depending on the spacing between births and circumstances. The strength of this relationship is indicated by Terry's thoughts below.

"The relationships that the health visitor had built over the years in the community were formidable."

Terry, 2nd-year children's nursing student

The service is highly valued by parents and a real lifeline in times of crisis, as shown by the quotation below. This was a mother's response when asked, 'What is a health visitor?'

"I was lost and in a scary place and my health visitor was the rock I needed to help guide me ..."

Child, Unite/CPHVA Twitter feed, 12 July 2016

THE VALUE OF UNIVERSAL SCREENING AND THE EVIDENCE THAT UNDERPINS PRACTICE

SEE ALSO
CHAPTER 14

Universal screening is the main way in which health visitors fulfil many of the principles outlined above. The purpose of screening is to monitor children's health and development and detect early on deviations from normal development or physical abnormalities (Lipkin and Macias, 2020). The regular contact with children and families provided by screening programmes is also used to promote health and wellbeing (Emond, 2019). There is evidence that these activities significantly improve long-term health, social and educational outcomes for the individual child, communities and the nation (Marmot, 2010).

Much of the knowledge underpinning screening activities has been provided by David Hall and David Elliman in their series of publications (1989–2003), commonly referred to as 'The Hall Report'. The fourth edition (Hall and Elliman, 2003) was controversial because it suggested a more targeted approach whereby health visiting was primarily offered to those in most need. This would have fundamentally changed the universal nature of the service and was met with strong opposition by health visitors at that time. As well as moving away from the universal nature of the service, health visitors and other health professionals were concerned that it would be difficult to identify those most in need without universal screening (illustrated by the case study of Angharad later). There was much debate about this in 2003, and more recently. The potential impact of this was researched (see 'What's the evidence?' below). The lessons learned from this and similar research on an international level presented by Emond (2019) has led to the graded levels of service set out in the Healthy Child Programme (see 'Theory stop point' below) which is underpinned by Key Performance Indicators in relation to the core contacts offered to families in the four countries of the UK.

All families continue to be allocated a health visitor but the level of need is identified at the start of the child's life and regularly reviewed via the Family Health Needs Assessment, discussed in more depth later.

WHAT'S THE EVIDENCE?

King (2015) examined health visitors' accounts of the impact of 'Hall 4' (Hall and Elliman, 2003) on their practice and profession. The trigger for the study was health visitors' strong reaction to the major change in service delivery. This was a qualitative study which used interviews to collect data and found that the implementation of 'Hall 4' had impacted negatively on health visiting practice and morale. The researcher concluded that health visitors play a crucial role in policy implementation and their feelings can shape how families experience the service. Recommendations were made to engage health visitors in consultations about changes to policy.

- What do you think may be the consequences of targeted rather than universal health visiting practice?

UNIVERSAL SCREENING PROGRAMMES IN THE UK

Universal screening activities are delivered via a variety of frameworks across the UK. These differ slightly due to devolved government in Wales, Scotland and Northern Ireland. In England, the Healthy Child Programme sets out the screening activities and developmental checks undertaken by the health visitor (Department of Health (DH), 2009) and the Healthy Child Wales Programme (Welsh Government, 2016) is similarly configured. In England there is also an intensive visiting model call the Family Nurse Partnership. Similarly, the significant challenges of child poverty in some areas of Wales have been recognised by the Welsh Government which has invested in Flying Start programmes (Welsh Government, 2016) that aim to enhance life chances for children living in deprived circumstances. In Scotland, the framework is The Scottish Child Health Programme (NHS National Services Scotland, 2015). Northern Ireland also has its own version of the Healthy Child Programme, called Healthy Child, Healthy Future (Department of Health, Social Services and Patient Safety Northern Ireland, 2010). All four of these frameworks include fundamental visits such as the new birth visit (10–14 days post-delivery) and development checks (at ages predetermined by each framework). The case studies used in this chapter relate to universal screening activities carried out as part of these frameworks. These (fictitious) case studies are not framed within any particular country of the UK, as the principles of health visiting are central to practice, whichever framework is used. This chapter is structured around these case studies to demonstrate universal screening in action. The 12-month review is covered in most depth as this is considered the end of infancy, the period in which the most dramatic trajectories of growth and development occur (Sharma et al., 2022). Many aspects of this assessment apply to other developmental checks.

ACTIVITY 13.1: EVIDENCE-BASED PRACTICE

Read the Marmot Review, *Fair Society, Healthy Lives* (2010) and write a brief summary of the report and how it will impact on your practice.

Family health needs assessment

As part of the Healthy Child Programme, health visitors complete a robust Family Health Needs Assessment (FHNA) with each family for each new birth. This occurs sometime between the 28th and 36th weeks of the antenatal period and the New Birth Visit, which is conducted 10–14 days post-delivery. This assessment may also be completed at the 6/8 week contact if appropriate.

A needs assessment by health visitors is a continuing process and is essential to home visiting and the professional–client relationship. It can be commenced at the antenatal contact and completed by the 6/8 contact to account for changes that are occurring within the family unit. The main skills and knowledge required for making these assessments and professional judgements are observation, empathy, application of knowledge and highly developed interpersonal skills (Cowley et al., 2015). The FHNA should therefore be reviewed by the health visiting team at every contact and/or change in family dynamics. The contact is preferably face to face and in the new parent's home. The health visitor promotes sensitive parenting to include sustaining good emotional care and good mother–father–infant relationships, relationship development with the practitioner and a thorough assessment of growth and development in the infant. The family situation is assessed in order to decide the most appropriate service provision – the categories are fully explained in the 'Theory stop point' below and represent a combination of universal and targeted services once the level of need has been assessed.

THEORY STOP POINT: FOUR LEVELS OF HEALTH VISITING SERVICE

Health visiting teams offer four levels of service to families with children under 5:

Your community offers a range of services, including children's centre services and the services families and communities provide for themselves. Health visitors work to develop these and make sure local families know about them.

Universal services from the health visitor team working with GPs to ensure that families can access the Healthy Child Programme, that parents are supported at key times and have access to a range of community services.

Universal plus offers a rapid response from the local health visiting team when specific expert help is needed – for example, because of postnatal depression, a sleepless baby, weaning or concerns about parenting.

Universal partnership plus provides ongoing support from the health visiting team and a range of local services to deal with more complex issues over a period of time. These include services from children's centres, other community services including charities and, where appropriate, the Family Nurse Partnership. Social care services are also available as are specialist support services for children with disabilities.

Source: Adapted from *Health Visitor Implementation Plan 2011-15* (Department of Health, 2011)

Table 13.1 shows the 4, 5, 6 health visiting model (Public Health England (PHE), 2018) which includes the 4-level service model outlined above, the 5 mandated visits within the Healthy Child Programme, England, and the 6 high-impact areas of the model together with the underpinning aims of this approach.

Table 13.1 4, 5, 6 health visiting model (PHE, 2018)

4-level service model	5 mandated elements	6 high-impact areas
• Your community • Universal • Universal plus • Partnership plus	• Antenatal health-promoting visits • New baby review • 6-8-week assessment • 1-year assessment • 2-2 ½ year review	• Transition to parenthood and the early weeks • Maternal (perinatal) mental health • Breastfeeding • Healthy weight • Managing minor illness and reducing accidents • Health, wellbeing of child aged 2 and support to be 'ready for school'
Improved access Improved experience Improved outcomes Reduced health inequalities		

Used with permission under the terms of the Open Government-licence.

HOW SCREENING ACTIVITIES ARE USED TO MONITOR DEVELOPMENT AND PROMOTE HEALTH

The 12-month review

Health visitors in England and Scotland conduct developmental assessments at 12 months and 2–2½ years (these are two of the five 'core' contacts in England and two of the 11 'core' contacts in Scotland). These contacts give the practitioner an opportunity to further explore the dynamics within a family, revisit the FHNA, assess the growth and development of the child against evidence-based assessment tools – for example, Mary Sheridan (Sharma et al., 2022), Denver Developmental Screening Test (Frankenburg and Dodds, 1967), Ages and Stages Questionnaire [ASQ] (Brookes, 2021) and Schedule of Growing Skills [SOGS] (GL Assessment, 2015). During these visits, routine assessments of parental mental health and wellbeing are also made.

The 12-month review should take place in a mutually agreed venue such as a clinic, children's centre, nursery or the child's home. Both parents are encouraged to attend and participate in the review, giving them time to discuss their concerns and aspirations for their child. If the parents do not accept the invitation, a second appointment will be sent. If the family fail to attend a second time, where there are concerns regarding the child's social or medical development or evidence of poor engagement with services, the health visitor is responsible for contacting the family to decide future action. This may be in liaison with members of the team or other relevant agencies.

The 12-month review is a face-to-face contact with a child to systematically assess growth, social and emotional development and detect possible abnormalities; while reviewing the family's strengths, needs and risks. This will include actions to address any needs identified and agreeing future contact with the service.

This review aims to:

- Improve emotional and social wellbeing
- Improve learning, speech and language development
- Ensure early detection of and action to address developmental delay or abnormalities, ill health and growth impairments
- Maximise protection against communicable disease
- Prevent obesity and promote healthy behaviours

- Reduce the adverse impact on the child of poor parenting, disruptive family relationships, domestic violence, mental health issues and substance abuse
- Address parental concerns
- Review immunisation status
- Raise awareness of dental health and prevention, and give advice about healthy weaning, portion sizes, types of food and meal-time routines, feeding cups, Healthy Start and vitamin supplements, obesity risk factors and iron deficiency
- Give practical advice about sensitive parenting, healthy sleep practices and managing crying
- Promote age-appropriate local activities
- Raise awareness of injury and accident prevention, including car safety
- Review the health needs of the family, give advice about smoking cessation and preventing inhalation of second-hand smoke
- Promote interaction between parent and child via reading through the Bookstart scheme (see www.bookstart.org.uk)
- Raise awareness of skin cancer prevention
- Discuss as appropriate referral of families whose first language is not English to relevant local services

There are many competencies required to undertake this and other developmental and family assessments. Practitioners are expected to be trained in and have an understanding of child development and of factors that influence health and wellbeing. This knowledge needs to be applied so that health visitors can recognise the range of normal development and identify deviations from it, together with possible causes. Practical skills such as being adept at using scales, measuring length and head circumference and completing growth charts are essential for the accurate recording of measurements. In addition, practitioners need consultation skills, purposeful listening skills and an ability to use guiding questions (motivational interviewing skills) in order to interact and gain maximum benefit from the contact for the parents of the child. Knowledge of care pathways, the Common Assessment Framework, safeguarding, child protection procedures and an awareness of domestic abuse/intimate partner violence risks are also key to the role as this will enable identification of major stressors and risks in a timely manner.

CASE STUDY 13.1: BEAU

Teenage parents Jade and John have been invited to an appointment for Beau's 12-month review at the local children's centre. The appointment is sent well in advance. The health visitor, Sally, sent a reminder text to Jade's mobile phone the day before. There was no response. On the morning of the appointment neither Jade nor John attend with their daughter, Beau.

Sally decided to complete an opportunistic home visit rather than invite them to another appointment because the parents had not brought Beau to clinic or been seen for some time. When Sally visited, she found Jade to be at home with Beau. Jade let Sally in and disclosed that her relationship with John had broken down. She was in debt and felt very low. Sally was able to actively listen to Jade, complete a mood assessment and signpost Jade to the local Depression and Anxiety service. Sally offered weekly listening visits whilst Jade awaited the appointment. Jade was encouraged to access the children's centre to support her in managing debt and to socialise with other mums.

Beau was assessed as meeting her developmental milestones and her growth was satisfactory. Sally offered visits by the community nursery nurse to support the relationship between Jade and Beau. Sally decided to defer some of the health promotion activities usually carried out during the 12-month review until future visits because she wanted to prioritise Jade's mental health and her relationship with Beau.

- How is health promotion defined by the World Health Organization?
- List the health promotion activities usually carried out at the 12-month review.

SEE ALSO
CHAPTER 11

Being flexible: Being truly needs led

There may be many occasions when health visitors need to defer matters until another visit. In some instances this may be to prioritise another health need as described in the case study above. It could also be that the main purpose for the visit – for example, a developmental check – is temporarily put on hold if there is a crisis occurring at the time of the visit. There would be little point in pressing on with a development check if the parents/carers are experiencing a highly stressful situation such as eviction or disconnection of utility services. Similarly, efforts to promote health by encouraging smoking cessation may fall on deaf ears if the parent is using smoking as a stress reliever. Decisions to delay activities which are a key part of a screening activity must be taken carefully and not suspended indefinitely; otherwise the welfare of the child may be compromised. However, even when universal screening is carried out in line with local frameworks, issues can arise. The section below describes such an instance.

The two-and-a-half year review

Many developmental review frameworks include an assessment at around the age of 2½ years. Since many children start school soon after this time the term 'school readiness' is often used (UNICEF, 2012) to describe what is being assessed. This is an area where early years practitioners can have a significantly positive effect on outcomes for children who are vulnerable and living in disadvantaged circumstances (Ofsted, 2014). There is no national definition of school readiness but in the Ofsted (2014) document *Are You Ready?* a primary school teacher suggests that the child should:

- Be able to separate from their parent/carer
- Demonstrate listening skills – that is, show interest and pay attention
- Have sufficient language to express their needs
- Say their name, age and something about their family
- Be able to interact with an adult
- Be able to interact with their peers – for example, take turns in play
- Take responsibility for their actions
- Show interest in what is around them
- Notice things and ask questions
- Hold a book
- Understand the narrative of an age-appropriate book
- Respond to boundary setting

The case study below outlines issues identified during a 2½ year review.

CASE STUDY 13.2: ANGHARAD

Angharad is 2½. She lives in a deprived area with her mother, Sian, and sibling, Tom, aged 9. Angharad was last reviewed by the health visitor, Jane, when she was aged 18 months. At that time her development was satisfactory. At the 2½ review Angharad's development is significantly delayed. She says very few words. She grunts and points to make herself understood but she appears to understand what is asked of her. Her fine motor skills development is delayed; she is unable to hold a pen and is still using a 'palmar grasp' to pick up small objects, rather than the 'pincer grasp' expected at age 2½-3 years (Sharma et al., 2022). Her gross motor skills are also delayed. The health visitor discusses her concerns with Sian. She is mindful of using a non-judgemental and supportive approach. Sian is unconcerned, stating that Angharad is lazy. However, she agrees to referrals to the community paediatrician and speech and language therapist (SALT). Jane discusses ways in which Sian and Tom can encourage Angharad's speech development in the meantime.

The community paediatrician advises Jane that her assessment identified global developmental delay due to insufficient stimulation.

Sian does not take Angharad to the SALT appointment. The SALT offers another appointment but they do not attend this either. Sian tells Jane that she doesn't see the point as she is not worried about Angharad's speech.

- Explain the value of universal services in this case study.
- Why is a non-judgemental and supportive approach essential when working with families who have failed to meet their child's needs?

This case study shows that parents are not always willing to work in partnership with the health visitor, even when a need has been clearly identified. In some cases this may be a minor issue. In others it may present a real cause for concern about the wellbeing of the child.

SEE ALSO
CHAPTER 9

SAFEGUARDING STOP POINT

Physical, sexual and emotional abuse together with neglect and fabricated illness are categories of abuse (HM Government, 2018).

Based on the circumstances outlined above it could be argued that Sian has neglected Angharad and continues to do so by not attending appointments. Neglect is defined by the NSPCC (2021) as 'the ongoing failure to meet a child's basic needs'. Although Angharad has her food, shelter and clothing needs met, other basic needs identified in the UN Convention on the Rights of the Child (United Nations, 1989) are lacking. Keeping in mind the primary principle of the Children Act 1989 that the welfare of the child is paramount, if this situation continues or deteriorates, the health visitor may need to escalate the matter so that further support can be provided.

CHAPTER SUMMARY

- Evidence exists to underpin universal screening activities for the under-5s and the role of the health visitor in implementing evidence-based frameworks
- Universal screening provision in the UK is wide ranging and these activities are used to monitor development and promote health
- Universal screening is used to identify level of need and facilitate appropriate targeted interventions
- The role and responsibilities of the health visitor are diverse and are much more than drinking tea and weighing babies
- Health visitors work in collaboration with other professionals and services to ensure health and wellbeing for children and families

BUILD YOUR BIBLIOGRAPHY

Books

- Burrows, P. and Cowie, J. (2022) *Health Visiting: Specialist Community Public Health Nursing*, 3rd edn. London: Elsevier.

  FURTHER
  READING

  A comprehensive and practice overview of contemporary health visiting. The sections on inter-personal skills and the therapeutic relationship are particularly valuable.
- Luker, K.A., McHugh, G. and Bryar, R.M (2016) *Health Visiting: Preparation for Practice*, 4th edn. Chichester: Wiley-Blackwell.

  A critical exploration of health visiting practice in the current social and policy context.
- Sharma, A. and Cockerill, H. (2022) *From Birth to Five Years: Practical Developmental Examination*, 2nd edn London: Routledge.

  A key text in guiding practitioners through early-years assessments.

Journal articles

- Cowley, S., Kemp, L., Day, C. and Appleton, J. (2012) 'Research and the organisation of complex provision: conceptualising health visiting services and early years programmes'. *Journal of Research in Nursing*, 17 (2): 108-24.

  FURTHER
  READING:
  ONLINE
  JOURNAL
  ARTICLES

  This article discusses universal and targeted provision, so it links with the article in 'What's the evidence?' and to the format of the Healthy Child Programme.
- Kemp, L., Bruce, T., Elcombe, E., Anderson, T., Vimpani, G., Price, A., Smith, C. and Goldfield, S. (2019) 'Quality of delivery of "right@home": implementation evaluation of an Australian sustained nurse home visiting intervention to improve parenting and the home learning environment'. *PLoS ONE*, 14(5): e0215371. https://doi.org/10.1371/journal.pone.0215371

  Useful in gaining an understanding of the challenges of implementing changes in practice and evaluating them.

- Aston, M., Price, S., Etowa, J., Vukic, A., Young, L., Hart, C., MacLeod, E. and Randel, P. (2015) 'The power of relationships: exploring how public health nurses support mothers and families during postpartum home visits'. *Journal of Family Nursing*, 2 (1): 11-34.

  An insight into one of the key areas of health visiting practice.

Weblinks

FURTHER
READING:
WEBLINKS

- Community Practitioner and Health Visitors Association (CPHVA) www.unitetheunion.org/how-wehelp/list-of-sectors/healthsector/healthsectoryourprofession/cphva/cphvaaboutus Unite/ CPHVA is the leading professional body and union representing health visitors, school nurses and commu nity nursery nurses.
- Institute of Health Visiting (iHV) http://ihv.org.uk The Institute of Health Visiting is a new professional body. It provides many educational resources and professional development opportunities.
- Healthy Child Programme www.gov.uk/government/uploads/system/uploads/attachment_data/file/167998/Health_Child_Programme.pdf Different countries of the UK have their own version of the Healthy Child Programme. The link above is to the one produced by the Department of Health for England.
- BMJ Blogs, Anna's student nursing-experience https://blogs.bmj.com/ebn/2015/08/26/annas-student-nursing-experience/ A children's nursing student perspective on the health visitor placement.

REFERENCES

Adams, C. (2012) 'The history of health visiting'. *Nursing in Practice, 68.* Available at: www.nursinginpractice.com/article/history-health-visiting (accessed 4 February 2021).

Baldwin, S. (2012) 'Exploring the professional identity of health visitors'. *Nursing Times, 108* (25): 12–15.

Black, D. (1980) *Inequalities in Health: Report of a Research Working Group.* London: DHSS.

Brookes, P. (2021) *Ages and Stages Questionnaires.* Available at: http://agesandstages.com (accessed 4 February 2021).

Clark, J. (2020) 'Fifty years on: reflections on research on the role of the health visitor'. *Nursing Standard, 35* (10): 15–18. doi.10.7748/ns.35.10.15.s23.

Cowley, S. and Frost, M. (2006) *The Principles of Health Visiting: Opening the Door to Public Health Practice in the 21st Century.* London: CPHVA.

Cowley, S., Whittaker, K., Malone, M., Donetto, S., Grigulis, A. and. Maben, J. (2015) 'Why health visiting? Examining the potential public health benefits from health visiting practice within a universal service: a narrative review of the literature'. *International Journal of Nursing Studies, 52*: 465–80.

Department of Health (DH) (2009) *Healthy Child Programme: Pregnancy and the First Five Years of Life.* London: DH.

Department of Health (DH) (2011) *Health Visitor Implementation Plan 2011–15: A Call to Action.* London: DH.

Department of Health, Social Services and Patient Safety Northern Ireland (DHSSPSNI) (2010) *Healthy Child, Healthy Future: A Framework for the Universal Child Health Promotion Programme in Northern*

Ireland. Available at: www.health-ni.gov.uk/publications/healthy-child-healthy-future (accessed 4 February 2021).

Emond, A. (2019) *Health for All Children,* 5th edn. Oxford: Oxford University Press.

Frankenburg, W.K. and Dodds, J.B. (1967) 'The Denver Developmental Screening Test'. *Journal of Paediatrics, 77:* 181.

GL Assessment (2015) *Schedule of Growing Skills.* Available at: www.gl-assessment.co.uk/products/schedule-growing-skills (accessed 4 February 2021).

Hall, D.M.B. and Elliman, D. (2003) *Health for All Children,* 4th edn. Oxford: Oxford University Press.

HM Government (2018) *Working Together to Safeguard Children: A Guide to Inter-agency Working to Safeguard and Promote the Welfare of Children.* London: DfE. Available at: https://assets.publishing.service.gov.uk/government/uploads/system/uploads/attachment_data/file/942454/Working_together_to_safeguard_children_inter_agency_guidance.pdf (accessed 4 February 2021).

Holland, A., Phillips, K., Moseley, M. and Joomun, L. (2022) *Fundamentals for Public Health Practice.* London: Sage.

King, C. (2015) 'Health visitors' account of the impacts of "Hall 4" on their practice and profession: a qualitative study'. *Community Practitioner, 88* (2): 24–7.

Lipkin, P. and Macias, M. (2020) Promoting optimal development: identifying infants and young children with developmental disorders through developmental surveillance and screening. *Pediatrics, 145*(1): e20193449. doi: 10.1542/peds.2019-3449 (accessed 9 February 2021)

Marmot, M. (2010) *Fair Society, Healthy Lives: Strategic Review of Health Inequalities in England Post 2010.* London: Department for International Development. Available at: www.instituteofhealthequity.org/resources-reports/fair-society-healthy-lives-the-marmot-review (accessed 4 February 2021).

NHS National Services Scotland (2015) *Child Health Programme: Child Health Systems Programme Pre-School (CHSP Pre-School).* Available at: www.isdscotland.org/Health-Topics/Child-Health/Child-Health-Programme/Child-Health-Systems-Programme-Pre-School.asp (accessed 4 February 2021).

NSPCC (National Society for the Prevention of Cruelty to Children) (2021) *Neglect: What Is Neglect?* Available at: www.nspcc.org.uk/preventing-abuse/child-abuse-and-neglect/neglect (accessed 4 February 2021).

Nursing and Midwifery Council (NMC) (2022) *Standards of Proficiency for Specialist Community Public Health Nurses.* London: NMC.

Ofsted (2014) *Are You Ready? Good Practice in School Readiness.* Manchester: Ofsted.

Public Health England (2018) *Healthy Child Programme: The 4-5-6 Approach for Health Visiting and School Nursing.* London: PHE. Available at: https://app.box.com/s/i0b4d3zhkpaltpau641nrbsu0t7s8qkn/file/99823814810 (accessed 9 February 2021).

Robinson, K. (2016) 'Managing knowledge in health visiting', in K.A. Luker, G. McHugh and R.M. Bryar (eds), *Health Visiting: Preparation for Practice,* 4th edn. Chichester: Wiley–Blackwell.

Sharma, A., Cockerill, H. and Sanctuary, L. (2022) *Mary Sheridan's From Birth to Five Years: Children's Developmental Progress,* 5th edn. London: Routledge.

UNICEF (2012) School Readiness: A Conceptual Framework. New York: UNICEF.

United Nations (1989) *United Nations Convention on the Rights of the Child (UNCRC).* Available at: www.unicef.org.uk/what-we-do/un-convention-child-rights (accessed 6 June 2023).

Welsh Government (2016) *An Overview of the Healthy Child Wales Programme* Cardiff: Welsh Government. Available at: https://gov.wales/sites/default/files/publications/2020-12/an-overview-of-the-healthy-child-wales-programme.pdf (accessed 4 February 2021).

PART 3 CARING FOR CHILDREN AND YOUNG PEOPLE WITH ACUTE HEALTHCARE NEEDS AND INJURY

ASSESSMENT AND CARE OF CHILDREN AND YOUNG PEOPLE WITH ACUTE NEEDS

14

RACHAEL BOLLAND

THIS CHAPTER COVERS

- Assessment and treatment of a child with a fever
- Assessment and care of a child with a gastrointestinal disturbance
- Assessment and care of a child having a seizure
- Assessment and care of a child with sepsis
- Unintentional injury in children

> "William Mead was born on the 27th November 2013. He died on the 14th December 2014. The coroner's inquest identified missed opportunities in relation to earlier diagnosis and escalation which could probably have prevented William's death."
>
> NHS England, 2016

INTRODUCTION

Children become ill. This is a predictable and normal occurrence. In most instances the child's illness will be self-limiting and resolve in a couple of days. However, there are a number of illnesses and injuries that can have devastating consequences for the child and their family. William Mead died of sepsis in December 2014 when he was only 12 months old. In this chapter we will look at some of the most common illnesses and injuries and how you can assess which children are acutely unwell and need urgent care and treatment.

It is important that all children who present with an acute care need are thoroughly assessed using a structured ABCDE approach. Poor assessment contributes to avoidable deaths (Hogan, 2014). A child's physiological parameters often deviate from the normal in the hours before they collapse. Serious case reviews have highlighted that critical conditions are not always recognised by healthcare professionals and this leads to children being only partially treated or not treated at all (Roland, 2015). This includes attention to electrolyte imbalance, specifically hyponatraemia, the subject of a recent critical national report (Report of the Inquiry into Hyponatraemia-related Deaths, 2018). It is highly recommended that all nurses in practice caring for children and young people make themselves familiar with this report and its findings.

SEE ALSO
CHAPTER 26

Assessment needs to take into account the age and developmental level of the child and any underlying health need. You need to observe the child, record vital signs but most important of all you need to listen to the child and their parent/carer. What are they worried about? What changes have they noted in their child? Parents often feel that their concerns are not heeded or they may lack the confidence to raise their fears (Roland, 2015). Parents and carers generally know and understand their child best.

SEE ALSO
CHAPTER 6

Do not be lulled into a false sense of security. Just because a child is talking doesn't mean that they aren't sick.

> "In a younger child I would have been concerned about their observations if they were scoring red on the early warning scoring system. But she was a teenager and she was talking. I was really shocked when I heard she had died."
>
> **Aaravshah, children's nurse**

ACTIVITY 14.1: CRITICAL THINKING

In the case of William Mead his parents contacted healthcare professionals on numerous occasions but the professionals did not hear and react appropriately to his parents' concerns (NHS England, 2016). NHS England has developed the ReACT tool to encourage a collaborative approach between healthcare professionals and parents/carers and to empower parents to speak up.

Listen to the talks on Improving Communication with Families on the ReACT - the Respond to Ailing Children Tool (Roland, 2015) accessible via the links below.

- How to spot the sick child https://www.youtube.com/watch?v=N35J3NLJW_s&list=PL6IQwMACXkj1jaPoRVmEQaruL13sBlNok&index=9
- Spotting Sepsis in The Sick Child https://www.youtube.com/watch?v=H3_SeLC3O7M&list=PL6IQwMACXkj1jaPoRVmEQaruL13sBlNok&index=10
- Families as Partners in Achieving Safer Care https://www.youtube.com/watch?v=Gm793UYy8uA&list=PL6IQwMACXkj1jaPoRVmEQaruL13sBlNok&index=4

Reflect on how you communicate and engage with parents and carers. How good are you at listening to families? How could you improve your skills?

Various assessment frameworks have been developed to help you assess and recognise the child with an acute care need and guide you in their care management. We will look now at how you can apply these in practice.

ASSESSMENT AND TREATMENT OF A CHILD WITH A FEVER

As a children's nurse you will see many children who present with a fever. Feverish illness is one of the most common reasons for a child to be taken to see a healthcare professional and is the second most common reason for a child to be admitted to hospital (NICE, 2019a). Fever can distress a child and cause anxiety in their parent/carer (Purssell, 2009, 2014; Bertille et al., 2018) because although the cause is usually a viral infection that is self-limiting, it can also be a sign of more serious illness such as bacterial meningitis (see Table 14.1). NICE (2019a) has developed guidance on the assessment and initial management of children younger than 5 years. You should follow this guidance until a clinical diagnosis of the underlying condition has been made.

Table 14.1 Summary of symptoms and signs suggestive of specific diseases (NICE, 2019a)

Diagnosis to be considered	Symptoms and signs in conjunction with fever
Meningococcal disease	Non-blanching rash, particularly with one or more of the following:
	an ill-looking child
	lesions larger than 2 mm in diameter (purpura)
	capillary refill time of ≥3 seconds
	neck stiffness
Bacterial meningitis	Neck stiffness
	Bulging fontanelle
	Decreased level of consciousness
	Convulsive status epilepticus
Herpes simplex encephalitis	Focal neurological signs
	Focal seizures
	Decreased level of consciousness

(Continued)

Table 14.1   (Continued)

Diagnosis to be considered	Symptoms and signs in conjunction with fever
Pneumonia	Tachypnoea (RR >60 breaths/minute, age 0-5 months; RR >50 breaths/minute, age 6-12 months; RR >40 breaths/minute, age >12 months)
	Crackles in the chest
	Nasal flaring
	Chest indrawing
	Cyanosis
	Oxygen saturation ≤95%
Urinary tract infection	Vomiting
	Poor feeding
	Lethargy
	Irritability
	Abdominal pain or tenderness
	Urinary frequency or dysuria
Septic arthritis	Swelling of a limb or joint
	Not using an extremity
	Non-weight bearing
Kawasaki disease	Fever for more than 5 days and may have some of the following:
	bilateral conjunctival injection without exudate
	erythema and cracking of lips; strawberry tongue; or erythema of oral and pharyngeal mucosa
	oedema and erythema in the hands and feet
	polymorphous rash
	cervical lymphadenopathy

RR= respiratory rate

NICE (2019a) defines fever as 'an elevation of temperature above the normal daily variation'. The normal daily variation or normal child range is 36.6–37.7°C.

Measuring fever in children

As part of your assessment it is important that you accurately measure body temperature using the most appropriate route and device (Table 14.2). Forehead chemical thermometers are unreliable and should not be used by healthcare professionals (Foley, 2018; NICE, 2019a). Parental perception of fever must be taken seriously by healthcare professionals (NHS England, 2016).

Table 14.2   Sites and devices to be used when measuring body temperature in infants and children

Age	Site and device
<4 weeks	Electronic thermometer in the axilla The oral and rectal route must not be routinely used
4 weeks to 5 years	Electronic thermometer in the axilla Chemical dot thermometer in the axilla Infra-red tympanic thermometer The oral and rectal route should not be routinely used
5 years upwards	Electronic thermometer in the axilla or mouth Chemical dot thermometer in the axilla or mouth Infra-red tympanic thermometer

Assessing children with feverish illness

It is important that you identify any immediately life-threatening features. Use the ABCDE approach.

A: Is the airway patent? Do you need to support the airway?

B: Is the child breathing? – Look, listen and feel

C: Check circulation. Measure pulse: rate, rhythm, strength

D: Check temperature, blood glucose (if possible), ascertain if they are on any regular medications, have a history of seizures or could have had access to any drugs/poisons

E: Whilst respecting the child's dignity carry out an examination to see if the child has any rashes, bruises or visible injuries

Once you have completed your ABCDE assessment look for the presence or absence of any signs and symptoms that could predict the risk of serious illness. NICE (2019a) has developed a traffic-light system to help identify the risk factors. For children with a learning disability, you must take account of the child's learning disability when interpreting the traffic-light table.

Caring for the child according to risk of serious illness

Once you have assessed the child using the traffic-light system your actions should be guided by the level of risk of serious illness (Table 14.3).

Table 14.3 Management according to risk of serious illness (NICE, 2019a)

Risk	Management
Life-threatening signs and symptoms	If outside the hospital setting, refer for immediate medical care by the most appropriate means of transport (usually 999 ambulance)
Red features but not considered immediately life threatening	Referred urgently to paediatrician
Amber features with no diagnosis	Can either be cared for at home by parents/carers or referred to a paediatrician for further assessment. If the child is cared for at home, the parents should be given a 'safety net'. This should include verbal and written information on warning symptoms and how further healthcare can be accessed. They should be advised: • To offer cool oral fluids regularly and continue breastfeeding if the child is breastfed • To encourage the child to drink more fluids • Not to underdress or overwrap the child • Not to use tepid sponging to cool the child
Green features only	Can be cared for at home with appropriate advice (see advice under amber features) including when to seek further help

Antipyretic interventions

Due to parental anxiety leading to 'fever phobia', parents/carers tend to treat fever in children aggressively and use over-the-counter medication inappropriately (Purssell, 2009, 2014; Purssell and While, 2013; Bertille et al., 2018). When assessing the child's temperature, it is important to check with their parents/carers what medication they have given and when they last gave it. Antipyretic measures do not prevent febrile convulsions and so should not be used specifically for this purpose (NICE, 2019a).

Physical interventions

It is important not to over-cool a child with fever as this can cause the child to shiver and raise the set point. *Tepid sponging is contra-indicated*. The environment should be kept cool by opening a window and *not* pointing a fan directly onto the child.

Pharmacological interventions

Ibuprofen and paracetamol should only be used if the feverish child is distressed. They should not be used simultaneously unless the child's distress continues or recurs before the next dose of the chosen medication is due.

ACTIVITY 14.2: CRITICAL THINKING

• Are there any potential benefits for a child having a fever?

Think about what effect a temperature has on a child's immune system and tissue repair. Does a temperature increase or decrease the rate of pathogen replication?

CASE STUDY 14.1: ZAC

Zac is 4 years old. His nursery contacted his mother earlier today as he was irritable and had a fever of 37.8°C per axilla. The nursery had given him a dose of paracetamol (which he vomited) and were encouraging him to drink, although he was reluctant to do so and said he his tummy hurt.

His parents collected him from nursery and took him to their local urgent care centre as they were anxious about the temperature as Zac had previously had a febrile convulsion.

At the urgent care centre he was found to have a temperature of 38.2°C per axilla, heart rate of 142 beats/minute, respiratory rate of 28 breaths per minute and oxygen saturations of 96%. Zac was sleepy and not smiling at his parents, he was reluctant to drink and had not had a wee since the morning. He said his tummy hurt. There is no obvious source of infection.

Using the traffic-light system (NICE, 2019a) for identifying risk of serious illness, describe what level of risk Zac is displaying.

• What actions would you take and why?
• Zac is seen by a paediatric consultant in the rapid review clinic at the local hospital and the decision is made to admit him. With reference to the NICE guidelines what further investigations would need to be performed?
• How often would you record Zacs's observations (vital signs in hospital)?
• What anti-pyretic interventions will Zac require?

SEE ALSO CHAPTER 26 AND 27

ASSESSMENT AND CARE OF A CHILD WITH A GASTROINTESTINAL DISTURBANCE

Diarrhoea and vomiting are common symptoms in children, especially in children under 5 years of age. Ten per cent of all children under the age of 5 will present to healthcare services each year with diarrhoea and vomiting (NICE, 2009). The child develops loose or watery stools and/or a sudden onset of vomiting usually as a result of gastroenteritis. The vomiting usually resolves after 1–2 days whilst the diarrhoea usually resolves after 5–7 days. Whilst the majority of children can be cared for at home, some children will need admission to hospital because of the risk of dehydration and shock (NICE 2009, 2019b). Children admitted to hospital pose an infection risk to other vulnerable hospitalised children, therefore it is important that good infection control practices are practised at all times.

Which children are most at risk of dehydration?

Infants under 6 months of age are especially at risk. The signs of dehydration may be less obvious in this age group, leading to a risk of rapid and severe deterioration (NICE, 2020a). Children are also at risk of hypernatraemic dehydration – a life-threatening condition requiring immediate treatment (Powers, 2015). You should suspect hypernatraemia in any child who presents with jittery movements, increased muscle tone, hyperreflexia, convulsions or drowsiness (NICE, 2009).

To help you identify which children are most at risk of dehydration it is important that you assess the child fully to identify any specific risk factors such as:

- passing six or more diarrhoeal stools in the previous 24 hours
- vomiting three or more times in the previous 24 hours
- not tolerating supplementary feeds
- infants who have stopped breastfeeding during this illness
- children showing signs of malnutrition (assess using a validated tool such as STAMP, PYMS, Growth Charts [RCPCH, 2012])

To help you gain this information you need to ask the parent/carer the following questions:

- How long has your child had diarrhoea and vomiting?
- How frequent is their diarrhoea and/or vomiting?
- What does their stool look like – for example, colour, smell, consistency? Did it contain any blood, mucus, pus or undigested food?
- Does your child have any other symptoms such as abdominal pain, vomiting or bloating?
- Has your child had/got a fever? (Assess using NICE [2019a] Traffic Light table).
- Has your child had any recent infections?
- Has your child lost weight recently? (This could be an indication of gut dysfunction alongside failure to thrive and symptoms of anaemia.)
- Has your child travelled abroad recently?
- Are any other family members or other contacts unwell at the moment?

NICE (2009) recommends that in children under 5 you use the table below (Table 14.4) to assess the severity of dehydration.

SEE ALSO
CHAPTER 26

When should you take a stool specimen from a child with diarrhoea and vomiting?

Financial constraints in the NHS have led us to question which investigations are necessary. You need to ask – how will the results of the investigation influence the child's care and treatment? For the majority of children, stool culture is unnecessary and will not influence the child's care and treatment.

Table 14.4 Assessing dehydration in children under 5 years (NICE, 2009)

	Increasing severity of dehydration		
	No clinically detectable dehydration	**Clinical dehydration**	**Clinical shock**
Symptoms (remote and face-to-face assessments)	Appears well	**Red flag** Appears to be unwell or deteriorating	-
	Alert and responsive	**Red flag** Altered responsiveness (e.g., irritable, lethargic)	Decreased level of consciousness
	Normal urine output	Decreased urine output	-
	Skin colour unchanged	Skin colour unchanged	Pale or mottled skin
	Warm extremities	Warm extremities	Cold extremities
Signs (face-to-face assessments)	Alert and responsive	**Red flag** Altered responsiveness (for example, irritable, lethargic)	Decreased level of consciousness
	Skin colour unchanged	Skin colour unchanged	Pale or mottled skin
	Warm extremities	Warm extremities	Cold extremities
	Eyes not sunken	**Red flag** Sunken eyes	-
	Moist mucous membranes (except after a drink)	Dry mucous membranes (except for 'mouth breather')	-
	Normal heart rate	**Red flag** Tachycardia	Tachycardia
	Normal breathing pattern	**Red flag** Tachypnoea	Tachypnoea
	Normal peripheral pulses	Normal peripheral pulses	Weak peripheral pulses
	Normal capillary refill time	Normal capillary refill time	Prolonged capillary refill time
	Normal skin turgor	**Red flag** Reduced skin turgor	-
	Normal blood pressure	Normal blood pressure	Hypotension (decompensated shock)

A stool specimen for stool microbiology should be obtained if the child meets one of the following criteria:

- There is a suspicion that the child may have septicaemia
- The child has blood and/or mucous in the stool
- The child is immuno-compromised

Consider performing stool microbiology if

- The child has recently travelled abroad, or
- The child's diarrhoea has not improved by day 7, or
- There is uncertainty about the diagnosis of gastroenteritis

If stool microbiology is performed you should collect, store and transport to stool as advised by your hospital laboratory. The relevant clinical information must be included on the request form. A blood culture should also be performed if antibiotic therapy is given (NICE, 2019b).

ACTIVITY 14.3: EVIDENCE-BASED PRACTICE

Do all children with diarrhoea and vomiting need intravenous fluids? You will remember that we said earlier that most children can be cared for at home. Most children who are not displaying signs of dehydration can be cared for at home - therefore the answer is no, not all children need intravenous fluids. Parents caring for their child at home will need advice on what food and fluids their child can have, infection control measures and when a child can go back to school/nursery.

- What advice regarding food and fluids would you give to a parent caring for their child at home?

What fluids would you give to a child who has diarrhoea and vomiting and is dehydrated?

These children also do not need intravenous therapy as first-line treatment unless they have any red flag symptoms (Table 14.4). They should be given a low osmolarity oral rehydration salt (ORS) solution (NICE, 2019b, 2020a). The ORS solution should be reconstituted according to the instructions on the packaging. Rehydration should be rapid over 3–4 hours (except in hypernatraemic dehydration where rehydration should occur more slowly over 12 hours). A dose of 50ml/kg of ORS solution plus maintenance volume should be given (NICE, 2019b). If the child is unable to drink the ORS or persistently vomits you will need to consider passing a nasogastric tube through which to give the ORS. Breastfeeding can be continued alongside the ORS solution.

You must maintain an accurate record of the child's input and output. It is important that you regularly reassess the child and look for signs of improvement or deterioration.

When should intravenous therapy be commenced?

You should commence intravenous fluids if the child has any Red Flag symptoms (Table 14.4), shows signs of clinical deterioration (despite ORS rehydration therapy) or shock (suspected or confirmed) or if the child persistently vomits the ORS solution via the oral or nasogastric route.

It is vital that the most appropriate intravenous fluids are used (NICE, 2009, 2015). Suspected or confirmed shock should be treated with a glucose-free, isotonic crystalloid such as 0.9% sodium chloride given as a raid bolus (20ml/kg). Routine maintenance fluids should be an isotonic crystalloid solution that contains sodium in the range of 131–154 mmol/litre. To ensure that each child receives the most appropriate fluids you must monitor their blood plasma regularly and ensure that the medical team adjusts their fluids accordingly.

Once a child has been rehydrated they can start back on full-strength milk straight away and their usual solid food. It is a myth that they must have half-strength milk or a light diet only. The only fluids that they need to avoid until their diarrhoea stops are fruit juices and fizzy drinks (including carbonated drinks that have been allowed to go 'flat').

Any child whose diarrhoea lasts for longer than 2 weeks needs to be further investigated. There are a number of reasons that the child could have prolonged diarrhoea. Non-specific toddler diarrhoea is the commonest cause of loose stools in children. Parents and carers may report that the child has undigested vegetables in their stool. Non-specific toddler diarrhoea is thought to be due to the immaturity of the toddler's GI tract with rapid intestinal motility. The toddler appears well and thrives, showing no other signs of gut dysfunction.

Prolonged diarrhoea may be due to infections such as rota virus and adenovirus. It can also occur after a child has had a bout of gastroenteritis and is known as post-gastroenteritis syndrome. Prolonged diarrhoea may also indicate a more serious underlying condition leading to malabsorption such as coeliac disease, cystic fibrosis, cow's milk protein intolerance or irritable bowel disease (IBD).

SEE ALSO
CHAPTER 19

ASSESSMENT AND CARE OF THE CHILD HAVING A SEIZURE

Seizures may also be referred to as convulsions and fits. Most seizures are generalised, usually last 2–3 minutes and stop by themselves. Epilepsy is a term used when fits recur and is usually diagnosed by a neurologist.

The commonest cause of seizures in children is a high temperature. Febrile convulsions are most common in toddlers. Other causes include:

- Epilepsy
- CNS infection
- Aspiration/gastro-oesophageal reflux disease
- Metabolic – hypoglycaemia, hyperglycaemia, hyponatraemia, hypernatraemia or hypomagnesaemia
- Vitamin D deficiency (Arundel and Shaw, 2018)
- Cerebral hypoxia
- Head trauma/non-accidental injury
- Toxins/poisoning

Immediate assessment and care in the community setting

Seizures can appear frightening to parents and bystanders so it is important that you remain calm. Call 999 to request an ambulance/assistance. Children should be assessed and managed using the ABCDE approach we discussed earlier in the chapter.

Assessment and care in the emergency department

The more detailed ABCDE approach is suitable for the emergency department setting and should be used to assess the child and direct their management (see Table 14.5).

Table 14.5 Assessment and management of the fitting child/status epilepticus

AIRWAY

Apply oxygen via a non-rebreathe mask
Support airway
Consider nasopharyngeal airway
Monitor oxygen saturations

BREATHING

Assess effort and efficacy of breathing
Support breathing as required

CIRCULATION

Secure IV/IO access
Monitor heart rate and blood pressure
Check venous blood gas, urea and electrolytes (U&E), bone profile, magnesium, blood glucose, anticonvulsant levels (if appropriate)

DISABILITY

Correct hypoglycaemia 2ml/kg of 10% dextrose
Correct electrolyte abnormalities slowly
If seizure > than 5 minutes give:
Lorazepam IV/IO 0.1mg/kg Max dose 4mg **or**
Diazepam IV/IO 0.25mg/kg Max dose 10mg **or**
Rectal diazepam 0.5mg/kg Max dose 10mg **or**
Buccal midazolam 0.5mg/kg Max dose 10mg

If seizure lasts for a further 10 minutes
give a second dose of benzodiazepine

Check if the child received a dose of benzodiazepine before coming to the hospital. Do not give more than two doses.

Start to prepare the phenytoin

Senior review

Reconfirm that it is an epileptic seizure

Phenytoin 20mg/kg IV or IO over 20 minutes. Max dose 2 g.
Caution: risk of thrombophlebitis with peripheral infusion. Give via large vein.
Phenytoin can cause dysrhythmias and hypotension: monitor ECG and BP
If already on phenytoin give:
Phenobarbitone 20mg/kg (max dose 1 g) IV or IO over 5 minutes

20 minutes from start of infusion:
Rapid sequence induction
Inform Paediatric Intensive Care Unit (PICU)

ASSESSMENT AND CARE OF A CHILD WITH SEPSIS

CASE STUDY 14.2: TOBIAS (1)

Tobias is 2 years old. He is usually fit and healthy. However, for the last couple of days he has not been his usual self. He looks pale and is very lethargic, wanting to sleep all the time. He is reluctant to drink and is not weeing as much as normal. Despite it being a warm day, his hands feel cold to touch.

Initially his mum thought that he just had a virus and would be better in a couple of days. Now she is very concerned about him as she recently read in the newspaper about a toddler who died of sepsis and thinks he has some of the signs. She decides to take him straight to the emergency department at her local hospital. At the emergency department she tells the receptionist that she thinks he has sepsis and needs to be seen straight away.

Sepsis is defined as a life-threatening organ dysfunction caused by a dysregulated host response to infection (Ashton, 2020). Sepsis affects 10,000 children each year in the UK (UK Sepsis Trust, 2019). It can be hard to diagnose because the signs and symptoms can mimic other childhood illnesses. Not all children will present with a fever and children are able to compensate during the early stages. Therefore, you should have a high index for suspicion in children particularly those showing any of the following signs and symptoms.

Any child who:

- Is breathing very fast
- Has a 'fit' or convulsion
- Looks mottled, bluish or pale
- Has a rash that does not fade when you press it
- Is very lethargic or difficult to wake up
- Feels abnormally cold to touch

(UK Sepsis Trust, 2019)

Any child under 5 years of age who:

- Is not feeding
- Is vomiting repeatedly
- Hasn't had a wee or a wet nappy for 12 hours

(UK Sepsis Trust, 2019)

As discussed earlier in the chapter, William Mead died of sepsis aged 12 months in December 2014. At the inquest into William's death the coroner identified missed opportunities for an earlier diagnosis and escalation that might have prevented his death (NHS England, 2016). To aid early recognition and treatment of sepsis, NICE published a guideline in July 2016 (NICE, 2016a).

Table 14.6 Risk stratification tool for a 2-year-old with suspected sepsis (adapted from NICE, 2016a)

	High risk criteria	Moderate to high risk criteria	Low risk criteria
Behaviour	No response to social cues Appears ill to a healthcare professional Does not wake, or if roused does not stay awake Weak high pitched or continuous cry	Not responding normally to social cues No smile Wakes only with prolonged stimulation Decreased activity Parent or carer concern that child is behaving differently from usual	Responds normally to social cues Content or smiles Stays awake or awakens quickly Strong normal cry or not crying
Respiratory	Grunting Apnoea Oxygen saturation less than 90% in air or increased oxygen requirement over baseline Raised respiratory rate: 50 breaths per minute or more	Oxygen saturation of less than 92% in air or increased oxygen requirement over baseline Nasal flaring Raised respiratory rate: 40-49 breaths per minute	No high risk or moderate to high risk criteria met
Circulation and hydration	Bradycardia: heart rate less than 60 beats per minute Rapid heart rate: 150 beats per minute or more	Capillary refill time of 3 seconds or more Reduced urine output For catheterised children - pass less than 1ml/kg of urine per hour Raised heart rate: 140-149 beats per minute	No high risk or moderate to high risk criteria met

	High risk criteria	Moderate to high risk criteria	Low risk criteria
Skin	Mottled or ashen appearance Cyanosis of skin, lips or tongue Non-blanching rash of skin	Pallor of skin, lips or tongue	Normal colour
Other		Leg pain Cold hands or feet	No high risk or moderate to high risk criteria met

CASE STUDY 14.2: TOBIAS (2)

Tobias is seen by the triage nurse in the emergency department. He listens to Tobias's mother's concerns and assesses Tobias using the age-appropriate risk stratification tool for children with suspected sepsis guideline and algorithm (NICE, 2016a) (Table 14.6).

Tobias is found to have a core temperature of 38.4°C, a heart rate of 155 beats per minute, a respiratory rate of 38 per minute, oxygen saturations of 92% in air, capillary refill >3 seconds and systolic blood pressure of 95mmHg. He is sleeping but responds to his mother's voice. However, he falls straight back to sleep. He appears pale.

Tobias is graded as having a high risk of sepsis. The nurse fast bleeps the paediatric registrar.

- You are the nurse who has assessed Tobias. Outline the conversation you would have with the registrar using the SBAR (Situation, Background, Assessment, Recommendation) tool.

SEE ALSO
CHAPTER 6

Screening for Red Flag Sepsis

The table below outlines the next steps to take in screening for Red Flag Sepsis, which in our case is performed by the registrar.

Table 14.7 Emergency department Red Flag Sepsis criteria for children aged under 5 years (Nutbeam and Daniels, 2020)

Doesn't wake when roused/won't stay awake
Looks very unwell to healthcare professional
Weak, high-pitched or continuous cry
Severe tachypnoea
Severe tachycardia
Bradycardia (<60 beats per minute)
Non blanching rash/mottled/ashen/ cyanotic
Temperature <36°C
If under 3 months, temperature 38°+
Oxygen saturation <90% or increased O_2 requirements

CASE STUDY 14.2: TOBIAS (3)

The registrar comes straight to the emergency department to review Tobias. She assesses Tobias using the emergency department Red Flag Sepsis Criteria for Children under 5 years (Table 14.7).

Tobias has several red flags (review his observations against the criteria) and urgent intervention is required. The registrar informs her consultant and paediatric intensive care unit (PICU).

Management: urgent intervention

In cases that need urgent intervention, the emergency department team will normally implement the Paediatric Sepsis 6 procedures (as in Table 14.8). All elements must be completed within 1 hour.

Table 14.8 Example of Paediatric Sepsis 6 chart: Complete all elements within 1 hour (Nutbeam and Daniels, 2020)

	Date/Time	Sign
1. Ensure senior clinician attends to review.		
2. Oxygen if required. Start if oxygen saturations less than 92% or evidence of shock		
3. Obtain IV/IO access and take blood tests: a Blood cultures b Blood glucose - treat low blood glucose c Lactate, FBC, U&E, CRP and clotting d Lumbar puncture if indicated		
4. Give IV or IO antibiotics: - Maximum dose broad-spectrum therapy		
5. Consider IV/IO fluids: - If lactate is above 2 mmol/l give fluid bolus of 20ml/kg without delay - If lactate >4 mmol/l call PICU		
6. Consider inotropic support: - Consider inotropic support if normal physiology is not restored after ≥20ml/kg fluid. Call PICU or a regional referral centre urgently		
Record Additional Notes Here: allergy status, arrival of specialist teams, de-escalation of care, delayed antimicrobial decision-making, variance from Sepsis 6		

CASE STUDY 14.2: TOBIAS (4)

After the emergency department team have implemented Paediatric Sepsis 6 procedures, Tobias is moved to the Paediatric Intensive Care Unit for further observation and treatment.

Sadly, despite the development and implementation of the NICE Sepsis guidelines children have continued to die due to missed opportunities to diagnose and effectively manage and treat.

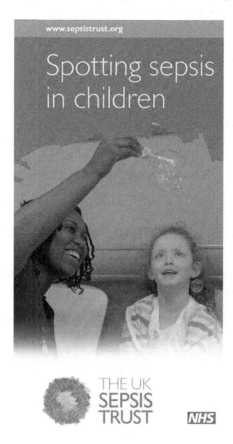

Figure 14.1 Poster from the UK Sepsis Trust who provide support and advice to healthcare professionals and families

UNINTENTIONAL INJURY IN CHILDREN

The term 'unintentional injury' is the term we now use to describe 'accidents' to recognise that these injuries are the result of events that can be prevented. Unintentional injury, in and around the home, is a leading cause of preventable death in children under 5 years with an average of 55 children under 5 years dying each year from such an injury. On average, each year 370,000 children attend Accident and Emergency and 40,000 children are admitted as an emergency (Public Health England, 2018).

Which children are most at risk of unintentional injury?

Risk is affected by a number of factors:

- Age
- Developmental level
- Underlying medical condition(s)

- Behaviour – for example, risk taking
- Physical environment in the home
- Knowledge and behaviour of parents and other carers
- Overcrowding and homelessness
- Availability of safety equipment
- New consumer products in the home

NICE (2010, 2013) reports that:

- Children under 5 years old are more vulnerable to unintentional injuries in the home
- Children over the age of 11 years are more vulnerable to unintentional injuries on the road

In this chapter we will focus on falls, fractures and head injury.

———— PROMOTING HEALTH ————

How can we prevent unintentional injury in children? The following publications outline how we might prevent unintentional injury in children:

- Child Accident Prevention Trust (2020) Keeping Children Safe From a Serious Fall
- NHS Choices (2019) Baby and Toddler Safety
- NICE (2016b) Preventing Unintentional Injury in Under 15s
- Public Health England (2018) Reducing Unintentional Injuries in and around the Home Among Children under Five Years
- World Health Organization (2018) Children and Falls

The key messages are:

- Preventing unintentional injury is an important factor in improving public health outcomes. It is important that healthcare professionals and the NHS work with local government and the voluntary sector.
- Parents need advice on maintaining safety in the home. Simple measures can significantly reduce risk. For example, stairgates can reduce the number of children falling downstairs when fitted securely at the top and bottom of stairs. The introduction of window restrictors saw a 96% reduction in falls from windows admissions to emergency departments.
- Information leaflets on prevention and safety in the home should be available in all healthcare settings. They need to be engaging and colourful to appeal to parents and carers.

Assessment and care of a child or young person following a fall

Children under 5 are most at risk of being admitted to hospital for treatment of injuries following a fall (Public Health England, 2018). They fall over and get knocks and bruises while learning to walk, but serious injuries can be avoided. The World Health Organization (WHO) (2018) defines a fall as 'an event which results in a person coming to rest inadvertently on the ground or floor or other lower level'.

Most cuts and grazes are minor and can be treated at home. The parent/carer should be advised to clean the cut or graze thoroughly and cover with a plaster or dressing. However, parents/carers should be advised to dial 999 to request an ambulance if their child:

- Stops breathing or is struggling to breathe
- Is unconscious or seems unaware of what is happening around them
- Won't wake up
- Has a fit for the first time, even if they seem to recover

They should be advised to take their child to the emergency department if their child has:

- A leg or arm injury and can't use the limb
- A cut that may have something in it such as a piece of glass

SAFEGUARDING STOP POINT

All children who present following a fall out of windows or from buildings should be assessed under your safeguarding children processes.

SEE ALSO
CHAPTER 9

Assessment and care of a child or young person with a fracture

A fracture is a partial or complete break in the bone. It can be an open (compound) fracture where the bone breaks through the skin. Or it can be a closed (simple) fracture where the bone is broken but the skin is still intact.

SEE ALSO
CHAPTER 23

Although fractures are common in children (approximately 66% of boys and 40% of girls will sustain a fracture by the age of 15) we should still try to reduce the rate of unintentional injuries. In children over 5 years, 85% of fractures are due to unintentional injuries.

SAFEGUARDING STOP POINT

Fractures can also be an indication of child abuse and indicate a serious assault on a child (NSPCC, 2012a).
When should you be concerned that a child may have been abused?
Look up your local safeguarding guidelines including those on the management of bruises or marks in non-ambulant babies/children, and the following leaflets by the NSPCC:
NSPCC (2012a) Core-Info: Fractures in Children
NSPCC (2012b) Core-Info: Bruises on Children

SEE ALSO
CHAPTER 9

If you see any of the following signs or symptoms you should suspect that the child may have a fracture:

- Pain or swelling in the injured area
- Obvious deformity in the injured area

- Difficulty using or moving the injured area in a normal manner
- Warmth, bruising or redness in the injured area

First aid

Parents/carers should be advised to seek medical care immediately. If the child has an open fracture or a neck or spinal injury they should not be moved because unnecessary movement can cause paralysis. For other fractures, if a parent/carer cannot easily move the child without causing them pain, they should be advised to call an ambulance. If it is possible for them to move their child, they should do so gently, putting one hand above the injury and the other below it to stabilise the fracture. Blankets or clothing can be used to support it. They should also be advised to give their child some painkillers, following the instructions on the label, comfort the child and take them to the emergency department.

How are fractures in children treated?

On arrival at the emergency department the nurse practitioner or doctor will examine the injured area(s) for tenderness, redness and swelling, and order diagnostic imaging tests.

SEE ALSO
CHAPTER 15
AND 16

Specific treatment for a fracture depends on the type of fracture, its severity and the child's age. In the majority of cases the fracture can be treated with a splint or cast. These immobilise the injured bone, promoting healing and reducing pain and swelling (see NHS Choices (2018) 'How should I care for my plaster cast?').

Some children will require surgery and the insertion of metal rods or pins. Neurovascular observations should be performed, examining colour, warmth, sensation and movement of the affected limb.

The child's pain should be assessed and appropriate analgesia administered. Some doctors have expressed concerns about the use of NSAIDs (non-steroidal anti-inflammatory drugs) as they believe that they may inhibit new bone growth following surgery. There are no studies to support this view (Association of Paediatric Anaesthetists of Great Britain and Ireland, 2012). If it is a fracture to a lower limb, then the nursing team should liaise with the orthopaedic surgeon to ascertain whether the child can weight-bear and along with the physiotherapists support the child to learn to use crutches and be able to walk up and down stairs.

SEE ALSO
CHAPTER 3

Assessment and early management of a child with a head injury

A head injury is any trauma to the head other than superficial injuries to the face (NICE, 2014). Head injury is the commonest cause of death and disability of people aged 1–40 years in the UK. The majority of people attending the emergency department will have minor or mild head injuries but we need to ensure that all patients are assessed to identify those who will develop serious acute intracranial complications (Mulryan, 2018).

SEE ALSO
CHAPTER 19

SAFEGUARDING STOP POINT

It is estimated that 25–30% of children under the age of 2 who are admitted to hospital will have an abusive head injury (NICE, 2014). Those who survive the injury may have significant long-term disabilities such as cerebral palsy, visual impairment, epilepsy, learning and behavioural problems (NSPCC, 2014).

A clinician who has been trained in safeguarding children should be involved in the assessment of any child presenting in the emergency department with a head injury. It is important to examine them for other injuries such as retinal haemorrhages, bruises, burns, bites, oral injuries or fractures. Any concerns should be identified and documented and local safeguarding procedures followed (NICE, 2014).

SEE ALSO
CHAPTER 9

Assessment and treatment of head injuries

The NICE guidelines *Head Injury: Assessment and Early Management* (2014) should be followed. These cover:

- Pre-hospital assessment, advice and referral to hospital
- Immediate management at the scene and transport to hospital
- Assessment in the emergency department
- Investigating clinically important brain injuries
- Investigating injuries to the cervical spine
- Information and support for families and carers
- Transfer from hospital to a neuroscience unit
- Admission and observation
- Discharge and follow-up

WHAT'S THE EVIDENCE?

NICE first produced a head injury guideline in 2003. It was updated in 2007 and again in 2014. Each update is based on up-to-date evidence and key NHS changes such as the introduction of regional trauma networks with major trauma triage tools within NHS England. The guidelines have resulted in CT scanning replacing skull radiography and have led to an increase in the proportion of people being cared for in specialist centres. This has been associated with a decline in fatality among patients with a severe head injury. In 2019, NICE reviewed but did not update the guideline, they did however change their advice in relation to children on anti-coagulants – advising that they should have a CT head scan within 8 hours of head injury.

- Read the NICE guidelines and think about what you have seen in practice. Does the Trust follow these guidelines? How are policies developed in the Trust to ensure they are based on the best available evidence?

CHAPTER SUMMARY

- When assessing children with acute needs it is crucial to remember to select an appropriate assessment tool and to adopt an ABCDE approach
- It is essential that as a children's nurse you should listen to and involve parents in the assessment of children

- You should use a child-centred approach when assessing and managing a child with acute health needs
- Particular vigilance is required to ensure signs of sepsis and electrolyte imbalance are spotted early and acted upon immediately

---

BUILD YOUR BIBLIOGRAPHY

Books

FURTHER
READING

- Carter, B., Bray, L., Dickinson, A., Edwards, M. and Ford, K. (2014) *Child-centred Nursing: Promoting Critical Thinking.* London: Sage.

  Read Chapter 6 on 'Understanding children's and young people's experience of illness'. This will help you to gain further insight into the impact that illness and hospitalisation has on a child.
- Standing, M. (2020) *Clinical Judgement and Decision Making in Nursing.* London: Learning Matters.

  Read Chapters 3 and 4 on 'Using observations to inform decisions' and 'Systematic clinical decision-making'. These reinforce key messages from this chapter.

Journal articles

FURTHER
READING:
ONLINE
JOURNAL
ARTICLES

- Richard, M. and Purssell, E. (2015) 'Who's afraid of fever?' *Archives of Disease in Childhood*, 100 (9): 818-20.

  Read this article to see how research and evidence-based practice are incorporated into national fever guidelines.
- Powers, K. (2015) 'Dehydration: isonatremic, hyponatremic and hypernatremic recognition and management'. *Pediatrics in Review*, 36 (7): 274-85.

  The article links with the section of the chapter entitled 'How do we assess and care for a child with a gastrointestinal disturbance?' and looks at the different types of dehydration a child is susceptible to.

REFERENCES

Arundel, P. and Shaw, N. (2018) *Vitamin D and Bone Health: A Practical Clinical Guideline for Patient Management in Children and Young People.* National [Royal] Osteoporosis Society. Available at: https://theros.org.uk/media/54vpzzaa/ros-vitamin-d-and-bone-health-in-children-november-2018.pdf (accessed 9 November 2020).

Ashton, J. (2020) 'Sepsis and children: what should the message be?' *Nursing Children and Young People*, 32 (4): 12.

Association of Paediatric Anaesthetists of Great Britain and Ireland (APA) (2012) *Good Practice in Postoperative and Procedural Pain Management*, 2nd edn. *Paediatric Anaesthesia*, 22 (Suppl 1): 1–79.

Bertille, N., Purssell, E., Hjelm, N., Bilenko, N., Chiappini, E., de Bont, E.G.P.M., Kramer, M.S., Lepage, P., Lava, S.A.G., Mintegi, S., Sullivan, J.E., Walsh, A., Cohen, J.F and Chalumeau, M. (2018) 'Symptomatic management of febrile illnesses in children: a systematic review and meta-analysis of parents' knowledge and behaviors and their evolution over time'. *Frontiers in Pediatrics*, 6. doi:10.3389/fped.2018.00279.

Child Accident Prevention Trust (2020) *Safety Advice: Falls*. London: Child Accident Prevention Trust. Available at: www.capt.org.uk/falls (accessed 26 August 2020).

Foley, V. (2018) 'Clinical measurement', in C. Delves-Yates (ed.), *Essentials of Nursing Practice*, 2nd edn. London: Sage.

Hogan, H. (2014) 'The scale and scope of preventable hospital deaths'. PhD dissertation, London School of Hygiene and Tropical Medicine. Available at: https://researchonline.lshtm.ac.uk/id/eprint/1776586/44/2014_PHP_PhD_Hogan_H.pdf (accessed 25 August 2020).

Mulryan, C. (2018) 'First aid', in C. Delves-Yeates (ed.), *Essentials of Nursing Practice*, 2nd edn. London: Sage.

NHS Choices (2018) How Should I care for my plaster cast? Available at: www.nhs.uk/chq/Pages/2543.aspx?CategoryID=72&SubCategoryID=721 (accessed 26 August 2020).

NHS Choices (2019) Baby and toddler safety. Available at: www.nhs.uk/Conditions/pregnancy-and-baby/pages/baby-safety-tips.aspx (accessed 26 August 2020).

NHS England (2016) Root Cause Analysis Investigation Report 2014/41975. Available at: www.england.nhs.uk/south/wp-content/uploads/sites/6/2015/03/root-cause-analysis-wm-report.pdf (accessed 25 August 2020).

NICE (National Institute for Health and Clinical Excellence) (2009) *Diarrhoea and Vomiting in Children. Diarrhoea and vomiting caused by gastroenteritis: diagnosis, assessment and management in children younger than 5 years*. Available at: www.nice.org.uk/guidance/cg84/resources/diarrhoea-and-vomiting-caused-by-gastroenteritis-in-under-5s-diagnosis-and-management-pdf-975688889029 (accessed 25 August 2020).

NICE (National Institute for Health and Clinical Excellence) (2010) Public Health Guidance 29, 30, 31: *Strategies to Prevent Unintentional Injuries among Children and Young People Aged under 15*. Available at: www.nice.org.uk/guidance/ph29/resources/unintentional-injuries-prevention-strategies-for-under-15s-pdf-1996245405637 (accessed 26 August 2020).

NICE (National Institute for Health and Care Excellence) (2013) Evidence Update 29: *Strategies to Prevent Unintentional Injuries among Children and Young People Aged under 15*. Available at: www.nice.org.uk/guidance/ph29/evidence/strategies-to-prevent-unintentional-injuries-among-under15s-evidence-update-67472317 (accessed 26 August 2020).

NICE (National Institute for Health and Care Excellence) (2014) *Head Injury: Assessment and Early Management*. Available at: www.nice.org.uk/guidance/cg176/resources/head-injury-assessment-and-early-management-pdf-35109755595493 (accessed 26 August 2020).

NICE (National Institute for Health and Care Excellence) (2015) *Intravenous Fluid Therapy in Children and Young People in Hospital*. Available at: www.nice.org.uk/guidance/ng29/resources/intravenous-fluid-therapy-in-children-and-young-people-in-hospital-pdf-1837340295109 (accessed 25 August 2020).

NICE (National Institute for Health and Care Excellence) (2016a) *Sepsis: Recognition, Diagnosis and Early Management*. Available at: www.nice.org.uk/guidance/ng51/resources/sepsis-recognition-diagnosis-and-early-management-pdf-1837508256709 (accessed 25 August 2020).

NICE (National Institute for Health and Care Excellence) (2016b) *Preventing Unintentional Injuries in under 15s*. NICE quality standard (QS107). Available at: www.nice.org.uk/guidance/qs107 (accessed 26 August 2020).

NICE (National Institute for Health and Care Excellence) (2019a) *Fever in under 5s. Assessment and Inititial Management*. Available at: www.nice.org.uk/guidance/ng143/resources/fever-in-under-5s-assessment-and-initial-management-pdf-66141778137541 (accessed 25 August 2020).

NICE (National Institute for Health and Care Excellence) (2019b) *Diarrhoea and Vomiting in Children: Overview*. Available at: https://pathways.nice.org.uk/pathways/diarrhoea-and-vomiting-in-children (accessed 25 August 2020).

NICE (National Institute for Health and Care Excellence) (2020a) *BNF for Children*. Available at: https://bnfc.nice.org.uk/ accessed 29/10/2020

NICE (National Institute for Health and Care Excellence) (2020b) *Intravenous fluid therapy in hospital overview*. Available at: https://pathways.nice.org.uk/pathways/intravenous-fluid-therapy-in-hospital (accessed 25 August 2020).

NSPCC (National Society for Prevention of Cruelty to Children) (2012a) *Core-Info: Fractures in Children*. Available at: https://learning.nspcc.org.uk/media/1038/core-info-fractures-children.pdf (accessed 26 August 2020).

NSPCC (National Society for Prevention of Cruelty to Children) (2012b) *Core-Info: Bruises on Children*. Available at: https://learning.nspcc.org.uk/media/1046/core-info-bruises-children.pdf (accessed 26/ August 2020).

NSPCC (National Society for Prevention of Cruelty to Children) (2014) *Core-Info: Head and Spinal Injuries in Children*. Available at: https://learning.nspcc.org.uk/media/1062/core-info-head-spinal-injuries.pdf (accessed 26 August 2020).

Nutbeam, T. and Daniels, R. (2020) *Sepsis Screening Tool: Acute Assessment*. On behalf of the UK Sepsis Trust. Available at: sepsistrust.org/professional-resources/clinical/ (accessed 12 November 2020).

Powers, K. (2015) 'Dehydration: isonatremic, hyponatremic and hypernatremic recognition and management'. *Pediatrics in Review*, 36 (7): 274–85.

Public Health England (2018) *Reducing Unintentional Injuries in and around the Home among Children under Five Years*. Available at: www.gov.uk/government/uploads/system/uploads/attachment_data/file/322210/Reducing_unintentional_injuries_in_and_around_the_home_among_children_under_five_years.pdf (accessed 26 August 2020).

Purssell, E. (2009) 'Parental fever phobia and its evolutionary correlates'. *Journal of Clinical Nursing*, 18: 210–18.

Purssell, E. (2014) 'Fever in children – a concept analysis'. *Journal of Clinical Nursing*, 23: 3575–82.

Purssell, E. and While, A. (2013) 'Does the use of anti-pyretics in children who have acute infections prolong febrile illness? A systematic review and meta-analysis'. *Journal of Paediatrics*, 163: 822–7.

RCPCH (Royal College of Paediatrics and Child Health) (2012) *UK-WHO Growth Charts*. Available at: www.rcpch.ac.uk/resources/growth-charts (accessed 25 August 2020).

Report of the Inquiry into Hyponatraemia-related Deaths (2018) Available at: www.ihrdni.org/Full-Report.pdf (accessed 22 February 2023).

Roland, D. (2015) *Re-ACT – the Respond to Ailing Children Tool*. NHS England. Available at: https://webarchive.nationalarchives.gov.uk/20161104070852/https://www.england.nhs.uk/patientssafety/re-act/ (accessed 25 August 2020).

UK Sepsis Trust (2019) *The Sepsis Manual*, 5th edn. Available at: https://sepsistrust.org/wp-content/uploads/2020/01/5th-Edition-manual-080120.pdf (accessed 12 November 2020).

World Health Organization (WHO) (2018) Falls. Available at: www.who.int/news-room/fact-sheets/detail/falls (accessed 09 November 2020).

PREPARING CHILDREN AND YOUNG PEOPLE FOR HOSPITALISATION

15

NICKY VARLEY AND ELENA HIGGINSON

--- THIS CHAPTER COVERS ---

- History of hospitalisation for children
- The importance of emotional health and wellbeing
- The role of the children's nurse
- Family-centred care

> "Children's nurses should always have big smiles and talk to me in a way I understand"
>
> **Isla – aged 10**

INTRODUCTION

As the opening quotation suggests, children's nurses, where possible, ensure that encounters between children admitted to hospital and health professionals are not intimidating, anxiety-inducing or frightening. Considering the child's age and stage of development is vital to these interactions; however, children and young people are individual and should not be generalised. Considering their specific needs is crucial to their experience at the time but, importantly, also to future interactions.

Within this chapter we will consider how children being admitted into hospital has changed over time and, importantly, investigate how children's nurses can make the interactions between nurses and other health professionals a better experience for children and their families. Nurses should endeavour to educate and promote best practice, demonstrating the importance of family-centred, holistic care for children at every stage of their development. With this in mind we also investigate the importance of Making Every Contact Count (MECC) when considering health promotion.

The importance of emotional health and wellbeing

When a child goes into hospital for a planned procedure or emergency admission it can be a frightening experience (Robertson, 1958; Coyne, 2006; Livesley and Long, 2013). As children's nurses we must endeavour to ease this anxiety through preparation and/or, in emergency situations, appropriate communication. Anxiety can present in many forms but often emotions such as shouting, crying and agitation are commonplace. This is due to the lack of control over the environment the child is presented with, a world that is unfamiliar to them with different noises, sights, smells, people in uniforms, monitors and other medical equipment which can look, sound and smell very different and frightening (NICE, 2021). Evidence suggests that positive interactions between health professionals and children and their families builds more trusting relationships (Roberts et al., 2015), and therefore will speed up both the treatment and recovery process which is crucial to a child's health outcomes (Lerwick, 2016).

ACTIVITY 15.1

It is difficult to comprehend that just 70 years ago when children went into hospital for a procedure or as an emergency patient, that their parents/carers were allowed only restricted visits and were not permitted to stay overnight with their child. It is imperative as children's nurses that we recognise the importance of these relationships and adopt a family-centred, holistic approach. Robertson (1958) highlighted the significance of this and produced several films in which he captured the distress of a 2-year-old girl during her hospital admission (Robertson, 1952). Though the film is upsetting, it is an important learning point for all children's nurses.

View the Robertson film discussed above through the URL provided, then consider the following points:

- What do you notice about the interactions between the nurse and the little girl?
- How does the girl appear during the film?
- How does the film make you feel?
- How is this practice different to your own practice or practice you have seen?

Go to: www.youtube.com/watch?app=desktop&v=s14Q-_Bxc_U "Two Year Old Goes to Hospital" (Robertson Films) – YouTube (accessed 20 March 2023).

The role of the children's nurse

Children's nurses are advocates for children within their care and should always consider the thoughts and feelings of both the child and family (Nursing and Midwifery Council, 2018). This is known as family-centred care and has been practised by children's nurses since the 1980s and incorporates the thoughts, feelings and considerations of the whole family whilst keeping the child at the centre of the care (Webb, 1993). Too often the child is lost within the communications and the focus of discussion shifts to health professionals and family/carers, therefore it is essential that we value the child or young person's voice and as a nurse advocate for their voice to be heard (Office of the Children's Commissioner, 2013). If we are to maintain trusting relationships with children when they meet health professionals, priority needs to be given to this essential part of communication.

Whilst it is important that the child remains the focus, ensuring family-centred care is maintained and communicating with parents or carers appropriately enables families to fully understand the care and treatment of their child, so they can also support in preparing their child effectively for hospitalisation (He et al., 2015). This has positive outcomes for both the child and their parents or carers, empowering them within their parental role to have an important and influential role in encouraging their child to feel comfortable and safe (Healy, 2013). The CARE acronym provided by Lerwick (2016) provides a good framework for students and children's nurses to deliver care to children and young people (CYP) in all healthcare settings. Below is a breakdown of the abbreviation and examples and explanations.

CARE

Choices

Give CYP choices in their care, this gives children an element of control back when they feel at their most vulnerable. An example of this might be to ask the child or young person which arm they would like the blood pressure measurement to be taken from, this simple question enables the patient to feel empowered and as health professionals this must be the goal, too often we 'do' nursing to our patients rather than offering a choice.

Agenda

It is important to discuss all aspects of the child's care with them, when children have a plan, and they know what is going to happen next through careful discussions with them and the family it will ease their anxieties around the unknown. Taking a few moments to discuss next steps with CYP will build rapport and secure trust that could potentially last throughout a child's lifetime of engaging with healthcare professionals and health settings.

Resilience

By focusing on the positives and reframing negatives we can attempt to elevate worry and anxiety within the medical setting. For example, talking about who is important to them, what they are good at and putting a positive slant on negative emotions will help with the current situation and, importantly, future interactions with the health professionals and settings.

(Continued)

Emotions

Children like to feel validated and validating their emotions is a key factor in building trusting relationships between the child and the nurse or healthcare provider. Allowing children to express their emotions in their individual ways will not only build positive, trusting relationships but also anchor their sense of security in an environment that is strange and frightening (Lerwick, 2016).

Consider cultural differences when using the CARE concept. Some cultures will avoid any kind of emotion whilst others will embrace it. As mentioned above, we should not try to inflict more distress and anxiety onto children, young people and their families at a time that may be difficult for them (Twycross and Stinson, 2014). If in doubt, ask the child or young person and their family; by doing this you are fully involving them in their care and, more often than not, families are more than happy to discuss their ideas of care with health professionals (Smith et al., 2015).

How can we better prepare children and young people?

Over the last few years alone, hospital preparation for children, young people and their families has changed significantly. A key part of preparation in some hospitals was to encourage hospital visits, where CYP and their parents/caregivers were invited to the clinical area to help reduce anxiety and stress, allowing them to become familiar with the clinical environment and equipment prior to hospitalisation. When asking children about hospital, many associate this with negative thoughts and feelings, such as pain and not being in their safe place, which then creates fear. The rationale behind the hospital visits was to attempt to address these negative preconceptions by CYP and their families by experiencing the environment for themselves. These visits targeted children who had a planned admission or who were high risk for admission; for example, it was part of the neonatal discharge process for families. Whilst this approach helps support planned admissions and acute admission for high-risk admissions, it did not support emergency admissions for a large proportion of acutely unwell CYP who present to hospital. During the coronavirus pandemic, which began in late 2019, hospital visits were no longer possible due to infection risk, and in many Trusts these visits have not been reintroduced. Some of the resources available to children, young people, and their families to aid with preparation for hospitalisation will be explored later within the chapter.

Health promotion

Making Every Contact Count (MECC) is an initiative which is seen across healthcare settings that aims to engage and empower frontline staff to contribute to health improvement by making health promotion 'everyone's business'. This strategy is particularly important within children and young people's nursing and is an opportunity to empower and improve the lives of children and their families and help foster positive health outcomes. The underlying principle of MECC is behaviour change, which is important when considering the child or young person and hospital admissions. As seen above, children can feel many different emotions when they attend any healthcare setting, fear and a lack of control being central to these emotions. As children's nurses we have an opportunity to allow children to 'play' with some of the equipment they may see when they come into hospital; ideally this needs to start at a young age. This activity is particularly important in breaking down barriers that may exist in relation to the fear and anxiety children and young people may feel prior to visiting a healthcare setting. We are aware of the importance of children and young people having a significant other with them when they visit healthcare settings; however, we must understand and appreciate that the environment itself is very different to their normal. The sights, noises and smells associated with healthcare settings are unique and can assault the senses, triggering feelings of being unwell and sometimes this can lead to negative feelings. This activity can be done on a pre-planned visit to the hospital before a planned procedure or as a Teddy Bear Clinic when nursing students along with university staff attend primary schools and nurseries taking equipment and empowering children to touch, see and hear some of the medical devices they may encounter when visiting a healthcare environment. This will be discussed later in the chapter.

THEORY STOP POINT

The importance of brain development in both young children and adolescents is central to interactions with their caregivers, it is also important that children's nurses understand this when considering hospital admissions.

Review the '1001 Critical Days' manifesto (Leadsom et al., 2014) and critically consider the implications for nursing practice.

www.nspcc.org.uk/globalassets/documents/news/critical-days-manifesto.pdf (accessed 20 March 2023)

Consider the implications of what you have read for your role as a children's nurse.

You may already be aware of the importance of early interactions, but can spend time looking further into this by looking at the website of the WAVE Trust:

https://www.wavetrust.org/understanding-the-adolescent-brain (accessed 31 October 2023)

SEE ALSO
CHAPTER 11

UNDERSTANDING THE LEGISLATION

Within this section the needs of children coming to hospital will be considered through exploring the relevant legislation.

United Nations Convention on the Rights of the Child (UNCRC)

The United Nations Convention on the Rights of the Child (UNCRC) is legislation which was universally agreed in 1989 and sets out the obligations and standards for the rights of children and young people (United Nations, 1989). The UNCRC came into force in the UK in 1992 and applies to children and young persons under the age of 18. The UNCRC addresses the human rights of a child or young person in relation to civil, political, economic, social, cultural, and environmental rights. It is also recognised that childhood is a key developmental stage, and as a result the UNCRC also recognises the importance of a child's right to grow, learn, play, develop and flourish with dignity, which is an additional consideration when compared to the rights of adults. These rights are reflected throughout the 54 articles which make up the Convention. Through the UNCRC recognising a child/young person's rights, it enables care to be delivered holistically to improve outcomes and recognise them not only as an individual but also on a wider level, as a member of a family and a community. UNCRC rights are often grouped into four areas:

- Protection – a child or young person has the right to be protected from exploitation and abuse
- Promotion – a child or young person has a right to grow and develop, this includes their right to have adequate housing, food, education, childcare and play
- Participation – a child or young person has the right to have an opinion and be involved in making decision which involve or impact them
- Prevention – This enables prevention systems to be implemented to ensure children and young people are protected from abuse or to avoid violation of their rights.

SEE ALSO
CHAPTER 8

When considering hospitalisation of a child or young person it is essential that as nurses we consider and protect their rights as outlined within the UNCRC, when preparing them and their family.

THEORY STOP POINT

Access a copy of the United Nations Convention on the Rights of the Child. This can be accessed through the UNICEF website at:

www.unicef.org.uk/what-we-do/un-convention-child-rights

Look at the document and try to decide to which of the categories above, the following articles belong:

- Article 9
- Article 12
- Article 28

Once you have done this, make some notes on how each of these articles might impact your day-to-day practice as a student nurse.

It would improve your understanding further if you are able to consider the other articles in this way too, considering how they will impact a children's nurse's practice.

Gillick competence

The Children Act 2004 suggests that once a person reaches the age of 18, they are an adult, and with this have the right to autonomy just as any other adult, suggesting that before the age of 18 they would be unable to make decisions legally. The Family Law Reform Act 1969 states that young people aged 16 and 17 can consent to medical treatment, if they have capacity to do so, despite not yet being classed as an adult. Following a legal case in the 1980s, Gillick competency was introduced to recognise that young people under the age of 16 years should be able to express their wishes and give consent to treatment.

whether or not a child is capable of giving the necessary consent will depend on the child's maturity and understanding and the nature of the consent required. The child must be capable of making a reasonable assessment of the advantages and disadvantages of the treatment proposed, so the consent, if given, can be properly and fairly described as true consent. (*Gillick* v. *West Norfolk and Wisbech AHA* [1985])

If a young person is deemed to be Gillick competent and refuses treatment, then parental consent can overrule. However, if a young person is Gillick competent and consents to treatment, but parents or carers disagree with this decision, then the young person's consent is respected, and treatment can go ahead. However, consent is not valid if the young person is being influenced or pressured.

The Academy of Medical Royal Colleges (2020) recognises the importance of Gillick competency and its place in recognising and respecting a child's individuality and ability to make decisions.

There is no standardised set of questions used to assess Gillick competency; however, professionals must consider:

- a child's age, maturity, and mental capacity
- their understanding of the advantages, disadvantages, and the long-term impact of the proposed treatment
- their understanding of risks, implications, and consequences as a result of their decisions
- their understanding of alternative treatment options
- their ability to provide and explain their rationale behind their decision

A young person may be deemed as Gillick competent to make one decision, but not when making another decision.

SEE ALSO
CHAPTER 8

WHAT'S THE EVIDENCE?

Further guidance around Gillick competency and consent has been published by the Department of Health (2009), which you can view here:

https://www.gov.uk/government/publications/reference-guide-to-consent-for-examination-or-treatment-second-edition

ACTIVITY 15.2: REFLECTIVE PRACTICE

Consider the emergency admission of a 15-year-old girl who has taken an overdose of paracetamol. She tells you she wants to end her life because she is being bullied at school.

- What should you do in these circumstances to ensure her safety and emotional and physical well-being?
- Considering the importance of Gillick competence, what should you do in these circumstances?

──────── SAFEGUARDING STOP POINT ────────

Considering the case study above, it is essential that the need for this 15-year-old to be safeguarded is recognised.

It is vitally important that children's nurses can identify potential issues in relation to interactions with their family/carers. Healthcare staff must be competent to recognise signs of maltreatment and therefore take appropriate actions to safeguard children, keeping up to date with mandatory training policies and procedures is not only the responsibility of the employing organisation but equally of the employee.

HOW DOES HOSPITALISATION IMPACT THE CHILD AND THEIR FAMILY?

──────── CASE STUDY 15.1: JESSICA ────────

Jessica is a 6-year-old girl who has quadriplegic cerebral palsy and epilepsy. She is non-verbal and has a gastrostomy tube due to having an unsafe swallow. She is fully dependent on her caregivers for all her needs and is fully wheelchair-bound. Jessica has been having increasing seizure activity at home over the last month. Jessica's mum, Lucy, has contacted Jessica's neurology consultant to inform them of her concerns. Lucy has received a letter stating a date for a planned admission for Lucy to have her current management and medications reviewed.

- What preparation do you think both Jessica and her Lucy might need?
- What would your concerns be here?

Lucy has expressed her worries about the upcoming planned admission, as she is anxious about what the planned admission will involve and does not feel that hospital is the appropriate environment for Jessica as she feels her needs will not be met. Lucy also states that she will struggle to reside with Jessica whilst caring for her other children, and the staff within the hospital do not understand Jessica like she does. As a result, Lucy is reluctant to attend with Jessica for the planned admission.

A multidisciplinary team (MDT) meeting has been arranged to prepare for the upcoming admission and offer some reassurance to Jessica's mum.

- Who do you think should attend the MDT meeting to ensure effective preparation for Jessica's planned admission, and what would their role be?
- What is important within this case study to ensure effective MDT working, and what are potential challenges to this?
- What are the principal needs of Jessica and her mum?
- How could the situation be improved?
- What are the consequences if we do not get preparation for hospitalisation right in this situation?

ACTIVITY 15.3: CRITICAL THINKING

Consider the advantages and disadvantages of bringing children/young people and their families to the clinical area prior to admission.

As previously identified within the chapter, pre-arranged visits to clinical areas only supports certain groups of children and young people and is largely related to planned admissions. Therefore, it is important to consider how those excluded from these groups, for example acute admissions, are prepared for hospitalisation and whether this is effective. We have a growing range of resources available to support in the preparation of CYP for hospitalisation which encourage conversations and questions, such as story books and role play.

Play can be extremely beneficial, particularly for younger children, as it is a key part of everyday life (Ofsted, 2022), helping to normalise some of the clinical experiences and equipment they may see in healthcare environments, with the Care Quality Commission (2015) recommending play as an important part of hospitalisation and treatment for children and young people. The concept of play as a method of providing information is utilised by play therapists who have a range of equipment to provide accurate and informed information to CYP both in the hospital setting but also within the community to facilitate effective preparation. However, these are essential skills which nurses can also possess to help support CYP within the healthcare environment (NICE, 2021).

If there is limited access for children, young people and their families to support prior to hospitalisation then misunderstanding could develop, leading to ineffective support being cascaded. For example, if a child's negative expectations around injections are being inappropriately reinforced then is effective preparation being achieved?

Despite young people recognising that social media is not an accurate source for health information, young people find themselves accessing information in this way, which causes concern as often the online content available is biased, with those with poor health perceptions being most likely to share their views, which can negatively impact perspectives around medical procedures (Hausmann et al., 2017). In view of this, e-health methods are being developed and used to support young people in accessing effective and appropriate health information (Treadgold and Grant, 2014). If the parent or carer of the child or young person is supported by healthcare professionals to develop a detailed and accurate understanding of what to expect, then this enables them to be able to prepare their child appropriately. It is important to remember that generally it is the parents who will be responding to questions the child or young person might have when in the home environment prior to hospitalisation, which reinforces the importance of family-centred care in preparing the whole family for hospitalisation (Institute for Patient– and Family-Centered Care, 2017). By equipping parents/caregivers to support their child in this way, it helps them make an important and valuable contribution to keeping their child as calm and comfortable as possible in what will be a strange environment. However, this family-centred approach is an evolving educational approach which takes time, therefore cannot be a short-term conclusion to hospital preparation.

A developing approach to preparing younger children for hospitalisation within the community is the 'Teddy Bear Clinic', which also utilises the valuable concept of play to provide education associated with medical equipment and environments, a scheme which was first introduced in 1994 to help overcome and reduce some of the anxieties and challenges around hospitalisation of young children

(Santen and Feldman, 1994). The 'Teddy Bear Clinic' consists of children being exposed to a clinical environment through role play with their 'sick' teddy bears, where they can familiarise themselves with various medical equipment and medical unforms to help develop positive experiences within these settings, seeking to make their soft toys better (Rashid et al., 2021).

CRITICAL THINKING STOP POINT

- Is a 'Teddy Bear Clinic' approach available locally to you for children and young people?
- Do you think it should be something which is built into the curriculum for children?

STUDENT TIPS

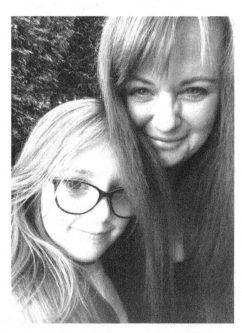

Figure 15.1 Erica (nursing student) and child

There are some simple ways we can put children and young people at ease:

Smiling, saying hello, saying their name, and using a gentle voice and touch (where appropriate) to also calm and reassure parents/carers helps to settle a child

Involving siblings can also help settle the situation for everyone and giving people a 'job' to do (such as recording the numbers or reading them out) can make everyone feel like they are helping

Having a ready stock of bubbles, story books and stickers for younger children can help build the therapeutic relationship

As discussed throughout this chapter, hospitalisation of a child can be a very scary time for children, young people and their families. Whilst it is important that we consider the family, it is equally as important to keep the child at the centre of care to ensure that holistic care is provided.

The impact of separation from a caregiver is well recognised as being detrimental, which over the years has led to advances in hospital care for children and young people to recognise the importance of family-centred care. Wherever possible, caregivers are now supported and encouraged to reside with their child to reduce further disruption and distress. The separation from siblings, friends, and pets creates additional disturbance to daily life. Younger children are particularly susceptible to routine disturbances, which can further impact their response to hospitalisation. It is important that nurses try to reduce this impact where possible by promoting and encouraging family-centred care and empowering parents/carers to be involved in caring for their child and continuing a familiar routine to reduce disturbance. An effective therapeutic relationship between the nurse and the child/young person and their parent/carer helps facilitate this effectively. Early preparation can support families to plan appropriately for instances of hospitalisation; however, emergency admissions can make this more difficult for parents who find themselves having to manage siblings, employment, and an unwell child.

As nurses, we want to help wherever possible, although this can lead to frustration with certain patients and their families. When considering the care of older children, nurses can unintentionally create feelings of powerlessness or loss of control, which can cause breakdown in trust and the therapeutic relationship. It is essential we are aware of this and empower young people as much as possible.

In times of stress, parents may be unable to be emotionally available to their child to provide care and reassurance as discussed above, particularly in emergency situations. As expressed by parents, their emotions reflect on their child, therefore a key role for us as nurses when providing care to children and young people in hospital is considering the emotional wellbeing of their parents/caregivers and having an awareness of the challenges they may be facing during the period of hospitalisation.

CHAPTER SUMMARY

- Emotional health and wellbeing
- Therapeutic relationships and family-centred care
- Preparing children for healthcare settings
- Health promotion
- Legislation

BUILD YOUR BIBLIOGRAPHY

Consider hospitalisation from the family's point of view – it can lead to a lot of anxiety and stress as we have explored within the chapter.

Journal articles

- Jensen, C.S., Jackson, J., Kolbæk, R. and Glasdam, S. (2012) 'Children's experiences of acute hospitalisation to a paediatric emergency and assessment unit – A qualitative study'. *Journal of Child Health Care*, 16(3) 263-73.

  This journal article presents a qualitative study which looks into children's experiences first hand of acute hospitalisation.
- Kennedy, M. and Howlin, F. (2022) 'Preparation of children for elective surgery and hospitalisation: A parental perspective'. *Journal of Child Health Care*, 26(4) 568-80.

  Preparation of children for elective surgery and hospitalisation: a parental perspective.

FURTHER
READING:
ONLINE
JOURNAL
ARTICLES

Weblinks

FURTHER
READING:
WEBLINKS

- What? Why? Children in Hospital, Preparing for Hospital, is a valuable resource which provides a range of different videos to help prepare for various different situations that may be faced within a hospital environment: www.whatwhychildreninhospital.org.uk
- To target younger children, a series on CBeebies seeks to discover and share facts about health and hospitals. Songs and videos are available to view through the link below and target both children and parents in relation to hospitalisation and hospital treatment: www.bbc.co.uk/cbeebies/shows/get-well-soon
- Great Ormond Street Children's Hospital (GOSH) is one of the world's leading children's hospitals and their website helps prepare children and families for hospitalisation, including a virtual tour of the hospital: www.gosh.nhs.uk/your-hospital-visit/take-virtual-tour-great-ormond-street-hospital/

REFERENCES

Academy of Medical Royal Colleges (2020) Academy of Medical Royal Colleges statement on Gillick Competency. [online] Available at: www.rcpch.ac.uk/resources/academy-medical-royal-colleges-statement-gillick-competency (accessed 13 June 2023).

Care Quality Commission (2015) *Children and Young People's Inpatient and Day Case Survey 2014: Key findings*. Newcastle upon Tyne: Care Quality Commission.

Children Act 2004, c. *31*. Available at: www.legislation.gov.uk/ukpga/2004/31.

Coyne, I. (2006) 'Children's experiences of hospitalization'. *Journal of Child Health Care*, 10 (4): 326–36.

Family Law Reform Act 1969, c. *46*. Available at: www.legislation.gov.uk/ukpga/1969/46.

Gillick v. *West Norfolk and Wisbech AHA* [1985] 1 All ER 533.

Hausmann, J.S., Touloumtzis, T., White, M.T., Colbert, J.A. and Gooding, H.C. (2017) 'Adolescent and young adult use of social media for health and its implications'. *Journal of Adolescent Health*. 60 (6), 714–19.

He, H-G., Zhu, L-X., Chan, W-C.S., Liam, J.L.W., Ko, S.S., Li, H.C.W., Wang, W. and Yobas, P. (2015) 'A mixed-method study of effects of a therapeutic play intervention for children on parental anxiety and parents' perceptions of the intervention'. *Journal of Advanced Nursing*, 71 (7): 1539–51.

Healy, K. (2013) 'A descriptive survey of the information needs of parents of children admitted for same day surgery'. *Journal of Pediatric Nursing*, 28: 179–85.

Institute for Patient- and Family-Centered Care (IPFCC) (2017) *Advancing the Practice of Patient and Family-Centered Care in Hospital Settings*. Bethesda, MD: Institute for Patient- and Family-Centered Care. Available at: www.ipfcc.org/resources/getting_started.pdf.

Leadsom, A., Field, F., Burstow, P. and Lucas, C. (2014) *The 1001 Critical Days: The Importance of the Conception to Age Two Period*. A Cross-Party Manifesto. WAVE Trust/NSPCC. Available at: www.wavetrust.org/1001-critical-days-the-importance-of-the-conception-to-age-two-period; and www.nspcc.org.uk/globalassets/documents/news/critical-days-manifesto.pdf (accessed 20 March 2023).

Lerwick, J.L. (2016) 'Minimizing pediatric healthcare-induced anxiety and trauma'. *World Journal of Clinical Pediatriacs*, 85 (2):143–50.

Livesley, J. and Long, T. (2013) 'Children's experiences as hospital in-patients: voice, competence and work. Messages for nursing from a critical ethnographic study'. *International Journal of Nursing Studies*, 50: 1292–303.

National Institute for Health and Care Excellence (NICE) (2021) *Babies, Children and Young People's Experience of Healthcare*. Available at: www.nice.org.uk/guidance/ng204 (accessed 13 June 2023).

Nursing and Midwifery Council (NMC) (2018) *The Code: Professional Standards of Practice and Behaviour for Nurses, Midwives and Nursing Associates*. London: NMC. Available at: www.nmc.org.uk/standards/code/.

Ofsted (2022) *Best start in life Part 1: Setting the scene*. Available at:www.gov.uk/government/publications/best-start-in-life-a-research-review-for-early-years/best-start-in-life-part-1-setting-the-scene (accessed 29 March 2023).

Rashid, A.A., Cheong, A.T., Hisham, R., Shamsuddin, N.H. and Roslan, D. (2021) 'Effectiveness of pretend medical play in improving children's health outcomes and well-being: a systematic review'. *BMJ Open*. 11 (1):e041506. Doi: 10.1136/bmjopen-2020-041506.

Roberts, J., Fenton, G. and Barnard, M. (2015) 'Developing effective therapeutic relationships in children, young people and their families'. *Nursing Children and Young People*, 27 (4): 30–5.

Robertson, J. (1952) *A 2-year-old Goes to Hospital*. Film, Concord Video and Film Council.

Robertson, J. (1958) *Young Children in Hospital*. London: Tavistock.

Santen, L. and Feldman, T. (1994) 'Teddy bear clinics: a huge community project'. *MCN The American Journal of Maternal/Child Nursing*, 19(2), 102-6.

Smith, J., Cheater, F., Bekker, H. and Chatwin, J. (2015) 'Are parents and professionals making shared decisions about a child's care on presentation of a suspected shunt malfunction: a mixed method study?' *Health Expectations*, 18 (5): 1299–315.

Treadgold, P. and Grant, C. (2014). Evidence Review: what does good health information look like? *Report commissioned by the Patient Information Forum*. Available at: www.pifonline.org.uk/wp-content/uploads/2015/03/What-does-good-health-information-look-like-October-2014.pdf.

Twycross, A. and Stinson, J. (2014) 'Physical and psychological methods of pain relief in children', in A. Twycross, S. Dowden and J. Stinson (eds), *Managing Pain in Children: A Clinical Guide for Nurses and Healthcare Professionals*, 2nd edn. Chichester: Wiley–Blackwell.

United Nations (1989) *Convention on the Rights of the Child (UNCRC)*. Available at: www.unicef.org.uk/what-we-do/un-convention-child-rights (accessed 6 June 2023).

Webb, B. (1993) 'Trauma and tedium: an account of living on a children's ward', in J. Walmsley, J. Reynolds, P. Shakespeare and R. Wolf (eds), *Health, Welfare and Practice: Reflecting on Roles and Relationships*. London: Sage.

CARE OF CHILDREN AND YOUNG PEOPLE IN THE PERI- AND POSTOPERATIVE RECOVERY PERIOD

16

KAREN PATTRICK

THIS CHAPTER COVERS

- Types of paediatric surgery
- Perioperative preparation
- Postoperative care
- The role of the nurse
- Transferring the child or young person to theatre
- Discharge

INTRODUCTION

"Where other specialties are concerned with a particular technique or area of the body, paediatric surgery is the only surgical specialty that is defined by the patient's age rather than by a specific condition and deals with the diseases, trauma and malformations from the foetal period to teenage years."

Royal College of Surgeons, 2022

Paediatric surgery was not considered specialised until first half of the 20th century but it encompasses a wide range of procedures and nursing care of children ages 0–15 years of age, including preterm neonates weighing 500–600g to adolescents (Royal College of Surgeons, 2022). This chapter will cover just some of the different types of paediatric surgery that may be seen though it is not inclusive to all specialties. It will include perioperative preparation including the importance of play and age-appropriate approaches, consent, fasting and the role and responsibilities of the nurse preparing the child and young person for theatre. Postoperative care will discuss the frequency of observations required, pain assessment and preparation for discharge home. Although different specialities will have their own specific requirements, the general principles of nursing care can be applied to most surgical situations requiring surgical care both peri- and postoperatively. However, it is the specific knowledge and skills in relation to age and stage of development, cognitive emotional and anatomical differences, careful fluid and drug calculations, and the availability of specialist equipment and access to staff with the appropriate skills that enables the delivery of high-quality family-centred care within the specialist field of children's nursing.

TYPES OF PAEDIATRIC SURGERY

Surgical procedures as day case surgery is suitable for most healthy children but in recent years this has increasingly included those who have chronic illnesses. Most patients are able to undergo day case surgery unless there is a valid reason why an overnight stay would be required (Bailey et al., 2019). In these cases, an overnight admission in a designated high dependency area or tertiary centre may need to be considered (see Table 16.1).

Table 16.1 Children and young people who would not be suitable for day surgery in a District General Hospital as suggested by British Association of Day Surgery (2018)

Ex-premature babies < 60 weeks post conceptual age

Difficult airway

Extreme obesity

Previous anaesthetic problems leading to delayed recovery

Metabolic disorder that cannot tolerate starvation

Haemoglobinopathy

Obstructive sleep apnoea

Poorly controlled chronic disease

There are many surgical procedures that may be required by the infant, child or adolescent. Table 16.2 provides an example of a surgical procedures undertaken by each specialty.

Table 16.2 Examples of surgical procedures undertaken by each specialty

Specialty	Presenting Problem	Intervention
Ophthalmology: Strabismus	Strabismus: About 2-3% of children develop a squint, which is lack of coordination of the eyes meaning they point in different directions. If left untreated then this can become permanent.	Surgery may be required under general anaesthetic where the muscle that connects to the eye is detached and moved to a new position allowing the eye to point in the same direction.
Urology: Hypospadias	Hypospadias occurs during development before birth and is present in 3:1000 and is characterised by the hole in the penis at the end of the ureter not in the correct place.	The surgery required under general anaesthetic would depend upon severity, but in most cases the urethra is moved to the tip of the penis.
Plastic Surgery: Otoplasty	Otoplasty or ear correction due to protruding or prominent ears. This is usually undertaken by plastic surgeons as it is considered cosmetic.	Surgical procedure under general anaesthetic aims to reposition the elastic cartilage and to achieve a natural position.
General surgery: Appendicitis	Appendicitis is inflammation of the appendix. It is a common reason for abdominal surgery, particularly in older children and teenagers.	Whilst conservative management is considered a safe and effective management strategy, surgical intervention under general anaesthetic for the removal of the appendix may be required. The appendix is cut off from the caecum and the hole is closed with stitches.
Ear, Nose and Throat (ENT): Tonsillectomy	Recurrent tonsillitis. Tonsils are two mounds of lymphatic tissue which help fight infection, but are only important during the first few years of life. These can become infected causing tonsillitis. Usually children grow out of recurrent tonsillitis, however, removal may be at the discretion of the surgeon and the criterion for surgical intervention is met.	Under general anaesthetic the surgeon removes the tonsils through the mouth and seals the blood vessels around them.
Neurosurgery: Hydrocephalus	Hydrocephalus occurs when excess cerebrospinal fluid (CSF) collects in the brain's ventricles. It affects 1:1000 children and may be congenital or due to illnesses such as meningitis.	The shunt (long silicon tube) will be inserted into the ventricles leading to the abdomen. This will then allow for excess CSF to be drained away into the abdomen.
Orthopaedic: Fractures	Fractures are common in children and severity depends on how the bone has broken and the damage to the surrounding tissue.	Severe fractures may require surgical intervention under general anaesthetic to realign the bone, or manipulation under anaesthetic (MUA) and may require the use of wires, plates, screws or rods to assist with the realignment and healing process.
Cardiology: Atrial Septal Defect (ASD)	ASD is a congenital heart defect, so occurs during foetal development, where there is a hole in the septum between the atria.	Treatment will depend on the size of the hole, and may require surgical intervention by either cardiac catheterisation or open-heart surgery.

SEE ALSO
CHAPTER 20

SEE ALSO
CHAPTER 29

SEE ALSO
CHAPTER 19

SEE ALSO
CHAPTER 23

PERIOPERATIVE PREPARATION

SEE ALSO
CHAPTER 15

Approaches to preparation in the perioperative period is aimed at providing the child, young person and family with good-quality preoperative information, opportunity for pre-admission visits and provision of written information or booklets for the child and parents. This provides opportunity for education and to establish a rapport between the patient, family and healthcare professionals and information provided should include fasting, what to do if the child becomes unwell on the day of surgery, and discharge advice (RCN, 2020b).

Play

> "Play prepares children at their level to what is going to happen. It gives them opportunities to work through their feelings, build confidence and coping mechanisms. It also helps the MDT find out if they have any fear or anxiety such as to needles so this can be worked around. Ultimately it gives the child a choice."
>
> **Gina, play specialist**

Play is an essential part of preparing the child for surgery. The Royal College of Nursing (RCN) (2020a) support this stating 'a play specialist should be available to provide preparation and support to the child or young person'. Preparation for surgery can be challenging and may require specific preparation if the child or young person has a chronic illness, learning difficulties or communication impairments which must be considered. Children learn through play, developing creativity imagination, dexterity, physical, cognitive and emotional strength and play allows the child to engage in the world around them from an early age (Ginsberg, 2006; Early Years Foundation Stage, 2022). Piaget's stages of development suggest that cognitive understanding develops as the infant, child and young person develop through age (Piaget, 1936). Vygotsky (1978) suggests children learn through social interactions, and it is these interactions that provide learning opportunities for the child to build knowledge from peers and adults. Understanding the stages of cognitive development in children is therefore fundamental to understanding children's perceptions of health-related events and their information-processing abilities. Ultimately, children's questions and behavioural adjustments can provide cues regarding appropriate timing for information to be given before an invasive procedure.

From birth to 2 years of age the infant develops an awareness that people and things exist when out of sight and limitations in conceptual abilities at this developmental age mean pre-procedure preparation focuses on the parents or carers. Between the ages of 2 to 7 years cognitive development is characterised by egocentric and concrete thinking. Therefore, children now view external events as the cause of illness but cannot conceptualise internal body parts. Unguided play is important at this stage, using dolls, doctor kits, or simple hospital props such as surgical hats, masks, syringes and stethoscopes, to provide the child opportunity to express anxiety, process information, and become familiar with equipment. This should be supported by a trained healthcare provider who can offer simple explanations. From 7 years onwards, children have increased awareness of internal body parts, body functions, and fear loss of body parts. Whilst some methods described previously are beneficial at this age, now the optimum time to provide children information regarding upcoming surgery is approximately 1 week beforehand. Older children in this age range may benefit from pre-procedure preparation at 2–4 weeks beforehand.

ACTIVITY 16.1: REFLECTIVE PRACTICE

Reflect on how you implement play when communicating with infants and children in clinical practice. What play activities have you encouraged, and how has this benefited your professional relationship with the child and their family?

Consent

Consent is law and the Nursing and Midwifery Council (2018) states consent should be obtained before undertaking any treatment or care, upholding people's rights to be fully involved in their care, respecting their right to accept or decline treatment. Though the United Nations Convention on the Rights of the Child (1989) and the Children Act 1989 state a child is a person below the age of 18 years, young people age 16–17 years can give consent to surgical procedures, as there is now a presumption of capacity in this age group. Autonomy underpins informed consent and the information given to the patient or family from which they make their decision. There are instances where children under the age of 16 years may give valid consent for treatment based on the fact they have the cognitive ability to demonstrate sufficient understanding of the proposed surgery and the implications of their decision, and Gillick competence recognises this (RCN, 2022). Therefore, when nursing children it is important an appropriate healthcare professional explains the treatment or care; the expected benefits; the material risks and side effects; the alternative courses of action; and likely consequences of not receiving the treatment. Legally this underpins the appropriateness of the treatment but clinically consent can increase the success of treatment which depends on the child's cooperation. When a child relies on a person with parental responsibility to make decisions about their healthcare, the ethical and legal rationale for all treatments is based on the fact decisions made should be in the best interests of the child (Children Act 2004).

SEE ALSO
CHAPTER 8

CASE STUDY 16.1: ELLIE

Ellie is a 4-year-old girl admitted with a 2-day history of vomiting, fever, abdominal pain, lethargy and clinical signs suggesting mild dehydration. Ellie has had an ultrasound scan (USS) confirming her diagnosis of appendicitis and which her mum (who was accompanying Ellie) was informed of and the need for surgery. Ellie's mum left the ward to 'quickly' return home, which was close by and collect some items for Ellie and herself needed for the expected stay in hospital. However, further reporting of the USS showed Ellie had fluid in her abdomen suggesting her appendix had perforated and blood test results demonstrated a raised CRP (C reactive protein), indicating the severity of infection. Ellie needed to be taken to theatre immediately and the consultant surgeon arrived on the ward to gain informed consent from Ellie's mum. As Ellie's mum was not present the consultant waited on the ward for the mother to return. This took longer than anticipated; nursing staff attempted to contact her to request she return to the ward, but was unsuccessful. The consultant decided Ellie should be taken to theatre without consent as this was in Ellie's best interest, to prevent further widespread infections, sepsis and possibly death. Ellie was prepared for theatre by nursing staff (as per Table 16.3), at which point her mum returned and informed consent was gained for the appendicectomy.

Question: Can the consultant take Ellie to theatre for the surgical procedure without obtaining informed consent from her mother?

Fasting

Preoperative fasting in children undergoing surgery follows the 2-4-6 rule (RCN, 2020). This means solid food, cow's milk or infant milk can be consumed up until 6 hours before surgery, breast milk up to 4 hours and the intake of water and other clear fluid up to 2 hours before induction of anaesthesia. The period of fasting prior to surgery is important to avoid pulmonary aspiration, although the incidence of aspiration is suggested to be low in children (Disma et al., 2021). When the administration of regular medication is required, where possible this should be continued, especially those medications considered time-critical, meaning they need to be taken at the same time each day, such as anti-epileptic medications. The anaesthetic team should consider further interventions for children at higher risk of regurgitation and aspiration, such as emergency surgery when fasting guidelines may not have been implemented. However, when there is a delay in the infant child or young person going to theatre the resulting period of prolonged fasting can lead to increased irritability, hypoglycaemia, dehydration, headaches, delayed wound healing and increased likelihood of postoperative nausea and vomiting.

WHAT'S THE EVIDENCE?

Fasting times have been an ongoing debate. Andersson et al. (2018) suggested that the introduction of a 0-4-6 fasting regime reduced the number of children subjected to extended fasting. Disma et al. (2021) recognise the fact that fasting guidelines are intended to reduce pulmonary aspiration; however they also recognise fasting guidelines have consequences, such as discussed previously, which may exacerbate parental dissatisfaction. Therefore, should the 2-4-6 rule be reduced to 1-4-6?

The role of the nurse

The nursing role is to prepare the child for theatre and to support the child and family through the surgical journey. Courtman et al. (2022) suggest that where possible preparation should commence at least 2 weeks before, which may be in a nurse-led pre-assessment clinic. However, surgery is not always planned and can be required as a result of an acute illness or injury, but in either situation the assessment should be undertaken by an appropriately trained paediatric nurse. Prior to surgery the nurse will need to ensure that the relevant documentation is completed and that the child's perioperative condition is assessed. This includes activities as outlined in Table 16.3.

Table 16.3 Perioperative nursing procedures

Nursing intervention	Consideration
Obtain baseline observations (ABCDE Assessment))	**Airway assessment** This should include: Is the airway patent or at risk of obstruction? Does the patient have a tracheostomy or other airway conditions that could affect patency of the airway? **Breathing (respiratory) assessment** Obtain and document the following: respirations per minute, note ventilatory requirements preoperatively, any specific conditions (i.e., asthma or recurrent chest infections), obtain oxygen saturations, documenting any oxygen requirements and any observed use of accessory muscles or recession (sternal, intercostal or subcostal). **Circulatory assessment** Obtain and document the following: heart rate per minute (obtained appropriately for age). Are there any specific conditions (i.e., cardiac) to be aware of? Blood pressure, capillary refill time, urine output (ml/kg/hour) or noted difference in frequency of wet nappies/going to the toilet. **Disability assessment** Obtain and document the Glasgow Coma Scale assessment, check blood glucose if required. **Environment** Temperature (obtained appropriately for age) and consider thermoregulation requirements (i.e., hats for neonates), skin assessment (rashes, injuries, pressure ulcers or moisture-associated skin damage present).
Weight and height	Should be obtained on admission or in nurse-led preoperative clinic.
Identification: refer to local policy	All patients should wear identity bands displaying the core identifiers for the patient. This includes first and last name, date of birth, NHS number and barcode. A white wristband is used for identity and red identity band is used to identify a potential risk.
Perioperative bloods	Full blood count, cross match, urea and electrolytes, C-reactive protein (CRP) test, blood cultures, blood gas, blood sugar.
Intravenous access	Peripheral cannula in working order, or numbing cream applied for intravenous cannulation in theatre.
Intravenous fluids	If requires intravenous fluids, check appropriate fluids in situ dependent on blood results if available, rate and type of fluid is correctly prescribed and infusing as per prescription.
Nil by mouth	Fasting guidelines have been adhered to where possible, or check when last ate and drank to assist with the prevention of pulmonary aspiration.
Regular prescribed medications	Regular medications can be taken with water. The recommended amount of water is up to 0.5ml/kg to a maximum amount of 30ml. However other routes of administration could be considered if applicable. Intravenous or oral antibiotics and pain relief may be required perioperatively.
Informed consent	Consent form is signed by an appropriate person with parental responsibility, their signature confirmed on the form and signature of the person providing the information. Check the procedure is clearly stated along with the potential risks.
Documentation	Documentation should be clear and accurate, identifying any risks or problems that have arisen. Documentation should be gathered and accompany the patient to and from theatre including PAWS/PEWS charts; fluid balance charts, fluid prescription chart, prescription chart, nursing evaluation and medical notes. Other information such as blood results and X-rays should be widely available to staff via the Trust's own intranet services and as per Trust policies.

Adapted from Royal College Nursing (2020b)

Transferring the child or young person to theatre.

The Royal College of Nursing *Day Surgery for Children and Young People* guidance (RCN, 2020b) states there is no agreed standard for transferring children to and from theatre, but the main focus is patient safety and involving the family, which helps reduce anxiety. Therefore, family members are actively encouraged to accompany their child to theatre and into the anaesthetic room, remaining with them until the child is asleep. It is recognised that some parents or carers will not feel comfortable accompanying their child to theatre and should be supported in their decision not to be present. The method of transport to the anaesthetic room could be walking, being carried, using a special car, on a trolley, and own pushchair or wheelchair whilst considering any premedication administered and patient safety. National Institute for Health and Care Excellence (NICE, 2020) guidance for prevention and treatment of surgical site infections, which includes children and young people, states theatre wear should be appropriate, provide easy access to the operative site and for placing devices, whilst maintaining patient comfort and dignity. The child should therefore be offered the choice of what to wear for theatre having been advised of appropriate clothing in the preoperative consultation (RCN, 2020b). However, local policy may supersede this and in such cases the child should be offered a hospital theatre gown.

POSTOPERATIVE CARE

Postoperative care begins when the child or young person leaves the post-anaesthetic care unit (PACU), when it is suggested that at this point children are at a higher risk of developing postoperative complications (Gormley-Fleming, 2018), and ends when they are discharged home. Although parents or carers should have the information they need to continue to provide care at home, it is essential parents or carers feel comfortable about going home. Whilst different specialties will have specific requirements related to the surgical procedure they have performed and follow-on care required, there are fundamental principles which can be applied to any surgical procedure. Communication is one of the 6 Cs and is influential on patient treatment and care and upon returning to the ward from the PACU the nurse handing over the care should provide a well-communicated, detailed handover, using the SBAR communication tool (Situation, Background, Assessment, Recommendation).

SEE ALSO
CHAPTER 6

SBAR is suggested to be a standardised, structured form of communication between healthcare professionals to ensure concise and focused information is given and received (Dougherty and Lister, 2015).

Observation of vital signs, wounds, monitoring equipment

CYP nurses must be able to undertake a comprehensive nursing assessment and recognise deterioration and respond appropriately (NMC, 2018), therefore suggesting surgical nursing care aims to identify early any potential complications. All vital signs can be affected by surgery and anaesthesia and the frequency of observations should reflect the child's level of instability both peri- and post-surgery, and in all cases include a level of consciousness and pain assessment (RCN, 2020b). Observations should be recorded continually whilst the child or young person is being cared for in the PACU, though once they are able to maintain their own airway and present with respiratory stability then the frequency can, if needed, be reduced as detailed in Table 16.4.

Table 16.4 Frequency of postoperative vital signs (Royal College of Nursing, 2020)

Surgical procedure	Frequency of observations
For non-complex procedures	Every 30 minutes for 2 hours then hourly for 2–4 hours until the child is fully awake, eating and drinking
Following adenotonsillectomy	Every 30 minutes for 4 hours, or more frequently if there is any evidence of bleeding

For more complex procedures
    Theatre time greater than 6 hours
    Significant fluid loss
    Under 1 year of age
    Physiological instability preoperatively
    Physiological instability during the recovery period
	Continuous monitoring should be in situ for a minimum of 4 hours
	
	If the child is stable after continuous monitoring for 4 hours, routine 4-hourly observations can then be undertaken

Children may be discharged more quickly, in which case a full set of vital sign observations should be undertaken on discharge. Vital signs obtained should include heart rate, respiratory rate, oxygen saturation, non-invasive blood pressure and temperature, wounds and dressings. Other considerations include eating and drinking, or are intravenous fluids required, in which case there should be a fluid balance chart detailing their input and output. When considering output, it is also important to acknowledge any drains or catheters which may be in situ and how the output from these is measured and recorded to ensure it is included in the overall fluid balance.

Pain assessment

"Always pain score and check the anaesthetic and operative notes to ascertain what medications are prescribed and what has been given but, really importantly, when."

Eve, 3rd-year children's nursing student

Paediatric anaesthetists may initiate postoperative analgesia using a multidisciplinary approach including patients and their families, surgeons and nursing staff providing ongoing postoperative care. Pain assessment in children can be challenging as it varies greatly with their age and stage of development, but this is the most important factor to consider when choosing an appropriate pain tool for assessment. For neonates and infants or cognitively impaired children, the Faces, Legs, Arms, Cry, Consolability (FLACC) scale may be used, consisting of five components, observed for at least a minute each.

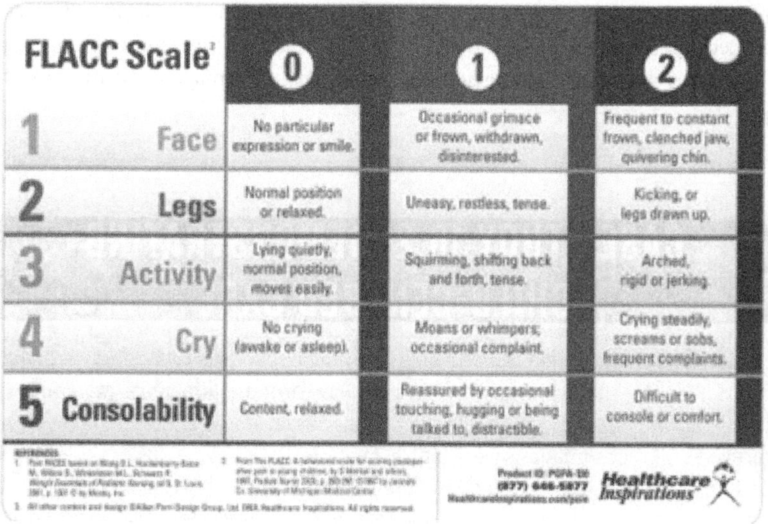

FLACC Scale		0	1	2
1	Face	No particular expression or smile.	Occasional grimace or frown, withdrawn, disinterested.	Frequent to constant frown, clenched jaw, quivering chin.
2	Legs	Normal position or relaxed.	Uneasy, restless, tense.	Kicking, or legs drawn up.
3	Activity	Lying quietly, normal position, moves easily.	Squirming, shifting back and forth, tense.	Arched, rigid or jerking.
4	Cry	No crying (awake or asleep).	Moans or whimpers; occasional complaint.	Crying steadily, screams or sobs, frequent complaints.
5	Consolability	Content, relaxed.	Reassured by occasional touching, hugging or being talked to, distractible.	Difficult to console or comfort.

Figure 16.1 FLACC Scale

The Wong–Baker FACES Scale can be used for verbal children including toddlers and pre-schoolers (ages 2–4), although is validated for ages 3 and above (Murphy, 2020). Verbal and behavioural indicators can be observed to assess pain in this age group; however, these indicators may be influenced by the approach to the child, meaning good communication skills with knowledge of age-appropriate approaches should be used to enhance the accuracy of assessment.

PAIN SCALE LEVEL

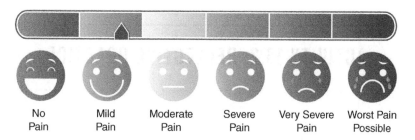

| No Pain | Mild Pain | Moderate Pain | Severe Pain | Very Severe Pain | Worst Pain Possible |

Figure 16.2 Pain rating scale (https://www.freepik.com/free-vector/diagram-showing-pain-scale-level-with-different-colors_19377144.htm#query=pain%20scale&position=4&from_view=keyword&track=ais)

The pain rating scale can be used in children aged 3 and above, and may be the most appropriate; however, the numerical pain scale can be used for children and young people at the older end of this age bracket who can rate their pain on a scale of 1–10. Pain should be assessed, recorded and treated with prescribed postoperative analgesia appropriate for the developmental age of the child, and surgical procedure. It should be administered within a safe environment by appropriately trained nursing staff and pain should be reassessed following any pharmaceutical or non-pharmaceutical interventions.

CASE STUDY 16.2: DEMONSTRATING CHILD-CENTRED CARE

A 10-year-old boy, Joe, had returned from theatre following appendicectomy, division of adhesions and wash-out of pus from the abdomen. On his return he was responsive to voice, maintaining his airway, self-ventilating in air with saturations of 95%, and further assessment of breathing highlighted no concerns. His cardiovascular observations were stable, he had intravenous fluids in situ, and a nasogastric tube in situ on free drainage and aspirates from the stomach were being replaced millilitre for millilitre. He was able to follow commands, move spontaneously, and eyes were opening to speech as he was still sleepy. Temperature was recorded and was within normal range and pain assessment was undertaken; his score was moderate and it was noted his prescribed analgesia was due for administration. He had an epidural in situ which was prescribed as patient controlled analgesia (PCA), as he was deemed to have cognitive ability to be able to use this appropriately. However, as he had arrived back from theatre he needed a full skin check and position change. When he was informed of this, he was scared and worried that movement would hurt. Time was spent with him preparing him for the change of position, intravenous paracetamol was administered as per British National Formulary Guidelines (2022) and prior to the turn he pressed the button for his PCA. Although this was explained and reassured him, the most effective reassurance was offered by the nurse who demonstrated a step-by-step approach, took the time he needed for each movement and when asked would it hurt, was honest in her answer which was appropriate for age and reassuring, developing a trusting professional relationship and the position change was successful and skin assessment was undertaken.

ACTIVITY 16.2: REFLECTIVE PRACTICE

Reflect on your clinical practice experiences and when pain scales have been implemented.

How effective were these?

What influenced the effectiveness of the tool?

DISCHARGE AND ADVANCE PLANNING

Timely discharge of children and young people requires children's nurses to have knowledge and experience of the protocols. Advance discharge planning should include three aspects, physical, psychological and social, as can be seen in Table 16.5.

Table 16.5 Discharge criteria (Royal College of Nursing, 2020b)

Physical criteria	<ul><li>Consciousness level should be consistent with pre-anaesthetic and preoperative state</li><li>Vital signs should be consistent with pre-anaesthetic and preoperative vital signs</li><li>Pain, nausea and vomiting should be assessed, well controlled and manageable by medication administered orally where possible</li><li>Oral intake should be assessed and recorded</li><li>Passing urine successfully is only a requirement if the child has undergone a urological or penile procedure or received a caudal block. However, the child should have passed urine within 6-8 hours of the procedure</li><li>Wound site should be clean with no bleeding</li><li>Mobility should be consistent with pre-anaesthetic status unless surgery has impacted this</li></ul>
Psychological criteria	<ul><li>A responsible adult should escort the child home and provide care in the first 48 hours following anaesthetic</li><li>Families should not be expected to use public transport</li><li>Parents should be made aware of specific information related to the recovery at home in relation to the procedure their child has undergone</li><li>Written information with specific instructions should be available</li><li>Discharge advice should be detailed to facilitate ongoing care by parents</li><li>Contact telephone numbers should be made available for both emergency and continuing care</li><li>Communication with primary healthcare through prompt discharge letter to the GP</li><li>Community children's nursing teams notified in a timely manner of the child's needs if appropriate</li></ul>
Social criteria	<ul><li>All families should have access to a telephone and someone who can communicate their concerns in English</li><li>Families should have in place suitable transportation home prior to admission</li><li>Assessment of the home environment including access to bathroom and toilet facilities</li><li>Support should be sought from local Social Services for parents where time off work is difficult and will incur financial difficulties</li><li>Criteria for returning to school and participating in sporting activities should be included in the discharge information</li></ul>

CHAPTER SUMMARY

- Different types of surgery performed by various specialites, including day case and inpatient requirements, alongside the debate on fasting requirements
- The importance of preparation via play and knowledge of the stages of cognitive development, alongside parental responsibility, Gillick competence and consent
- Role of the nurse and required preoperative nursing interventions, including transferring the child to theatre
- Postoperative nursing interventions, including pain assessment and discharge criteria

BUILD YOUR BIBLIOGRAPHY

Books

- Glasper, E.A., Richardson, J. and Randall, D. (2021) *A Textbook of Children's and Young People's Nursing*, 3rd edn. London: Elsevier.

FURTHER
READING

Chapter 38, 'Children and surgery', provides further insight into the nature of paediatric surgery, family-centred care, legal and ethical principles and the patient journey from preparation for admission to discharge home.

- Henry, M.M. and Thompson, J.N. (2012) *Clinical Surgery,* 3rd edn. Edinburgh: Elsevier Saunders.

Chapter 36, 'Principles of paediatric surgery', discusses the general principles of paediatric surgery, identifying the main differences and also common surgical conditions found in children.

- Lister, S.E., Hofland, J., Grafton, H., Wilson, C. and The Royal Marsden NHS Foundation Trust (2021) *The Royal Marsden Manual of Clinical Nursing Procedures,* 9th student edn. 10th edn. Chichester: Wiley-Blackwell.

Chapter 16, 'Perioperative care', includes pre-, intra- and post-operative care, including procedures and the evidenced-based approaches to implementing care.

Journal articles

FURTHER READING: ONLINE JOURNAL ARTICLES

- Bray, L., Appleton, V. and Sharpe, A. (2019) 'The information needs of children having clinical procedures in hospital: Will it hurt? Will I feel scared? What can I do to stay calm?'. *Child: Care, Health & Development,* 45 (5): 737–43.

A study that aimed to identify what information children felt was important to them prior to attending hospital for a procedure and identify three types of information that was recognised to be important.

- Haynes, N. et al. (2022) 'Persistent post-operative pain in children – an argument for a transitional pain service in pediatrics'. *Pain Management Nursing,* 23 (6): 784–90.

Recognises that postoperative pain is still a problem in paediatrics, despite increasing literature, and this study suggests that the identifying of the risk factors and strategies for prevention is needed, and could be implemented by a transitional pain service.

- Dai, Y. and Livesley, J. (2018) 'A mixed-method systematic review of the effectiveness and acceptability of preoperative psychological preparation programmes to reduce paediatric pre-operative anxiety in elective surgery'. *Journal of Advanced Nursing,* 74 (9): 2022–37.

This mixed-method systematic review recognises preoperative preparation is aimed at reducing anxiety and draws on a number of studies exploring the use of preparation material.

- Disma, N., Frykholm, P., Cook-Sather, S.D. and Lerman, J. (2021) 'Pro-con debate: 1- vs 2-hour fast for clear liquids before anesthesia in children'. *Anesthesia Analgesia,* 133 (3): 581–91.

Provides arguments in favour of reducing the fasting times of clear fluids to 1 hour in children.

Weblinks

FURTHER READING: WEBLINKS

- Royal College of Nursing: Day Surgery for Children and Young People: www.rcn.org.uk/Professional-Development/publications/rcn-guidance-day-surgery-for-children-and-young-people-pub-009330 Highlights care required by children and young people in the perioperative and postoperative phase, including preparation and the involvement of the families and planning towards discharge.
- British Association of Paediatric Surgeons: www.baps.org.uk/resources/childrens-surgery-guidelines/ Presents standards of care for children requiring non-specialist emergency care from pre-admission to discharge.
- What? Why? Children in Hospital: Preparing for Hospital www.whatwhychildreninhospital.org.uk/videos Has a video library of short videos aimed at helping to prepare the child and young person and their family requiring admission or attendance to hospital for a procedure.

REFERENCES

Andersson, H., Hellström, P.M., Frykholm, P. and Veyckemans, F. (2018) 'Introducing the 6–4-0 fasting regimen and the incidence of prolonged preoperative fasting in children'. *Pediatric Anesthesia*, 28 (1): 46–52.

Bailey, C.R., Ahuja, M., Bartholomew, K., Bew, S., Forbes, L., Lipp, A., Montgomery, J., Russon, K., Potparic, O. and Stocker, M. (2019) 'Guidelines for Day-Case Surgery 2019: Guidelines from the Association of Anaesthetists and the British Association of Day Surgery'. *Anaesthesia*, 74: 778–92.

British National Formulary (2022). Available at: https://bnf.nice.org.uk/.

Children Act 1989 c 41. Available at: www.legislation.gov.uk/ukpga/1989/41/section/2.

Children Act 2004, c 31. Available at: www.legislation.gov.uk/ukpga/2004/31/contents.

Courtman, S., Babb, M., Black, S., Deacon, R., Endean, E., Gildersleve, C., Hulatt, L., Ladak, N., Lambert, B., Moganasundram, S., Norrington, A., Perkins, R., Riley, C., Sivaprakasam, J. and Tomas, M. (2022) *Best Practice Guidance: Preassessment Services for Children Undergoing Surgery or Procedures*. Association of Paediatric Anaesthetists of Great Britain and Northern Ireland. Available at: www.apagbi.org.uk/sites/default/files/2022-05/Best%20Practice_Preassessment%20 standards%20in%20Children%20%202022%20-%20Published.pdf (accessed 9 November 2023).

Disma, N., Frykholm, P., Cook-Sather, S.D. and Lerman, J. (2021) 'Pro-con debate: 1- vs 2-hour fast for clear liquids before anesthesia in children'. *Anesthesia and Analgesia*, 133 (3): 581–91.

Dougherty, L. and Lister, S. (2015) *The Royal Marsden Manual of Clinical Nursing Procedures*, 9th edn. Chichester: Wiley–Blackwell.

Early Years Foundation Stage (2022) *Early Years Matter*. Available at: www.earlyyearsmatters.co.uk/ eyfs/a-unique-child/play-learning/ (accessed 13 June 2023).

Ginsberg, K.R. (2006) 'The importance of play in promoting healthy child development and maintaining strong parent-child bonds'. Clinical Report. American Academy of Pediatrics. Available at: www.waldorflibrary.org/images/stories/Journal_Articles/playpediatricsreport.pdf (accessed 13 June 2023).

Gormley-Fleming, E. (2018) *Children and Young People's Nursing Skills at a Glance*. Hoboken, NJ: Wiley–Blackwell.

Murphy, C (2020) Paediatric analgesia and pain assessment. Don't Forget the Bubbles. Available at: https://dontforgetthebubbles.com/paediatric-analgesia-pain-assessment/ (accessed 13 June 2023).

National Institute for Health and Care Excellence (2020) Surgical site infections: prevention and treatment. NICE guideline [NG125]. Available at: www.nice.org.uk/guidance/ng125 (accessed 13 June 2023).

Nursing and Midwifery Council (NMC) (2018) *The Code: Professional Standards of Practice and Behaviour for Nurses, Midwives and Nursing Associates*. London: NMC. Available at: www.nmc.org.uk/standards/code/.

Piaget, J. (1936) *Origins of Intelligence in the Child*. London: Routledge & Kegan Paul.

Royal College of Nursing (2020a) *Caring for Children and Young People: Guidance for Nurses Working in the Independent Sector*. Available at: www.rcn.org.uk/professional-development/publications/rcn-caring-for-cyp-uk-pub-009405 (accessed 13 June 2023).

Royal College of Nursing (2020b) *Day Surgery for Children and Young People: RCN Guidance*. Available at: www.rcn.org.uk/Professional-Development/publications/rcn-guidance-day-surgery-for-children-and-young-people-pub-009330 (accessed 13 June 2023).

Royal College of Surgeons (2022) *Paediatric Surgery*. Available at: www.rcseng.ac.uk/news-and-events/ media-centre/media-background-briefings-and-statistics/paediatric-surgery/ (accessed 13 June 2023).

Vygotsky, L.S. (1978) *Mind in Society: The Development of Higher Psychological Processes*. Cambridge, MA: Harvard University Press.

CARE OF CHILDREN AND YOUNG PEOPLE WITH RESPIRATORY PROBLEMS

17

ZOË VEAL, ORLA McALINDEN AND DOREEN CRAWFORD

THIS CHAPTER COVERS

- Respiratory assessment
- Common respiratory conditions
- Nursing care and management
- Discharge planning and continuing care in the community

REQUIRED KNOWLEDGE

An understanding of respiratory anatomy and physiology is recommended before you start this chapter.

> "A lot of nurses describe respiratory support and oxygen administration as the bread and butter of children's nursing. I have begun to understand this since my placement on a general medical ward. Most children on the ward require some sort of respiratory support."
>
> **Sarah, children's nursing student**

INTRODUCTION

The respiratory system is vital for life, supplying oxygen to the body and removing carbon dioxide. Respiratory illnesses such as coughs and colds and other upper respiratory tract infections are very common, especially in young children (Lissauer and Carroll, 2022). Respiratory conditions can, however, be life-limiting and life-threatening, with a major impact on lifestyle, affecting both the child and their family. As a nursing student, you are highly likely to provide care to children with respiratory conditions, both in hospital and in the community.

RESPIRATORY ASSESSMENT

Respiratory assessment is a key aspect in identifying the child's physical status and although respiratory distress usually occurs due to respiratory illness, it can also be seen in other conditions where the child is acutely unwell (Samuels and Wieteska, 2016). Respiratory assessment involves more than counting the rate of respiration, although frequently that is all that is indicated in the respiratory section of a vital signs observation chart.

Table 17.1 Normal respiratory rates

Age	Respiratory rate at rest (breaths per minute)
Birth	25-50
3 months	25-45
6-12 months	20-40
18 months	20-35
2-7 years	20-30
8-11 years	15-25
12 years and over	12-24

Adapted from Samuels and Wieteska, 2016

Respiratory assessment involves assessment of rate, depth, effort, sounds and physical appearance (see Table 17.2). By carrying out a thorough respiratory assessment, you will be able to identify children who are at risk of further deterioration and respiratory failure. Although cardiorespiratory arrest is uncommon in children, the primary cause is often respiratory failure (Samuels and Wieteska, 2016), and consequently, the survival of children experiencing cardiorespiratory arrest is low (Resuscitation Council (UK), 2021). Early recognition that a child is seriously unwell through thorough observation and assessment is therefore vital.

Assessment should follow a structured approach in the unwell child, assessing ABCDE – Airway, Breathing, Circulation, Disability and Exposure in that order. Patency of the airway is of primary importance. Talking and crying provide an indication that the airway is patent, but this may be compromised in the child who is snoring, has stridor, is drooling or showing signs of reduced responsiveness.

SEE ALSO
CHAPTER 14

Table 17.2 Respiratory assessment and signs of respiratory distress

Respiratory assessment	Rationale and associated signs of respiratory distress
Rate	Varies according to age. Indicates if breathing is too fast/slow or within normal range. For accuracy, assess over a full minute, without the child's knowledge to avoid subconscious rate changes

(Continued)

Table 17.2 (Continued)

Respiratory assessment	Rationale and associated signs of respiratory distress
Depth and expansion	Shallow, moderate or deep? Gives an indication of breathing efficacy. The chest should expand equally on both sides
Regularity	Each breath should be equally spaced and rhythmical (infants may have a mildly irregular pattern). Observe for paradoxical 'seesaw' breathing where the chest and abdomen move opposite to each other
Effort (work of breathing)	Respiration should be effortless. Recession or the use of accessory muscles to improve gas exchange indicates that the child is working hard to breathe. Intercostal recession, head bobbing and/or nasal flaring involve accessory muscle use and indicate respiratory distress, resulting in tiredness and potential collapse
Sounds	Breathing should be quiet. Noises include stridor, a high-pitched noise on inspiration, or grunting and wheezing on expiration. Grunting is a sign of severe respiratory distress. Sounds heard on auscultation (listening with a stethoscope) include crackles, crepitations, wheezes, rhonchi and friction rub and may be of use in diagnosis. A silent chest is a pre-terminal sign and requires immediate attention
Physical appearance	
• Position	Sitting forward with neck extended indicates respiratory difficulty
• Skin colour	Observe skin for pallor, which indicates low oxygenation. If central cyanosis is present, respiratory arrest is close
• Level of consciousness	Inappropriate drowsiness/reduced responsiveness may indicate tiredness and deterioration. Agitation may indicate hypoxia
• Facial expression	Respiratory distress can cause children to appear tense and anxious
Oxygen saturation (pulse oximetry)	Normal oxygen saturation is above 97%, but can be lower in children with congenital heart disease. Provides a good indication of breathing efficacy

As a nursing student, you should learn the medical terminology related to normal and abnormal respiration so that you are able to understand nursing handover, medical/nursing notes and treatment instructions. Some of the common terminology is listed below, but you may also find the use of a medical/nursing dictionary helpful.

Table 17.3 Common terminology and descriptors

Term used	Description
Inspiration	The act of breathing in
Expiration	The act of breathing out
Tachypnoea	Faster respiratory rate than expected for the child's age
Bradypnoea	Slower respiratory rate than expected for the child's age
Apnoea	Absence of respiration
Hyperpnoea	Rapid, deep breathing
Dyspnoea	Difficulty in breathing
Hypoventilation	Slow, shallow breathing
Air trapping	Usually associated with the presence of a wheeze, this is difficulty in breathing out
Hypoxia	Deficiency of oxygen in the tissues

Term used	Description
Hypoxaemia	Deficiency of oxygen in the blood
Cyanosis	Bluish discoloration of the skin and mucous membranes caused by an increase in deoxygenated haemoglobin
Silent chest	Absence of breath sounds, indicating a lack of airflow in and out of the lungs. This is a pre-terminal sign
Compensation	The body's ability to cope with functional deficiency. Children frequently compensate when unwell
Decompensation	Occurs when the body is no longer able to cope with functional deficiency. When a child tires, they lose the ability to compensate and rapidly deteriorate
Grunting	Occurs by exhaling against a partially closed glottis in an attempt to prevent airways from collapsing at the end of expiration. Sign of severe respiratory distress
Nasal flaring	Flaring of the nostrils. Seen in respiratory distress in infants
Stridor	High-pitched noise on inspiration, indicating laryngeal or tracheal obstruction
Wheeze	Indicates lower airway narrowing. Usually more evident on expiration
Recession	Drawing in of the rib cage on inspiration. Can be intercostal, subcostal, sternal or suprasternal (tracheal tug) and indicates increased work of breathing. Degree of recession (mild, moderate, severe) indicates the severity of respiratory distress
Head bobbing	The head bobs up and down with each breath due to the use of the sternomastoid muscle. Seen in infants and indicates increased work of breathing
Auscultation	The act of using a stethoscope to listen to breath sounds within the chest
Crackles/crepitations (rales)	Crackling sounds heard on inspiration or expiration. Can be fine or coarse and may indicate the reopening of a small airway, or the presence of fluid, mucus or pus
Rhonchi	Low-pitched noise, sounds similar to snoring and may indicate presence of secretions in the larger airways
Friction (pleural) rub	Harsh grating sound caused by inflamed pleural surfaces rubbing against each other during respiration

Auscultation

Auscultation involves using a stethoscope to listen to the chest, so that breath sounds can be heard more clearly. This is a skill that takes practice. Interpretation of breath sounds is not easy but it is a useful skill to add to your repertoire as a student. All children have breath sounds that can be heard on auscultation and these can be very loud in young children as their chest wall is thin, and difficult to hear in the crying child. The aim of auscultation is to ascertain if the chest is clear, in which case only normal breath sounds will be heard, or if there are any adventitious sounds, such as crackles, wheezes or rhonchi. Listen first for normal breath sounds, then listen for adventitious sounds.

The deteriorating child

Children, especially young children, can deteriorate very quickly when unwell and their survival depends on prompt recognition of the situation (Miall et al., 2016). Rapid assessment of the acutely ill child should identify 'red flags' that raise a concern and these should be reported to your practice assessor/supervisor or a doctor immediately. Using a Paediatric Early Warning System (PEWS) can help to identify the child in need of urgent medical review, but it is also important that you use your knowledge and skills in alerting appropriate personnel. Prompt recognition and intervention alert nursing and medical staff to impending respiratory failure and can prevent cardiorespiratory arrest.

COMMON RESPIRATORY CONDITIONS

Bronchiolitis

Usually caused by the respiratory syncytial virus (RSV), bronchiolitis is an infectious lower respiratory tract disease seen most commonly in children under 1 year. Bronchiolitis is seasonal, with the peak incidence occurring between October and March (Harding, 2018). Most children will recover in the community with no specific treatment, but severity can vary and some children will require admission to hospital, with a small percentage needing admission to intensive care. As a nursing student, you will almost certainly care for children with bronchiolitis during at least one hospital-based placement. Premature babies and those under 3 months of age have an increased risk of severe bronchiolitis, as do children with chronic lung disease, congenital heart disease, neuromuscular disorders and immunodeficiency (NICE, 2021).

Bronchiolitis presents initially as coryza (runny or stuffy nose), followed by cough, low fever, increased respiratory rate and wheeze. The virus results in cell debris that blocks and irritates the bronchioles, causing inflammation and mucus production. Current guidelines from the National Institute of Health and Care Excellence (NICE) recommend taking a pulse oximetry reading in children where bronchiolitis is suspected and any child who presents to the GP with difficulty feeding, clinical dehydration, a respiratory rate above 60 breaths/minute or an oxygen saturation persistently below 92% in air should be referred to hospital for further assessment (NICE, 2021). Children must be referred to hospital immediately for emergency care and admission if they present with any of the following:

- Severe respiratory distress – for example, grunting, marked chest recession, respiratory rate above 70 breaths/minute
- Observed or reported apnoea
- Difficulty in feeding, taking 50–75% of usual feed volume
- Appearing seriously unwell
- Central cyanosis

(NICE, 2021)

Treatment for bronchiolitis in hospital is supportive and involves oxygen therapy if the oxygen saturations are persistently below:

- 90% in babies over 6 weeks of age
- 92% in air in babies under 6 weeks of age or there are other underlying health conditions

(NICE, 2021)

Suctioning the upper airway (nasal cavities and pharynx) is only recommended if the child has respiratory distress, apnoea or difficulty feeding, and enteral feeding is advised if the child is unable to take adequate feeds orally. Intravenous (IV) fluid therapy is only recommended for children unable to tolerate enteral feeding, or where respiratory failure is a concern (NICE, 2021). The use of bronchodilators, antibiotics and saline nose drops is no longer recommended.

Most children with bronchiolitis can safely be cared for at home, but their caregiver should be advised of 'Red Flags' that indicate deterioration and how to get help – known as safety netting.

'Red Flags' include increased work of breathing, decrease in fluid intake, apnoea or cyanosis, and signs of exhaustion such as difficulty in waking. The caregiver should also be aware that smoking in the child's home increases the risk of severe symptoms developing (NICE, 2021). Finally, the caregiver should be advised of how to get immediate help if 'Red Flag' signs develop and arrangements for any follow-up made (NICE 2021).

Asthma

Asthma is the most common chronic condition in children in the UK (Lissauer and Carroll, 2022), affecting 1 in 11 children (Asthma + Lung UK, 2022a). Asthma is difficult to diagnose in preschool children, with wheezing seen in approximately half of all children under 3 years, either in response to a trigger such as dust or cold air, or as a symptom of viral upper respiratory tract infection (Lissauer and Carroll, 2022). As the child grows, wheezing often self-resolves, but many children presenting with a trigger wheeze are later diagnosed with asthma. Asthma symptoms include cough, wheeze and difficulty in breathing due to mucosal inflammation and narrowing of the bronchi and bronchioles (Miall et al., 2016). In asthma, the airway is more sensitive and an asthma attack can be triggered by a number of factors (see Table 17.4). During an asthma attack, the lining of the bronchioles become swollen, causing epithelial cells to slough away from the airway walls. The cells then mix with mucous and thick plugs form, resulting in bronchoconstriction which causes wheezing, coughing, shortness of breath and difficulty in breathing (Glasper et al., 2015). Status asthmaticus occurs when asthma fails to respond to inhaled reliever medication, steroid and oxygen therapy (Dixon, 2012).

Asthma can be life-threatening – it is amongst the top ten reasons for emergency admission to hospital for children (RCPCH, 2020) and the UK has one of highest death rates in Europe for childhood asthma (NHS England, 2019), with around 20 deaths per year (Lissauer and Carroll, 2022). It is for these reasons that the NHS Long Term Plan (2019) committed to developing a nationwide clinical network for asthma, and the Royal College of Paediatrics and Child Health (RCPCH) include the establishment of an asthma clinical network as one of their key policy recommendations from their *State of Child Health* report (RCPCH, 2020).

Table 17.4 Examples of asthma triggers

Cold and flu	Cigarette smoke
House dust mites	Cleaning products
Mould spores	Aerosols and sprays
Animal hair	Paint, glue, varnish
Pollution	Pollen
Stress/anxiety	Cold, damp weather

Adapted from Asthma + Lung UK, 2022b

There is no cure for asthma, so the focus is on treatment and management. The current *British Guideline on the Management of Asthma*, jointly produced by the Scottish Intercollegiate Guidelines Network (SIGN) and the British Thoracic Society, states all children and their families should be offered education in self-management of their asthma, with a written personalised asthma action plan (PAAP) alongside regular review by a healthcare professional (SIGN, 2019). A clinical audit on childhood asthma published in 2021 by the National Asthma and Chronic Obstructive Pulmonary Disease Audit Programme, identified review or issue of a PAAP was only recorded in 45.5% of cases (NHS England, 2022). Ensuring that 95% of children and young people have a PAAP as part of their discharge bundle is now a national quality improvement priority within the National Bundle of Care for Children and Young People with Asthma (NHS England, 2022).

In managing asthma, the aim is to control the disease with minimal medication side effects, increasing treatment when necessary to achieve control and decreasing when control is good, using a stepped approach (SIGN, 2019).

Most asthma treatments involve the use of inhalers. A bronchodilator ('reliever') is used on an 'as needed' basis to relax the smooth muscle, making it easier to breathe during an asthma attack (Glasper et al., 2015). There are two types of bronchodilator – β2 (Beta-2) agonists, which work on the β2 receptors, and antimuscarinics (also known as anticholinergics), which block the actions of muscarinic receptors in the parasympathetic nervous system. Salbutamol and terbutaline are examples of short-acting β2 agonists (SABA), and salmeterol is an example of a long-acting β2 agonist (LABA), which can be used as an add-on therapy. Ipratropium bromide is an example of an antimuscarinic bronchodilator, which is used for babies and young children when β2 agonists are ineffective. Inhaled corticosteroids ('preventers'), such as budesonide, or beclometasone, work by reducing the reactivity of the airway to triggers and should be used twice daily initially, dropping to daily once good control is established. In the UK preventer inhalers come in a range of colours, whereas reliever inhalers are usually colour-coded blue (Asthma + Lung UK, 2022c). In addition, there are other add-on asthma therapies, such as leukotriene receptor antagonists (for example, montelukast) that can be used to improve control of asthma, and once control has been gained, these therapies would be reduced and stopped (SIGN, 2019).

Inhaler technique is important in ensuring correct delivery of asthma medication. Use of a pressurised metered dose inhaler and a spacer device is recommended for children, alongside training in their use. In young children, a facemask is required until the child is old enough to use the spacer device mouthpiece (SIGN, 2019). Compliance with preventative inhalers is improved if built into the child's daily routine.

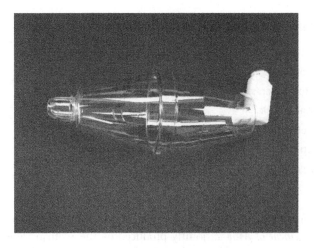

Figure 17.1   Spacer device with pressurised metered dose inhaler

SAFEGUARDING STOP POINT

You are on placement in the children's emergency department when 8-year-old Noah is brought in by ambulance from school. Noah has asthma and this is his third admission to the ED in 4 weeks. On Noah's last admission, his mum admitted that she hadn't collected his prescription for the 'brown' inhaler as it 'doesn't do anything'. Noah also uses a 'blue' inhaler, but forgot to take it to school today. Noah's teacher says that he often forgets his inhaler and when you check his previous ED admission card, you notice that he had not taken his inhaler to school then either.

- What are the differences between the 'brown' inhaler and the 'blue' inhaler?
- Should Noah be taking a preventative inhaler as well as a reliever?
- Is Noah's current asthma management a potential safeguarding concern?
- What health promotion could be put in place to improve control of Noah's asthma?

Cystic fibrosis

Cystic fibrosis (CF) is a recessive genetic disease, caused by gene mutations found on chromosome 7, causing the CF transmembrane conductance regulator protein to be defective (Lissauer and Carroll, 2022). As a nursing student, it is one of the most common life-limiting conditions you will see in children of European heritage. Alongside increased sodium levels in sweat, CF causes the body to produce excessively sticky secretions, resulting in obstruction to the airways and recurrent chest infections. Although CF predominantly affects the lungs, other organs can be involved, including the liver, gastrointestinal tract, pancreas and the reproductive system where again, sticky secretions cause obstruction or reduce the organ's ability to work efficiently. For a child to have cystic fibrosis they must inherit the faulty gene from both parents. Carriers of the faulty gene are unaffected and there is a 1 in 4 chance of a child having CF when both parents are carriers. 1 in 25 people are carriers for CF, with 1 in 2500 babies born with the condition each year (Lissauer and Carroll, 2022).

All babies are screened for CF as part of the Newborn Screening Programme. This involves taking a small amount of blood via a heel prick test at 5 days of age and is usually carried out by a midwife. Newborn screening can be carried out up to a year of age, but if the child is over 8 weeks old when their heel prick test is carried out, the test for CF is excluded, as the results are unreliable (NHS, 2021). Approximately 1 in 10 newborns with CF present with meconium ileus (bowel obstruction) shortly after birth, although most children with CF are diagnosed following newborn screening. A small number of children are diagnosed later, presenting with recurrent chest infections, malabsorption and failure to thrive from infancy. Diagnosis is confirmed via a sweat test and genetic testing (Lissauer and Carroll, 2022).

Treatment for CF depends on the severity of the disease and the presence of infection (see Table 17.5). One aim of treatment is to maintain lung health and prevent scarring which can lead to deterioration in lung function. Two bacteria in particular are of concern – *Pseudomonas aeruginosa* and *Burkholderia cepacia*. Colonisation with either can result in chronic respiratory infection and rapid lung function deterioration. For this reason, segregation within hospital and at respiratory clinics is recommended to reduce the risk of cross-infection (Miall et al., 2016).

Table 17.5 Treatment for cystic fibrosis

Treatment	Rationale
Daily oral antibiotic therapy	Prophylactic to prevent infections which result in lung scarring
Twice daily physiotherapy, which may increase in frequency during infections	Helps to break down secretions and clear the airways
Nebulised DNAse/hypertonic saline	Helps to break down mucus in the lungs
Bronchodilators	Relaxes the smooth muscle to open the airways
Fat-soluble vitamin supplementation	Pancreatic failure leads to failure to break down fatty foods and may result in malnutrition and vitamin A, D, E and K deficiency
Intravenous antibiotics	Used when symptomatic of infection. Hospitalisation may be required
Pancreatic enzyme replacement therapy (PERT) e.g., Creon⁻	Aids digestion of fats and absorption of vitamins and minerals
Salt supplementation	Abnormal sweat gland function leads to the loss of excessive amounts of sodium (salt). High salt foods can be used instead of salt supplements.
Ursodeoxycholic acid	May help bile flow if the bile ducts become sticky and the bile flow is sluggish
Steroid therapy	Suppresses lung inflammation
High-calorie diet	A high-calorie diet may be required to meet the high metabolic demand created by CF
Enteral feeding overnight	Enteral feeding may be required to maintain a good weight
Glucose monitoring and treatment for CF-related diabetes	Some children develop CF-related diabetes, which requires glucose monitoring and control of blood sugars with either diet or insulin
Oxygen therapy	24-hour oxygen therapy may be needed in advanced CF
CFTR modulators	CF is caused by a faulty gene that affects the production of a protein called CFTR, which acts as a chloride channel. CFTR modulators help to make the CFTR protein work more effectively, reducing the overall impact of CF

WHAT'S THE EVIDENCE?

In 2015 the first CFTR modulator treatment was licensed for use in the UK, and although evidence for this treatment appeared to demonstrate significant effectiveness in modifying the faulty CFTR protein, it was extremely expensive. Pharmaceutical companies spend millions in discovering, developing and testing new treatments and the process can take a number of years. Once a treatment has been granted a licence for use in the UK, it is then appraised for its clinical and cost effectiveness. In England, Scotland and Wales, licensing is carried out by the Medicines and Healthcare products Regulatory Agency (MHRA), and by the European Medicines Agency in Northern Ireland. Appraisal is conducted by NICE in England, the All Wales Medicines Strategy Group in Wales, NICE and the Department of Health and Social Care in Northern Ireland and in Scotland, the Scottish Medicines Consortium. In deciding on whether a treatment should be available on the NHS, the price the pharmaceutical company are asking is weighed up against the data for clinical effectiveness and this is done within the context of the available NHS budget.

Once knowledge of CFTR modulator treatment began to circulate, it was natural that families wanted access to this treatment. Initially, cost and the lack of evidence on its long-term effectiveness meant the treatment was not approved for use on the NHS. According to a BBC report (BBC, 2019), the original cost from the pharmaceutical company was £100,000 per patient per year, but campaigning by the families and negotiations on price with the pharmaceutical companies meant that agreements for availability on the NHS have since been reached. There is now a rollout programme in place for all those eligible for the treatment, but long term funding remains uncertain.

ACTIVITY 17.1: CRITICAL THINKING

- Using the British National Formulary (BNF) for Children, look up Orkambi, Symkevi and Kaftrio and look at the NHS indicative price for each. Compare this price to other medications you have administered as a nursing student.
- What are the ethical concerns surrounding expensive, but innovative, life-saving treatments?

Management of CF requires a high level of commitment from the family and compliance with treatment from the child. Families may find their lives revolve around the child with CF and the disease can be isolating because segregation is advised. This is done to reduce the risk of cross-infection, but it means that children with CF cannot meet face-to-face and gain support from each other. With the advent of Internet technology, support has become easier using social media. One of the hardest times is during adolescence as the young person begins to develop independence from their parents and adopts responsibility for managing their condition. During this period, young people may find adherence challenging as they juggle to maintain their treatment regime and a social life with their peers.

ACTIVITY 17.2: CRITICAL THINKING

- Using your knowledge of cystic fibrosis and its treatment regime, make a list of the ways in which living with the condition impacts on the child and their family.

There is currently no cure for CF, although with aggressive nutritional and respiratory treatment life expectancy has improved greatly in the last few decades, and is set to improve further with the advent of CTFR modulation therapy. Currently, over half of children living with CF today are expected to reach their 47th birthday and life expectancy continues to increase (Cystic Fibrosis Trust, 2022a). Lung, heart–lung or liver transplants can be offered when CF results in respiratory or liver failure, but due to a scarcity of organs, a third will die whilst waiting on the transplant list (Cystic Fibrosis Trust, 2022b).

SEE ALSO
CHAPTER 32

CASE STUDY 17.1: MIA

You are on placement with a cystic fibrosis nurse specialist. You and your mentor are going to visit Mia, who is 14 years old and has recently been discharged home on IV antibiotics for a chest infection. During the visit, Mia's mother asks to talk to you and your mentor in private. She discloses that Mia has been refusing to comply with her daily physiotherapy routine and she is worried about Mia's long-term health.

- Why is a daily physiotherapy routine important for young people with cystic fibrosis like Mia?
- Why might Mia refuse to comply with treatment?
- What could be the impact on Mia's long-term health?
- What could you do to encourage Mia to comply with treatment?

Other respiratory conditions

As a nursing student, you may also care for children with other respiratory disorders. The most common of these are summarised in Table 17.6.

Table 17.6 Other respiratory conditions

Condition	Description
Croup	Mainly affects children from 6 months to 3 years old. The main cause is parainfluenza infection of the upper airway, causing inflammation and potential obstruction. Symptoms include coryza, stridor, wheeze and a barking cough. Most cases self-limit, but severe croup may require hospital admission. Ventilator support is rare, but necessary in severe airway oedema
Acute epiglottitis	Medical emergency, due to life-threatening nature of the illness. Caused by *Haemophilus influenzae*, it presents in children aged 2–5 years, but is now rare since the introduction of the Hib vaccine. Inflammation of the epiglottis creates difficulty in swallowing and drooling. Symptoms include high fever, tachycardia and tachypnoea, with signs of sepsis. Do not lay the child down as this will obstruct the airway
Viral induced wheeze	Caused by viral infection. Symptoms similar to asthma, but only occur when the child has a respiratory infection. A reliever inhaler may be prescribed
Inhaled foreign body	Present with stridor and difficulty in breathing. Sudden onset and signs, such as a wheeze, may be one-sided. Treatment involves identification of object and bronchoscopy to remove
Pneumonia	Bacterial or viral lower respiratory tract infection. Presents with fever, cough and respiratory distress, tachypnoea and intercostal recession. Treatment usually involves antibiotics. Oxygen therapy may also be required
Pertussis (whooping cough)	Coughing spasms during expiration, followed by a sharp intake of breath, causing a 'whoop' sound. Can cause apnoea in infants. Coughing can continue for several months and is known as the 100-day cough. Affects young infants and children who are not fully vaccinated against the disease

ACTIVITY 17.3: REFLECTIVE PRACTICE

Think back over your placements so far and make a list of the respiratory conditions you have encountered.

- Which conditions did you encounter most frequently?
- What nursing care did these conditions require?
- Which diagnostic tests did you see carried out?

Common diagnostic tests

As a nursing student, you will be involved in assisting healthcare professionals to carry out diagnostic tests and collecting specimens for examination by biomedical scientists in the pathology, biochemistry and haematology departments. See Table 17.7.

Table 17.7 Common diagnostic tests

Diagnostic test	Purpose
Chest X-ray	May show lung changes which can assist in diagnosis
Full blood count (FBC)	Raised neutrophils in bacterial pneumonia Raised lymphocytes in pertussis
Blood cultures	Isolate bacteria, so antibiotic treatment can be targeted
Sputum	Isolate causative organisms so treatment can be targeted
Nasopharyngeal aspirate (NPA)	Diagnose RSV bronchiolitis
Bronchoscopy	Used to perform diagnostic bronchio-alveolar lavage or to remove a foreign body
Per-nasal swab	Isolate *Bordetella pertussis* and diagnose whooping cough
Peak expiratory flow rate (see Figure 17.2)	Measures the ability to breathe out. May be recorded in a peak flow diary to monitor changes over time
Allergy tests	Identify allergy triggers in asthma
Sweat test	Diagnostic test for CF in which the sodium concentration in sweat is high. Measurements made by passing a small electric current across the skin

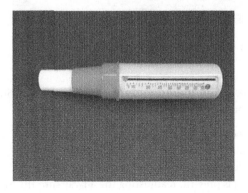

Figure 17.2 Peak expiratory flow meter

NURSING CARE AND MANAGEMENT

Alongside respiratory assessment, the main nursing care you will be involved in is the delivery of respiratory support. This involves oxygen therapy, suctioning and positioning.

Oxygen therapy: Includes head boxes, nasal cannula (see Figure 17.3), facemasks, continuous positive airway pressure (CPAP) and high-flow nasal cannula. A nasal cannula delivers an oxygen flow of less than 2 litres, whereas head boxes, facemasks, CPAP and high-flow nasal cannulas can be used to deliver higher concentrations of oxygen. A non-rebreathe facemask (see Figure 17.4) is the most effective method of oxygen delivery in the acutely unwell child.

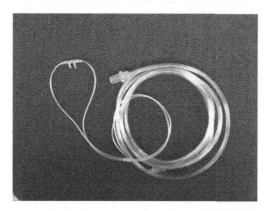

Figure 17.3   Infant size nasal cannula

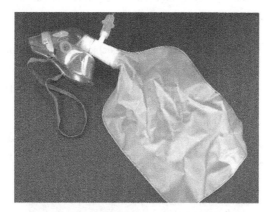

Figure 17.4   Child size non-rebreathe facemask

Suctioning: May be required to help clear secretions from the airway. Suctioning can be traumatic, causing desaturation, and should only be used when necessary.

Positioning: Can help open the airways and improve oxygenation and children will sometimes adopt the optimum position themselves. Positions known to be effective include lying prone (face down), sitting upright, leaning forward over the back of a chair, or for infants, lying over someone's shoulder. If snoring is present, readjusting the airway into the 'sniffing' or 'neutral' position can relieve the obstruction.

DISCHARGE PLANNING AND CONTINUING CARE IN THE COMMUNITY

As with all discharge planning, this should start on admission. As a student, you may be involved in helping the child and their family prepare for discharge. If inhalers are to be continued in the community, inhaler technique should be taught and assessed to ensure the child receives maximum benefit.

Other considerations for discharge include:

- Medication management – times, amounts, repeat prescriptions
- Outpatient appointments
- Specialist nursing input – for example, asthma nurse at GP practice, CF nurse specialist
- Contact with support groups
- When to seek medical advice – often called safety netting
- Maintenance of peak expiratory flow rate diary

—————————— **CHAPTER SUMMARY** ——————————

- The ability to accurately assess the respiratory status of the child is a vital aspect in children's nursing
- Early recognition of the deteriorating child in relation to respiratory status is essential
- Ensuring an effective transition to community care requires early planning and partnership working with the family

—————————— **BUILD YOUR BIBLIOGRAPHY** ——————————

Books

- Fergusson, D. (2008) *Clinical Assessment and Monitoring in Children.* Oxford: Blackwell.

  Very useful book containing two chapters on respiratory assessment and monitoring.
- Dixon, M., Crawford, D., Teesdale, D. and Murphy, J. (2009) *Nursing the Highly Dependent Child or Infant: A Manual of Care.* Chichester: Blackwell.

  Detailed chapter on respiratory nursing of the high dependency child.
- Glasper, A., Coad, J. and Richardson, J. (eds) (2015) *Children and Young People's Nursing at a Glance.* Chichester: Wiley-Blackwell.

  Easy to use for quick reference. Contains pages on respiratory conditions, monitoring and assessment.

FURTHER READING

Journal articles

- Ference, E.H., Min, J., Chandra, R.K., Schroeder, J.W. Ciolino, J.D., Yang, A., Holl, J and Smith, S.S. (2016) 'Antibiotic prescribing by physicians versus nurse practitioners for pediatric upper respiratory infections'. *Annals of Otology, Rhinology & Laryngology,* 125 (12): 982-91.

  This American article explores the prescribing rate differences between doctors and nurse practitioners and is transferable to the UK.

FURTHER READING: ONLINE JOURNAL ARTICLES

- Hughes, M., Savage, E. and Andrews, T. (2018) 'Playing the game: How young people moderate influences in accommodating asthma in their lives'. *Journal of Child Health Care*. 22 (3): 309-16.

  This research article explores how young people manage their daily lives alongside their asthma management, exploring how behaviour is impacted by social influences.

- Gathercole, K. (2019) 'Managing cystic fibrosis alongside children's schooling: Family, nurse and teacher perspectives'. *Journal of Child Health Care*, 23 (3): 425-36.

  This UK-based research article provides insight into how families manage CF alongside their child's education, and the challenges this brings.

Weblinks

FURTHER
READING:
WEBLINKS

- Easy Auscultation - *Easy Auscultation: Lessons, Quizzes and Guides* www.easyauscultation.com This website contains audio material of different breath sounds to help you learn what to listen for on auscultation.
- Asthma + Lung UK - *How to use your inhaler* www.asthma.org.uk/inhalervideos Selection of videos on inhaler technique according to each type of inhaler
- Spotting the Sick Child https://spottingthesickchild.com/ Supported by the Department for Health and Royal College of Paediatrics and Child Health, this website is a training tool for healthcare professionals. You can use this to learn about respiratory assessment and management of the acutely unwell child.

REFERENCES

Asthma + Lung UK (2022a) *What is Asthma?* Available at: www.asthma.org.uk/advice/understanding-asthma/what-is-asthma/ (accessed 23 July 2022).

Asthma + Lung UK (2022b) *Asthma Triggers*. Available at: www.asthma.org.uk/advice/triggers (accessed 25 July 2022).

Asthma + Lung UK (2022c) *Reliever Inhalers*. Available at: www.asthma.org.uk/advice/inhalers-medicines-treatments/inhalers-and-spacers/reliever/ (accessed 25 July 2022).

BBC (2019) *Cystic Fibrosis Drug Given Green Light in England*. Available at: www.bbc.co.uk/news/health-50144742 (accessed 14 August 2022).

Cystic Fibrosis Trust (2022a) *CF in Adulthood*. Available at: www.cysticfibrosis.org.uk/life-with-cystic-fibrosis/growing-old (accessed 22 August 2022).

Cystic Fibrosis Trust (2022b) *Transplants*. Available at: www.cysticfibrosis.org.uk/what-is-cystic-fibrosis/cystic-fibrosis-care/transplant-information-and-resources (accessed 22 August 2022).

Dixon, M. (2012) 'Care of an infant or child with a respiratory illness and/or the need for respiratory support', in M. Dixon and D. Crawford (eds), *Paediatric Intensive Care Nursing*. Chichester: Wiley–Blackwell.

Glasper, A., Coad, J. and Richardson, J. (2015) *Children and Young People's Nursing at a Glance*. Chichester: Wiley–Blackwell.

Harding, M. (2018) *Bronchiolitis*. Available at: https://patient.info/doctor/bronchiolitis-pro (accessed 16 July 2022).

Lissauer, T. and Carroll, W. (2022) *Illustrated Textbook of Paediatrics,* 6th edn. London: Elsevier.

Miall, L., Rudolf, M. and Smith, D. (2016) *Paediatrics at a Glance*, 4th edn. Chichester: Wiley–Blackwell.

NHS (2019) *The NHS Long Term Plan*. Available at: www.longtermplan.nhs.uk/publication/nhs-long-term-plan/ (accessed 23 July 2022).

NHS (2021) *Newborn Blood Spot Test*. Available at: www.nhs.uk/conditions/baby/newborn-screening/blood-spot-test/ (accessed 27 July 2022).

NHS England (2019) News: NHS warning to to parents as 'asthma season' hits. Available at: www.england.nhs.uk/2019/09/nhs-warning-to-parents-as-asthma-season-hits/ (accessed 23 July 2022).

NHS England (2022) *National Bundle of Care for Children and Young People with Asthma*. Available at: www.england.nhs.uk/publication/national-bundle-of-care-for-children-and-young-people-with-asthma/ (accessed 23 July 2022).

NICE (National Institute for Health and Care Excellence) (2021) Bronchiolitis in children: diagnosis and management. NICE guideline [NG9]. Available at: www.nice.org.uk/guidance/ng9 (accessed 13 June 2023).

Resuscitation Council (UK) (2021) *Paediatric Advanced Life Support Guidelines*. Available at: www.resus.org.uk/library/2021-resuscitation-guidelines/paediatric-advanced-life-support-guidelines (accessed 16 July 2022).

Royal College of Paediatrics and Child Health (RCPCH) (2020) *State of Child Health*. London: RCPCH. Available at: stateofchildhealth.rcpch.ac.uk (accessed 23 July 2022).

Samuels, M. and Wieteska, S. (2016) *Advanced Paediatric Life Support: A Practical Approach to Emergencies*, 6th edn. Chichester: Wiley–Blackwell.

Scottish Intercollegiate Guidelines Network (SIGN). (2019) *British Guideline on the Management of Asthma*. SIGN publication no. 158. Available at: www.sign.ac.uk/our-guidelines/british-guideline-on-the-management-of-asthma/ (accessed 23 July 2022).

CARE OF CHILDREN AND YOUNG PEOPLE WITH CARDIOVASCULAR PROBLEMS

JO BAILEY AND ZOË VEAL

THIS CHAPTER COVERS

- Congenital heart disease
- Acquired heart disease
- Arrhythmias
- Nursing considerations

REQUIRED KNOWLEDGE

It would be helpful to have an understanding of 'normal' cardiac anatomy and the conduction pathway of the heart, and cardiac embryology before you start this chapter.

> "As first-time parents [we] had to learn about it all in front of an audience of nurses and doctors. Every private moment, giggle, cry, nappy change and milestone, which should have been just us three, had many onlookers. The kindness, humour and friendliness of the nurses has meant we not only felt comfortable sharing these experiences, but actually enjoyed it. We have been in hospital for several months and I feel the nurses are aunts and uncles to our boy. We feel we can be silly without being self-conscious. It can be very lonely in hospital, in a room just you and your child. The nurses have made this feel like a home to raise our child in."
>
> **Parent of a 6-month old cardiac patient**

INTRODUCTION

The heart is not only necessary for life, but is also associated with emotion, love and affection, and we describe ourselves and others as being 'led by the heart', 'wearing our hearts on our sleeves', being 'broken hearted' or 'heartless'. The ancient Egyptians considered the heart to be our soul, the very centre of our being and, alongside the brain, the heart is probably considered to be the most significant of all our organs. In reality, of course, the heart is nothing more than a physical organ and the emotional side that we attribute to the heart is really part of our very complex brain and nervous system. In children, heart disease can be either congenital or acquired, the most common being congenital heart disease (CHD), which affects 8 children in every 1000 live births (Lissauer and Carroll, 2022). Where children are concerned, the heart can malfunction in three areas: its structure (plumbing), its function (mechanics) and its conduction (wiring). Although significant advances in cardiac care and surgery have occurred, some cardiac conditions remain life-limiting with palliative treatment rather than curative. You may care for children and their families at various stages of their cardiac journey, perhaps supporting them emotionally when they receive a diagnosis, preparing them for surgery, caring for them after surgery, or educating, informing and supporting them as they transition to adult services and start taking more ownership of their health needs.

ACTIVITY 18.1: CRITICAL THINKING

Think about how you view the heart and the image that the word 'heart' conjures in your mind. Do you see the heart as physical, emotional or both?

In the opening quote to this chapter, a parent explains how the nursing staff helped hospital feel like home. Think about how family-centred care can be used to address the emotional needs of children and their families and answer the questions below.

- Why is a holistic understanding of the child and their family so important?
- What concerns do you think the child and family might have when receiving a new diagnosis, or preparing for surgery?

Think about how you may need to adapt the care you provide to families based on their specific needs and social situation. This chapter will consider some of the cardiovascular problems that children can have, and will guide you to develop the knowledge needed to care for them.

CONGENITAL HEART DISEASE

Congenital heart disease (CHD) is the most common congenital malformation (Miall, 2016), and although it is associated primarily with children, adults with CHD now outnumber children as survival rates have increased (Ávila et al., 2014), with a need for transitional care as the young person moves into adulthood.

The cause of CHD is thought to be primarily idiopathic, but it is also associated with certain environmental factors, chromosomal defects, syndromes or other congenital birth defects. Approximately 30% of children born with a chromosomal abnormality will have CHD (Horrox, 2002). Cardiac services, both adult and paediatric, have undergone a thorough review in recent years, which resulted in the Congential Heart Disease Standards and Specifications (NHS England, 2016), which provide a framework for provision of cardiac services throughout England. Networks have been formed with Level 1 surgical centres, liaising closely with linked Level 2 and Level 3 centres to provide equitable care for all CHD patients under their care. These standards give a clear framework for service provision within these networks and cover aspects such as foetal support, transition to adult services and access to dental care. In addition, the Royal College of Nursing has recently updated its nursing guidelines for caring for children and young people with cardiac conditions (Royal College of Nursing, 2021).

Although cardiac care is carried out in a specialist setting, increased susceptibility to illness leads to frequent admissions to hospital and you could care for a child with CHD in a general ward setting. Similarly, the physical and psychological impact of CHD means children and their families have increased contact with health visitors, school nurses and community children's nurses. Community support is an important aspect in supporting the child and family with CHD.

All congenital cardiac defects are present from birth, and the foetal heart is routinely scanned at the 20-week anomaly ultrasound scan, which detects up to 70% of all serious CHD (Lissauer and Carroll, 2022). However, where antenatal screening has not detected CHD, a diagnosis may be made shortly after birth, but some children will be discharged home before a diagnosis is made. For those not diagnosed at birth, a cardiac murmur, respiratory concerns or failure to gain weight may be identified by the GP or health visitor, depending on the severity of the defect. For more serious CHD, as the remnants of the foetal circulation close, the infant may present in a collapsed state to their GP or local emergency department.

Management of the child with CHD is likely to be multifactorial. Many require open heart surgery involving cardiopulmonary bypass. Medical management will often be utilised both before and after surgery. Some heart defects can be corrected through cardiac catheterisation, which is less invasive. Other conditions may be medically managed, and some children will have to adhere to certain lifestyle restrictions to manage their cardiac health. Most children will need regular check-ups with a cardiologist, and some will require additional surgery later in childhood. Table 18.1 provides a brief overview of four surgical cardiac conditions you may encounter.

Table 18.1 Four common congenital heart defects requiring surgery

Ventricular septal defect (VSD)	Brief explanation:	Hole in the wall (septum) separating the two ventricles. Due to the higher pressure in the left side of the heart, oxygen-rich blood passes from the left to the right ventricle causing increased pressure in the lungs
	Presentation:	Increased work of breathing, respiratory infections and faltering weight
	Treatment:	Open-heart surgery to close the hole with a patch. Some infants will have an initial stage surgery, where a band is placed around the pulmonary artery to reduce the flow of blood to the lungs, until they are a sufficient weight for surgery.
	Prognosis:	Most children will not require further surgery and should be able to live normal, active lives

Coarctation of the aorta	Brief explanation:	A narrowing of the aorta, usually just after the branches which supply the upper part of the body (which then have increased blood pressure) whilst the lower part of the body receives insufficient blood
	Presentation:	Dependent upon the severity of the narrowing. Often absent or faint femoral pulses. Lethargy and faltering weight
	Treatment:	Usually in infants, this is corrected by cardiac surgery – the narrowing is removed and the aorta sewn back together. This is known as an end-to-end anastomosis. Surgery is usually via a thoracotomy without the need for bypass
	Prognosis:	Narrowing may develop over time, which may require ballooning via a cardiac catheter procedure. High blood pressure may also develop in later life requiring medication
Tetralogy of Fallot (TOF)	Brief explanation:	A large VSD and a narrowing of the pulmonary valve (pulmonary stenosis) that causes the right ventricle to become overworked and thicker (hypertrophied). There is also an overriding aorta: the aorta sits above the VSD resulting in deoxygenated blood getting pumped around the body
	Presentation:	Sometimes identified during pregnancy scans. Babies may appear blue, depending on the severity of the pulmonary stenosis. Some babies have hypercyanotic 'spells' where they become blue very suddenly. These can be life-threatening
	Treatment:	Open heart surgery via a sternotomy and bypass to correct the VSD and pulmonary stenosis. This is often done at 6 months of age. Some infants may require additional blood flow to their lungs and require further intervention before corrective surgery.
	Prognosis:	In later life, further intervention may be required if there is pulmonary valve regurgitation. Arrhythmias are also a possible complication due to scarring from surgery near the conduction pathway of the heart
Transposition of the great arteries (TGA)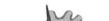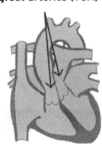	Brief explanation:	The positioning of the pulmonary artery and the aorta are transposed: the pulmonary artery arises from the left ventricle instead of the right, and the aorta arises from the right ventricle instead of the left
	Presentation:	Often diagnosed antenatally, allowing for planned delivery at an appropriate centre. Post-natal diagnosis – may present in a collapsed state as unless there is a means of mixing blood (through a patent ductus aterious or patent foramen ovale) the infant may be at risk of death.
	Treatment:	Dinoprostone is given to keep the ductus arteriosus open to enable sufficient oxygenated blood to circulate. Babies may also require a balloon septostomy (cardiac catheter procedure) which creates a hole between the two atria of the heart, ensuring sufficient oxygen circulation. Usually within the first 3 weeks of life the child will require a 'switch procedure' to correct the transposition. Sometimes a switch procedure is not possible and other palliative routes must be considered
	Prognosis:	In later life the pulmonary artery and coronary arteries may narrow and there may be regurgitation from the aortic valve – all of which may require further intervention

SEE ALSO
CHAPTER 16

For more information on congenital heart disease, including diagrams, go to www.bhf.org.uk /informationsupport/conditions/understanding-your-congenital-heart-condition.

It is important to understand that there are risks associated with both cardiac surgery and anaesthesia. Surgeons will cover this with families when they obtain consent from parents.

CASE STUDY 18.1: OLIVER

You are overseeing the admission of Oliver with your practice assessor. Oliver is a 3-month-old baby with a VSD who has been admitted for surgical repair. Oliver's heart defect was identified following concern from his health visitor that his weight was faltering. Oliver's mum, Katie, appears very anxious.

- During the admission process, what information would you need to gain from Katie?
- What concerns might Katie have?
- What members of the interprofessional team can help support Oliver and Katie?

SAFEGUARDING STOP POINT

Whilst you are doing Oliver's baseline observations (vital signs), you overhear Katie having a heated conversation on her mobile phone. Katie leaves the ward briefly and, on return, she is visibly upset and appears to be more agitated and anxious than previously. You ask Katie if everything is all right – she smiles and tells you that Oliver's father will be visiting. You notice Katie is shaking.

- What concerns might you have?
- What would you say to Katie?
- Who would you tell?
- Where would you document your concerns?
- How would you promote family-centred care?

WHAT'S THE EVIDENCE?

Quality of life is an important consideration for children with cardiovascular problems. The World Health Organization defines quality of life (QOL) as 'an individual's perception of their position in life in the context of the culture and value systems in which they live and in relation to their goals, expectations, standards and concerns' (WHOQOL group, 1993. p.153). Within healthcare, QOL measurement is important in understanding the everyday lived experience of people with chronic health conditions, but how or what to measure is contentious (Wray et al., 2009). Generic QOL measures enable comparisons with the general population (e.g., CHD versus non-CHD) whereas disease-specific measures enable discrimination between disease subgroups (e.g., VSD versus TGA) but do not allow for comparison with the general population. In 2009, a systematic review of 33 studies into QOL and psychological adjustment identified significant risk of psychological maladjustment in children following open-heart surgery and impaired QOL for those with severe CHD (Latal et al., 2009). Further research was recommended, with the impact of parental wellbeing on the child's psychological adjustment being highlighted.

- What aspects of childhood/adolescence do you think would be important when measuring QOL?
- How might the QOL aspects you identified above be affected by a cardiovascular problem?

ACQUIRED HEART DISEASE

Acquired heart disease is normally associated with adults, but a small percentage of children will acquire heart disease in infancy or childhood. Although most children with CHD are at increased risk of developing infective endocarditis (Tidy, 2021), acquired heart disease can affect all children and is a serious diagnosis. The acquired heart diseases you may encounter are explained below.

Table 18.2 Acquired heart diseases

Infective endocarditis	Brief explanation:	Infection of the heart lining/valves usually caused by bacteria entering the bloodstream. Platelets and fibrin adhere to the heart lining/valves to create vegetation (thrombosis)
	Presentation:	Mainly flu-like symptoms for over a week – fever, lethargy, headache, weight loss, pallor, aching muscles and joints. May be a heart murmur
	Treatment:	A prolonged hospital stay for intravenous antibiotics. Occasionally surgery may be required to remove the vegetation or repair damaged valves
	Prognosis:	Despite medical advances, prognosis is poor with an overall mortality of 30% (Cahill and Prendergast, 2015)
Cardiomyopathy (picture depicts dilated cardiomyopathy with a large baggy left ventricle)	Brief explanation:	Disease of the heart muscle which reduces the ability to pump blood around the body. Most common types are dilated and hypertrophic. Cause is often unknown
	Presentation:	Cardiac failure, arrhythmias, respiratory difficulties, fatigue, weakness and reduced exercise tolerance
	Treatment:	Management of cardiac failure and arrhythmias with prevention of thromboembolism and sudden death, using beta-blockers, vasodilators, inotropes, anticoagulation and diuretic therapy, depending on clinical need. Transplantation may also be required

(Continued)

Table 18.2 (Continued)

	Prognosis:	Varies considerably. Some children may improve, others may need long-term medical treatment, others may require heart transplantation, or palliation. Risk of sudden death is a concern
Kawasaki disease (diagram depicts coronary artery aneurysms)	Brief explanation:	Acute, febrile systemic vasculitis, a major complication of which is coronary artery aneurysm formation
	Presentation:	Fever lasting ≥ 5 days, irritability, bilateral conjunctivitis, inflamed mucus membranes, rash, peeling skin on hands and feet, enlarged lymph nodes, tachycardia or gallop rhythm. Symptoms often missed or misinterpreted
	Treatment:	Management of the inflammatory process with aspirin and intravenous immunoglobulin, to reduce fever and myocardial inflammation with the aim of preventing coronary aneurysm formation
	Prognosis:	Discovered in 1967, long-term follow-up results are not yet known (Jarvis, 2020). Prognosis is dependent on the depth of cardiac impairment, but generally appears to be good if diagnosed early and treated appropriately

ARRHYTHMIAS

The final type of cardiovascular problem in children is arrhythmia which means that the heart is beating either irregularly or abnormally fast/slow. Arrhythmias can occur at any life stage, including during foetal life, and can be seen in children with cardiomyopathies, or during the pre- and postoperative period following cardiac surgery, caused either by the structural defect itself, or by the surgical intervention (Dhillon et al., 2009). A number of inherited cardiac conditions can also cause arrhythmias, the most common being cardiomyopathies and channelopathies, such as Long QT and Brugada syndrome. Families of affected patients will be offered screening and genetic testing if appropriate.

You may be involved in caring for children with arrhythmias in a number of settings. They may present in ED and require synchronised electrical cardioversion or treatment with medication to restore a regular rhythm. You may have a cardiology placement and care for children undergoing a cardiac catheter procedure to ablate an accessory electrical pathway, which is causing their arrhythmia. Some children need to have an implantable cardioverter–defibrillator (ICD) fitted if they are at risk of having a life-threatening arrhythmia. Some children may also require a permanent pacemaker to be fitted. These children will need to be appropriately supported within school, and school nurses will often liaise with nurse specialists to ensure appropriate healthcare plans are in place.

Sinus rhythm

This is the 'normal' expected rhythm – deviations from this are known as arrhythmias.

The heart rate and rhythm are normal for the age of the patient. The electrical impulse originates in the sinoatrial node and is conducted to the atrioventricular node and through to the bundle of His, bundle branches and Purkinje fibres. It is important to recognise normal before looking at abnormal rhythms.

Sinus bradycardia

Characteristic of sinus rhythm, but the rate is too slow for the age of the patient, potentially affecting cardiac output and oxygenation, requiring prompt investigations and treatment for the underlying cause.

Sinus tachycardia

Characteristic of sinus rhythm, but the rate is too fast for the age of the patient. In sinus tachycardia, cardiac output may be affected, which can be detrimental in the ill child. As well as a potential indication of a serious underlying issue, such as cardiac failure, myocardial disease, hypovolemia or circulatory shock, sinus tachycardia is also a common response to pain, anxiety and fever. Treatment involves treating the underlying cause.

Supraventricular tachycardia (SVT)

SVT is caused by abnormal electrical impulses which arise in the atria ('supra' means 'above', hence a high heart rate originating above the ventricles). It is often referred to as a 'short circuit', because there is an accessory tissue/pathway which allows the electrical current to repeatedly travel in a loop causing a fast heart rate. Parents of babies born with this condition are given training on how to listen to their child's heart rate, and given advice on when to escalate care. If a child experiences persistent episodes, then medication such as a beta-blocker may be considered. Older children may be able to restore a normal heart rhythm by performing the Valsalva manoeuvre. Any non-resolving episodes of SVT would require assessment in the emergency department. For older children who are experiencing significant symptoms a catheter procedure, involving an electrophysiology study and ablation of the accessory pathway, may be considered. Wolff–Parkinson–White syndrome is a heart condition associated with SVT.

Long QT syndrome

This is a genetic condition affecting around 1 in 2000 people (British Heart Foundation, 2022), in which the time between depolarisation and repolarisation of the heart (the QT interval) is lengthened due to faulty potassium or sodium channels affecting the electrical activity. Although for some children this diagnosis may occur as an incidental finding or through screening of a family member, appropriate counselling is required due to the risk of sudden death. Symptomatic patients may be treated with medication, or may require an ICD (implantable cardioverter–defibrillator) or permanent pacemaker to be fitted. Some lifestyle adjustments may be necessary and certain 'over-the-counter' medication may need to be avoided.

Heart block

This occurs when there is a delay in conduction, usually at the site of the AV node, resulting in a slow heart rate.

It is classified according to severity as either first-, second- or, more severely, third-(complete) degree heart block, which would necessitate a permanent pacemaker to be fitted. Complete heart block can be congenital (if the mother has certain antibodies present), or it can be acquired, and is a potential complication post cardiac surgery.

CASE STUDY 18.2: MALACHI

Malachi is 14 years old and has Wolff-Parkinson-White syndrome. Malachi enjoys sport and has had several recent episodes of SVT that have required hospital treatment. Malachi has been admitted for catheter ablation of his extra pathway to prevent further episodes of SVT.

- Who should be approached to give consent for Malachi's procedure?
- What care would Malachi require following his catheter procedure?
- What might be the challenges in providing Malachi with privacy and dignity during his admission?
- What are the issues that need to be considered as Malachi transfers between child and adult services?

NURSING CONSIDERATIONS

You may care for a child with a cardiac condition in a variety of settings. For example:

Working with a community team who visits an infant at home awaiting cardiac surgery, and whose condition requires careful monitoring and liaison with their cardiac team

Preparing a child for a cardiac procedure, such as a cardiac catheter or surgery

Caring for a child post procedure, either in intensive care or in a cardiac ward setting

Caring for a child with CHD who has been admitted to a general children's or non-cardiac ward for a non-cardiac reason

It is important that you have a good understanding of how to care for them appropriately. This section covers what monitoring they will require, what tests may need to be performed, what types of medication may be prescribed, and key members of the interprofessional team who you will work with.

ACTIVITY 18.2: REFLECTIVE PRACTICE

Reflect on a young person that you have cared for recently.

- How did their heart condition impact on their daily activities and on family life?
- What long-term considerations or worries might they have?
- How could you support them during their stay in hospital?
- What resources or support groups are available for young people with a cardiac condition?

General nursing considerations

Vital sign observations are a major aspect of cardiac nursing and all patients will have regular observations taken. This will be an opportunity for you to refine and perfect your skills in this area. Following an increase in medication or post cardiac catheter/surgery, observations need to be completed more frequently.

Table 18.3 Vital signs in cardiac nursing

Vital sign	Rationale
Oxygen saturations 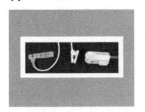	Indicates the level of oxygen perfusion in the circulating bloodstream and can be significantly reduced in children with CHD. The expected parameters should be clearly documented.
Respiration	Visual inspection of respiration for rate, noting any increased work of breathing such as head bobbing, nasal flaring, subcostal and intercostal recession. Increased respiratory effort may be a sign of worsening heart failure.
Heart rate/pulse 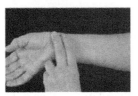	Although bedside monitoring will automatically provide you with a heart rate and electrical trace, useful information can also be obtained from palpating a pulse, such as rhythm (regular or irregular) and pulse volume (weak/thready or bounding). In the neonate/infant an apex pulse is more accurate than a peripheral pulse. (Note – when listening to an apex pulse, a heart murmur may be heard, making it harder to count the pulse until you have become familiar with the sound.) Femoral pulses are checked if coarctation of the aorta is suspected. Pedal pulses are checked post cardiac catheterisation.
General appearance	Observe for any pallor, mottling, and duskiness, particularly around the lips and extremities, which may indicate poor perfusion, low saturations or low cardiac output. Sweating, oedema and clamminess of the skin may indicate worsening heart failure. It is important to have an understanding of what is a 'normal' presentation for each child.
Capillary refill	Prolonged capillary refill times indicate poor systemic perfusion.
Blood pressure 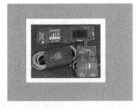	For accuracy, use the right arm wherever possible. Blood pressure is not a reliable indicator of cardiac output in children due to their ability to compensate and a low BP may be a pre-terminal sign. Four limb blood pressures may be required if coarctation of the aorta is suspected.
Temperature 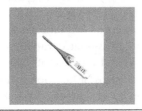	A high temperature may indicate an infection, which can be a possible complication post surgery/cardiac catheter. It is also important to note any differences between core and peripheral temperatures. Cool peripheries may indicate a low cardiac output state.

Children with cardiac conditions can deteriorate quickly, therefore any concerns must be escalated in a timely manner.

Child safety

It is vital to ensure that all bedside safety equipment is present and in good working order at the start of each shift. Bedside monitoring alarms must be set at appropriate levels specific for each child. Any unnecessary clutter should be cleared from the bedspace so as not to impede medical assistance should an emergency arise.

Positioning

Ensure the child is positioned to ensure optimal respiratory, circulatory and neurological function appropriate for their age and diagnosis. Children unable to move themselves should be turned regularly to avoid pressure area deterioration and scrupulous tissue viability recording must be documented and monitored at prescribed intervals.

Mobilisation

Mobilisation is a key aspect of a child's recovery post surgery. Nursing considerations include pain assessment and adequate pain relief, and appropriate support for drains and lines.

Nutrition and fluid

Prior to surgery/cardiac catheter, appropriate nil by mouth times must be adhered to according to local evidence-based policy. Many children are fluid-restricted in the postoperative period, or if in cardiac failure to avoid placing the heart under increased pressure. Regular weight checks are important; a sudden gain could indicate fluid retention which would need investigation and treatment. Some children awaiting cardiac surgery may struggle to gain weight and may require dietetic input to allow them to grow.

Post-surgery care

Following surgery, admission to paediatric intensive care is common, as support and management of airway, breathing and circulation is often required. Length of stay depends on the surgery and the child's recovery. On return to the cardiac ward, they may have drains and pacing wires in situ. Drains could be placed in the pleural or mediastinal spaces and will require hourly observations of the entry site and drainage volume. Familiarise yourself with local policy and safety procedures, including infection control matters regarding drain care. Children occasionally experience abnormal rhythms post surgery, such as junctional ectopic tachycardia. Postoperative temporary pacing wires are attached to the atria and ventricles and these wires can be attached to an external pacing box to override any abnormal rhythms. Surgical wounds, particularly thoracotomies, are very painful, and appropriate pain management is a key component of your nursing care. Good pain management reduces child and parent anxiety and increases the likelihood of early mobilisation, thus reducing the incidence of complications associated with immobility, so accurate pain assessment using appropriate pain assessment tools is vital (Twycross et al., 2021).

Postoperative wounds require regular visual assessment and recording for signs of infection (pain, redness, swelling, signs of non-healing, abnormal/excessive exudate or bad odour) and wound swabs may need to be taken and treatment commenced if infection is suspected or present. Parents need to be shown how to hold their child post surgery, for example, avoiding any underarm lifting which would cause unnecessary stress across the child's sternal area.

Discharge planning and ongoing health promotion

It is important that discharge planning commences early, particularly for children with a complex diagnosis or complex social family background. Sometimes children may be under a number of specialties so discharge planning meetings with the multidisciplinary team will be essential for a safe discharge. Patient/parental education is an important part of the nursing role and, as a nursing student, you may be involved in assessing parental clinical competence and providing information. Below are some key aspects that will need to be considered prior to discharge:

- Wound care: caring for the wound, Red Flags for potential infection and/or inadequate pain management/symptom relief.
- Medication: it is important that parents are aware of what each medication is for, when they should be given and are aware of any medications that cannot be given together.
- Nutrition: some infants are discharged home on nasogastric feeds and so would need to be linked in with local dietetic support. Parents will also need to be trained and assessed as competent to safely deliver the feed, and if appropriate, competently place the feeding tube. Chylothorax is a potential complication post cardiac surgery, which would result in the child being prescribed an MCT (medium-chain triglyceride) diet for a period of time.
- Promotion of regular dental treatment/immunisation schedules.
- Things to look out for, when to worry and who to contact, including out of hours – for example, some children will be discharged home pending a surgical date. It is important parents are trained to visually assess their child and escalate concerns accordingly.
- Follow-up appointments: as well as an initial review post surgery, most cardiac children will require lifelong follow-up. It is important that families understand the importance of regular follow-up – there may be subtle changes noted on echocardiogram requiring monitoring that would not necessarily result in any physical symptoms.
- Returning to nursery/school: Post surgery, children will usually require 6–8 weeks off school. Post cardiac catheter recovery should be just a couple of days. Children who have had internal cardiac devices or pacemakers inserted will require specific information to support their return to school.

As a nursing student caring for a child with a cardiac condition and their family, it is important you take every opportunity to maximise their long-term health outcomes by promoting healthy lifestyle choices. Although there may be some children who have restrictions on the amount and type of exercise they can do, for the majority of CHD patients, some form of exercise will be beneficial. Parents may feel anxious about their child undertaking exercise with their peers, so it is important they receive appropriate advice on what would be acceptable for their child. Children with CHD are at higher risk of endocarditis and therefore should be counselled to avoid piercings and tattoos as they get older, as well as being encouraged to have good dental hygiene to reduce the risk of infection.

These children and families also need to be supported psychologically. Many centres have dedicated psychology teams who can help support children and families come to terms with a new diagnosis or help prepare them for a forthcoming admission. Children and families can also gain a great deal of support from other families managing a similar diagnosis, and would benefit from being signposted to local support groups.

SEE ALSO
CHAPTER 28

SEE ALSO
CHAPTER 11

SEE ALSO
CHAPTER 3 & 16

ACTIVITY 18.3: CRITICAL THINKING

Some of the children you care for may have a diagnosis of hypoplastic left heart syndrome (HLHS). These children will require three surgical interventions, one shortly after birth, one around 3-6 months and another around 4 years of age. These operations cannot fully correct the heart, but are considered as a long-term palliative process. A shorter lifespan would be expected, with likely increased health complications in later life.

- Explore what these three stage interventions involve (the interventions are known as Norwood, Glenn, and Fontan).
- Think about what impact this diagnosis would have for a child and their family.
- How as a nurse can you support this child and family?

Common diagnostic tests

Alongside patient history and physical examination, cardiologists will also request diagnostic tests to assess and monitor the child's ongoing cardiac status to assist them in ongoing clinical decision-making.

ACTIVITY 18.4: REFLECTIVE PRACTICE

Using your previous knowledge and learning from placement, reflect on the purpose of each of the following diagnostic tests:

- Chest X-ray
- Echocardiogram (echo)
- ECG (electrocardiogram)
- Cardiac MRI (magnetic resonance imaging)
- CT (computed tomography) scan
- Cardiac catheterisation and angiography

What psychological preparation might the child undergoing a diagnostic test require?

Medication

The majority of children with cardiovascular problems will be prescribed medication to help their heart function more efficiently and prevent further damage. Table 18.4 includes some common examples of medications used in the care of cardiac conditions.

Table 18.4 Common medications used in cardiology

Type	Use	Common examples
Diuretics	Treat/prevent fluid retention and heart failure	Furosemide, spironolactone
Angiotensin-converting enzyme (ACE) inhibitors	Treat hypertension/heart failure	Captopril, enalapril
Beta-blockers	Treat hypertension and arrhythmias	Propranolol, nadolol
Vasodilator antihypertensive drugs	Reduce blood pressure	Hydralazine, sildenafil
Antibiotics	Treat bacterial infections; 24 hours of antibiotic treatment post-surgery is common	
Anticoagulants	Reduce clotting – often used when children have had a mechanical valve/shunt fitted	Heparin, warfarin, aspirin
Inotropes	Affect the contractility of the myocardium	Milrinone, dopamine, dobutamine

INTERPROFESSIONAL TEAM

As well as nurses, medical staff and surgeons, a number of other professionals are involved in the care of the child with cardiovascular problems. Below are some examples of other healthcare professionals who have expert input to children's cardiac care.

Dietician: Ensures optimum calorie intake is received for growth and healing and provides a specific feeding regime or supplements. Dieticians also liaise with community teams prior to discharge.

Play specialist: Provides appropriate toys/activities to help promote a sense of normality; provides distraction during painful procedures and can be successfully employed in preparing a child psychologically for procedure or interventions which are required.

Physiotherapist: Provides chest physiotherapy post surgery and gives advice on positioning and mobilising the child, and suctioning secretions.

Children's cardiac nurse specialist: Provides additional in-house and outreach expertise and support, liaising with children and families pre admission and as a point of expert contact between hospital visits.

Speech and language therapist: Assists with babies struggling to establish successful oral feeding regimes following a period of tube feeding.

Psychologists: Provide emotional support for the child and/or their family following a diagnosis or in preparation for a surgical admission.

Cardiac physiologists: Healthcare professionals who perform cardiac diagnostic tests such echocardiogram or ECG. They may also assist in the cardiac catheter lab.

ACTIVITY 18.5: TEAM WORKING

Imagine you are taking verbal handover of a patient from the paediatric cardiac intensive care unit.

- What questions will you need to ask prior to the child arriving on the unit?
- What information will you need to obtain and from whom when the child arrives?
- What non-medical information might you need in order to provide appropriate holistic care to the child and family?

Reflect on handovers that you have observed or participated in. Were they performed in a structured manner to ensure all aspects were covered? Was a tool such as SBAR utilised (Situation, Background, Assessment, Recommendation)?

CHAPTER SUMMARY

- CHD is the most common congenital abnormality, but it is not the only cause of cardiac disease in children and young people. A cardiac specialty placement will bring you into contact with cardiac conditions affecting structure, function and conduction of the heart
- Providing effective care for a child/young person with a cardiac diagnosis requires a number of clinical skills as well as knowledge of cardiac anatomy and physiology
- Care of the child/young person with CHD is complex and involves input from a wide range of healthcare professionals
- It is vital that nurses caring for children and their families with a cardiac diagnosis remain cognizant of the impact that such a diagnosis can have for them, both in the short and long term

BUILD YOUR BIBLIOGRAPHY

Books

FURTHER
READING

- Chamley, C.A., Carson, P., Randall, D. and Sandwell, M. (2005) *Developmental Anatomy and Physiology of Children: A Practical Approach.* London: Elsevier Churchill Livingstone.

  Contains a very useful chapter on the development of the cardiovascular system.
- Gleason, M.M., Rychik, J. and Shaddy, R.E. (2012) *Pediatric Practice: Cardiology.* New York: McGraw-Hill Medical.

  American textbook which covers foetal development and detailed explanations of heart defects, as well as aspects of care.
- Lissauer, T. and Carroll, W. (2022) *Illustrated Textbook of Paediatrics*, 6th edn. London: Elsevier.

  Contains an informative chapter on cardiology, including diagrams of some cardiac defects.
- Hampton, J. and Hampton, J. (2019) *The ECG Made Easy*, 9th edn. London: Elsevier Churchill Livingstone.

  User-friendly guide to understanding ECG and heart rhythms.

Journal articles

- Etoom, Y. and Ratnapalan, S. (2014) 'Evaluation of children with heart murmurs'. *Clinical Pediatrics*, 53 (2): 111–17.

  Useful article on heart murmurs, a frequent physiological finding in children with CHD.
- Leslie, C.E., Schofield, K., Vannatta, K. and Jackson, J.L. (2020) 'Perceived health competence predicts anxiety and depressive symptoms after a three-year follow-up among adolescents and adults with congenital heart disease'. *European Journal of Cardiovascular Nursing*, 19 (4): 283–90.

  Interesting research study on the correlation of competency in manging health needs and anxiety and depressive symptoms in adolescents and adults with CHD.
- van der Mheen, M., van der Meulen, M.H., den Boer, S.L., Schreutelkamp, D.J., van de Ende, J., de Nijs, P.F.A., Breur, J.M.P.J., Tanke, R.B., Blom, N.A., Rammeloo, L.A.J., ten Harkel, A.D.J., du Marchie Sarvaas, G.J., Utens, E.M.W.J. and Dalinghaus, M. (2020) 'Emotional and behavioural problems in children with dilated cardiomyopathy'. *European Journal of Cardiovascular Nursing*, 19 (4): 291–300.

  Research study exploring emotional and behavioural issues in children with dilated cardiomyopathy, highlighting the need for psychosocial support for children with chronic illness.

FURTHER READING: ONLINE JOURNAL ARTICLES

Weblinks

- Cincinnati Children's, Heart Institute Encyclopedia www.cincinnatichildrens.org/patients/child/encyclopedia/defects/default The Cincinnati Children's Hospital website offers comprehensive information for both health professionals and patients/families.
- The Children's Heart Foundation www.chfed.org.uk The Children's Heart Federation website has annotated diagrams of heart conditions, useful fact sheets which can be printed off and links to other useful sites such as the British Heart Foundation and Great Ormond Street Hospital.
- The British Heart Foundation www.bhf.org.uk/informationsupport/conditions/understanding-your-congenital-heart-condition This section of the British Heart Foundation website focuses on congenital heart disease and offers information useful for your learning, and for families.
- Arrhythmia Alliance http://arrhythmiaalliance.org.uk/ This organisation works to improve the quality of life in children and adults with cardiac arrhythmias. Their website contains lots of useful information about conditions that impact on the heart's electrical activity.

FURTHER READING: WEBLINKS

REFERENCES

Ávila, P., Mercier, L.A., Dore, A., Marcotte, F., Mongeon, F.P., Ibrahim, R., Asgar, A., Miro, J., Andelfinger, G., Mondésert, B., de Guise, P., Poirier, N. and Khairy, P. (2014) 'Adult congenital heart disease: a growing epidemic'. *Canadian Journal of Cardiology*, 30 (12): S410–19.

British Heart Foundation (2022) Long QT syndrome. Available at: www.bhf.org.uk/informationsupport/conditions/long-qt-syndrome (accessed 3 October 2022).

Cahill, T.J. and Prendergast, B.D. (2015) 'Infective endocarditis'. *The Lancet*, 387 (100210): 882–93.

Dhillon, R., Sharland, G., Robinson, A., Clay, C. and Bearne, C. (2009) 'Presentation and diagnosis', in K. Cook and H. Langton (eds), *Cardiothoracic Care for Children and Young People: A Multidisciplinary Approach*. Chichester: Wiley–Blackwell.

Horrox, F. (2002) *Manual of Neonatal and Paediatric Heart Disease.* London: Whurr Publishers.

Jarvis, S. (2020) *Kawasaki Disease.* Available at: https://patient.info/doctor/kawasaki-disease-pro#nav-8 (accessed 3 October 2022).

Latal, B., Helfricht, S., Fischer, J.E., Bauersfeld, U. and Landolt, M.A. (2009) 'Psychological adjustment and quality of life in children and adolescents following open-heart surgery for congenital heart disease: a systematic review'. *BMC Pediatrics,* 9 (6).

Lissauer, T. and Carroll, W. (2022) *Illustrated Textbook of Paediatrics,* 6th edn. London: Elsevier.

Miall, L., Rudolf, M. and Smith, D. (2016) *Paediatrics at a Glance,* 4th edn. Chichester: Wiley–Blackwell.

NHS England (2016) *Congenital Heart Disease Standards & Specifications.* Available at: www.england.nhs.uk/wp-content/uploads/2018/08/Congenital-heart-disease-standards-and-specifications.pdf (accessed 17 September 2022).

Royal College of Nursing (2021) *Children and Young People's Cardiac Nursing: RCN Guidance on Roles, Career Pathways and Competency Development.* London: Royal College of Nursing.

Tidy, C. (2021) *Infective Endocarditis Causes, Symptoms and Treatment.* Available at: https://patient.info/doctor/infective-endocarditis-pro (accessed 3 October 2022).

Twycross, A., Stinson, J. and Saul, R. (2021) 'The management of pain in children and young people', in A. Glasper, J. Richardson and D. Randall (eds), *A Textbook of Children's and Young People's Nursing,* 3rd edn. London: Elsevier.

WHOQOL Group (1993) 'Study protocol for the World Health Organization project to develop a quality of life assessment instrument (WHOQOL)'. *Quality of Life Research,* 2 (2): 153–9.

Wray, J., Green, C. and Kennedy, F. (2009) 'Impact of heart disease on young people and their families: an introduction', in K. Cook and H. Langton (eds), *Cardiothoracic Care for Children and Young People: A Multidisciplinary Approach.* Chichester: Wiley–Blackwell.

CARE OF CHILDREN AND YOUNG PEOPLE WITH NEUROLOGICAL PROBLEMS

STUART HIBBINS

THIS CHAPTER COVERS

- Intracranial physiology in infants and children
- Late signs of raised intracranial pressure (ICP)
- Recording neurological observations
- Acute and long-term neurological conditions

REQUIRED KNOWLEDGE

It would be helpful to have an understanding of the anatomy and physiology of the nervous system before you start this chapter.

> "I have really enjoyed learning more about the care of children with neurological problems that I can honestly say it has opened my eyes to the complexities of neurosurgical and neurology nursing and also made me realise how much I like my job."
>
> **Fiona, children's nurse**

INTRODUCTION

The chapter will provide information useful to children's nurses working with patients with a neurological illness. The opening quotation highlights the complex nature of caring for children with neurological problems and their families. Thus, before studying this chapter the reader should gain an awareness of a range of practical knowledge and skills in managing a child with a neurological illness during the acute and long-term phase, whether in hospital or a community setting.

INTRACRANIAL PHYSIOLOGY IN INFANTS AND CHILDREN

Many children and young people who present with an acute neurological condition have raised intracranial pressure (ICP), a potentially life-threatening situation. An understanding of intracranial physiology and early recognition is a prerequisite for managing patients with raised ICP.

Intracranial pressure

The intracranial vault (skull) is filled with three components. Brain tissue constitutes approximately 80% of the volume, cerebral blood accounts for approximately 10% and CSF makes up the remaining 10%. These components coexist within the rigid confines of the skull and exert a pressure known as intracranial pressure (Mestecky, 2011).

Raised intracranial pressure (RICP)

A good way to understand the concept of RICP is by using the Monro–Kellie Doctrine. This states that the volume of the three components of the rigid skull (brain, blood and cerebrospinal fluid [CSF]) remain relatively constant. According to the Monro–Kellie Doctrine there are compensatory mechanisms that allow an increase in one component and a corresponding reduction in one or two of the other components. If this does not occur, there will be an increase in ICP.

Compensatory mechanisms

There are several compensatory mechanisms that occur to maintain normal ICP. These include the displacement of CSF and the compression of CSF spaces (arachnoid spaces); the compression of cerebral venous sinuses and large veins and the displacement of venous blood. Anatomical features that allow greater compensation in neonates and young infants include greater pliability of the skull; open fontanelles and patent cranial sutures. This is why the signs of RICP differ through the age groups from infancy through to the ages where the skull sutures are fixed and cannot accommodate a rise in ICP without disastrous results.

The brain is able to withstand small increases in intracranial pressure using the compensatory mechanisms outlined above. However, if the cause of the intracranial volume is not treated (see section on medical management) then the compensatory mechanisms will eventually run out and the brain will be in a decompensated state and extremely vulnerable to further increases in volume. Brain tissue itself is capable of significant distortion to allow increases in volume but will eventually give way to the high intracranial pressure and in extreme cases will herniate through the foramen magnum (the opening at the lower part of the skull). This is referred to as coning and is considered a terminal state.

WHAT'S THE EVIDENCE?

The Monro-Kellie Doctrine is one of the fundamental principles on which the treatment of raised ICP is based. It was first developed and named after two Scottish doctors, Alexander Monro (1733-1817) and George Kellie (1770-1829).

Table 19.1 Causes of raised intracranial pressure

Cause	Pathology
Head injury, stroke	Intracerebral bleed
Brain swelling (cerebral oedema)	Infection (e.g., meningitis), head injury, hypoxic brain injury, metabolic abnormality (e.g., diabetic ketoacidosis)
Space-occupying lesion	Brain tumour
Hydrocephalus (blocked VP [ventriculoperitoneal] shunt)	Congenital or acquired

Early signs and symptoms of RICP

Early signs and symptoms of RICP can be subtle and include the following: excessive drowsiness; decreased consciousness; confusion; vomiting; headache and visual disturbances. In infants and young children there can be 'sun-setting' eyes, where the eyes appear to be in a permanent downward gaze and the sclera is observable between the upper eyelid and the iris.

Late signs of RICP

Changes to vital signs are generally thought of as late and indicate that the progression of the rising intracranial pressure is at a critical and life-threatening stage which needs effective and speedy management in order to preserve life. Cushing's triad is the name given to a situation where there is a 'triad' of signs: raised blood pressure, abnormal breathing patterns and pronounced bradycardia. It is usually preceded by the early signs and symptoms of RICP.

Table 19.2 Signs and symptoms of raised intracranial pressure

All or some features may be present with the last three signs regarded as very late features:

- Poor feeding and vomiting/nausea
- Tense bulging anterior fontanelle in infants
- High-pitched cry (cerebral cry)
- Irritability, especially on handling
- Lethargy
- Headaches
- Seizures

(Continued)

Table 19.2   (Continued)

- Changes in the level of consciousness
- Changes in pupil reaction, impaired, upward gaze (sun-setting eyes), new or evolving symptoms or signs such as unequal pupils, asymmetry of limb or facial movement
- Cushing's triad (irregular respiration, bradycardia and hypertension). This is a very late sign and at this stage the child is already extremely unwell
- False localising signs which reflect dysfunction distant or remote from the expected anatomical locus (site) of pathology (disease)

Adapted from NICE, 2019

WHAT'S THE EVIDENCE?

Harvey Cushing (1869–1939) was an American surgeon working in Berne, Switzerland who studied the effects of increasing intracranial pressure on vital signs. His paper was published in 1903 and remains one of the fundamental principles on which the management of raised ICP is based.

Raised blood pressure

Blood pressure is relatively stable in both infants and children during the early stages of RICP. Changes in vital signs are related to the medulla oblongata (lower part of the brainstem) being directly compressed as a result of RICP. This causes the capillaries of the medulla to become ischaemic. This initiates a sympathetic response where vasoconstriction occurs and the systemic blood pressure increases to restore the blood supply to the medulla at the same time as overcoming the high ICP. If the raised ICP is not treated and further rises occur and BP cannot match it then brain herniation (often known as 'coning') occurs and the medulla becomes terminally ischaemic and the patient will die (Brunker, 2011).

Abnormal breathing pattern

Changes in respiration usually follow a decrease in conscious levels. When ischaemic changes to the medulla occur, breathing becomes slow and irregular. Breathing will cease completely if blood supply to the medulla is not restored. Signs of increased effort of breathing often associated with respiratory distress are not usually evident with RICP.

Pronounced bradycardia

Like blood pressure, the heart rate is relatively stable in both infants and children during the early stages of RICP. However, in cases where ICP increases to dangerous levels there is a parasympathetic slowing of the heart which is counter-productive as it reduces cardiac output (Brunker, 2011).

Investigations for RICP

Computed tomography (CT scan) is the preferred choice of investigation (NICE, 2019). It is fast, widely available and generally well tolerated by infants and young children. It is very sensitive and good for detecting the presence of RICP; the cause, size and location of lesions; and for seeing enlarged ventricles in hydrocephalus. However, one of the disadvantages of the CT scan is it that it uses radiation, which is known to be harmful to the developing brain. Repeated use should therefore be avoided (NICE, 2019). Cranial ultrasound is the preferable method of investigation in neonates and infants. Performing a lumbar puncture is contraindicated if RICP is suspected as it can cause a serious pressure gradient (a sudden change from high to low pressure) resulting in an acute brain herniation where the brain stem is forced through the foramen magnum (the opening at the base of the skull). The neural pathways in the brain stem for blood pressure, heart rate and breathing can become irreparably damaged and can result in death.

Medical management

Severe or complex cases should be managed in the paediatric intensive care unit (PICU). Treatment may include the use of intravenous (IV) osmotic agents such as hypertonic saline or mannitol. Both of these work by drawing fluid from the cerebral tissues and into the circulatory system. Surgical removal of the cause may be another option (e.g., tumours, lesions, blood clots). If the RICP is due to hydrocephalus, the surgical insertion of a shunting device, an external ventricular drain or a CSF tapping device would be considered.

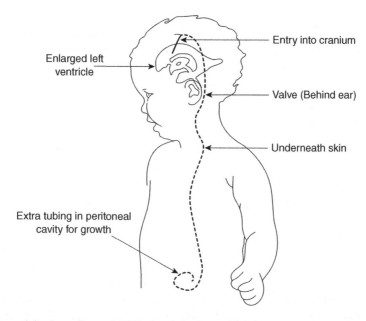

Figure 19.1 A ventriculoperitoneal (VP) shunt device, which is commonly used to treat raised intracranial pressure in hydrocephalus. Cerebral spinal fluid (CSF) drains from the enlarged ventricles into the peritoneal cavity via valve and tube

Nursing management

This will depend on how acutely ill the patient is and on the cause of RICP. Initial management would be based on a structured approach to assessment and intervention of airway, breathing and circulation (Advanced Paediatric Life Support Group, 2016). If RICP is suspected, senior clinical help should be sought immediately. Positioning the patient at 30 degrees with the child's head up and in the midline may help alleviate intracranial pressure by allowing venous drainage from the cranial vault. Temperature should be kept within normal parameters and seizures should be controlled with

SEE ALSO
CHAPTER 26

anti-convulsant drugs. Careful management of IV fluids will be required if the patient is hypertensive. All nurses need to be aware of the hazards of fluid management therapy, in particular risks associated with hypo- and hypernatraemic states. Scrupulous record-keeping and regular blood levels should be maintained.

ACTIVITY 19.1: REFLECTIVE PRACTICE

Reflect on the care management of a patient you have looked after who had signs of raised intracranial pressure. Discuss with your practice assessor/supervisor the expected steps to be taken and why these are necessary.

NEUROLOGICAL OBSERVATIONS

Neurological deterioration can be caused by various conditions (see Table 19.1) and the need for close neurological observation is important. In infants, children and young people neurological assessment usually comprises of the assessment of consciousness; pupil response; limb power and vital signs. The next section will focus on neurological assessment as this is an area which can cause students most concern regarding accurate measurement, interpretation, and reporting.

What is consciousness?

Philosophers and scientists have been discussing the complex nature of consciousness for centuries (Malik, 2000). For nurses carrying out neurological observations the concept of consciousness is about the ability of an individual to be aware of themselves and their surrounding environment. Because of developmental constraints, young children have an incomplete understanding of these concepts. Assessing consciousness in children under 5 (particularly infants) can therefore be difficult. Nurses need to use their knowledge of child development, play and diversion as well as rely on information from the family. Listening to the parents is very important as they will pick up very quickly on the often subtle changes in their child's behaviours. This is one of the key skills of a children's nurse, working alongside the parents.

Consciousness relies on the functioning of the reticular formation, which is a network of ascending and descending nerve fibres that extend from primitive areas located in the brain stem to the higher functioning areas of the cerebral cortex (Cole et al., 2005). When a healthy individual is awake and conscious the reticular formation is intact and functional. In the context of brain damage (e.g., RICP) an interruption of the reticular formation occurs and consciousness is affected. This is why assessing consciousness is considered as an assessment of brain function and an important part of neurological observations.

The Glasgow Coma Scale (GCS)

The GCS was originally developed to assess consciousness in adults and has been modified for use with children (Kirkham et al., 2005). It is based on the nurse's observation of the patient's ability to perform three activities: best eye opening, best motor response and best verbal response Each activity is given a score and added together to produce a coma score. The lowest score is 3 and indicates the patient is in a deep coma and 15 is the highest score and indicates the patient is fully conscious. For more information on the Glasgow Coma Scale go to their website. https://www.glasgowcomascale.org/

Modified forms of the Glasgow Coma Scale for use with children

Modified Glasgow Coma Scales are more suitable for use in children aged over 5 years because they assess verbal response and motor response which rely on a child's ability to understand and respond to verbal instructions. For example, an infant will not talk or obey commands; a newborn baby demonstrates reflexive movement; the expected best motor response at 6 months is flexion with spontaneous movement. Observations of infants and young children under 5 years should be performed by staff with appropriate experience (NICE, 2019).

Eye opening is the only activity that can be measured in all age groups. There have been various adapted versions of the GCS for use in children (Kirkham et al., 2008). The Adelaide Scale, Pinderfield Scale and James Coma Scale are all examples in use but none is as widely used as the PGCS.

Which brain structures are being tested?

Eye opening

Eye opening tests a primitive response initiated by the reticular activating system (RAS). This is a network of neural circuitry extending from the brain stem through the thalamus to the cerebral cortex.

Best verbal response

The best way to determine whether someone is orientated is to ask them their name, where they are and what time of day it is. Younger children will respond better to the sound of their mum's voice. This activity tests two areas of the cerebral cortex associated with speech. The first is Wernicke's area in the left temporal lobe which processes what has been said (reception of speech). The other area is Broca's area in the frontal lobe which is linked with the ability to articulate a reply (expression of speech). The nerve pathway called the internal arcuate fasciculus, which connects these two structures, is also being tested.

Best motor response

Asking a child to move their limbs also tests nerve pathways for several higher neurological functions in the brain. For example, neural circuitry for movement is associated with the motor strip in the cerebral cortex as well as the cerebellum and basal ganglia.

Physical stimulus

If a child is not responding to a tactile or verbal stimulus you will need to apply a physical stimulus. Various types of physical stimulus can be used and the specific age of the child will determine which method is used. The National Paediatric Neuroscience Benchmarking Group recommends use of supraorbital pressure to test for localisation, and nail bed pressure to test for flexion (NICE, 2019). While there is generally a consensus on which methods are appropriate, there is no universal agreement as to which method is optimal (Hibbins, 2009; Teasdale et al., 2014). In the context of children this is complicated further by the fact that some methods are better suited for older children than for younger ones. Physical stimulus should be applied forcefully and cause no injury. The general principle of 'do no harm' applies here and the nurse should ensure that he or she applies the least painful method possible to achieve a result. Always listen to what the parents have to say as well as they are best placed to know what is usual for their child and may well pick up sooner on more subtle changes. Local guidance should also be sought in the clinical setting.

Assessment of pupils

Assessment of pupils and limbs are not part of the coma scale but can potentially detect damage to specific nerve pathways that lead to focal signs of neurological deterioration. Assessment of pupils tests cranial nerves II and III. Cranial nerve II is responsible for vision and cranial nerve III controls pupillary constriction and eye movement. Both may become compressed by increased intracranial pressure and in extreme cases the pupils can become fixed and dilated.

Assessment of limb response

Assessment of limbs or posture identifies any focal neurological deficits caused by damage to specific nerve pathways. Focal signs of neurological problems could include damage to the motor pathways (e.g., hemiplegia, hypertonia and hypotonia).

Assessment of vital signs

See above section on the late signs of RICP (Cushing's triad).

Frequency of observations

NICE (2023) recommend that observations for head-injured patients should be performed and recorded half-hourly until the GCS is 15. The frequency of observations after the initial assessment for patients with GCS equal to 15 should be as follows: half-hourly for 2 hours; then hourly for 4 hours; 2-hourly thereafter. If the patient deteriorates after the initial 2-hour period, observations should revert to half-hourly and follow the original frequency schedule (NICE, 2023). If these observations are indicated in a child's care they should be assiduously carried out as ordered and not omitted because, for example, the child is sleeping. The child may not be sleeping. They may in fact have a deteriorating level of consciousness. Always seek senior advice when considering whether CNS sign measurement is to be altered in frequency.

ACUTE AND LONG-TERM CONDITIONS

Hydrocephalus

Hydrocephalus is the most common paediatric neurosurgical disorder. Most cases present in infancy during the first year and in children within the first decade (Hibbins, 2011). It is caused by a number of different disease processes, which can be either congenital or acquired (see Table 19.3). It occurs because of an imbalance between the production of cerebrospinal fluid (CSF) in the cerebral ventricles and its absorption by the arachnoid villi in the subarachnoid space, which creates an over-accumulation of CSF within the CSF pathways. This results in the dilatation and enlargement of the ventricles and can result in RICP.

Non-communicating and communicating hydrocephalus

Hydrocephalus is commonly described as having either a non-communicating or a communicating cause. Non-communicating hydrocephalus is caused by an abnormal anatomical obstruction within the CSF pathways. For example, in aqueduct stenosis, infants are born with a narrowing of the cerebral aqueduct which blocks the flow of CSF and results in hydrocephalus. In communicating hydrocephalus there is a functional obstruction to the sites of CSF reabsorption. For example, in meningitis the arachnoid villi are damaged by infection and CSF absorption is impaired, resulting in hydrocephalus. It is also thought that in some cases it is possible to have a combination of both types. For example, infants with intraventricular haemorrhage (IVH) have large blood clots that obstruct CSF pathways and blood in the CSF which impairs reabsorption (Hibbins, 2011).

Table 19.3 Congenital and acquired causes of hydrocephalus

Congenital causes	Acquired causes
Spina bifida aperta (e.g., myelomeningocele)	Subarachnoid haemorrhage
Aqueduct stenosis	Intraventricular haemorrhage
Dandy-Walker syndrome	Brain tumours
Chiari malformations	Head injury
	Meningitis

Treatment

CSF shunt devices are the principal method of treating hydrocephalus. These devices shunt CSF from its site of production within the cerebral ventricles past the site of obstruction to an area where the CSF can be reabsorbed. The ventriculoperitoneal (VP) shunt is the most commonly used system used today.

Another method which avoids the use of shunt devices is third endoscopic ventriculostomy. This has become more popular in recent times because it avoids the complications associated with VP shunts (infection, blockage and displacement).

CASE STUDY 19.1: SIMON

Simon, aged 9 years, had a 3-week history of vomiting and headaches. He had visited the GP four times and was diagnosed with childhood migraines and given painkillers. His parents were unhappy with his diagnosis and took Simon to his local emergency department. He was seen by the on-call paediatrician and sent for a head CT scan. This showed a large posterior fossa lesion (brain tumour) and dilated ventricles (hydrocephalus) with signs of RICP. Simon was transferred to a paediatric neurosurgical unit.

- How would you describe Simon's raised ICP using the Monro-Kellie Doctrine?
- Does Simon have a non-communicating (obstructive) or a communicating type of hydrocephalus?

Acquired brain injury

Many children are admitted to hospital with acquired brain injury (ABI) each year, and for some the consequences can be very severe, requiring ongoing care in the community or at a residential rehabilitation centre. 'Acquired' refers to the way the injury occurred – as a result of either an accident or illness that happened after birth.

ABI is classified into two main types:

- Traumatic brain injury (TBI)
- Non-traumatic brain injury

Traumatic brain injury (TBI)

A TBI is caused by an impact to the head and there are three types:

Closed head injury: This refers to a severe head injury where the skull is not fractured. It can result from a deceleration injury (e.g., car accident) where the brain has become severely damaged as a result of movement within the skull. Damage is usually widespread and is referred to a diffuse brain injury (Cartwright and Wallace, 2017). The most common cause of severe head injury in infants under 12 months is non-accidental injury (NAI). It is often referred to as 'shaken baby syndrome', but now known as abusive head trauma (AHT).

SAFEGUARDING STOP POINT

To learn more about abusive head trauma (AHT) and non-accidental injury (NAI) read the BBC article on the dangers of shaking babies: www.bbc.co.uk/news/uk-england-york-north-yorkshire-49906916

'Shaken baby syndrome' is an area of ongoing controversy and debate within the scientific community. You can hear the view of a doctor who is openly critical of the science behind shaken baby syndrome.

- Consider the different arguments presented.
- What impact does this have for the future role of the expert witness?

Open or penetrating injury: A head injury where the skull is fractured and the brain exposed. It can be caused by deceleration injury, explosion or gunshot.

Crushing injuries: This is the least common type of brain injury. It can be caused by falling heavy objects such as furniture or a walled-mounted television. Younger children who have more pliable skulls are most at risk.

For further reading on head injuries in children, see Pennington (2009).

Non-traumatic brain injury

A non-traumatic acquired brain injury is caused by an illness rather than an impact to the head. The following are all examples of possible causes: brain tumours, meningitis, encephalitis, hypoxic brain injury, stroke, arteriovenous malformation, cerebral aneurysm (see Table 19.4).

"After he came out of PICU he was moved to a chest unit with a ratio of one nurse to eight patients and they could not cope ... he was waking up from his coma and was confused, agitated and required constant attention and care. We were relieved when he was eventually transferred to the rehabilitation centre ... the doctors and nurses there understood his injuries better there because they'd looked after other head injured children. They didn't take his disinhibited behaviour to heart."

Sofia, parent

"One characteristic common to many people after an ABI is lack of self-awareness ... I have no memory of the initial post-injury weeks, and my recollections of the subsequent months and years of recovery are fragmentary."

Sheena, an adult who recovered from an early ABI (McDonald, 2008)

Long-term outcome

Children with severe ABI are likely to need some form of rehabilitation. This may take place either at the hospital or in a residential rehabilitation centre. Rehabilitation can be a slow and complicated journey for both the affected children and their families. Recovery may be ongoing and last for years. The aim is not to cure the individual but to help the child compensate for any changes to their abilities and promote independence through different therapies with help from the multidisciplinary team (MDT) (Woodward and Waterhouse, 2009).

Problems after ABI are complex and result from widespread neurological damage, and no two individuals will present with the same clinical symptoms. Damage to the immature or developing nervous system means that although the initial damage to the brain does not progress, symptoms may appear to worsen as the brain matures and problems become more evident as the child gets older (NICE, 2017).

Symptoms vary and can include: problems with mobility; disturbances in balance and coordination abilities; difficulty in controlling and maintaining posture; epilepsy and intellectual development. The rehabilitation team includes different therapies and may include the following: physiotherapy, occupational therapy, speech and language therapy (SLT), play therapy, music therapy, social work, clinical psychology, neuropsychology, educational psychology and family therapy. Nurses are in a unique position as they are the most consistent carers and provide continuity of care (May, 2001). This means they play a key role within the rehabilitation programme by coordinating care while providing family support as well as leadership of the MDT.

ACTIVITY 19.2: REFLECTIVE PRACTICE

Reflect upon a patient with an ABI you have looked after and make a list of the things you found challenging. Try to identify what made this care challenging.

Epilepsy is the most common neurological condition found in children. It is often perceived as a single condition but there are many different types of epilepsy and conditions which cause it. Most have their epilepsy controlled with anti-epilepsy drugs (AEDs). However, those whose epilepsy is not controlled with AEDs can have other forms of treatment (e.g., surgery). The management of epilepsy in children is aimed at improving their health and general quality of life as well as minimising the detrimental impact on educational, social and family life. This can be achieved by effective clinical management and enabling the family to manage their child's epilepsy.

Table 19.4 Terminology associated with epilepsy and seizures

Term	Definition
Seizure	A seizure can be a single event that results in an altered state of brain function. Seizures occur because of abnormal neuronal activity in the brain. The appearance of the seizure depends on the site of the abnormal electrical activity. It can occur in a specific area (focal seizure) or it can occur throughout the brain (generalised seizure) (May, 2001)
Epilepsy	An individual can be diagnosed as having epilepsy if repeated and unpredictable seizures occur. Epilepsy can be caused by a variety of disorders (see below)
Seizure disorder	This term is sometimes used as an alternative to 'epilepsy'
Epilepsy syndrome	Epilepsy syndrome is a term that refers to various types of epilepsy which can be grouped together because of shared characteristics (e.g., benign rolandic epilepsy, childhood absence epilepsy and juvenile myoclonic epilepsy)
Febrile convulsion	The most common form of epileptic seizure seen in children under 4 years. It occurs following a fever arising from an infection outside of the central nervous system (e.g., an upper respiratory infection)
Movement disorder	Movement disorders are neurological conditions, caused by damage to the brain that result in uncontrolled abnormal movement such as excessive or involuntary movements (e.g., ataxia). Movement disorders are not considered to be a form of epilepsy
Status epilepticus	A generalised convulsion lasting 30 minutes or longer or when successive convulsions occur without a period of recovery in between (APLSG, 2016)

ACTIVITY 19.3: CRITICAL THINKING

NICE have produced guidelines for the diagnosis and management of epilepsy in children and adults, which you can access via https://www.nice.org.uk/guidance/ng217

Using these guidelines, answer the following questions:

- How is epilepsy diagnosed?
- Which investigations do the guidelines recommend for those with suspected epilepsy?
- How should those with complex or intractable epilepsy be managed and which alternative treatment other than anti-epilepsy drugs (AEDs) are available?

CASE STUDY 19.2: SARAH

Sarah is 15 years old and has a history of runny nose and headache. Her mother reported that she has had a fever for the past 3 days. While waiting in A&E she had a generalised tonic clonic seizure.

- What action would you initially take?
- How would you manage Sarah's seizure?
- How would you explain to Sarah and her mother what is happening?

Table 19.5 Neurological conditions, age of presentation, and signs and symptoms

Condition	Average age of presentation	Signs and symptoms
Seizure and epilepsy	Seizures can occur at any age and most cases of epilepsy are diagnosed under 18 years of age	Focal or generalised seizures
Spinal cord abnormalities Encephaloceles Arachnoid cysts Dandy-Walker syndrome Arnold Chiari malformation Spina bifida aperta (e.g., myelomeningocele) Spina bifida occulta (e.g., tethered cord)	Present at birth (origins are congenital)	Hydrocephalus, nerve damage resulting in neurological, orthopaedic and urological dysfunction
Cerebral palsy (movement disorder)	Diagnosis before 5th birthday	Motor and sensory problems
Neurodegenerative disorders Neurometabolic (e.g., Batten's disease)	Birth and pre-birth, or any stage of childhood	Presenting features are commonly loss of motor and cognitive abilities. Other signs and symptoms include: epilepsy, regression of skills, visual disturbances, spasticity and muscle spasm, hypotonia
Spinocerebellar (e.g., Huntington's disease) Neuromuscular (e.g., Duchenne muscular dystrophy) Acquired (e.g., Rasmussen's encephalitis)		Gastro-oesophageal reflux, feeding difficulties, aspiration, chest infections, constipation, change in sleep patterns, excessive oral secretions, change in behaviour, irritability
Brain tumours (Most common solid tumour in children, usually confined to the CNS) Types: Astrocytoma Medulloblastoma Ependymoma brain stem tumour Midline tumour (e.g., craniopharyngioma)	Can present during infancy or childhood	Focal neurological signs (symptoms vary and depend on the location in the brain of the tumour), signs of raised ICP, headache, endocrine disturbances, hemiparesis, seizures, changes in behaviour, seizures, ataxia, hydrocephalus
Cerebral vascular abnormalities Occlusive arteriopathies (e.g., Moya Moya syndrome) Neurovascular abnormalities (e.g., AVM and aneurysms, Vein of Galen malformation) Cerebrovascular (e.g., acute stroke)	Can present during infancy or childhood	Focal neurological signs (symptoms vary and depend on the location in the brain of the bleed), deterioration in consciousness, sudden collapse, severe headache, signs of raised ICP, hemiparesis

CHAPTER SUMMARY

A sound understanding of the nervous system – and the impact that disease and injury can have on it – is a prerequisite for nurses caring for children with acute or long-term neurological problems. More importantly, for nurses working in this area, having a basic grasp of the complexities not only enhances performance but also enjoyment of their role. This results in a more rounded, empathetic and fulfilled carer. Having an appreciation of this can only be positive for children and families. In this chapter you will have:

- Reviewed intracranial physiology in infants and children
- Considered the dynamics of raised intracranial pressure and identified early and late change in children's condition
- Reviewed neurological observations tools and observations and how to record these
- Identified acute and long-term neurological conditions and their associated care (hydrocephalus, acquired brain injury and epilepsy)

─── BUILD YOUR BIBLIOGRAPHY ───

Books

FURTHER
READING

- Costandi, M. (2013) *50 Ideas You Really Need to Know: The Human Brain*. London: Quercus Publishing.

  An easy-to-read book that includes good introductory sections on A&P as well as chapters explaining many contemporary findings of neuroscience.
- Crossman, A. and Neary, D. (2019) *Neuroanatomy: An Illustrated Colour Text*. Edinburgh: Churchill Livingstone.

  A book dedicated to neuroanatomy for students who want to explore the nervous system in more depth. The introductory chapter provides an excellent overview.
- Smith, J. and Martin, C. (2008) *Paediatric Neurosurgery for Nurses: Evidence-based Care for Children and Their Families*. London: Routledge.

  This text provides accessible and evidence-based information for nurses working in paediatric neurosurgery.

Journal articles

FURTHER
READING:
ONLINE
JOURNAL
ARTICLES

- Khoo, T.-B. (2012) 'Classification of childhood epilepsies in a tertiary pediatric neurology clinic using a customized classification scheme from the International League against Epilepsy 2010 Report'. *Journal of Child Neurology*, 28 (1): 56-9.

  For further reading on the classification of seizures.
- Bui, A.D., Alexander, A. and Soltesz, I. (2015) 'Seizing control: from current treatments to optogenetic interventions in epilepsy'. *The Neuroscientist*, 23 (1): 68-81.

  For a review of current and future treatments.
- Moseley, B.D., Nickels, K. and Wirrell, E.C. (2011) 'Surgical outcomes for intractable epilepsy in children with epileptic spasms'. *Journal of Child Neurology*, 27 (6): 713-20.

  For more information on epilepsy surgery.

Weblinks

FURTHER
READING:
WEBLINKS

- Neuroscience for Kids https://faculty.washington.edu/chudler/neurok.html This site has been created for all students and teachers who would like to learn about the nervous system.

- Young Epilepsy (The National Centre for Young People) www.youngepilepsy.org.uk This site provides information about epilepsy for young people, parents and professionals.
- Headway: the Brain Injury Association www.headway.org.uk For information about support services for families with children with acquired brain injury.
- The Glasgow Coma Scale www.glasgowcomascale.org/ This site provides excellent resources to help clinicians develop their neurological assessment skills.
- Royal College of Paediatrics and Child Health (RCPCH) (2019) *Management of Children and Young People with an Acute Decrease in Conscious Level: Clinical Guidance* www.rcpch.ac.uk/resources/management-children-young-people-acute-decrease-conscious-level-clinical-guideline For comprehensive evidence-based guidance on the management of decreased consciousness in children and young people.

REFERENCES

Advanced Paediatric Life Support Group (APLSG) (2016) *The Practical Approach*, 6th edn. Chichester: Wiley–Blackwell.

Brunker, C. (2011) 'Assessment, interpretation and management of altered cardiovascular status in the neurological patient', in S. Woodward and A.-M. Mestecky (eds), *Neuroscience Nursing: Evidence-based Theory and Practice*. Oxford: Wiley–Blackwell.

Cartwright, C. and Wallace, D. (2017) *Nursing Care of the Pediatric Neurosurgery Patient*. New York: Springer.

Cole, M., Levitin, K. and Luria, L. (2005) *The Autobiography of Alexander Luria*. New York: Psychology Press.

Hibbins, S. (2009) 'Painful stimulus in the paediatric setting'. *British Journal of Neuroscience Nursing*, 5 (5): 215.

Hibbins, S. (2011) 'Management of patients with hydrocephalus', in S. Woodward and A.-M. Mestecky (eds), *Neuroscience Nursing: Evidence-based Theory and Practice*. Oxford: Wiley–Blackwell.

Kirkham, F., Newton, C. and Whitehouse, W. (2008) 'Paediatric coma scales'. *Developmental Medicine and Child Neurology*, 50: 267–74.

Malik, K. (2000) *Man, Beast and Zombie: What Science Can and Cannot Tell Us About Human Nature*. London: Weidenfeld and Nicolson.

May, L. (2001) *Paediatric Neurosurgery: A Handbook for the Multidisciplinary Team*. London: Whurr Publishers.

McDonald, S. (2008) 'Travels in the land of no self awareness'. *British Journal of Neuroscience Nursing*, 4 (10): 510.

Mestecky, A.-M. (2011) 'Intracranial physiology', in S. Woodward and A.-M. Mestecky (eds), *Neuroscience Nursing: Evidence-based Theory and Practice*. Oxford: Wiley–Blackwell.

NICE (National Institute for Health and Care Excellence) (2023) Head injury: assessment and early management. NICE guideline [NG232] Available at: https://www.nice.org.uk/guidance/ng232 (accessed 11 July 2023).

Pennington, N. (2009) 'Head injuries in children'. *Journal of School Nursing*, 26 (1): 26–32.

Teasdale, G. et al. (2014) 'Forty years on: updating the Glasgow Coma Scale'. *Nursing Times*, 110 (42): 12–16.

Woodward, S. and Waterhouse, C. (eds) (2009) *Oxford Handbook of Neuroscience Nursing*. Oxford: Oxford University Press.

CARE OF CHILDREN AND YOUNG PEOPLE WITH URINARY AND RENAL PROBLEMS

20

MARY BRADY AND LINDA MOORE

THIS CHAPTER COVERS

- A review of normal anatomy of the renal system
- Acquired renal conditions in childhood
- Care of a child or young person with a renal condition

REQUIRED KNOWLEDGE

It would be helpful to have an understanding of the anatomy and physiology of the renal system before you start this chapter and associated learning. Read Gormley-Fleming, E. (2021) 'The renal system', in I. Peate and E. Gormley-Fleming, *Fundamentals of Children and Young People's Anatomy and Physiology*. Chichester: Wiley–Blackwell. pp.280–303.

> "Having a child who suffers from repetitive UTIs caused by an overactive bladder and dysfunctional voiding is challenging. As a parent I find the juggle of her physical and emotional needs challenging. The emotional consequences of her condition at present outweigh the physical side and I often feel under supported in relation to this. The nurse specialists are a very good point of contact for me as a parent when I don't understand what is happening or I need support myself, they are very patient with me as a parent."
>
> **Marsha, parent**

INTRODUCTION

The kidneys are important organs that maintain homeostasis, control waste elimination, and maintain fluid levels within the body. This chapter will guide you with the nursing assessment of a child or young person (CYP) with a renal condition. Renal conditions can be divided into congenital or acquired disorders. This chapter will explore the aetiology as well as the manifestation of the physical signs of ill health linked to renal pathophysiology such as pyrexia, hypertension, weight gain due to oedema, skin condition, the monitoring of urinary output and urinalysis. Thereafter, aspects of holistic nursing care provision will be discussed covering the early detection of deterioration and cascading that information succinctly and efficiently to other members of the healthcare team. The specific nursing care required for relatively common renal conditions will be discussed, such as in maintaining appropriate fluid and dietary input (in particular fluid volumes, sodium, potassium and protein intake), alongside the observation of fluid output. Medication that is commonly used (antibiotics, steroids and analgesia) will be mentioned but for issues related to the administration of medication you should refer to Chapter 4.

SEE ALSO
CHAPTER 4
AND 26

The manifestation of renal disorders can have a wide-reaching effect on the child since the disorder can affect body image, school education and family life (Clavé et al., 2019), as indicated in the opening quotation from a parent. Aspects of caring for a child with an altered body image due to oedema or a chronic renal condition will be discussed as well as the impact of ill health on their school education, alongside the nurse's role in facilitating education. The psychosocial impact of having a child with a renal condition will also be covered as well as any related renal educational provision that is required for the family.

NORMAL ANATOMY

The renal system consists of two bean-shaped kidneys, each connected by a muscular tube (called the ureter) to the bladder. The kidneys produce a waste product called urine that collects in the bladder and in the continent child passes along the urethra for elimination at a convenient time. Internal and external sphincter muscles at either end of the urethra control when this occurs (Gormley-Fleming, 2021). The amount and constituents of the child's urine can provide information on renal function and the presence of disease (see Chapter 26).

SEE ALSO
CHAPTER 26

Table 20.1 Normal average volume of urine (Gormley-Fleming, 2015)

Stage of childhood	Normal average urine output ml/kg/hr
Infant	1.0-3.0
Child	1.0-2.0
Adolescent	0.5-1.0

Table 20.2 Constituents of urine (Gormley-Fleming, 2015)

Characteristic	Normal findings	Abnormal findings
Colour	Amber due to the presence of urochrome	Dark orange - concentrated urine, fluid deficit as kidneys are conserving water
	Pale urine - normal for neonates, or dilute urine for older child	Very pale - dilute urine due to excessive fluid intake or renal disease where there is an inability to concentrate urine

(Continued)

Table 20.2   (Continued)

Characteristic	Normal findings	Abnormal findings
Transparency	Clear when first voided. Will become cloudy if allowed to stand	Very cloudy urine may indicate the presence of white blood cells
Odour	Ammonia or mildly aromatic odour	Fishy smell – putrefaction occurs due to the decomposition of protein by bacteria
Protein	Small amount of protein may be present due to immaturity of nephrons	Proteinuria >1000mg/day is indicative of renal impairment
Glucose	Negative	Glycosuria indicates that renal threshold has been reached and the plasma glucose is >11mmol/l. This is indicative of diabetes type 1 or gluconeogenesis from steroid therapy
Ketones	Negative	Ketonuria – ketones are produced when fat is metabolised
Blood	Negative	Haematuria indicates active bleeding in the renal system or renal disease
Bilirubin	Negative	May indicate jaundice secondary to liver disease
Specific gravity	Neonate: 1.002–1.008 Child: 1.002–1.030	Low specific gravity: excessive fluid intake High specific gravity: dehydration, glycosuria
pH	Neonate: 5–7 Child: 4.5–8	A decrease in pH occurs as hydrogen ions are excreted in urine and metabolic acidosis is present

Congenital renal conditions

The renal system develops during the third week of uterine life from the mesoderm and subsequently embryological errors can result in a variety of conditions:

- Total absence of both kidneys (agenesis), which is often incompatible with life although in the absence of other conditions could be treated with dialysis
- Unilateral absence of a kidney
- Fusion of the two kidneys into one horseshoe-shaped kidney
- Duplex ureters
- Ureteric stenosis
- Malposition of the ureter at the ureteric junction with the bladder or pelvis of the kidney
- The development of valves along the internal urethral walls that prevent the flow of urine
- Reimplantation of ureters

  It is possible to surgically re-implant the ureters either at the pelviureteric junction or the bladder depending on the defect. However, it is important that postoperatively the urinary output is monitored closely, and the nurse is vigilant for signs of infection and blood loss and that these are escalated quickly to the surgical team.

- Bladder exstrophy

Bladder exstrophy is a very rare condition where the abdominal wall has failed to close in utero leaving an exposed bladder (Kumar et al., 2015). It often coexists with epispadias and requires surgery during the neonatal period within a specialist centre.

- Hypospadias and epispadias

In some male infants, the urinary meatus exits the penis on the ventral (hypospadias) or dorsal (epispadias) side of the penis. Surgical repair is usually done when the child is about 1 year of age.

- Differences of Sex Development (DSD) formally refered to as Ambiguous genitalia

This condition requires sensitive handling and consideration. Genetic information and endocrine tests are required to ascertain the best plan of treatment. During this difficult time for the parents and family, support needs to be collaborative amongst a multidisciplinary team of professional experts.

With antenatal scanning, some of these defects can be diagnosed and corrected or potential damage to the kidneys minimised with intrauterine surgery (Ruano et al., 2015). After birth, various surgical techniques (described later) may be used to prevent further damage to the kidneys and maximise renal function.

ACQUIRED RENAL CONDITIONS

Urinary tract infections

A urinary tract infection (UTI) is a relatively common childhood condition that requires immediate diagnosis, treatment, and investigative management. A small infant may present with a fever or febrile convulsion and a clean urine sample is a routine test. Indeed, a UTI is commonly found in 8% of girls and 2% of boys, and if untreated the ensuing renal scarring may lead to hypertension and renal morbidity (Brandström and Hansson, 2015) and chronic kidney disease (Diaz Kane, 2022). Diagnosis and treatment are therefore important, so much so that the National Institute for Health and Care Excellence (NICE) (2022) has produced guidance and a quality standard to minimise kidney damage, which covers diagnosis, assessment of risk factors for underlying causes, treatment and subsequent management including surgery. Assessment and care should centre round the individual needs of the child and be carried out in partnership with the family. Care, treatment, and management can impact the child in the long term as indicated by Melanie's voice below.

"I have an overactive bladder and recurrent UTIs which have caused permanent renal damage. I take medicine which stops me from having to go to the toilet as much but my bladder is still naughty and makes me feel desperate every time I need to go. I don't like going into hospital as I don't like blood tests because it hurts and makes me sad. I like the big hospital where I go to see the nurses and doctors, they put jelly on my belly and we look at my insides, it's gross. There is a big slide there and I love it, I go round and round a hundred times but then I have to go and listen to the doctors and that's boring as there aren't many fun things to do in the rooms only in the bit where we wait. I like the lady who plays with me best, we do colouring together and I tell her when I'm sad about my bladder and kidneys. I sometimes wish I wasn't poorly as it annoys me when I have to be in hospital and I miss my friends, but it's not too bad as I always make new friends and the nurses are always really nice, they give me jelly and I love that."

Melanie, child

CASE STUDY 20.1: DANNY

Danny is 14 months old. He was admitted again following a second febrile convulsion thought to be induced by a urinary tract infection (UTI). On admission it was noted that although his length is on the 75th centile his weight is on the 50th centile. He was generally irritable, especially when voiding urine.

Urine testing on the ward revealed some proteinuria. He was prescribed a 5-day course of antibiotics.

- What care will Danny require for this hospitalisation and why?
- Danny's parents are worried. What short- and long-term consequences might they be worried about?

Children who present with urinary tract infections are often assessed for the extent of renal damage using radioactive isotopes such as DMSA (dimercaptosuccinic acid) and MCUG (mercapto acetyltriglycine) scans.

ACTIVITY 20.1: CRITICAL THINKING

The consultant arranged for Danny (Case study 20.1) to have a DMSA scan as a day case and this revealed that he has vesico-ureteric reflux on his left kidney with some renal scarring. The consultant decided that Danny will require surgery to re-implant his left ureter and has referred Danny to a paediatric renal surgeon.

- What can the nurse do to allay parental fears?

Hydronephrosis

Normally the ureter is a muscular tube that has a funnel-shaped opening which connects with the pelvis of the kidney. In some cases, there is an obstruction due to a kink in the ureter, an aberrant blood vessel or a renal stone. This causes dilation above the obstruction with subsequent scarring and damage to the kidney.

Glomerulonephritis

CASE STUDY 20.2: BILLY

Billy is 6 years old. Two weeks ago, he had a sore throat and was given some antibiotics by his GP. Over the past few days his mother has noticed that when he wakes up his eyes are puffy, and he doesn't seem to be as energetic as he used to be. He has mentioned that his head hurts sometimes. His mother was worried that he might have tonsillitis again and need to take more time off school, so she took him back to the GP who asked for him to be admitted to hospital because he has 'inflamed kidneys'. On admission to the ward a urine test shows that he has blood and protein in his urine. The medical staff have commenced intravenous antibiotics. What other treatment will Billy require?

Glomerulonephritis tends to affect more boys than girls and of age range between 6 and 7 years old and is an autoimmune condition where the body reacts to toxins produced following a streptococcal infection elsewhere in the body (e.g., 10–14 days after a β-haemolytic streptococcal throat infection). The antigen–antibody–antigen response results in swelling of endothelial cells in glomeruli that leak blood cells and protein out of the body. The child develops oedema which is peri-orbital in the morning but becomes more generalised around the body as the day progresses, plus, cloudy, smoky brown urine of reduced volume. They may also complain of headaches and have slight pyrexia with a slight rise in blood pressure.

Treatment involves intravenous antibiotics and input from a dietician when low potassium, low protein diet and reduced fluids are required. It is important that the nurse also supports the child who will be feeling unwell and will have an altered body image. The family will also be concerned about the long-term outcome since glomerulonephritis may cause permanent damage to the glomeruli with subsequent renal failure. See Table 20.4 for details of further care.

Nephrotic syndrome

This condition, which is also more prevalent in boys, affects 1:50,000 children. The epithelial cells of the glomeruli become swollen, causing protein to leak out into the filtrate, resulting in oedema with a low circulating blood volume and serum albumin. The child may be prone to coagulation issues (thrombosis) and will be susceptible to infection due to a low level of gamma globulin. Blood pressure monitoring may show blood pressure to be normal or reveal slight hypotension due to low serum albumin (see Table 20.3 for differentiation).

Treatment includes steroids, low sodium diet and accurate monitoring of fluid balance and weight measurements. Support is required for the child and family who will be concerned about future renal function, although with nephrotic syndrome the condition may resolve with or without future exacerbations and compromised renal function.

Table 20.3 Differentiation between glomerulonephritis and nephrotic syndrome

	Glomerulonephritis	Nephrotic syndrome
Cause	Post β-haemolytic streptococcal infection	Unknown
Urine	Haematuria, proteinuria	Proteinuria
	Cloudy, smoky brown urine	Dark opalescent frothy urine
	Reduced urine output	Reduced urine output
Blood test		High levels of cholesterol, phospholipids and triglycerides
		Low level of albumin
		Hypovolaemia
Blood pressure	Mild to moderate rise	Normal to slightly low
Temperature	Pyrexia	
Oedema	Periorbital-generalised	Periorbital-generalised
Weight	Weight gain	Weight gain
Further infection		Susceptibility to infection due to loss of gamma globulins
Other symptoms	Headaches	General malaise
Prognosis	May lead to permanent damage and chronic renal failure	

Haemolytic uraemic syndrome (HUS)

There are three main aspects to this syndrome:

- Haemolytic anaemia caused by the destruction of red blood cells
- Acute kidney failure
- Low platelet count (thrombocytopenia)

HUS usually occurs in children under 5 years old and is the main reason children present with acute kidney failure and often occurs after a gastrointestinal infection with bloody diarrhoea caused by ingesting bacteria such as *Escherichia coli*, *Shigella*, or *Campylobacter*. The toxins these bacteria produce affect the lining of the glomerulus triggering kidney failure. Whilst most children make a full recovery, some will develop chronic kidney failure and require dialysis. There is also a 5–10% mortality rate.

Henoch Schönlein purpura (HSP)

HSP is more common in 3–10-year-old boys and tends to occur in the winter months. Often the child has had a respiratory illness and it is thought that immunoglobulins (IgA and IgG) interact to trigger inflammatory responses. Typically, the child may present with:

- An initially urticarial rash that becomes purpuric
- A rash mainly over the buttocks and extensor surfaces of the legs
- Painful and swollen joints
- Colicky abdominal pain
- Glomerulonephritis with microscopic or macroscopic haematuria

As well as supportive nursing care, the child needs to be monitored for proteinuria, hypertension, oedema and renal deterioration. Those children with renal involvement must be monitored for a year to detect ongoing and long-term urinary abnormalities.

SEE ALSO
CHAPTER 31

Wilms tumour

This is an embryonic tumour and is the commonest renal tumour seen in children. It is believed to have a genetic link and usually presents between 5 and 10 years of age when the child develops an abdominal mass with or without other symptoms such as weight gain and poor appetite. After radiological diagnosis, treatment usually includes chemotherapy and a nephrectomy.

Table 20.4   Care of the child with an acute renal condition

Care	Rationale
Skin care: keep skin clean and dry	Due to oedema the skin may be fragile and prone to breakdown and sores
Avoid excessive use of tapes	
Change positions and use a pressure-relieving mattress	
Monitor for pyrexia	Hypoalbuminaemia may render the child susceptible to infection due to reduced immunoglobulins

Care	Rationale
Blood pressure	Hypotension may indicate a low circulating fluid volume. Child must be assessed for dehydration and fluid requirements adjusted accordingly (see Chapter 26)
Full blood count, urea and electrolytes	Patients with renal problems may not produce sufficient erythropoietin to stimulate the bone marrow to produce red blood cells
	Proteinuria results in low serum protein levels such as low albumin which moderates osmotic pressure and will have an ensuing effect on blood pressure
	Low serum gamma globulin which will reduce the immune response
Monitor weight	Oedema will cause weight to increase. Ultimately weight gain due to fluid will affect how much of any drug needs to be given. In children, medication is calculated according to weight so monitoring weight is vital to ensure that therapeutic doses are given. The dose for some drugs must be modified with children in renal failure
Body image/self-esteem	Excess weight gain and facial oedema will alter how the child views him/herself
Boredom due to inability to move due to tiredness and general malaise	Access to a hospital play specialist and a variety of age-appropriate toys Plan care to enable rest periods
Morbidity and mortality	Depending on the age and maturity of the child, he/she will have a variable understanding of the impact of the condition on their life potential and invincibility. Access to a psychologist may be required

ESCALATION OF CONCERNS TO APPROPRIATE STAFF

As a nursing student, you will work alongside a registered nurse observing your patient's physiological data. Many hospitals now use age-related paediatric early warning score charts (PEWS) to document observations and facilitate the identification of unwell and deteriorating children. PEWS charts can also be used in conjunction with the Situation, Background, Assessment, Recommendation (SBAR) technique to escalate concerns so that accurate and relevant information can be conveyed succinctly to the senior nurse and medical staff.

Renal failure

Renal failure in children falls into two main categories – acute and chronic. In both conditions the kidneys do not filter out the waste or excess fluid from the body, leaving the child with waste and fluid overload and electrolyte imbalance. Treatment varies depending on the severity of kidney failure, ranging from fluid/diet restrictions to dialysis.

Acute renal failure

Also known as acute kidney injury (AKI), this condition lasts for a short time, and it is possible that the kidneys will recover and the child's kidney function may return to normal. The need for long-term treatment is therefore variable.

Causes of AKI include:

- Birth trauma
- Sepsis
- Obstructive uropathy
- Glomerulonephritis
- Nephrotic syndrome

Signs and symptoms can develop over hours/days and include:

- Poor/no urine output
- Oedema
- Nausea/vomiting
- Hypertension
- Confusion/seizures

Chronic renal failure

Chronic renal failure (CRF) is an irreversible condition resulting in permanent kidney damage and can be divided into five stages (I–V) depending on the severity of the damage with stage V covering end stage renal failure (ESRF) and these children will need dialysis.

Causes of CRF include:

- Obstructive uropathy
- Hypoplastic/dysplastic kidneys
- Reflux nephropathy

Signs and symptoms:

- Poor appetite
- Stunted growth
- Anaemia
- Low glomerular filtration rate

Dialysis options

Dialysis means 'removal of waste products/fluid' and this is done by filtering out the unwanted material through a semi-permeable membrane. There are two options for dialysis – peritoneal dialysis and haemodialysis.

Peritoneal dialysis

Here the child's semi-permeable peritoneal membrane is used by inserting a peritoneal dialysis catheter into the child's abdominal cavity. The catheter can remain in situ for many months and fluid is passed via this catheter into the child's abdominal cavity. By the processes of diffusion and ultra-filtration, waste is drawn across the peritoneum into the fluid. After 3–4 hours the fluid is drained out with the waste products/excess fluid, thereby removing waste/fluid from the body. Afterwards another cycle of exchange fluid is introduced into the abdomen and the process repeated with these exchanges running throughout the day. However, they can also be managed by a machine overnight, allowing the child to have a relatively uninterrupted daily routine which minimises the impact on the child's education and social life. There are complications associated with peritoneal dialysis, such as peritonitis and infections at the catheter exit site. For some children who have undergone extensive abdominal surgery or who have adhesions, peritoneal dialysis is contraindicated, and haemodialysis is the preferred option.

Haemodialysis

In contrast to peritoneal dialysis, an artificial filter external to the body provides the semi-permeable membrane. The child's blood is drawn out of their body and is transported via tubes to the filter and back to the child in a continuous loop. For this form of dialysis, it is essential to create special vascular access, such as a central line or an arteriovenous fistula. To obtain arteriovenous fistula access, the child undergoes a surgical procedure in which an artery and vein are joined together and the high pressure in the artery causes the vein to dilate which allows easy venepuncture for haemodialysis.

Haemodialysis is performed over 3–4 hours and needs to occur three or four times a week, depending on the child's individual needs. If a home dialysis machine is available, haemodialysis may be delivered in the child's home; otherwise, the child will need to travel to a dialysis centre.

There are complications that can arise associated with haemodialysis and these include hypotension, infection, blood clotting in the circuit and hypothermia. Ultimately these children will require transplantation to live independent lives.

WHAT'S THE EVIDENCE?

Swallow et al. (2014) describe caring for children with chronic illness, in this case kidney disease. It is likely that there will be many health professionals involved. Whilst each professional has their own area of expertise it is important to appreciate the value of the contribution others make in the education of the child and family to manage the condition. In this paper, a variety of professionals involved in the care of the child and family are interviewed to explore their experience of multidisciplinary involvement.

Read the paper and consider the different professionals that may be involved in the care of a child with a renal condition.

Enuresis: Childhood incontinence in children

CASE STUDY 20.3: BECKA

Becka is an 11-year-old girl who has enjoyed being a Brownie but has never been away on a weekend trip. She has recently moved up to be a Girl Guide and would like to be able to join in the Guide weekends and go on sleepovers with her friends. However, on occasions she has wet the bed at home, so her mother has refused to allow her to go until she 'grows out of this habit'.

- What help and support could be made available to enable Becka to participate in more independent activities?

Enuresis is a relatively common problem in childhood and early adolescence with about 3% of girls and 2% of boys experiencing daytime incontinence at least once a week. Night-time incontinence affects more children (about 8% of 9½-year-olds) and the problem may continue into adulthood. The causes may be multifactorial. Underlying problems such as urinary tract infections and diabetes (mellitus and insipidus) should be excluded. Other causes can be due to defects in the normal renal anatomy or innervation (e.g., with spina bifida), low levels of vasopressin (antidiuretic hormone) and bladder instability. Enuresis is a distressing condition that affects the child's self-esteem and future psychological development; however. there is a variety of help available such as alarms, medication, pelvic floor exercises and self-help groups via the ERIC website (see Weblinks below).

CHAPTER SUMMARY

- Renal conditions in childhood are wide-ranging
- You will be expected to explain the pathophysiology in age-appropriate terminology to children and their families as well as referring them to further sources of information
- As a children's nurse, you need to be aware of the psychological impact of renal conditions on the child and their family, and to be able to provide the necessary support
- Care of the child with a renal condition is carried out by a range of professionals using an interdisciplinary approach

BUILD YOUR BIBLIOGRAPHY

Books

FURTHER
READING

- Peate, I. and Gormley Fleming, E (2021) *Fundamentals of Children and Young People's Anatomy and Physiology: A Textbook for Nursing and Healthcare Students*. 2nd edn. Chichester: Wiley–Blackwell

This book will provide a useful foundation for your knowledge of normal anatomy and physiology so that you can develop your understanding of abnormal anatomy or pathophysiology.

Journal articles

FURTHER
READING:
ONLINE
JOURNAL
ARTICLES

- Hanson, C.S., Craig, J C. and Tong, A. (2017) 'In their own words: The value of qualitative research to improve the care of children with chronic kidney disease'. *Pediatric Nephrology,* 32 (9): 1501-7.

Family-centred care is fundamental to the delivery of high-quality pediatric care. This partnership between children, their families and healthcare providers is central to caring for children with chronic kidney disease (CKD), given the long-term and profound impact of the disease and its treatment on the development and quality of life of these children.

- Nicholas, D.B., Kaufman, M., Pinsk, M., Samuel, S., Hamiwka, L. and Molzahn, A.E. (2018) 'Examining the transition from child to adult care in chronic kidney disease: an open exploratory approach'. *Nephrology Nursing Journal,* 45 (6): 553-60.

For young people with chronic kidney disease (CKD) and their families, transitioning from children's services to adult systems of renal care can be challenging. This study explored the process experienced by young people and discusses the facilitators and barriers to effective transition.

- Poursanidou, K., Garner, P. and Watson, A. (2008) 'Hospital-school liaison: perspectives of health and education professionals supporting children with renal transplants'. *Journal of Child Health Care,* 12 (4): 253-67.

This paper explores how a multidisciplinary team of health and education staff can work collaboratively to ensure good educational provision for children following renal transplants.

- Roupakias, S., Sinopidis, X., Karatza, A. and Varvarigou, A. (2013) 'Predictive risk factors in childhood urinary tract infection, vesicoureteral reflux, and renal scarring management'. *Clinical Pediatrics,* 53 (12): 1119-33.

Over recent years there has been much debate over how best to manage urinary tract infections to minimise renal scarring. The authors acknowledge that since some renal issues resolve with age and others require surgery, and despite the current availability of scanning, further research is required to identify definitive risk factors.

Weblinks

- NICE: Urinary tract infection in under 16s: diagnosis and management. NICE guideline [NG224] www.nice.org.uk/guidance/ng224 Evidence-based research regarding best practice regarding urinary tract infection.
- Spotting the Sick Child www.spottingthesickchild.com/about A website to help healthcare professionals identify children who have serious illnesses. It incorporates national guidelines with videos and interactive material to increase the learner's knowledge.
- NHS Choices: Urinary tract infections in children www.nhs.uk/conditions/Urinary-tract-infection-children/Pages/Introduction.aspx The website gives access to information about the treatment and management of urinary tract infections.
- ERIC www.eric.org.uk/ A website that provides a variety of learning resources for healthcare professionals who care for children with continence issues.

FURTHER
READING:
WEBLINKS

REFERENCES

Brandström, P. and Hansson, S. (2015) 'Long-term, low-dose prophylaxis against urinary tract infections in young children.' *Pediatric Nephrology*, 30: 425–32.

Clavé, S., Tsimaratos, M., Boucekine, M., Ranchin, B., Salomon, R., Dunand, O., Garnier, A,. Lahoche, A., Fila, M., Roussey, G., Broux, F., Harambat, J., Cloarec, S., Menouer, S., Deschenes, G., Vrillon, I., Auquier, P. and Berbis, J. (2019) 'Quality of life in adolescents with chronic kidney disease who initiate haemodialysis treatment'. *BMC Nephrology*, 20 (1): 163.

Diaz Kane, M.M. (2022) 'Diagnosing and treating urinary tract infections in the outpatient setting'. *Pediatric Annals*, 51 (5): e175-e177.

Gormley-Fleming, E. (2021) 'The renal system', in I. Peate and E. Gormley-Fleming (eds), *Fundamentals of Children and Young People's Anatomy and Physiology: A Textbook for Nursing and Healthcare Students*, 2nd edn. Chichester: Wiley–Blackwell.

Kumar, S., Mammen, A. and Varma, K.K. (2015) 'Pathogenesis of bladder exstrophy: a new hypothesis'. *Journal of Pediatric Urology*, 11: 314–18.

NICE (National Institute for Health and Care Excellence) (2022) Urinary tract infection in under 16s: diagnosis and management. NICE guideline [NG224]. www.nice.org.uk/guidance/ng224.

Ruano, R., Sananes, N., Sanghi-Haghpeykar, H., Hernandez-Ruano, S., Moog, R., Becmeur, F., Zalosyc, A., Girons, M., Morin, A.M. and Favre, R. (2015) 'Foetal intervention for severe lower tract obstruction: a multicenter case-control study comparing foetal cystoscopy with vesicoamniotic shunting'. *Ultrasound Obsteteric Gynacology*, 45: 452–8.

Swallow, V., Smith, T., Webb, N.J.A., Wirz, L., Qizalbash, L., Brennen, E., Birch, A., Sinha, M.D., Krischock, L., van der Voort, J., Kind D., Lambert, H., Milford, D.V., Crowther, L., Saleem, M., Lunn, A. and Williams, J. (2014) 'Distributed expertise: qualitative study of a British network of multidisciplinary teams supporting parents of children with chronic kidney disease'. *Child: Care, Health and Development*, 41 (1): 67–75.

CARE OF CHILDREN AND YOUNG PEOPLE WITH ENDOCRINE PROBLEMS

21

KATE DAVIES

THIS CHAPTER COVERS

- Recognition and nursing management of children with type 1 diabetes
- Recognition and nursing management of children with short stature
- Recognition and nursing management of children with congenital hypothyroidism

---

REQUIRED KNOWLEDGE

It would be helpful to have an understanding of the endocrine system before you start this chapter.

> "Building a relationship and gaining trust with the patient and family is paramount. There is such satisfaction when you can see the difference in the patients and their families once this has been achieved, and how the care given improves outcomes on so many levels."
>
> **Paediatric endocrine specialist nurse**

INTRODUCTION

Endocrinology is the study of hormones, and the endocrine system is one of the most important systems in the body to maintain normal homeostasis (Davies and Bryan, 2021). Much of what is seen in a paediatric endocrine clinic focuses on growth and development, as growth problems are very common. Diabetes also is commonly seen within paediatric endocrinology, with an incidence of around 1 in every 500 children (Donaldson et al., 2019) and various factors will be highlighted here with signposting to other resources. The importance of neonatal screening will also be discussed with reference to congenital hypothyroidism. Growth, diabetes and congenital hypothyroidism are the most common conditions seen in paediatric endocrinology (Donaldson et al., 2019). Whilst investigating these conditions, even though there is a medical focus, the children's nurse must not lose sight of the nursing process of Assess, Plan, Implement and Evaluate (Emerson and Northway, 2015): these will be demonstrated within the case studies.

When caring for children with endocrine conditions and their families, a team approach is paramount. The role of the paediatric endocrine nurse (PEN) within such an approach is key, as indicated in the opening quotation. There are many conditions within this specialty, some of which can be seen in Table 21.1.

SEE ALSO
CHAPTER 6

Table 21.1 Conditions seen in paediatric endocrinology

Condition	Average age of presentation	Signs and symptoms	Key guidelines/references
Type 1 diabetes	11–14 years	Blood glucose >11.1mmol/l	Guidelines from the British Society for Paediatric Endocrinology and Diabetes cover the management of Diabetic Keto-Acidosis (DKA) in children for type 1 and type 2 diabetes: www.bsped.org.uk/clinical/docs/DKAguideline.pdf
			British guidelines for the management of diabetes: www.nice.org.uk/guidance/ng18
			International guidelines for the management of diabetes:
			http://web.ispad.org/resource-type/idfispad-2011-global-guideline-diabetes-childhood-andadolescence
Short stature	Childhood	Height <2 SD below the mean	(Savage et al., 2016; Davies, 2020)
Turner syndrome	Prenatal, birth, childhood, adolescence	Short stature, some dysmorphia, ovarian dysgenesis	www.tss.org.uk/ UK support group
			Clinical practice guidelines for the care of girls and women with Turner syndrome: Proceedings from the 2016 Cincinnati International Turner Syndrome Meeting (Gravholt et al., 2017)
Noonan syndrome	Childhood	Short stature, some dysmorphia, cardiac defects	www.noonansyndrome.org.uk/ (UK Support group)
			Noonan Syndrome Clinical Management Guidelines (DYSCERNE, 2010)

(Continued)

Table 21.1 (Continued)

Condition	Average age of presentation	Signs and symptoms	Key guidelines/references
Tall stature	Childhood	Height >2 SD above the mean	(Davies and Cheetham, 2014)
Early puberty	Before 8 years in girls, 9 years in boys	Early pubertal development	(Latronico et al., 2016)
Delayed puberty	Adolescence	No secondary sexual development in girls by age 13 years, and boys age 14 years	(Wei et al., 2017)
Congenital hypothyroidism	Birth	Guthrie test	(Peters et al., 2018) www.bsped.org.uk/patients/docs/NN_CONGENITAL_HYPOTHYROIDISM_June2011.pdf
Graves' disease	Adolescence	Goitre, thyroid storm	(Leger et al., 2018) www.bsped.org.uk/patients/docs/NN_GRAVES_DISEASE_(THYROTOXICOSIS)_june2011.pdf
Differences of sex development	Birth	Genital ambiguity	(Ahmed et al., 2021)
Adrenal insufficiency	Congenital or acquired	Hypoglycaemia, jaundice (newborn), tiredness, lack of energy (older children)	(Bowden and Henry, 2018) (Miller et al., 2020)
Congenital adrenal hyperplasia	Congenital	Birth (females), first 2 weeks of life (males) (21-OHD)	(Speiser et al., 2018)
Panhypopituitarism	Congenital or acquired	Combination of pituitary hormone deficiency symptoms	(Higham et al., 2016)
Obesity	Birth, acquired	Increased weight gain	www.nationalobesityforum.org.uk (Styne et al., 2017)
Endocrine effects of cancer treatment	After treatment for cancer	Post treatment testing for hormone deficiencies	www.aftercure.org (Urquhart and Collin, 2016a) (Urquhart and Collin, 2016b)
Vitamin D deficiency	Babies, childhood, adolescence	Poor growth, delayed walking, bone and muscle pain, muscle weakness	(Chan et al., 2019)

Adapted from Donaldson et al., 2019

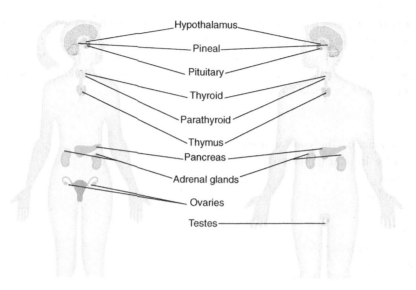

Figure 21.1   Major endocrine organs

RECOGNITION AND NURSING MANAGEMENT OF CHILDREN WITH TYPE 1 DIABETES

Diabetes mellitus is classified as a group of metabolic disorders, with the overall characteristic of chronic hyperglycaemia, or an increased blood glucose level. There are many types, with type 1 diabetes being the most commonly seen in childhood (Ng and Evans, 2021). Therefore, it is likely that there are at least one or two children per secondary school with type 1 diabetes, so it is likely that you as a children's nurse will come across a child with type 1 diabetes at some stage in your clinical practice.

In type 1 diabetes, the pancreas fails to make insulin, due to autoimmune destruction of the beta cells in the islets of Langherhans (Couper et al., 2018). This lack of insulin means the body fails to utilise the glucose, resulting in hyperglycaemia. The pancreas is about as big as your hand and is situated under the left rib cage towards the back of the abdominal cavity.

This hyperglycaemia leads to what is called an 'osmotic diuresis', which happens when the renal threshold for glucose is exceeded. This leads to polyuria – excessive urination – and polydipsia – excessive drinking. This can potentially lead to the child becoming dehydrated, especially if they have been vomiting. This lack of insulin also causes the breakdown of lipids – or fats – which causes an excess of free fatty acids and ketones, leading to ketones in the urine. This can cause metabolic acidosis: acetone is responsible for the sweet-smelling breath, a bit like pear drops. If left untreated, the combination of this dehydration, acidosis and hyperosmolality can cause 'diabetic ketoacidosis', or DKA, and the child may become unconscious, with the potential to lead to a coma and eventually death (Wolfsdorf et al., 2018).

ACTIVITY 21.1: CRITICAL THINKING

Critically reflect with a colleague on how a child may present with DKA. How would they be presenting, how would you assess them, and how would you plan their care? How would you explain what is happening to the child's parents?

Diagnosis of type 1 diabetes is confirmed in a symptomatic child with a raised blood glucose level: this would be classified as greater than 11.1mmol/l, alongside glycosuria – glucose in the urine, and ketonuria – ketones in the urine, which can be easily tested for by a dipstick urine test. Optimum diabetes management aims for a blood glucose level more than 3.9 mmol/l (Abraham et al., 2018). Signs and symptoms of hypoglycaemia – a low blood glucose – are:

- Early
  - Most common – the 'classical triad':
  - Excessive drinking (polydipsia)
  - Polyuria
  - Weight loss

- Less common:
  - Enuresis (secondary)
  - Skin sepsis
  - *Candida* (thrush) and other infections

- Late – diabetic ketoacidosis
  - Smell of acetone on breath
  - Vomiting
  - Dehydration
  - Abdominal pain
  - Hyperventilation due to acidosis (Kussmaul breathing)
  - Hypovolaemic shock
  - Drowsiness
  - Coma and death. (Dmitri, 2012)

As the pancreas is not making any insulin, insulin replacement is needed, and a child is started on a regime of subcutaneous insulin. This is always a big shock for the child and their family, as the therapy will be lifelong, so an intensive, thorough multidisciplinary team (MDT) educational programme is needed, which can involve the following members:

- Consultant paediatrician with a special interest in diabetes
- Consultant paediatric endocrinologist
- Paediatric diabetes specialist nurse
- Paediatric dietician
- Clinical psychologist
- Social worker
- Adult diabetologist for joint adolescent clinics
- Parent/patient support groups

Psychosocial factors play an important role in the management of children and young people with type 1 diabetes, and specialist psychologist input is recommended. Focus should be given to adjusting to the diagnosis and management, neurocognitive and school functioning, family functioning and other social support. Quality of life is at the height of optimum diabetes care, and input from patient support groups or behavioural interventions – either in clinic or at home – can enhance behaviours surrounding management, which can help improve glycaemic control (Delamater et al., 2018).

"The function of the diabetes MDT is to provide education, care and support that is evidence-based, culturally appropriate, meets the psychosocial needs of the child, young person and family, and offers equitable access to technology to support living with diabetes and achieving optimal outcomes. My role as a specialist dietician within the team is to provide education, advice, and support about the management of post prandial glucose levels, through education about nutrition, activity, and lifestyle which is essential for achieving glycaemic management goals.

Francesca Annan, Clinical Specialist Paediatric/Adolescent Diabetes Dietician"

Now have a look at case study 21.1.

CASE STUDY 21.1: FIONA

- Fiona is a 16-year-old girl with newly diagnosed type 1 diabetes. She was stabilised on subcutaneous insulin when hospitalised at diagnosis. A week after discharge, Fiona experienced nausea and anorexia. She was not really eating properly, but still took her insulin as usual in the morning. That afternoon, she experienced profuse sweating and started feeling very apprehensive, so she went to A&E with her mum. The initial diagnosis was hypoglycaemia due to taking insulin and not eating. She was admitted, and treated. After she rested and her glucose levels normalised, she was finally discharged home.
- What education should Fiona and her family receive before she leaves?
- Reflect on the stress that a newly diagnosed type 1 diabetic patient may undergo while trying to cope with the diagnosis and learning how to self-inject.
- What teaching could help Fiona to reduce her stress and to effectively plan her medical regimen?
- What sort of support would be useful for Fiona as she adjusts to her new life? What other members of the MDT do you think is important to be involved in Fiona's care?

Education needs to be child-focused as well as for the family. There are many resources available for children and families, and on how to manage diabetes in schools (Bratina et al., 2018; Smith et al., 2019).

There are various types of insulin available, with differences in the onset and duration of action. These include:

- Short-acting insulin, which starts working within 30–60 minutes, peaks at 2–4 hours, and lasts for 5–8 hours
- Rapid-acting analogues, which start working within 15 minutes, peak at 1–3 hours and last for up to 5 hours
- Intermediate-acting insulin, which starts to work after 2–4 hours, peaks at 4–12 hours, and lasts between 12 and 24 hours

There are also longer-acting insulins and analogues, which can last for 24 hours, and pre-mixed insulins which are a mix of short- and intermediate-acting insulins.

Commonly used regimes for insulin therapy include twice-daily injections three times a day, multiple daily injections, and more recently continuous subcutaneous insulin infusion, commonly known as 'pumps'. Pump therapy is now the recommended type of insulin therapy in children, delivering insulin throughout the day, as well as on-demand boluses when needed. By doing so, the insulin delivery is similar to normal physiological release, and therefore reduces the potential for hypo- or hyperglycaemic episodes. It is also more comfortable for children, giving parents more confidence in their child's care (Ziegler et al., 2020).

Hypoglycaemia or 'hypos'

Hypoglycaemia is classified as a blood glucose level less than 4mmol/l, and can happen occasionally (Abraham et al., 2018). There are many reasons why they can occur, alongside many symptoms that children may experience:

- Too little to eat, or a delayed meal
- Skipping a meal
- Neglecting to eat, despite symptoms of hypoglycaemia
- Physical exercise, which increases the risk of hypoglycaemia for the rest of the day and the following night
- Too much insulin
- New site for the injection – for example, from the thigh to the abdomen or to a site free of fatty lumps (lipohypertrophy)
- Recent hypoglycaemia – the glucose stores in the liver may be depleted, or there are fewer warning symptoms of hypoglycaemia (hypoglycaemic unawareness)
- Very low HbA1c (increased risk of hypoglycaemia awareness)
- Drinking alcohol
- Not mixing the cloudy insulin thoroughly enough
- Variable insulin absorption
- Gastroenteritis or tummy upset
- Certain drugs used for the treatment of high blood pressure

    (Hanas, 2015. Reproduced with kind permission of Class Publishing)

The way to manage a hypo is to raise the blood glucose level back to within normal limits, which is 4–7mmol/l. This can include giving glucose tablets, orange juice or a fizzy drink, and then some complex carbohydrates, such as a biscuit or bread. If it is more severe, then a sugary gel can be rubbed into lips or gums, or a glucagon injection may be needed. It is essential that children and their families are educated early on the importance of recognising symptoms and how to manage them.

Long-term management

The aim is for the child and family to live as normal a life as possible, both at home and at school, with good diabetic control. Education on diet is essential, avoiding too many sugary foods and optimum blood glucose measuring. Liaising with the diabetes team is essential, including regular contact in the outpatients' clinic, where discussion will focus on overall wellbeing, growth and development, adherence and assessing HbA1c. This is a small blood test measuring glycosylated haemoglobin, and can give a view of overall control from the previous 6–12 weeks (Abraham et al., 2018). Plans need to be in place with school, and diabetes nurse specialists can form and implement care plans, which will need to be evaluated regularly to ensure the child's continuing progress.

As the child enters adolescence, the diabetes can interfere with several elements (see Table 21.2).

Table 21.2 How diabetes interferes with normal adolescence (Dmitri, 2012)

Normal adolescence	How diabetes interferes with normal adolescence
Physical and sexual maturation	Delayed sexual development
	Invasion of privacy with frequent medical examinations
Conformity with peer group	Meals must be eaten on time
	Frequent injections and blood tests
Self-image	Hypoglycaemic attacks show that they are different
Self-esteem	Impaired body image
Independence from parents	Parental over-protection and reluctance to allow their child to be away from home
	Battles over diabetes
Economic independence	Loading of insurance premiums
	Discrimination by employers
	Statutory rules against becoming a pilot or driving heavy goods or public service vehicles

Children with diabetes need regular assessment and these assessments can help the child grow and develop optimally.

Some key aspects of diabetic assessment in children are:

- Any episodes of hypoglycaemia, diabetic ketoacidosis, hospital admission?
- Is there still awareness of hypoglycaemia?
- Absence from school? School supportive of diabetes care?
- Interference with normal life?
- HbA1c results – 58mmol/mol (7.5%) or less?
- Diary of blood glucose results – if monitoring, are they reacting to results?
- Insulin regimen – appropriate? Correction bolus doses given?
- Lipohypertrophy or lipoatrophy at injection sites?
- Diet – healthy diet, manipulating food intake and insulin to maintain good control?

General overview (periodic):

- Normal growth and pubertal development – check weight – under- or overweight? – measure each visit
- Blood pressure – check for hypertension yearly (age-specific centiles)
- Renal disease – screening for microalbuminuria yearly from 12 years
- Eyes – photography for retinopathy or cataracts, yearly from 12 years
- Feet – maintaining good care – yearly
- Screening for coeliac and thyroid disease at diagnosis, thyroid screening yearly, coeliac again after 3 years or if weight gain is poor
- Annual reminder to have flu vaccination

Knowledge and psychosocial aspects:

- Good understanding of diabetes – would participation/holidays with other diabetic children be beneficial? Member of Diabetes UK?

- Becoming self-reliant, but appropriate supervision at home, school, diabetic team?
- Taking exercise, sport? Diabetes not interfering with it?
- Leading as normal a life as possible?
- Smoking, alcohol?
- Is 'hypo' treatment readily available? Is stepped approach known?
- What are the main issues for the patient? Are there short-term goals to allow engagement with improving control (Dmitri, 2012)?
- Peer support
- Psychological support for the child/young person and their family

Surgery

Children with type 1 diabetes who need to undergo surgery should only have the surgery carried out in a centre that has dedicated facilities for children and young people with diabetes. Centres will have their own protocols and guidelines to follow, but surgical and anaesthetic teams need to liaise with the paediatric diabetes team before admission if the surgery is elective, or soon as possible if the surgery is not routine (NICE, 2022). Blood glucose may be more difficult to manage, due to physiological, emotional and metabolic stress, so close monitoring during surgery is essential. Special care should be taken if the perioperative is lengthy, as a variable rate insulin infusion may be needed (Tjen and Wilkinson, 2016).

WHAT'S THE EVIDENCE?

Study the guidelines developed by the British Society of Paediatric Endocrinology and Diabetes (BSPED) (www.bsped.org.uk/clinical/clini cal_endorsedguidelines.aspx). Here, you will find guidance for medical and nursing staff, as well as families, on DKA, and managing diabetes when a child is ill, and when they undergo surgery. See if these guidelines are in place in the clinical environment you are in. If not, what is in place instead and why do you think it is managed differently?

RECOGNITION AND NURSING MANAGEMENT OF CHILDREN WITH SHORT STATURE

To have a full understanding of the diagnosis of short stature, it is important to have an idea of normal growth in childhood. Growth is affected by an interaction of genetic, nutritional and hormonal factors. Adequate nutrition is mostly responsible for growth in infancy, whereas hormones such as growth hormone (GH), insulin-like growth factor (IGF-1) and thyroid hormones play more of a central role throughout childhood (Davies, 2020). Genetics are also important – short parents are more likely to have short children, and short stature is also associated with syndromes such as Turner syndrome and Down syndrome. Growth in childhood can be split into three categories: infancy, childhood and puberty (Donaldson et al., 2019) (see Table 21.3).

Growth assessment

This area is one of the most important aspects to consider when assessing a child, and it is important that it is done correctly. In the UK, children are measured in Reception class (age 4) and in Year 6 (at the end of primary school).

Table 21.3   Growth in childhood (Martin and Collin, 2015)

Infancy

- First two years of life
- Driven by nutrition
- Rapid growth
- Grow approximately 25cm in the first year

Childhood

- Dependent on growth hormone
- Period of time when children with growth hormone deficiency present with short stature
- Height velocity is around 4-8 cm/year
- Little difference in the growth rate between boys and girls

Puberty

- Height velocity doubles
- Pubertal growth spurt starts two years earlier in girls than boys
- Growth hormone and sex steroids now involved
- Girls grow around 8cm/year at their peak height velocity, and boys 10cm/year
- Puberty hormones also end growth, by fusing the growth plates at the ends of the bones

WHAT'S THE EVIDENCE?

What do you think about measuring all children in schools? Do you think it is a good idea? Some parents may refuse for their child to be weighed and measured. Why do you think they might do this? Do you think the focus is on how children are growing, or weight gain?

Many measurements are taken when assessing a child's growth, including length in babies, head circumference in babies (Figure 21.2), their height (Figure 21.3), their sitting height (most often usually done in paediatric endocrine clinics) and their weight.

Once the measurements are taken, they need to be properly plotted on an appropriate growth chart (Davies, 2020).

Specific centile lines on the charts can show you the percentage of measurements that have higher or lower values than the measurements you have plotted (Martin and Collin, 2015). It is important to take measurements over a period of time to show the child's height velocity – the speed at which they are growing – and whether it is in the normal limits for their age and sex, and in line with their parents' heights (Martin and Collin, 2015). Only now can the diagnosis of short stature be considered. Data can also be collected in the parent-held 'red books' for children under the age of 5.

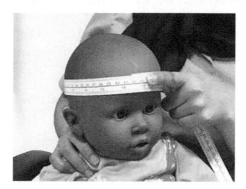

Figure 21.2   Correct measurement of head circumference

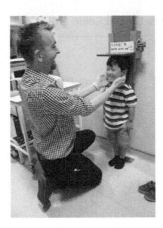

Figure 21.3 Measuring a child

Causes of short stature

Short stature is one of the most common reasons a child is referred to a paediatric endocrine clinic (Martin and Collin, 2015; Donaldson et al., 2019). There are many reasons why a child is smaller than their peers, as seen in Table 21.4:

Table 21.4 Causes of short stature

Non-pathological	Constitutional delay of growth and puberty
	Familial short stature
	Nutritional issues
	Emotional deprivation
	Intrauterine growth retardation
Intrauterine growth retardation/restriction	Syndromes – including Russell Silver syndrome
	Small for Gestational Age
	Non-syndromic
Systemic disorders	Cardiovascular disease
	Renal, including chronic renal failure
	Respiratory, including asthma and cystic fibrosis
	Gastrointestinal, including inflammatory bowel disease, Crohn's, coeliac disease
	Neurological
	Psychosocial, including anorexia, child abuse and neglect
Endocrine causes	Growth hormone-related causes
	Growth hormone deficiency, isolated or combined with multiple pituitary hormone deficiency
	Growth hormone resistance
	Hypothyroidism
	Cushing's syndrome
	Exogenous steroid administration and glucocorticoid excess
Chromosomal and genetic causes	Turner syndrome
	Noonan syndrome
	Down syndrome
	Skeletal dysplasia
	Prader-Willi syndrome

Source: Laing (2014). From *British Journal of Nursing*. 2015 MA Healthcare Ltd. Reproduced by permission of MA Healthcare Ltd

To ascertain the cause of the short stature, other investigations need to be performed, including blood tests. These blood tests can rule out other reasons why the child may be short – for example, anaemia, malabsorption, renal disease, Crohn's disease, or even Turner syndrome (Davies and Collin, 2015).

The most common endocrine reason for a child being short is growth hormone deficiency (Donaldson et al., 2019). This is seen in around 1 in every 4000 children (Martin and Collin, 2015). Treatment is currently given by a once-daily injection of growth hormone before bedtime, although new longer-acting injections which are given weekly have been developed. For children to be prescribed this treatment, they need to be investigated further beyond simple blood tests, by being admitted to a children's ward for day case investigations (Davies and Collin, 2015). This is because a simple one-off blood test to look at growth hormone levels would not work, as the levels in the blood are known as 'pulsatile' – that is, they go up and down throughout the day. The correct diagnosis is then made by examining the results of these tests in order for the child to receive the correct treatment.

CASE STUDY 21.2: SAM

Sam is an 8-year-old boy referred to the paediatric endocrine and growth clinic for poor growth. Sam was referred by his GP, via the school nurse and his parents, who noted that he has been the smallest in his class for a while. On assessment at his first clinic appointment, Sam was below the 2nd centile on his growth chart, but his projected height in accordance with his parents' heights was on the 50th centile.

Sam's growth was monitored by the GP for 6 months, resulting in the referral to the paediatric endocrine clinic. The team felt he warranted further investigation, so an admission was arranged to the day case unit for a glucagon stimulation test, showing his highest growth hormone (GH) level to be only 3 micrograms per litre (normal range: >7 micrograms per litre) which qualified him for GH treatment.

The paediatric endocrine nurse (PEN) then met with Sam's parents in clinic to demonstrate a range of GH delivery devices. There was discussion about the pros and cons of each device: some have to be refrigerated, and some are disposable, for example. Additional nursing and prescription support is also offered by each of the homecare delivery companies.

- Good adherence to GH treatment is essential for it to work effectively. What factors do you think will contribute to Sam's good adherence?
- Growth hormone is delivered by subcutaneous injection. What are some nursing considerations regarding subcutaneous injections in children?

Children should remain on growth hormone until they have stopped growing, and then sometimes even longer (Richmond and Rogol, 2016), especially if they are still growth-hormone deficient when final height is achieved. Children and their parents/carers can choose which growth hormone pen device to have: this has been shown to possibly increase adherence (Gilbert, 2018), as obviously children will not like taking an injection every day.

As there are so many causes for short stature, as a children's nurse you should keep up to date in your clinical practice. Children are weighed and measured as part of best practice not only within the outpatients' department during clinic visits, but also when they are admitted to children's wards. The nursing process is very clear during the assessment of short stature, as accurate growth assessment is vital to aid diagnosis.

"For so long we've been worried about Arthur's growth – he's always been the smallest in his class. He's always said it's never really worried him until recently. He's still in a car seat, whilst all his friends don't need one anymore, so he's really noticing a difference. It's difficult, you know … I've always been short, but his Dad is tall. We're looking forward to being assessed properly at the paediatric endocrine clinic, where we should be able to get some answers, and hopefully some treatment!"

Marie, parent

RECOGNITION AND NURSING MANAGEMENT OF CHILDREN WITH CONGENITAL HYPOTHYROIDISM

The diagnosis of congenital hypothyroidism is one of the most common conditions seen in a paediatric endocrine clinic, with an incidence of around 1 in every 4000 births in the UK (Donaldson et al., 2019). There are many causes, but the most common cause is where the thyroid gland has not positioned itself where it should be from foetal development, or 'maldescent of the thyroid' (Peters et al., 2018). Girls are twice as likely to be affected as boys, and there is an increased risk in babies born with Down syndrome.

Newborn screening

Testing for congenital hypothyroidism is undertaken on day 5 of life at the newborn blood spot (NBS) test – a heelprick blood test done by the midwife in hospital or at home (see Figure 21.4).

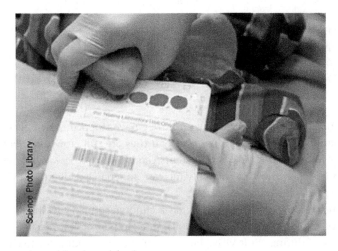

Figure 21.4 The newborn blood spot test

www.sciencephoto.com

ACTIVITY 21.2: CRITICAL THINKING

- Have a look at the NHS screening programme guide on testing for congenital hypothyroidism.
- What other conditions are screened for during the newborn screening test?
- What do you think might happen if a baby did not have the Newborn Blood Spot test?

Since babies are screened so early on in life, it is now unlikely that they will show any symptoms. Early detection, and therefore treatment, is vital as it can prevent neurodevelopmental disability and growth failure (Mondal et al., 2017). However, if babies are not tested, the symptoms described below may become apparent:

SEE ALSO
CHAPTER 13
AND 30

- Failure to thrive
- Feeding problems
- Prolonged jaundice
- Constipation
- Pale, cold, mottled, dry skin
- Coarse facies (for example a large bulging head or prominent scalp veins)
- Large tongue
- Hoarse cry
- Goitre (occasionally)
- Umbilical hernia
- Delayed development
- Wide posterior fontanelle
- Hypothermia
- Peripheral cyanosis
- Oedema (Donaldson et al., 2019)

Diagnosis is confirmed by a raised thyroid stimulating hormone (TSH) level in the blood from the blood spot test. Diagnostic limits vary around the UK, but if the TSH level is ≥10mU/l, a second sample is usually requested a week later. If this is still high, the baby's diagnosis is confirmed. A normal level of TSH in the blood is 0.27–4.20mU/l (Lee et al., 2020). Radioisotope scanning of the baby's thyroid gland is sometimes performed (Donaldson et al., 2019), which may show a kind of transient hypothyroidism, or sometimes an ultrasound scan.

Treatment is with levothyroxine, which comes in liquid or tablet formation, and is lifelong. Clinic visits will be necessary as the child grows for regular blood tests and dose changes.

ACTIVITY 21.3: REFLECTIVE PRACTICE

Think about the role of patient support groups whilst watching the BTF video (see Build your Bibliography Weblinks)

Endocrinology requires a robust knowledge of both anatomy and physiology, and the ability to support and educate children, young people and their families from referral and diagnosis, through treatment and often transitioning to adult services and living independent lives. This process can be very challenging for families, children and young people to understand and navigate. It is therefore the job of the PEN and the multidisciplinary team to support and educate in partnership; this will be very different for each family.

> "It takes many years to become an expert in endocrinology; hormones affect every body system and that takes time to learn, however placements offer the opportunity to acquire transferable skills including communication, recognising and treating hypoglycaemia, administering intramuscular and subcutaneous injections, tailoring interventions and education to families' specific needs and offering psychological support or onward referral. As a nurse relatively new to endocrinology I understand all too well the daunting prospect of all these challenges but the rewards and new opportunities more than overcome all of these."
>
> **Karen Thompson, Paediatric Endocrine Nurse Specialist**

CHAPTER SUMMARY

- Diabetes is one of the most common endocrine conditions in children with an incidence of around 1 in every 500 children
- Many of the endocrine conditions affecting children relate to growth and development
- Endocrine conditions have a wide-ranging impact on the child and family
- Team working is crucial and this should straddle hospital, school and home

BUILD YOUR BIBLIOGRAPHY

Books

FURTHER READING

- Hanas, R. (2015) *Type 1 Diabetes in Children, Adolescents and Young Adults.* Bridgwater: Class Health.

  This has been described as the 'bible' for everything you need to know about type 1 diabetes in children. It is written in a very easy to understand style, and is a useful resource for the whole multidisciplinary team.
- Llahana, S., Follin, C., Yedinak, C., Grossman, A., Davies, K. and Keil, M. (eds) (2019) *Advanced Practice in Endocrinology Nursing.* Cham: Springer.

  This is the first book aimed at nurses working in any area of endocrinology, at any level of expertise.

Journal articles

Read this article to learn more about psychological factors in type 1 diabetes management in young people:

FURTHER READING: ONLINE JOURNAL ARTICLES

- Martinez, K., Frazer, S.F., Dempster, M., Hamill, A., Fleming, H. and McCorry, N.K. (2018) 'Psychological factors associated with diabetes self-management among adolescents with type 1 diabetes: a systematic review'. *Journal of Health Psychology*. 23 (13): 1749–65.

  Read more information on initiating growth hormone therapy in children:

- Gilbert, J. (2018) 'Initiating growth hormone therapy in children'. *Nurse Prescribing*, 16 (6): 268–73.

Weblinks

These are the key support groups with excellent resources and societies providing care pathways and guidelines:

FURTHER READING: WEBLINKS

- Diabetes UK www.diabetes.org.uk www.jdrf.org
- Child Growth Foundation www.childgrowthfoundation.org
- The Pituitary Foundation www.pituitary.org.uk
- Living with CAH www.livingwithCAH.com
- Verity www.verity-pcos.org.uk
- British Thyroid Foundation www.btf-thyroid.org
- Turner Syndrome Support Society http://tss.org.uk
- DSD Families www.dsdfamilies.org
- British Society for Paediatric Endocrinology www.bsped.org.uk
- European Society for Paediatric Endocrinology www.eurospe.org
- Society for Endocrinology www.endocrinology.org
- https://assets.publishing.service.gov.uk/government/uploads/system/uploads/attachment_data/file/899485/Guidelines_for_Newborn_Blood_Spot_Sampling_March_2016.pdf You can read more on newborn screening here.

Acknowledgements

The author would like to thank the following practitioners for their assistance:

Francesca Annan, Clinical Specialist Paediatric/Adolescent Diabetes Dietician, University College London Hospitals, London

Lee Martin, Clinical Nurse Specialist in Paediatric Endocrinology, The Royal London Hospital, London

Karen Thompson, Endocrine Nurse Specialist, Royal Belfast Hospital for Sick Children, Northern Ireland

REFERENCES

Abraham, M.B., Jones, T.W., Naranjo, D., Karges, B., Oduwole, A., Tauschmann, M. and Maahs, D.M. (2018) 'ISPAD Clinical Practice Consensus Guidelines 2018: Assessment and management of hypoglycemia in children and adolescents with diabetes'. *Pediatric Diabetes*, 19 (Suppl 27): 178–92.

Ahmed, S.F., Achermann, J., Alderson, J. et al. (2021) 'Society for Endocrinology UK Guidance on the initial evaluation of a suspected difference or disorder of sex development (Revised 2021)'. *Clinical Endocrinology (Oxford)*, 95 (6): 818–40.

Bowden, S.A. and Henry, R. (2018) 'Pediatric adrenal insufficiency: diagnosis, management, and new therapies'. *International Journal of Pediatrics*, 2018:1739831.

Bratina, N., Forsander, G., Annan, F. et al. (2018)' ISPAD Clinical Practice Consensus Guidelines 2018: Management and support of children and adolescents with type 1 diabetes in school'. *Pediatric Diabetes*, 19 (Suppl 27): 287–301.

Candler, T.P., Mahmoud, O., Lynn, R.M., Majbar, A.A., Barrett, T.G. and Shield, J.P.H. (2018) 'Continuing rise of Type 2 diabetes incidence in children and young people in the UK'. *Diabetic Medicine*, 35 (6): 737–44.

Chan, Y.F., Milner, K.-L., White, C. and Musson, P. (2019) 'Vitamin D deficiency and treatment in children and adults', in S. Llahana, C. Follin, C. Yedinak, A. Grossman, K. Davies and M. Keil (eds), *Advanced Practice in Endocrinology Nursing*, Vol. 2. Cham: Springer. pp. 1037–62.

Couper, J.J., Haller, M.J., Greenbaum, C.J., Ziegler, A.G., Wherrett, D.K., Knip, M. and Craig, M.E. (2018) 'ISPAD Clinical Practice Consensus Guidelines 2018: Stages of type 1 diabetes in children and adolescents'. *Pediatric Diabetes*, 19 (Suppl 27), 20–2.

Davies, J.H. and Cheetham, T. (2014) 'Investigation and management of tall stature'. *Archives of Diseases in Childhood*, 99 (8): 772–77.

Davies, K. (2020) 'Biological basis of child health 7: growth, development and the reproductive system'. *Nursing Children and Young People*. [Online ahead of print] doi:10.7748/ncyp.2020.e1308.

Davies, K. and Bryan, S. (2021) 'Biological basis of child health 12: the endocrine system and common childhood endocrinopathies'. *Nursing Children and Young People*. [Online ahead of print] doi:10.7748/ncyp.2021.e1342.

Davies, K. and Collin, J. (2015) 'Understanding clinical investigations in children's endocrinology'. *Nursing Children and Young People*, 27: 26–36.

Delamater, A.M., de Wit, M., McDarby, V., Malik, J.A., Hilliard, M.E., Northam, E. and Acerini, C.L. (2018) 'ISPAD Clinical Practice Consensus Guidelines 2018: Psychological care of children and adolescents with type 1 diabetes'. *Pediatric Diabetes*, 19 (Suppl 27): 237–49.

Dmitri, P. (2012) 'Endocrine and metabolic disorders', in T. Lissauer and G. Clayden (eds), *Illustrated Textbook of Paediatrics*, 4th edn. Edinburgh: Mosby/Elsevier.

Donaldson, M.D.C., Gregory, J.W., Van-Vliet, G. and Wolfsdorf, J.I. (2019) *Practical Endocrinology and Diabetes in Children*, 4th edn. Oxford: Wiley–Blackwell.

DYSCERNE (2010) Management of Noonan Syndrome: a clinical guideline. Available at https://noonansyndrome.com.au/wp-content/uploads/2016/12/Clinical-Management-Guidelines.pdf (accessed 15 June 2023).

Emerson, K. and Northway, R. (2015) 'Patient, service user, family and carer perspectives', in C. Delves-Yates, (ed.), *Essentials of Nursing Practice*. London: Sage.

Gilbert, J. (2018) 'Initiating growth hormone therapy in children'. *Nurse Prescribing*, 16 (6): 268–73.

Gravholt, C.H., Andersen, N.H., Conway, G.S. et al. (2017) 'Clinical practice guidelines for the care of girls and women with Turner syndrome: proceedings from the 2016 Cincinnati International Turner Syndrome Meeting'. *European Journal of Endocrinology*, 177 (3): G1–G70.

Hanas, R. (2015) *Type 1 Diabetes in Children, Adolescents and Young Adults*, 6th edn. Bridgwater: Class Health.

Higham, C.E., Johannsson, G. and Shalet, S.M. (2016) 'Hypopituitarism'. *The Lancet*, 388 (10058): 2403–15.

Laing, P. (2014) 'Growth failure and hormone therapy'. *British Journal of Nursing*, 23: S3–S9.

Latronico, A.C., Brito, V.N., and Carel, J.-C. (2016) 'Causes, diagnosis, and treatment of central precocious puberty'. *The Lancet Diabetes and Endocrinology*, 4 (3): 265–74.

Lee, Y.L., Yap, F. and Vasanwala, R.F. (2020) 'Abnormal thyroid function in paediatric practice'. *Archives of Diseases in Childhood Education and Practice Education*, 105 (6): 361–3.

Leger, J., Oliver, I., Rodrigue, D., Lambert, A.S. and Coutant, R. (2018) 'Graves' disease in children'. *Annals of Endocrinology (Paris)*, 79 (6): 647–55.

Martin, L. and Collin, J. (2015) 'An introduction to growth and atypical growth in childhood and adolescence'. *Nursing Children and Young People*, 27: 29–37.

Miller, B.S., Spencer, S.P., Geffner, M.E. et al. (2020) 'Emergency management of adrenal insufficiency in children: advocating for treatment options in outpatient and field settings'. *Journal of Investigative Medicine*, 68 (1): 16–25.

Mondal, S., Mukhopadhyay, P. and Ghosh, S. (2017) 'Clinical approach to congenital hypothyroidism'. *Thyroid Research and Practice*, 14 (2): 45.

Ng, S.M. and Evans, M.L. (2021) 'Widening health inequalities related to type 1 diabetes care in children and young people in the UK: A time to act now'. *Diabetic Medicine*, 38 (11): e14620.

NICE (National Institute of Health and Care Excellence) (2022) Diabetes (type 1 and type 2) in children and young people: diagnosis and management. NICE guideline. Available at: www.nice.org.uk/guidance/ng18/resources/diabetes-type-1-and-type-2-in-children-and-young-people-diagnosis-and-management-pdf-1837278149317.

Peters, C., van Trotsenburg, A.S.P. and Schoenmakers, N. (2018) 'Diagnosis of endocrine disease. Congenital hypothyroidism: update and perspectives'. *European Journal of Endocrinology*, 179 (6): R297–R317.

Richmond, E. and Rogol, A.D. (2016) 'Treatment of growth hormone deficiency in children, adolescents and at the transitional age'. *Best Practice and Researchy Clinical Endocrinology and Metabolism*, 30 (6): 749–55.

Savage, M.O., Backeljauw, P.F., Calzada, R. et al. (2016) 'Early detection, referral, investigation, and diagnosis of children with growth disorders'. *Hormone Research in Paediatrics*, 85 (5): 325–32.

Smith, L.B., Terry, A., Bollepalli, S. and Rechenberg, K. (2019) 'School-based management of pediatric type 1 diabetes: recommendations, advances, and gaps in knowledge'. *Current Diabetes Reports*, 19 (7): 37.

Speiser, P.W., Arlt, W., Auchus, R.J., et al. (2018) 'Congenital adrenal hyperplasia due to steroid 21-hydroxylase deficiency: an Endocrine Society clinical practice guideline'. *Journal of Clinical Endocrinology and Metabolism*, 103 (11): 4043–88.

Styne, D.M., Arslanian, S.A., Connor, E.L., Farooqi, I.S., Murad, M H., Silverstein, J.H. and Yanovski, J.A. (2017) 'Pediatric obesity – assessment, treatment, and prevention: an Endocrine Society clinical practice guideline'. *Journal of Clinical Endocrinology and Metabolism*, 102 (3): 709–57.

Tjen, C. and Wilkinson, K. (2016) 'Perioperative care of children and young people with diabetes'. *BJA Education*, 16 (4): 124–9.

Urquhart, T. and Collin, J. (2016a) 'Understanding the endocrinopathies associated with the treatment of childhood cancer: part 1'. *Nursing Children and Young People*, 28 (8): 37–44.

Urquhart, T. and Collin, J. (2016b) 'Understanding the endocrinopathies associated with the treatment of childhood cancer: part 2'. *Nursing Children and Young People*, 28 (9): 36–43.

Wei, C., Davis, N., Honour, J. and Crowne, E. (2017) 'The investigation of children and adolescents with abnormalities of pubertal timing'. *Annals of Clinical Biochemistry*, 54 (1): 20–32.

Wolfsdorf, J.I., Glaser, N., Agus, M. et al. (2018) 'ISPAD Clinical Practice Consensus Guidelines 2018: Diabetic ketoacidosis and the hyperglycemic hyperosmolar state'. *Pediatric Diabetes*, 19 (Suppl 27): 155–17.

Ziegler, R., Waldenmaier, D., Kamecke, U., Mende, J., Haug, C. and Freckmann, G. (2020) 'Accuracy assessment of bolus and basal rate delivery of different insulin pump systems used in insulin pump therapy of children and adolescents'. *Pediatric Diabetes*, 21 (4): 649–56.

CARE OF CHILDREN AND YOUNG PEOPLE WITH IMMUNOLOGICAL PROBLEMS

22

KATIE WARBURTON

THIS CHAPTER COVERS

- Anatomy and physiology of the immune system
- How do childhood immunisations work?
- Nursing care of children with primary immune deficiencies
- Nursing care of children with human immunodeficiency virus (HIV)

REQUIRED KNOWLEDGE

It would be helpful to have an understanding of the anatomy and physiology of the immune system before you start this chapter.

"The trembling fear of 'Will I be neglected by the ones I call my friends?' Will I meet the end? Or will I be trapped by the stigma? My strength is only becoming stronger, not weaker. I fight my emotions with a smile on front. When nobody knows the true feelings; how can I be happy when I can't be me? It seems like the only way of being happy is being free. I am a fighter and I've fought this long, soon, very soon, the happiness, it won't be long. It's me against the world. What could possibly go wrong?"

CHIVA Youth Committee, 2015

INTRODUCTION

The immune system must identify foreign agents and stimulate a defence to protect the body. An ineffective response may be caused by a deficiency of the immune system, whereas an inappropriate immune response may be a result of allergy, transplant rejection or autoimmune diseases. An ineffective immune system leaves the host susceptible to infections including viruses, bacteria, protozoa, fungi, parasites and tumours. Common infections seen in children's nursing include those caused by bacteria and viruses. Bacteria are organisms able to reproduce independently. In practice they are seen to cause disease such as pneumococcal meningitis and *Escherichia coli* (*E. coli*) urinary tract infection. However, viruses –such as measles, chickenpox and HIV – cannot replicate without the use of cells within the body. Infection is a common reason for hospitalisation and community nursing input. You should be able to assess, plan, implement and evaluate care with the necessary knowledge of the evidence base to underpin decision-making. It is important to remember that children with an immune deficiency may present with minimal symptoms of severe infection.

ANATOMY AND PHYSIOLOGY

It is important that you have a good understanding of the immune system to understand immunological problems. Table 22.1 will help you revise some important components of the immune system.

Table 22.1 Components of the immune system

Lymphocytes	White blood cells are produced in the bone marrow and travel in the lymphatic and circulatory systems, identifying or responding to foreign agents. B and T lymphocytes have important roles in the acquired immune response. They are found in circulating blood or lymph or at specific lymphatic sites. T lymphocytes travel to the thymus where they mature and later further divide into cytotoxic, helper or suppressor T cells. Cytotoxic T lymphocytes destroy infected cells and instruct phagocytes to support the destruction of pathogens. B lymphocytes can become plasma cells and produce antibodies to target antigens when instructed to do so by T lymphocytes
Antibodies	Also known as immunoglobulins. They are plasma proteins split into five main classes: IgM, IgA, IgG, IgE and IgD. Immunoglobulins are Y-shaped molecules that are able to bind to antigens. Antibodies, produced by B lymphocytes, respond to specific antigens. They may individually neutralise and destroy the antigen, be destroyed with the antigen by macrophages or neutrophils, or trigger the complement cascade to destroy the antigen
Major histocompatibility complex (MHC)	MHC is a group of genes; MHC molecules allow T lymphocytes to identify cells containing foreign organisms by expressing peptides on the outside of the invaded cell. MHC plays an important role in tissue typing and tissue rejection
Natural killer cells	Are a type of lymphocyte and capable of destroying virus-infected cells and some tumour cells. They work closely with cytokines as part of the initial response to viruses
Macrophages	Developed from monocytes. They are phagocytic cells, which means they can ingest foreign substances or damaged cells. Some macrophages relate to the specific tissue in which they are found (e.g., Kupffer cells are found in the liver). They are one of the body's first defence mechanisms when a foreign agent is seen
Cytokines	Small proteins initially released following the attempt of macrophages to destroy foreign agents. They have a key signalling role

Dendritic cells	These cells have the important role of presenting antigens to T lymphocytes. Langerhans cells are specific dendritic cells found in the skin
Complement	A cascade of proteins that highlight and support the destruction of antigens by following a pathway of triggers. Complement is often activated by antibodies. The complement system plays an important role in phagocytosis
Neutrophils	A type of white blood cell with phagocytic properties. They particularly attack bacteria

Immune system deficiencies may be described as innate or acquired. Primary immune deficiencies predominantly have a genetic cause and are evident from birth. Acquired immune deficiencies include human immunodeficiency virus (HIV), an infection the body is unable to eradicate.

Innate immunity

Innate immune responses are the body's natural defence mechanisms. These defences include the skin, gastric acid, cilia, cytokines, complement cascade and phagocytic cells. The innate immune system has no memory of exposure or response.

If this is not successful, the acquired immune response is stimulated through chemical signalling by cytokines, which work as part of the innate and acquired immune system.

Acquired immunity

Acquired immunity is developed through exposure to infection generated through disease or vaccination. Memory will be developed so further exposure will result in immediate defence. Young children are exposed to infection through socialisation, amongst other things, which also supports the development of the immune system. However, immunisations are a vital part of developing acquired immunity.

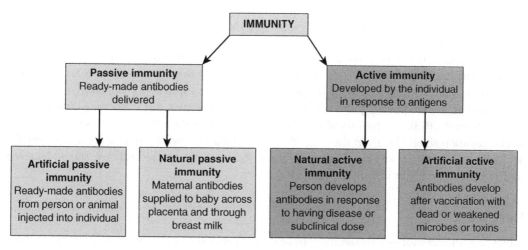

Figure 22.1 Types of immunity

HOW DO CHILDHOOD IMMUNISATIONS WORK?

The World Health Organization (WHO, 2020) highlighted that 19.7 million children under the age of 1 did not receive basic immunisations in 2019 despite recognition that immunisation prevents 2–3 million childhood deaths a year. The purpose of vaccines is to create long-term immunity, similar to that which would follow disease, but without illness. Health practitioners involved in the administration of vaccines must be competent, have the ability to provide current, accurate information to children and families and deliver safe, effective, high standards of care (Public Health England, 2018).

The history of vaccination could be said to commence with the development of the smallpox vaccine in 1798. Although Edward Jenner was not the first to identify the process of inoculation or immunisation, his work is described as instrumental in the eradication of the disease and development of the field of immunology (Riedel, 2005). The intention of all vaccines is to create adequate immunity to an infection without causing disease.

Vaccines have been traditionally produced using live attenuated or killed organisms. Live attenuated vaccines such as the Measles, Mumps and Rubella (MMR) vaccine have the ability to replicate within the body and create a response similar to that of infection. Inactivated vaccines, such as inactivated polio vaccine (IPV), do not always create a response as well as live attenuated vaccines. The live or killed organism, known as an antigen or an immunogen, creates an immune response. Vaccines can also contain antibiotics, stabilisers, adjuvants and preservatives in differing amounts to improve the stability and effectiveness of the vaccine.

Newer vaccines include viral vector vaccines that use a harmless virus as a carrier to deliver genetic material linked to the infection and cause the body to make an appropriate response to the antigen without causing infection (Van Riel and de Wit, 2020) such as the Ebola vaccine. Nucleic acid (DNA or mRNA) vaccines are made through synthetic production of the genetic template of an infection and instruct the body to make antigens against a virus (Van Riel and de Wit, 2020). Both of these vaccine platforms have resulted in the production of COVID-19 vaccines (British Society for Immunology, 2021).

The roll of T lymphocytes in vaccine response is crucial. T-helper lymphocytes instruct B lymphocytes to produce antibodies. The initial production of antibody is predominantly IgM antibody, which creates memory of the antigen. IgG production follows and will be the dominating antibody when a second dose of the same vaccine is administered; IgG is a longer-lasting antibody. When B lymphocytes are stimulated or recognise an antigen they will produce specific antibodies to target that antigen; they attach to the antigen through a lock-and-key technique. Re-exposure to an antigen results in a faster immune response.

Adverse reactions to vaccines are rare and anaphylaxis following vaccination is reported at a risk of one in a million (Public Health England, 2013). This is supported by a report on the Vaccine Safety Datalink data from the United States which states the risk of anaphylaxis following vaccination is 1.3 per million (McNeil et al., 2016). Despite the low risk the practitioner must be competent in anaphylaxis management.

Maternal antibodies provide protection for the newborn; however, this is not long lasting (Public Health England, 2013). Vaccines should not be delayed for premature infants. Babies born before 28 weeks' gestation should be given their first dose in hospital followed by respiratory monitoring for 48–72 hours. If there are any concerns when giving the first dose, the second dose should be given under observation (Public Health England, 2013).

Herd immunity

Individuals who cannot receive vaccinations or do not respond to vaccinations rely on 'herd immunity'. The term 'herd immunity' refers to the high number of individuals protected from infection through vaccination. This reduces the risk of infection to unimmunised individuals. Infections can be eliminated from populations through this process, as demonstrated by the elimination of smallpox.

Health promotion

Immunisation remains one of the most successful public health strategies. Every opportunity should be taken to promote the benefit of immunisation, ensure children receive the vaccine schedule and administer missed vaccines. In the case of all established vaccines, risk of adverse events following vaccination versus risk of complications from a vaccine-preventable disease make a clear case in support of vaccine. All practitioners must be able to clearly explain risk and benefit. Ensure you access the most up-to-date national schedule in the 'Green Book' online. Some parents remain concerned at their perception that vaccinations are harmful for children. Some parents are reluctant to expose their children to their perceived risk of harm. These parental views should be recognised, listened to attentively and the opportunity must be taken to provide evidence-based information to assist in allaying their fears. Ignoring their fears or dismissing their concerns is not an ethical or helpful approach in such cases. Working with parents using the best available scientific evidence is likely to be more effective in assuring parents that they are doing the best thing they can for their children by having them immunised. Always seek informed medical advice in such cases to inform and reassure the parents.

PRIMARY IMMUNE DEFICIENCIES

Primary immune deficiencies (PID) are disorders of the immune system that have a genetic link; the UK PID Registry provides key cohort information (Edgar et al., 2013). A number of signs and symptoms may be linked with an immune deficiency but can often also be assigned to a more common childhood illness, which can inevitably delay diagnosis. Included in this non-exhaustive list are: a family history of PID, frequent or recurrent infections, severe infections, failure to thrive and deep skin or organ abscesses.

The International Union of Immunological Societies Expert Committee for Primary Immunodeficiency (Al-Herz et al., 2014) classify primary immunodeficiencies in eight categories (see Table 22.2).

Table 22.2 Eight categories of primary immunodeficiencies as classified by the International Union of Immunological Societies Expert Committee for Primary Immunodeficiency

Classification	Example
Combined immunodeficiencies	X-linked severe combined immunodeficiency
Well-defined syndromes with immunodeficiency	DiGeorge syndrome
Predominantly antibody deficiencies	Common variable immune deficiency
Diseases of immune dysregulation	X-linked lymphoproliferative syndrome
Congenital defects of phagocyte number, function, or both	Chronic granulomatous disorder
Defects in innate immunity deficiency	NEMO
Auto-inflammatory disorders	Familial Mediterranean fever
Complement deficiencies	C1 inhibitor deficiency

Treatment is dependent on the diagnosis and may include:

- Prophylactic antibiotics given to prevent infections where there is susceptibility
- Additional vaccinations to improve response and acquired immunity

- Immunoglobulin therapy administered at regular intervals (this is a blood product made from the pooled plasma of donors providing short-lasting antibodies)
- Gene therapy, which involves replacing the faulty gene with a working copy of the faulty gene
- Bone marrow transplantation is required to cure some immune deficiencies such as severe combined immune deficiency (SCID); infants with this diagnosis are likely to present in the first year of life with severe infections

Antibody deficiencies are the most common primary immunodeficiency seen in clinical practice (Al-Herz et al., 2014).

Care plan for a child receiving routine IV immunoglobulin therapy on the day unit

Immunoglobulin therapy can be administered intravenously or subcutaneously for a child with an antibody deficiency. The benefits and disadvantages of both methods should be explored with the family. Clinical guidelines for immunoglobulin use (Department of Health, 2011, and subsequent updated information) must be consulted to guide practice as we are in an era of increasing demand and there is concern for supply. The nursing process as outlined in Table 22.3 should be adhered to.

Table 22.3 The nursing process

Assessment	Before therapy, blood tests will be requested by the clinical team. Baseline temperature, blood pressure, heart rate, respiration rate and weight must be recorded. Immunoglobulin therapy should not be administered if the child has a fever or is unwell without review by the immunology team
Planning	The prescription must be prepared in advance to ensure the product is available. It is essential that nurses are aware of the management of adverse reactions, including anaphylaxis. Ensure a name band is in situ. IV cannulation or insertion of a subcutanenous butterfly needle should be conducted following local policy, including aseptic non-touch technique and a choice of local anaesthetic cream or spray. Ensure the product is intact and check and record the batch number and expiry date
Implementation	Follow local medicine policy when administering medication and ensure safe administration. Observe the child closely throughout. Regularly measure vital signs, observe the cannula site and record rates and infusion balance
Evaluation	Evaluation is continuous and includes future investigations to assess the effectiveness of the therapy. Ensure the child and family are kept up to date. The cannula must be removed before discharge home and a follow-up appointment will be necessary for the child

CASE STUDY 22.1: ZARA

Zara is a 3-month-old baby who attended the GP surgery regularly with fever and infection. Zara received the BCG vaccine at birth, administered to the left upper arm. This was appropriate, as her grandparents were born in India, where the incidence of tuberculosis is reported at 188 per 100,000 (WHO, 2021). Zara was taken to A&E by her mother who was becoming increasingly concerned with the large lump under Zara's left arm and her worsening cough. Zara was admitted to the children's ward. A thorough medical history was taken.

Zara was born at 40 weeks' gestation by vaginal delivery. She was the second child of Sumaya and Mohammed, who reported no medical complaints. Sumaya was worried as some of her relatives had given birth to children who died in infancy, but as they lived in India there was limited additional information.

Zara appeared to feed well but was not gaining weight and had dropped from the 75th to 25th centile on a growth chart since birth. Blood results indicated that Zara had no B and T lymphocytes.

- What is the likely diagnosis in this case study?
- How will you nurse Zara on the children's ward before transfer to an immunology centre?

HIV

Human immunodeficiency virus (HIV) is a retrovirus that causes immune deficiency. In 2020, the World Health Organization (WHO, 2021) estimated that 37.7 million people were living with HIV around the world; 1.7 million of these were children under the age of 14 years. In the United Kingdom, approximately 489 children are accessing care for HIV infection at a recognised children's treatment centre (Collaborative HIV Paediatric Study [CHIPS], 2022).

HIV infection is transmitted through unprotected sexual intercourse when the person living with HIV does not have an undetectable viral load, from infected blood to uninfected blood, from mother to baby in utero, during childbirth and through breastfeeding when the mother does not have an undetectable viral load (WHO, 2020a). Nearly all children living with HIV in the UK acquired the virus from their mother and 41% of this cohort were born in the UK (CHIPS, 2022). The average age of the UK cohort is increasing, which is reflective of successful treatment and the prevention of mother-to-child transmission. It is important to note that HIV cannot be transmitted through every day activities such as sharing items, sharing food, holding hands, kissing or hugging.

HIV particularly affects T-helper lymphocytes that express the CD4 glycoprotein. The protein on the virus allows it to attach to and enter the cell via receptors on the cell wall. An enzyme, reverse transcriptase, allows the viral RNA to change into DNA and integrates into the cell nucleus. The virus is able to replicate and release more copies of HIV before it dies. Cytotoxic T lymphocytes expressing the CD8 glycoprotein increase in number as they try to respond to and control HIV.

Over time the CD4 cell count declines as a result of ongoing HIV replication. The CD4 cell count can be monitored by a blood test. HIV also infects other cells within the body. The lower the CD4 count the more severe the immune deficiency and consequent risk of infection.

Today, HIV should be discussed as a chronic health condition with life expectancy near normal when effective treatment is available, initiated in a timely manner and taken correctly (May et al., 2014). Today's effective treatment, monitoring and support demonstrates huge medical advances since the first reported cases of acquired immune deficiency syndrome (AIDS) in the 1980s. It is important to note that globally only 68% of adults and 53% of children are receiving treatment (WHO, 2020a).

The CD4 count and clinical staging have historically been the main indicators for initiating treatment to prevent the risk of severe infections. Today, it is recommended that treatment is started in all children diagnosed with HIV regardless of age or clinical indicators (PENTA, 2019). HIV treatment is often used in combination and described as highly active antiretroviral treatment (HAART).

The purpose of treatment is to prevent viral replication and reduce the amount of HIV in the body to an undetectable level. The measurement is referred to as the 'viral load'.

HIV treatment is currently lifelong therapy and adherence is crucial. Children must take the correct drugs at the same time every day. Poor adherence to treatment will result in a rising viral load, falling CD4 count and potentially permanent drug resistance. Challenges today include successful transition to adult care and lifelong treatment (Bamford and Lyall, 2015).

ACTIVITY 22.1: CRITICAL THINKING

The importance of adherence to treatment has been highlighted. This can be a challenge for children and young people with many different chronic health conditions. What would need to be considered before initiating treatment? What reasons may lead to poor adherence in children? How would you support a child and their family due to start lifelong treatment for a chronic health condition such as HIV?

Stigma

Stigma remains a significant challenge for anyone living with or affected by HIV. This affects the age at which children are informed they are HIV-positive. Children should be informed within primary school years by appropriately trained healthcare staff and with relevant education and support. Review the Children's HIV Association statement (CHIVA, 2015) on naming HIV to children to understand the challenges and importance.

ACTIVITY 22.2: REFLECTION

The chapter opened with a short piece of creative writing by a young person living with HIV and highlights the impact of stigma. Reflect on the impact of poor understanding of HIV and stigma in education.

The CHIVA Youth Committee has produced a list of important factors for practice to ensure care is appropriate. These are important points that a relevant across children and young people's nursing care:

1. Make sure you know what you're talking about. Misinformation or misunderstanding can affect me.
2. Please talk to me and not my parent or guardian.
3. If you have a private conversation (which seems to be about me) with a colleague when I'm in the same room, it makes me feel anxious.
4. Please take the time to explain my medicine and side effects.
5. Please treat me my age. Think about the language you use. Use simple words.
6. Don't make assumptions.

7. It doesn't matter how/when/why someone got HIV; don't focus on this.
8. HIV doesn't define me; I'll always be me first and can still achieve my ambitions.
9. Confidentiality is really important; my health isn't something to gossip about.
10. HIV affects my mental health just as much as my physical health; stigma hurts.

CASE STUDY 22.2: SUSAN

Susan is 13 years old. She was treated at an HIV specialist family clinic, where her mother also received her treatment and care. They both attended their appointments regularly, their HIV was well controlled with medication and they presented as essentially well.

The local children's social care team received a referral from Susan's school due to her poor attendance. A social worker made contact to arrange an assessment.

Mum was very reluctant to allow the social worker to visit. When the social worker visited, their home was found to be in an extremely poor state of hygiene. Medicine was scattered all over the floor and empty take-away food containers were piled high. It was evident that Susan slept in the same bed as her mother as her room was inaccessible due to piles of clothing and belongings. The assessment revealed that mum no longer cooked and they relied on take-away food.

The health information revealed that Susan's physical health had been consistently good. The high level of school absences appeared to be related to mum's need for her daughter to be at home. Susan's mother had become very dependent, and Susan presented little independent identity. It was clear that mum had mental health issues, which were previously unrecognised.

The family's health professionals collaborated in the safeguarding assessment and support plan, which included ongoing community visits to support the family in their home as well as clinic-based care.

- What would be the priorities for the care team supporting Susan and her mum in this case study?

The case demonstrates the complex social and psychological impacts HIV can bring to families where access to wider support and understanding of HIV can be difficult. It reinforces the importance of awareness of how in certain situations the welfare of the child is at risk and needs prompt intervention and support. (Amanda Ely, social worker and CEO, CHIVA)

CHAPTER SUMMARY

Understanding the immune system will help you to deliver appropriate high-quality evidence-based nursing care to children while also supporting their families. Immunisation remains an essential public health strategy internationally and it is important to note that everyone has a role to play in vaccine promotion. Development and progress are ongoing in the field of immune deficiencies, but some understanding can continue to positively influence clinical practice and wellbeing of the child and family.

In this chapter we have looked at the care of a child with immunological problems. We have highlighted:

- Principle components of the immune system
- Public health – immunisations
- Caring sensitively for a child with an immune deficiency disorder
- HIV awareness and ongoing education needs
- Safeguarding awareness and considerations for children

BUILD YOUR BIBLIOGRAPHY

Books

FURTHER
READING

- Randall, D. (2005) 'Development of the immune system and immunity', in C. Chamley, P. Carson, D. Randall and M. Sandwell, M. (eds), *Developmental Anatomy and Physiology of Children: A Practical Approach*. London: Elsevier Churchill Livingstone.

  It is important to have some knowledge of normal anatomy and physiology so that illness and changes can be understood.
- Public Health England and Department of Health (2020) *Immunisation against Infectious Disease*. London: TSO.

  Commonly known as The Green Book, this is essential for anybody involved in the care of children requiring immunisation.
- Playfair, J.H.L. and Chain, B.M. (2012) *Immunology at a Glance*, 10th edn. Chichester: Wiley-Blackwell.

  This book will help you develop your understanding of the immune system.
- Peate, I. and Gormley-Fleming, E. (eds) (2021) *Fundamentals of Children and Young People's Anatomy and Physiology: A textbook for Nursing and Healthcare Students*, 2nd edn. Chichester: Wiley-Blackwell.

  This book is good at exploring the immune system in children and young people.

Journal Articles

FURTHER
READING:
ONLINE
JOURNAL
ARTICLES

- Bamford, A. and Lyall, H. (2015) 'Paediatric HIV grows up: recent advances in perinatally acquired HIV'. *Archives of Disease in Childhood*, 100 (2): 183–8.

  This article highlights the important advances in children's HIV care in the UK since the 1980s.
- Hassan Abolhassani, H., Azizi, G., Sharifi, L., Yazdani, R., Mohsenzadegan, M., Delavari, S. et al. (2020) 'Global systematic review of primary immunodeficiency registries'. *Expert Review of Clinical Immunology*, 16 (7): 717–32.

  Prompt recognition and diagnosis of immune deficiency is important; this article gives some insight into the incidence and recognition globally.
- Wilder-Smith, A. and Qureshi, K. (2020) 'Resurgence of measles in Europe: a systematic review on parental attitudes and beliefs of measles vaccine'. *Journal of Epidemiology and Global Health*, 10 (1): 46–58.

This article highlights some of the challenges of vaccine uptake and the need for nurses to be ready to educate the public, have the knowledge to answer questions confidently and support vaccine uptake.

Weblinks

FURTHER
READING:
WEBLINKS

- World Health Organization – *Immunization, Vaccines and Biologicals* www.who.int/immunization/en Keep up to date with the recommended global immunisation programme.
- PID UK www.piduk.org.uk. Find out more about primary immune deficiencies.
- Children's HIV Association (CHIVA) www.chiva.org.uk Review children's HIV resources and guidelines in the UK
- AVERT www.avert.org Consult the excellent AVERT website for up-to-date global evidence and data on all aspects of HIV and AIDS across the age ranges.

REFERENCES

Al-Herz, W., Bousfiha, A., Casanova, J-L., Chatila, T., Conley, M.E., Cunningham-Rundles, C. et al. (2014) 'Primary immunodeficiency diseases: an update on the classification from the International Union of Immunological Societies Expert Committee for Primary Immunodeficiency'. *Frontiers in Immunology*, 5 (162): 1–33.

Bamford, A. and Lyall, H. (2015) 'Paediatric HIV grows up: recent advances in perinatally acquired HIV'. *Archives of Disease in Childhood*, 100 (2): 183–8.

British Society for Immunology (2021) Types of vaccine for COVID-19. Available at: www.immunology.org/coronavirus/connect-coronavirus-public-engagement-resources/types-vaccines-for-covid-19 (accessed 3 March 2021).

Children's HIV Association (CHIVA) (2015) CHIVA Statement on children's knowledge about their HIV. Available at: www.chiva.org.uk/professionals/support/chiva-position-statement/ (accessed 7 June 2017).

Children's HIV Association (CHIVA) Taking medication. Available at www.chiva.org.uk/parent/child-hiv/medication-support (accessed 22 May 2017).

Collaborative HIV Paediatric Study (2022) Summary Data. London: CHIPS. Available at: www.chipscohort.ac.uk/patients/summary-data/ (accessed 10 February 2023).

Department of Health (DH) (2011) *Clinical Guidelines for Immunoglobulin Use*, 2nd edn. London: DH.

Edgar, J.D.M., Buckland, M., Guzman, D., Conlon, N.P., Knerr, V., Bangs, C. et al. (2013) 'The UK Primary Immune Deficiency (UK-PID) Registry: a report of the first 4 years' activity 2008–2012'. *Clinical and Experimental Immunology*, 175: 68–78.

May, M.T., Gompels, M., Delpech, V., Porter, K., Orkin, C., Kegg, S. et al. (2014) 'Impact on life expectancy of HIV-1 positive individuals of CD+ cell count and viral load response to antiretroviral therapy'. *AIDS*, 28 (8): 1193–202.

McNeil, M., Weintraub, E.S., Duffy, J., Sukumaran, L., Jacobsen, S.J., Klein, N.P. et al. (2016) 'Risks of anaphylaxis after vaccination in children and adults'. *Journal of Allergy and Clinical Immunology*, 137(3): 868–78.

PENTA (2019) PENTA HIV first and second line antiretroviral treatment guidelines 2019. Available at: https://penta-id.org/hiv/treatment-guidelines/# (accessed 5 March 2021).

Public Health England (2013) *Immunisation Against Infectious Disease*. London: HMSO.

Public Health England (2018) *National Minimum Standards and Core Curriculum for Immunisation Training for Registered Healthcare Practitioners*. London: Public Health England

Riedel, S. (2005) 'Edward Jenner and the history of smallpox and vaccination'. *BUMC Proceedings*, 18: 21–5.

Van Riel, D. and de Wit, B. (2020) 'Next generation vaccine platforms for COVID-19'. *Nature Materials*, 19: 810–12.

World Health Organization (WHO) (2020) Fact Sheet: Immunizations. Available at: www.who.int/news-room/fact-sheets/detail/immunization-coverage (accessed 3 March 2021).

World Health Organization (WHO) (2021) Fact Sheet: HIV/AIDS data and statistics. Available at: www.who.int/news-room/fact-sheets/detail/hiv-aids (accessed 5 March 2022).

CARE OF CHILDREN AND YOUNG PEOPLE WITH MUSCULOSKELETAL PROBLEMS

23

JULIA JUDD

THIS CHAPTER COVERS

- Assessment of the child with a musculoskeletal problem
- Bone health
- Common orthopaedic conditions
- Care of children with fractures
- The role of the children's nurse in caring for a child with a musculoskeletal problem

---

REQUIRED KNOWLEDGE

It is helpful to have an understanding of the anatomy and physiology of the musculoskeletal system before you start this chapter.

> "Step into my shoes and walk the life I'm living and if you get as far as I am, just maybe you will see how strong I really am."
>
> Unknown, www.wisdomquotesandstories.com/stepinto-my-shoes-walk-my-life

INTRODUCTION

The children's orthopaedic specialism covers a wide range of disorders affecting the child's growing skeleton, and includes trauma, infection, syndromic and neoplastic conditions, known collectively as musculoskeletal (MSK) conditions. The challenge in nursing the orthopaedic child is to apply specific knowledge of children's orthopaedic conditions and encompass generic medical and surgical knowledge and skills. As a children's nurse working in this area, you will need a true understanding of the differences of a child's anatomy and be able to adapt the basic principles of orthopaedic management to meet their needs. Throughout this chapter you will see how this knowledge crosses the boundaries of specialisms. The chapter focuses on some common musculoskeletal problems, although you will need to read more widely to gain a fuller understanding of these conditions (see the 'Build your bibliography' section at the end of the chapter). The chapter will begin by looking at the first step for any nurse working with a child presenting with an MSK condition, which is a thorough assessment.

Assessment of the child with a musculoskeletal problem

There are key aspects to any assessment of a child who presents with an MSK problem, which are summarised in Table 23.1.

Table 23.1 The nurse's role in assessment of a child with an MSK problem

Listen to the history given by the child and family. Formulate in your mind a potential diagnosis Sometimes this is not obvious, hip pain is frequently manifested as knee pain (i.e., the pain is 'referred' pain)	• Focus on the child. Build a rapport with them • Assess the family and child's understanding. Is English their first language? • Is there a past or family history relevant to this assessment? • In your mind, consider what is normal for the child. What are the normal milestones for a young child? • If the child has an underlying diagnosis, for example cerebral palsy, their mobility and range of movement will be affected • Document the history
Look at the child	• Start looking as soon as possible - i.e., even before the formal assessment has begun. Children are often self-conscious, which can alter the true representation of the problem • Look at how they stand, sit down, stand up • Look at their leg alignment. Watch them walk (ideally when they walk into the clinic room or ward) • Look at their range of movement in their joints • Look and assess the colour of the limb • Look for swelling and compare with the contralateral side • Document your findings, e.g. grade a pressure ulcer - so comparison can be made in follow up assessment
Feel the affected area	• Feel for swelling, warmth. Feel for pain. Is there pain at a specific point/area? • Document your findings
Move the affected area	• Assess movement of the presenting problem and move the child's joints above and below the problem area (unless impossible due to immobilisation with a cast or traction). Does this induce pain? • Document your findings
Neurovascular assessment Investigations	• Depending on the reason for the assessment, the nurse performs a formal neurovascular assessment, to ensure normality and exclude acute limb compartment syndrome • Document your findings

You can use the Table 23.1 as a quick reference guide when working with a variety of MSK conditions. The chapter will explore a selection of these conditions in more detail, but first will look at key aspects of bone health that are essential to children's health and that you should be aware of.

SEE ALSO
CHAPTER 14

Bone health

Strong bones are essential for long-term health and wellbeing.

Childhood and adolescence are a very important time for the formation of the skeleton – the stage in which bones grow both in size and strength. This is the most important time to set a solid foundation for future bone health (Osteoporosis Foundation).

Children and young people should take part in moderate-to-vigorous intensity physical activity for an average of at least 60 minutes a day across the week. (NHS, Exercises for healthy bones – www.nhs.uk)

Vitamin D is essential to ensure the body's absorption of calcium. Inadequate serum levels of vitamin D have resulted in a prevalence of musculoskeletal symptoms, deformity, fractures and noticeably a rebirth of rickets (Horan et al., 2019). Table 23.2 shows the normal levels of vitamin D.

Table 23.2   Vitamin D values

Serum25-hydroxy vitamin D nmols/L (nanomoles per litre)			Recommended intervention
Serum 25(OH)D	< 25nmol/l	Deficient level	Treatment recommended
Serum 25(OH)D	30-50nmol/l	Insufficient level	Dietary advice on sources of vitamin D, plus a vitamin D supplement 400-600 IU (purchase over the counter)
Serum 25(OH)D	> 50nmol/l	Sufficient level	Reassurance and advice on maintaining adequate vitamin D status through diet and supplements

Source: The Royal Osteoporosis Society (2018) https://theros.org.uk/latest-news/2018-12-02-vital-vitamin-d-clinical-guidelines-updated-for-healthcare-professionals/

Typical presentations of vitamin D deficiency in children are those that describe a history of musculo-skeletal pain, which in essence is non-specific and termed as 'growing pains'. Normal variants such as physiological genu varum (bow legs) or valgum (knock knees) are commonly associated with vitamin D deficiency. Supplementation is usually beneficial in treating MSK symptoms and is recommended to facilitate resolution of bony deformity.

WHAT'S THE EVIDENCE?

There is growing evidence of the links between vitamin D deficiency and a variety of health problems. In children particularly, bony deformity, fractures and muscle pain are a feature.

You can find this evidence in a number of publications, including:

- NICE public health guidelines: www.nice.org.uk/guidance/ph56
- NHS Choices: www.nhs.uk/conditions/ricket
- Judd, 2013 (see reference list for details)

Read through one of the above articles and consider what this might mean for health promotion opportunities.

Rickets

Nutritional rickets in the UK is not a disease of the past and remains prevalent, particularly in children under 5 years. Although the majority are of Black or South Asian ethnicity, nutritional rickets is not exclusive to this population group (Julies et al., 2020).

Children's nurses and other healthcare professionals are responsible for identifying the problem early, initiating appropriate management and directing parents and carers to resource information regarding healthy dietary intake and recommendations for oral supplementation.

PROMOTING HEALTH

NICE have published an interactive flowchart on how to increase vitamin D supplement use among at-risk groups (Nice Guideline [PH56] 2014, updated 2017: Recommendation 8), which you can access from www.nice.org.uk/guidance/ph56 The key messages for you as a nurse to bear in mind when working with children and their families are:

Ensure health professionals recommend and record vitamin D supplement use, among at-risk groups (and other family members, as appropriate) whenever possible. This could take place during registration appointments with new patients in general practice, flu, other vaccine and screening appointments. It could also take place during routine appointments and health checks including, for example:

- NHS Health Check
- diabetes check-ups
- falls appointments and check-ups
- health assessments for looked-after children
- the first contact with someone who is pregnant
- antenatal and postnatal appointments
- medicine use and prescription reviews
- health visitor appointments
- developmental checks for infants and children.

These are not specific to children but take into account the importance of the role of the nurse in caring for the whole family.

Developers of standardised electronic and handheld maternity notes and developers of personal child health records (the 'Red Book') should add specific questions about the use of vitamin D supplements.

The classical picture of rickets is bony deformity, specifically noted at the wrists and lower limbs. Normalising the child's serum levels of 25-hydroxyvitamin D may rectify the deformity. However, in some cases, surgery is required to correct leg alignment. During this stressful time, the parents need vital support and reassurance from nurses.

ACTIVITY 23.1: EVIDENCE-BASED PRACTICE

Using your research skills to find appropriate evidence, list the factors that may be contributing to the growing problem of vitamin D deficiency in the UK.

Table 23.3 Common orthopaedic disorders affecting infants and children

Musculoskeletal disorder	Body part	Common age range	Signs/ symptoms	Investigations	Key guidelines/references
Developmental dysplasia of the hip – abnormal hip growth ranging from instability of the hip to a fixed dislocation	Hip	0–6 months Can be identified older – i.e., late presentation	Reduced hip abduction Leg length inequality	Ultrasound hip scan (under 8 months) Anteroposterior view (AP) hips and pelvis X-ray (over 8 months)	The website for the International Hip Dysplasia Institute contains lots of information and real patient stories: www.hipdysplasia.org Newborn and infant physical examination: clinical guidance: www.gov.uk/government/publications/newborn-and-infant-physical-examination-programme-handbook/newborn-and-infant-physical-examination-screening-programme-handbook Clarke et al (2016).
Legg-Calvé-Perthes disease (or Perthes) – a disruption of the blood supply to the head of the femur, causing it to collapse and deform	Hip	5–7 years	Persistent limp and pain Reduced hip abduction	AP and frog leg lateral views hips and pelvis X-ray MRI (if diagnosis equivocal)	The Perthes Association is a charitable organisation offering families help and advice: www.perthes.org.uk For the management of Perthes disease, see: www.ncbi.nlm.nih.gov/pmc/articles/PMC4292319 To see patient stories, see: Patient Stories (perthesdisease.org) from the International Perthes Study Group

(Continued)

Table 23.3 (Continued)

Musculoskeletal disorder	Body part	Common age range	Signs/ symptoms	Investigations	Key guidelines/references
Slipped capital femoral epiphysis – the femoral head slips off the neck of the femur, at the top, through the growth plate	Hip	Adolescence	Limp/unable to bear weight Pain Leg lies in external rotation	AP and frog leg lateral views hips and pelvis X-ray	For an overview of slipped capital femoral epiphysis see: http://emedicine.medscape.com/ article/91596-overview#a6 Judd (2023) and SCFE: https://patient.info/ doctor/slipped-capital-femoral-epiphysis-pro
Genu varum/ valgum (bow legs/knock knees)	Knees/ Tibia	6 months–6 years	Angular deformity (bowed legs –inward or outward)	Whole lower limb X-ray (i.e., both legs)	Medscape give a complete over view of bow legs and knock knees: http://emedicine.medscape.com/ article/1355974-overview#a2 http://emedicine.medscape.com/ article/1259772-overview
Bone deformity e.g., Infantile Blount/rickets	Knees/ Any bone	Newborn– adolescence	Angular leg deformity Rickets: affects any bone	X-ray	Medscape gives an overview of Blount disease: http://emedicine.medscape.com/ article/1250420-overview
Congenital talipes equinovarus ('club foot')	Feet	Newborn	Feet are turned inward, supinated and the heel is high	Clinical assessment	This website provides a wealth of information for health professionals and families: www.ponseti.info UK Guideline for the treatment of club feet, see: Clubfoot Consensus https:// bscos.org.uk/consensus/ consensus/clubfoot.php
Amplified pain (increased pain sensitivity)	Any	Adolescence	Abnormal pain sensitivity		Dr Sherry in Philadelphia has published extensively on amplified musculoskeletal pain. These two websites will give the reader a real insight into the condition: www.chop.edu/ conditionsdiseases/ amplifiedmusculoskeletal-pain-syndromeamps/about#. V3P6WLgrKW8 www.clinexprheumatol.org/ article.asp?a=1186
Trauma – a physical injury to bones, joints, or soft tissues, e.g., muscles, tendons, ligaments	Any	Any	Pain, deformity, neurovascular compromise	X-ray CT	Take a look at this website to better understand how children are different from adults: www.rch.org.au/paed_trauma/ manual/11_How_are_children_ different/ See also Clarke (2023)

COMMON CHILDREN'S ORTHOPAEDIC CONDITIONS

Caring for children with an orthopaedic problem requires medical and surgical nursing skills (Judd, 2010). Children may present with complex problems and often with comorbidities to manage. The common disorders affecting children require a variety of treatment interventions dependent on the child's age at presentation. Table 23.3 summarises these disorders, symptoms and the main guidelines that you should read and refer to when working with children and their families affected by these conditions. The chapter will then consider a selection of these in more detail.

There are a number of reasons why a child may present to the general practitioner or emergency department.

Some of these are represented in Table 23.3. For additional information not included in this chapter, see Perry and Bruce (2010).

Developmental dysplasia of the hip

Developmental dysplasia of the hip (DDH) is a descriptive term used to cover a spectrum of disorders affecting the infant hip. The UK incidence is 1–2 per 1000 live births, varying elsewhere to 4–20 per 1000 (Clarke et al., 2016). Presentation is either a dysplastic (abnormal development), subluxing (partial dislocation) or unstable hip (ligaments are loose, so the hip is not stable within the joint), or a frank (complete) dislocation. The cause is unknown, although there are a number of identified risk factors. The primary risk factors are those in bold type:

- **Family medical history of DDH**
- **Breech presentation (baby is born bottom first)**
- Twin delivery
- Reduced abduction (frog-leg position)

Other associated factors include:

- Oligohydramnios (reduced amniotic fluid in the uterus)
- Firstborn child
- Large baby for gestational age
- Packaging disorders (minimal room in the uterus) – for example, torticollis, positional/structural club foot
- Caesarean section delivery
- Cerebral palsy (Public Health England, 2016)

DDH is usually detected in the infant presenting at birth, or to their health visitor or GP with a hip click or reduced abduction.

Criteria for referral by a trained health professional include a positive clinical examination (hip has reduced abduction, hip clunk on testing – Ortolani or Barlow positive tests) and those with a true risk factor. In the UK a national infant hip screening programme exists, although there are geographical disparities (Aarvold et al., 2022). Ultrasound, however, is the gold standard in diagnosing hip dysplasia/dislocation in the cartilaginous hip joint (Eastwood and de Gheldere, 2010; Rhodes and Aarvold, 2022) (see Figure 23.1).

For an overview of DDH and treatment, see Judd and Clarke (2014); and see NIPE newborn hip screening positive pathway (Public Health England, 2021).

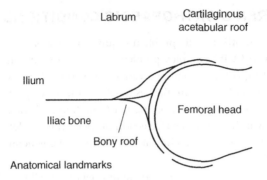

Figure 23.1 Hip ultrasound showing normal hip position

http://bonepit.com/Reference?Neonatal%20hip%20Ultrasound.htm

Treatment

Treatment is started when there is an abnormal clinical and ultrasound examination (Clarke and Castenada, 2012). In the infant, treatment is non-surgical, using a Pavlik harness (see Figure 23.3), with a success rate of 95%. A later diagnosis for an older child requires a closed or open hip reduction and possibility of subsequent reconstructive surgery (Young et al., 2020). Parents will seek information, so it is important that you have an understanding of the management options of DDH for the different age groups, as outlined in Table 23.4.

ACTIVITY 23.2: REFLECTIVE PRACTICE

Sometimes one of the hardest things to deal with emotionally is the fact that you assume you should handle this easily and well, because hip dysplasia is treatable (www.hipdysplasia.org).

- Look at the advice for parents and carers given by the International Hip Dysplasia Institute (www.hipdysplasia.org) and reflect on the support and reassurance you can give parents at this difficult time.
- See: Hip Dysplasia (DDH) – STEPS Charity (stepsworldwide.org) for parent information and YouTube videos.

Table 23.4 Treatment for developmental dysplasia of the hip (Clarke et al., 2016)

Newborn to 4 months	Pavlik harness (minimum 6 weeks, 24 hours/day and a further 6 weeks part-time wear until stable)
<18 months Failed Pavlik harness or late diagnosis	Closed or open hip reduction +/- preoperative gallows traction (using skin traction the baby's legs are suspended so that the buttocks are just clear of the bed).* Postoperative management: Hip spica 6-12 weeks +/- sequential broomstick and night splint casting (subsequent casts after the hip spica gradually enable more hip movement)
>18 months	Open hip reduction + femoral shortening Hip spica +/- sequential broomstick and night splint casting

*Gallows traction – patient information (www.uhs.nhs.uk/Media/UHS-website-2019/Patientinformation/Childhealth/Gallows-traction-2163-PIL.pdf).

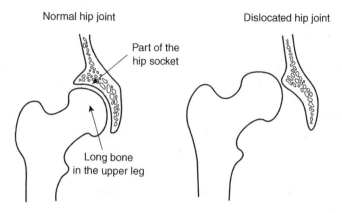

Normal hip joint

Dislocated hip joint

Part of the hip socket

Long bone in the upper leg

Figure 23.2 A normal and a dislocated hip

Pavlik harness

The Pavlik harness is a soft brace that places the baby's legs in an optimal position to facilitate normal hip development (Figure 23.3). The fabric straps secure the harness around the baby's chest and legs, allowing movement of the hip joint to encourage deepening of the hip joint socket. The legs straps are positioned to hold the hips in 90 degrees of flexion and 60 degrees of abduction. The role of the nurse is to support parents during this stressful time and ensure they have confidence in caring for their baby in the harness. Written information on hygiene, nappy care, clothing, handling, feeding and transporting should be provided. Further information can be found on the Steps website which has some great resources, including video links, to read and share with families caring for infants in Pavlik harnesses https://www.stepsworldwide.org/conditions/hip-dysplasia-ddh/

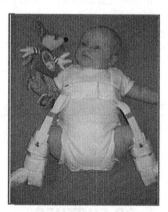

Figure 23.3 Pavlik harness. 90 degrees hip flexion/60 degrees hip abduction

Reproduced with permission from Clarke, S. and Santy-Tomlinson, J. (eds) (2014) *Orthopaedic and Trauma Nursing: An Evidenced-based Approach to Musculoskeletal Care.* Oxford: Wiley-Blackwell.

Further surgical procedures and hip spica care

The success of DDH treatment is dependent on age at diagnosis. Between 2 and 17% of children who are diagnosed will require subsequent surgical procedures to treat residual hip dysplasia (Cashman et al., 2002). This may be due to failure of the Pavlik harness or a late diagnosis of dysplasia (the harness is only effective before 4 months of age). A late diagnosis of hip dysplasia is the commonest reported risk factor for total hip replacement under the age of 40 years (Engesæter et al., 2011). Surgery for hip dysplasia varies depending on the severity of the condition and age of the child. Either a closed (manipulation) or an open procedure is performed to reduce the hip into the socket (acetabulum), with or without pelvic surgery to augment the shape of the socket. Postoperatively the child is managed in a hip spica cast for up to 3 months, with sequential cast changes to allow for growth and assessment of the hip. As a nurse, an important part of your role is to explain and support the family in postoperative care when the child is in a hip spica cast. Table 23.5 outlines some important considerations.

Table 23.5   The role of the nurse in caring for the child in a hip spica

Care aspect	Nursing support considerations
Support and information resources for the family	Provide written information on how to care for the child in a spica – for example, hygiene, sponge bathing, nappy care, toileting, seating and positioning, keeping the cast dry, preventing soiling and pressure sores
	It is helpful to show the family pictures of a child in a hip spica before the surgery, so they have an idea of what it looks like
	If possible introduce the parents to another family whose child has been in a spica
	Direct the family to appropriate websites – for example, IHDI (www.hipdysplasistepsworldwide.org).
	Liaise with the occupational therapy and physiotherapy teams to contact and meet with the family to give advice and reassurance regarding car seat (only certain models are suitable for children in spicas), manual handling, buggies and toileting
Child support	Make recommendations to the family regarding appropriate play for their child whilst in a spica. Consider the use of a hip spica table for the child to sit at (discuss with the occupational therapist and with the STEPS charity regarding a loan)
Pain relief and comfort	Ensure the child is comfortable and pain free. An epidural is commonly used for 48 hours after an open hip reduction. Once at home paracetamol is usually sufficient. Try alternative ways to console the child. They may be fretful because they are too hot or cold in the spica, need their position changed or are bored
Clothing	Suggest suitable clothing for a child in a spica. Some clothes can be adapted. More information is on the STEPS and IHDI websites

Source: Clarke and McKay, 2006; Judd, 2023

GO FURTHER

These books will give you the parents' perspective:

- Trice, N. (2015) *Cast Life: A Parent's Guide to DDH: Developmental Dysplasia of the Hip Explained.* Nell James Publishers. www.nelljames.co.uk
- Jay, G and Beattie, J. (2012) *Hope the Hip Hippo: a Story about Hip Dysplasia in Children.* Victoria, BC: Friesen Press.

LEGG-CALVÉ-PERTHES DISEASE

Legg–Calvé–Perthes disease (LCPD), named after the three orthopaedic surgeons who first described it in 1910, is a condition of unknown aetiology affecting the child's hip. The vascular supply to the femoral head (ball) of the hip joint is interrupted, causing bony necrosis (death of bone) and loss of hip joint congruency (ability to fit or work together). This results in a painful limp and reduced hip movement, and may also affect leg length, due to flattening of the head of the femur. During this time, the aim is to maintain movement within the hip joint, reduce pain and spasm, and with either non-surgical or surgical management, protect the deforming femoral head (Joseph, 2015).

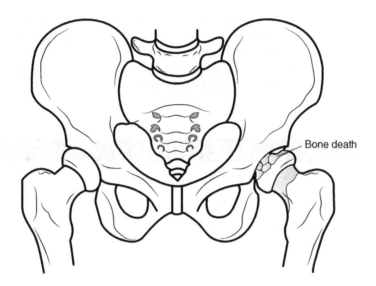

Figure 23.4 Perthes disease left hip

Perthes disease can last between two and four years, going through four distinct phases which are visible on the child's X-ray. This information gives guidance with regard to treatment and can inform parents of their child's progression through the disease process.

The stages of Perthes are:

- *Stage 1*: Necrosis (bone death)
- *Stage 2*: Fragmentation (the dead bone is replaced with softer, weak bone which breaks into pieces)
- *Stage 3*: Reossification (the blood supply returns to the head of the femur and new bone forms)
- *Stage 4*: Remodelling (the new bone heals; the shape of the head of the femur is dependent on the severity of the condition and the age of the child)

As a nurse, your support at diagnosis and throughout the duration of the disease process is vital for the parents and child. You should give guidance on avoiding activities that provoke pain and suggest or consider alternative activities to help reduce the child's symptoms. The condition is more prevalent in boys and helping them to understand the connection between impact activities (such as football) and their symptoms can be challenging.

ACTIVITY 23.3: CRITICAL THINKING

- What suggestions can you make to enable parents to help their child who has LCPD?

Think, for example, about switching activities, offloading the hip during painful episodes (crutches, bed rest).

Treatment

LCPD is one of many children's orthopaedic conditions in which the cause and the best treatment option continue to be debated by orthopaedic surgeons (Perry et al., 2022). However, the principles of management are agreed: to prevent further deformity of the head of the femur and to contain it within the socket of the hip joint. This will facilitate the best long-term outcome of a joint that has good movement and minimal symptoms (Bowen et al., 2011).

CASE STUDIES

For a patient's story see 'Will's Perthes story' on the STEPS Worldwide website www.stepsworldwide.org/our-stories/personal-stories/wills-perthes-story/
    For a case history see
    Daphne Dhas, Aparna Viswanath and Mark David Latimer, 'Perthes disease in a 2-year-old child'. BMJ Case Reports (2015) https://casereports.bmj.com/content/2015/bcr-2014-206731

Table 23.6 outlines the surgical options.

WHAT'S THE EVIDENCE?

Look at the latest evidence for the treatment of the condition and review the complexities in the decisions taken for best individual treatment options (Parmentier et al., 2016; Galloway et al., 2020).
    Consider the physical, emotional, and social core outcomes, patients' parents' and surgeons' view as essential when researching Perthes disease (Leo et al., 2020; Matsumoto et al., 2020).
    The two main surgical procedures are listed below (Table 23.6).

    Both aim to protect the deforming femoral head to achieve good remodelling by the final stage of the disease. Note that the roundness of the femoral head is dependent on it being located in the acetabulum (socket).
    As the disease worsens and the femoral head flattens, there is potential for it to extrude out of the acetabulum.

Table 23.6 Surgery for Perthes

Operation	Average age	Further reading
Shelf acetabuloplasty Aims: Bone graft provides additional cover for the extruding femoral head Femoral head remodels in the new hip socket	< 8 years (dependent on the stage of LCPD)	Parmentier et al., 2016 Carsi et al., 2015 (These two papers describe the surgery, non-operative management and discuss patient outcomes)
Varus derotation femoral osteotomy Aims: Realigns the proximal femur Redirects the force through the hip when weight bearing Achieves improved containment and facilitates femoral remodelling ability	Age not specific	Tripathy et al., 2010 Gives a complete overview of Perthes and treatment options

CONGENITAL TALIPES EQUINOVARUS OR CLUB FOOT

Congenital talipes equinovarus (CTEV), or club foot, is a deformity of the foot and ankle that can be present from birth. A club foot is diagnosed by the following features:

- Forefoot is turned inward (adducted)
- Sole is turned upward (supinated)
- Arch is high (cavus)
- Heel is high (equinus)

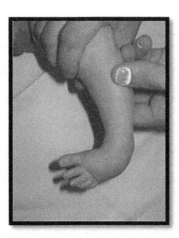

Figure 23.5 Left club foot

Reproduced with permission from Clarke, S. and Santy-Tomlinson, J. (eds) (2014) *Orthopaedic and Trauma Nursing: An Evidenced-based Approach to Musculoskeletal Care*. Oxford: Wiley-Blackwell.

Treatment

The gold standard for club foot treatment is the Ponseti method: gentle manipulation and serial casting to gradually correct the foot position, subsequently maintained with boots on an abduction bar until age 4 (see Table 23.7). Compliance with these is key to the success of the treatment and parent support is imperative. The Ponseti method is now an established treatment for infant clubfeet in the UK, although clinician expertise varies geographically. Some parents source practitioners via the Internet and travel long distances for their baby's treatment (Judd, 2004). Alternative management involves surgical correction of the foot deformity, resulting in a stiffer, less flexible foot with scars.

For national consensus guidelines of best practice see: Gelfer et al. (2021) and Clubfoot Consensus (bscos.org.uk).

The nurse's role in supporting parents at diagnosis, whether antenatally or at birth, is very important. Many parents are given the wrong impression by untrained and uniformed health practitioners – for example, that their child will have problems walking and not have normal function.

ACTIVITY 23.4: EVIDENCE-BASED PRACTICE

Browse the Internet to explore the information available to parents about club foot.
See: Clubfoot Consensus (bscos.org.uk)

- How would you as a nurse direct them to the appropriate information?
- Consider your opinion of social media information. For example, are Facebook groups helpful or otherwise?

Now explore the Global Clubfoot Initiative website (www.globalclubfoot.com).
This takes you straight to the home page with links on blogs from India, Pakistan, Solomon Islands, etc.
Look at how some of the low-income countries have advanced their ability to treat club foot through training. What can we learn from this?

Table 23.7 Ponseti method pathway

Club foot determined on ultrasound at 20 weeks
↓
Parents meet health professional to discuss treatment pathway
↓
Information pointers given to parents
↓
Baby seen by 2 weeks of age
↓
Deformity assessed (Pirani +/- Dimeglio score)
↓
Gradual correction with gentle manipulation and weekly serial casting (average five weeks)
↓
+/- Achilles tenotomy (70-85%)
↓
Final cast for 3 weeks in maximum ankle dorsiflexion
↓
Boots and bar full time (23 hours per day) for 3 months
↓
Boots and bar naps and night time up to 4 years of age

Note: Approximately 25% of children require tibialis anterior tendon transfer at approximate age 3

AMPLIFIED MUSCULOSKELETAL PAIN SYNDROME (AMPS)

Pain is:

> An unpleasant sensory and emotional experience normally associated with tissue damage or described in terms of such damage. (International Association for the Study of Pain, www.iasp-pain.org)

Amplified pain is a descriptive term for the problem. It is challenging to diagnose and treat, requiring the expertise of a multidisciplinary team to facilitate resolution.

Associated factors frequently identified with the initiation of AMPS are minor trauma, an episode of psychological stress and personal or family illness. The pain fails to settle within the expected time frame and dysfunction results due to muscle disuse. AMP is prevalent in female adolescents, who are frequently high achievers. The lower limbs are the most commonly affected and intrusive symptoms result in school non-attendance. The child may present with some of the following symptoms:

- Hyperalgesia – disproportionate extreme sensitivity to pain
- Allodynia – pain from light touch
- Swelling – may occur over the painful region
- Skin temperature changes
- Skin colour changes

(Logan et al., 2013)

The cause is unknown although associations between personality type and contributing factors have been made. Early recognition and prompt initiation of a therapy plan is vital to avoid functional deterioration.

Diagnosis requires exclusion of pathology with normal radiological and laboratory investigations. The child and the family need a clear explanation of the problem supported with evidence in a patient-information leaflet. This encourages their full commitment to the rehabilitation programme, facilitated by the whole MDT, which will address all the influencing factors to lead to the child's improvement and ultimate cure (Dougherty et al., 2021; Judd, 2023).

SEE ALSO
CHAPTER 5

ACTIVITY 23.5: CRITICAL THINKING

Think about how different people express or interpret pain.

- What does pain mean to you?
- How can we as nurses assess pain? What tools are available?
- What are the options for managing the child's AMP so they can participate in their physical therapy to regain normal function?

LIMB LENGTHENING

There are many reasons why a child may have either a short limb or a deformity.

Surgical options to treat these conditions include external devices such as a circular or monolateral frames (external fixators), internal magnetic/growing rods, or surgery to the 'normal' physis of the longer bone to stop bone growth, enabling the shorter limb to catch up. All are dependent on the underlying reason for length inequality.

See: 'Limb lengthening and reconstruction: Types of surgery' (aboutkidshealth.ca).

Table 23.8 outlines the main advantages to the patient in using internal versus external lengthening procedures

Table 23.8 Comparison of external lengthening device versus internal device

External fixator	Internal lengthening
Joint stiffness	Less joint stiffness
Muscle contracture	Less pain
Pin infection	No pin site infections
Malalignment	Improved activity level whilst lengthening
Re-fracture	Faster rehabilitation

An internal lengthening nail may be the patient's preferred option (Herzenberg et al., 2013), due to the non-requirement for pin site cleaning and the ease of returning to mobility without the encumbrance of an external frame. The nail is an intramedullary locked nail (a nail placed down through the middle (medulla) of the bone), which is lengthened by placing a magnet over osteotomised bone (bone that has been cut). However, this treatment option is usually reserved for children who are reaching skeletal maturity.

The external fixator may be used to correct length or deformity in the growing child. They may also be employed in the management of some fractures, particularly complex trauma and when loss of soft tissue is involved (enabling care of wounds).

For an overview of the use of external fixators see Hadeed et al. (2022).

The main priorities of nursing care of a child with an external fixator include:

1. Pain relief
2. Neurovascular compromise
3. Pin site care
4. Mobilisation

ACTIVITY 23.6: REFLECTIVE PRACTICE

Review these key aspects of care

Walker (2018) 'Assessing and managing pin sites in patients with external fixation'. www.nursingtimes.net/clinical-archive/tissue-viability/assessing-and-managing-pin-sites-in-patients-with-external-fixation-18-12-2017/

Royal College of Nursing (2022) Guidance on pin site care. www.rcn.org.uk/professional-development/publications/pub-004137

Royal College of Nursing (2022) 'Peripheral neurovascular observations for acute limb compartment syndrome'. RCN Consensus Guidance. www.rcn.org.uk/professional-development/publications/peripheral-neurovascular-observations-for-alcs-uk-pub-009-905

FRACTURE IN THE CHILD OR YOUNG PERSON

Children's fractures are different from those of adults. The causes for bone injuries in children are usually simple. The fact most fractures in children heal fairly well with indifferent treatment has led the unwary to neglect the fact that other fractures terminate disastrously unless expertly handled. (Blount, 1955, p.1)

This quotation is still relevant today: treating a child's fracture can be simple or necessitate significant expertise, depending on the nature of the fracture. Similarly, the nursing care of the child with a fracture requires knowledge and competence to detect signs of compartment syndrome, and manage pain, swelling and immobility.

The child's long bone is made up of the diaphysis, metaphysis, physis and epiphysis (Figure 23.6).

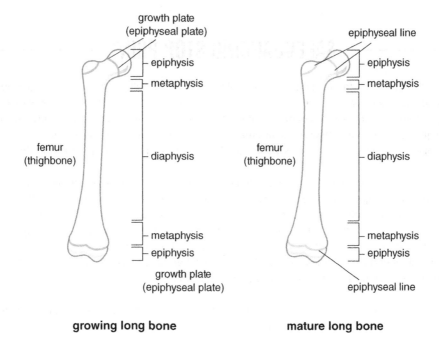

growing long bone   mature long bone

Figure 23.6 Growing long bone and mature long bone

http://kidshealth.org/en/growth-plate-injuries.html

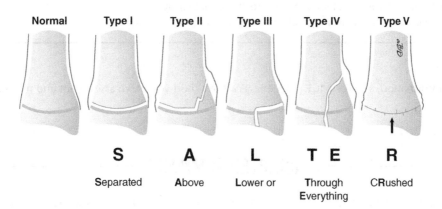

Figure 23.7 Salter Harris classification

A fracture through the physis (growth plate) will injure the growing cells of the bone. The severity of the injury is assessed using the Salter Harris (SH) classification (Figure 23.7). An SH 1 fracture is least likely to cause any long-term problems, whilst an SH 5 fracture will affect the growth of the bone and require follow-up.

Diagnosing a fracture in a child is not always straightforward. An X-ray of the injured limb may be ambiguous due to the cartilaginous components of the bone (dependent on the age of the child). It therefore requires a clear history and a thorough clinical examination, looking for reduced range of movement, deformity and pain. It is important to note whether the history fits the pattern of the fracture, and any discrepancies in the description of the injury should alert the practitioner. Any fracture sustained in the non-ambulant child requires careful investigation.

SAFEGUARDING STOP POINT

Every NHS Trust has a local child protection policy and lead consultant. As nurses it is our duty of care to appreciate the vulnerability of all children to potential abuse, in particular those with disability. A child who presents with an unexplained fracture requires investigation, but it is also important to recognise that disabled children are at greater risk of abuse than non-disabled children, and it is essential that safeguarding strategies are in place to protect them from harm and ensure their needs are met.

Treatment of the fracture is to realign the bone ends, and whilst a degree of angulation can be accepted (depending on the bone involved and the age of the child), rotational deformities require correction. Immobilisation of a fracture may be achieved by a plaster cast, traction, internal fixation with metal work, or external fixation such as a circular frame. Generally, the child will recover quickly following treatment for a fracture. Once out of immobilisation, when the fracture has healed, the child will self-limit their activities until confident. Physiotherapy is therefore rarely required.

The nurse's role in caring for the child with a fracture is to:

- Assess for peripheral neurovascular deficit (signs and symptoms of vascular problems to the limb) and report any concerns promptly
- Elevate the limb to reduce swelling
- Ensure the child receives optimal pain relief
- Reassure and explain the reason for immobilisation
- Educate the child and family in the care of the cast/splint
- Provide written family and child information and contact details

Further information, see: the NICE guideline 'Fractures (non-complex): assessment and management' (2016).

CHAPTER SUMMARY

- Musculoskeletal (MSK) conditions in children can be either acquired (e.g., trauma) or congenital/ developmental (e.g., clubfoot, hip dysplasia). The impact of MSK conditions may be short-lived

or lifelong, often with implications on the social, financial and daily living aspects for the child, family and carers
- Whilst specialist paediatric orthopaedic nursing is becoming centralised into the larger 'hub' hospitals, the generalist nurse in a district general hospital needs to have basic MSK knowledge and skills to provide safe and effective care
- The delivery of expert care for the child with a musculoskeletal disorder requires the nurse to be knowledgeable about the differences in the child's anatomy and the impact of growth on the structure and function of the MSK system. It is also key to have the skills to adapt orthopaedic interventions to meet the needs of the child or young person
- The differentiation between what is normal for a child and young person, versus the abnormal is paramount in the assessment; applying knowledge of normal milestones and gait pattern and understanding the impact a co-morbidity may have
- The nurse needs to have knowledge of their hospital's procedure for safeguarding concerns and bear these considerations in mind, especially when caring for the child presenting to the emergency department with musculoskeletal trauma

BUILD YOUR BIBLIOGRAPHY

Books

- Clarke, S. and Drozd, M. (eds) (2023) *Orthopaedic and Trauma Nursing. An Evidence-based Approach to Musculoskeletal Care*, 2nd edn. Oxford: Wiley-Blackwell.

    This book provides practitioners with up-to-date evidence and knowledge which underpins safe and effective nursing practice. It includes a specific section on the management of children.
- Judd, J. (2008) 'Application and care of traction', in J. Kelsey and G. McEwing (eds), *Clinical Skills in Child Health Practice*. London: Churchill Livingstone.

    This chapter gives a complete pictorial overview of the application of Thomas splint traction.
- Staheli, L.T. (2016) *Fundamentals of Pediatric Orthopedics*, 5th edn. Seattle, WA: Lippincott Williams & Wilkins.

    This book is an excellent resource covering children's orthopaedic conditions in a question and answer format.

FURTHER
READING

Journal articles

- Smith., S., Sumar, B. and Dixon., K. (2014) 'Musculoskeletal pain in overweight and obese children.' *International Journal of Obesity*, 38: 11–15. https://doi.org/10.1038/ijo.2013.187

    Read this article and reflect on the increasing problem of obesity in children and how it impacts on their growing skeleton. Obesity is also linked to slipped capital femoral epiphysis and vitamin D deficiency.

    Sherry, D., Sonagra, M. and Gmuca, S. (2020) 'The spectrum of pediatric amplified musculoskeletal pain syndrome'. *Pediatric Rheumatology Online Journal*, 18: 77.

    This paper examines the characteristics of the wide spectrum of amplified pain syndrome, that children may present with.

FURTHER
READING:
ONLINE
JOURNAL
ARTICLES

- Sims-Gould, J., Race, J., Hamilton, L., MacDonald, H., Mulpuri, K. and Mckay, H. (2016) '"I fell off and landed badly": Children's experiences of forearm fracture and injury prevention'. *Journal of Child Health Care*, 20 (1): 98–108.

  Using a research method called Photovoice this article presents children's views on their injury experience and reviews fracture prevention.

- Phelps, E.E., Tutton, E., Costa, M.L. et al. (2022) 'Protecting my injured child: a qualitative study of parents' experience of caring for a child with a displaced distal radius fracture'. *BMC Pediatrics*, 22 (1): 270. doi: 10.1186/s12887-022-03340-z

  This study looked at the child's and family's experiences after sustaining a displaced distal radius fracture. It discusses their participation in a research trial (CRAFFT) and highlights the importance of providing parents with information of surgical versus non-operative management of the injury. For further reading on the research project see: www.ndorms.ox.ac.uk/research/clinical-trials/current-trials-and-studies/crafft.

Weblinks

FURTHER
READING:
WEBLINKS

- RCN – *Benchmarks for Children's Orthopaedic Nursing Care* www2.rcn.org.uk/__data/assets/pdf_file/0007/115486/RCN_CYP_ortho_WEB.pdf
- RCN – *A Competence Framework for Orthopaedic and Trauma Practitioners* www.rcn.org.uk/library/Subject-Guides/orthopaedic-and-trauma-nursing Provides a framework for orthopaedic and trauma practitioners in clinical recognising the specific, specialist knowledge and skills required and reflecting different levels of practice and job roles. The document can be used as a self-assessment tool, ultising learning contracts.
- International Hip Dysplasia Institute www.hipdysplasia.org A wealth of evidence-based literature for the practitioner and essential information and advice for parents.
- RCN – *Guidance on Pin Site Care* www2.rcn.org.uk/__data/assets/pdf_file/0009/413982/004137.pdf Report and recommendations from the 2010 Consensus Project on pin site care (updated 2022).
- The child with a musculoskeletal alteration https://nursekey.com/the-child-with-a-musculo-skeletal-alteration/ An overview of the structure of the musculoskeletal system in children, assessment and evaluation and treatment modalities.

REFERENCES

Aarvold, A., Perry, D.C., Mavrotas, J., Theologis, T., Katchburian, M., on behalf of the BSCOS DDH Consensus Group (2023) 'The management of developmental dysplasia of the hip in children aged under three months'. *Bone and Joint Journal*, 105-B(2): 209–14.

Blount, W.T. (1955) *Fractures in Children*. Baltimore, MD: Williams & Wilkins.

Bowen, J.R., Guille, J.T., Jeong, C., Worananarat, P., Oh, C-W., Rodriquez, A., Holmes, L. and Rogers, K.J. (2011) 'Labral support shelf arthroplasty for containment in early stages of Legg-Calve-Perthes disease'. *Journal of Pediatric Orthopaedics*, 31 (2) Supplement: S206–11.

Carsi, B., Judd, J. and Clarke, N.M.P. (2015) 'Shelf acetabuloplasty for containment in the early stages of Legg-Calve-Perthes disease'. *Journal of Pediatric Orthopaedics*, 35 (2): 151–6.

Cashman, J.P., Round, J., Taylor, G. and Clarke, N.M.P. (2002) 'The natural history of developmental dysplasia of the hip after early supervised treatment in the Pavlik harness'. *Journal of Bone and Joint Surgery*, 84 (3): 418–25.

Clarke, N.M.P. and Castanada, P. (2012) 'Strategies to improve non-operative childhood management'. *Orthopaedic Clinics of North America*, 43: 281–9.

Clarke, N.M.P., Taylor, C.C. and Judd, J. (2016) 'Diagnosis and management of developmental dysplasia of the hip'. *Paediatrics and Child Health*, 26 (6): 252–6.

Clarke, S. (2023) 'Key issues in caring for the child and young person with an orthopaedic or musculoskeletal trauma condition', in S. Clarke and Drozd. M (eds), *Orthopaedic and Trauma Nursing: An Evidenced-based Approach to Musculoskeletal Care*, 2nd edn. Oxford: Wiley–Blackwell.

Clarke, S. and McKay, M. (2006) 'An audit of spica cast guidelines for parents and professionals caring for children with developmental dysplasia of the hip'. *Journal of Orthopaedic Nursing*, 10 (3): 128–37.

Clarke, S. and Santy-Tomlinson, J. (eds) (2014) *Orthopaedic and Trauma Nursing: An Evidenced-based Approach to Musculoskeletal Care*. Oxford: Wiley–Blackwell.

Dougherty, B.L., Zelikovsky, N., Miller, K.S., Rodriguez, D., Armstrong, S.L. and Sherry, D.D. (2021) 'Longitudinal impact of parental catastrophizing on child functional disability in pediatric amplified pain'. *Journal of Pediatric Psychology*, 46 (4): 474–84.

Eastwood, D.M. and de Gheldere, A. (2010) 'Clinical examination for developmental dysplasia of the hip in neonates: how to stay out of trouble'. *British Medical Journal*, 340: c1965.

Engesæter, I.Ø., Lehmann, T., Laborie, L.B., Lie, S.A., Rosendahl, K. and Engesæter, L.B. (2011) 'Total hip replacement in young adults with hip dysplasia. Age at diagnosis, previous treatment, quality of life, and validation of diagnoses reported to the Norwegian Arthroplasty Register between 1987 and 2007'. *Acta Orthopaedica*, 82 (2): 149–55

Galloway, A.M., van-Hille, T., Perry, D.C., Holton, C., Mason, L., Richards, S., Siddle, H.J. and Comer, C. (2020) 'A systematic review of the non-surgical treatment of Perthes' disease'. *Bone and Joint Open*, 1 (12): 720–30.

Gelfer, Y., Blanco, J., Trees, A., Davis, N., Buckingham, R., Peek, A.C., Wright, E. et al. (2021) 'Attaining a British consensus statement on managing idiopathic congenital talipes equinovarus (CTEV) through a Delphi process: a study protocol'. *British Medical Journal Open*, 11: e049212.

Hadeed, A., Werntz, R.L. and Varacallo, M. (2022) External Fixation Principles and Overview. [Updated 2021 Jul 31]. In: StatPearls [Internet]. Treasure Island (FL): StatPearls Publishing; 2022.

Herzenberg, J.H., Standard, S.C. and Specht, S.C. (2013) 'Limb lengthening in children with a new, controllable internal device'. Poster. *European Paediatric Orthopaedic Society (EPOS)*, April 17–20, 2013; Athens, Greece.

Horan, M.P., Williams, K. and Hughes, D. (2019) 'The role of vitamin D in pediatric orthopedics'. *Orthopedics Clinics of North America*, 50 (2): 181–91.

Joseph, B. (2015) 'Management of Perthes' disease'. *Indian Journal of Orthopaedics*, 49 (1): 10–16.

Judd, J. (2004) 'Congenital talipes equinovarus – evidence for using the Ponseti method of treatment'. *Journal of Orthopaedic Nursing*, 8 (3): 160–3.

Judd, J. (2010) 'Defining expertise in paediatric orthopaedic nursing'. *International Journal of Orthopaedic and Trauma Nursing*, 14 (3): 159–68.

Judd, J. (2013) 'Rickets in the 21st century: a review of the consequences of low vitamin D and its management'. *International Journal of Orthopaedic and Trauma Nursing*, 17 (4): 199–208.

Judd, J. (2023) 'Common childhood orthopaedic conditions, their care and management', in S. Clarke and M. Drozd (eds), *Orthopaedic and Trauma Nursing: An Evidenced-based Approach to Musculoskeletal Care*, 2nd edn. Oxford: Wiley–Blackwell.

Judd, J. and Clarke, N.M.P. (2014) 'Treatment and prevention of hip dysplasia in infants and young children'. *Early Human Development*, 90 (11) 2014. Available at: www.scribd.com/document/535450102/Early-Human-Development-Volume-90-Issue-11-2014-Doi-10-1016-j-earlhumdev-2014-08-011-Judd-Julia-Clarke-Nicholas-M-P-Treatment-and-Prevention# (accessed 19 June 2023).

Julies, P., Lynn, R.M., Pall, K., Leoni, M., Calder, A., Mughal, Z., Shaw, N., McDonnell, C., McDevitt, H. and Blair, M. (2020) 'Nutritional rickets under 16 years: UK surveillance results'. *Archives of Diseases in Childhood*, 105 (6): 587–92.

Leo, D.G., Jones, H., Murphy, R., Leong, J.W., Gambling, T., Long, A.F., Laine, J. and Perry, D.C. (2020) 'The outcomes of Perthes' disease'. *Bone and Joint Journal*, 102-B (5): 611–17.

Logan, D.E., Williams, S.E., Carullo, V.P., Claar, R.L., Bruehl, S. and Berde, C.B. (2013) 'Children and adolescents with complex regional pain syndrome: more psychologically distressed than other children in pain?' *Pain Research Management*, 18 (2): 87–93.

Matsumoto, H., Hyman, J.E., Shah, H.H., Sankar, W.N., Laine, J.C., Mehlman, C.T. et al. International Perthes Study Group (2020) 'Validation of Pediatric Self-Report Patient-Reported Outcomes Measurement Information System (PROMIS) Measures in different stages of Legg-Calvé-Perthes disease'. *Journal of Pediatric Orthopedics*, 40 (5): 235–40.

National Osteoporosis Society (2018) *Vitamin D and Bone Health: A Practical Clinical Guideline for Patient Management in Children and Young People*. Available at: https://ros-vitamin-d-and-bone-health-in-children-november-2018.pdf (theros.org.uk).

NDORMS: Children's Radius Acute Fracture Fixation Trial (2020) 'A multi-centre prospective randomised non-inferiority trial of surgical reduction versus non-surgical casting for displaced distal radius fractures in children'. Available at: www.ndorms.ox.ac.uk/research/clinical-trials/current-trials-and-studies/crafft (accessed 19 June 2023).

NICE (National Institute for Health and Care Excellence) (2016) Fractures (non-complex): assessment and management. Nice guideline [NG38]. Available at: www.nice.org.uk/guidance/ng38 (accessed 19 June 2023).

Osteoporosis Foundation (2017) Building Strong Bones in Youth. Available at: www.osteoporosis. foundation/sites/iofbonehealth/files/2019-03/2017_BuildingStrongBonesInYouth_Brochure_English.pdf

Parmentier, C., Madoki, A., Mercier, P. and Docquier, P. (2016) 'Shelf acetabuloplasty in Perthes disease: comparison with nonoperative treatment'. *Current Orthopaedic Practice*, 27 (4): 375–81.

Perry, D.C., Arch, B., Appelbe, D., Francis, P., Craven, J., Monsell, F.P., Williamson, P. and Knight, M.; BOSS collaborators (2022) 'The British Orthopaedic Surgery Surveillance study: Perthes' disease: the epidemiology and two-year outcomes from a prospective cohort in Great Britain'. *Bone and Joint Journal*, 104-B (4): 510–18.

Perry, D. C. and Bruce, C. (2010) 'Evaluating the child who presents with an acute limp'. *British Medical Journal*, 341: c4250. Available at: www.bmj.com/content/bmj/341/7770/Clinical_Review. full.pdf (accessed 19 June 2023).

Public Health England (2016) Newborn and Infant Physical Examination Screening Programme Standards 2016/17. Available at: http://www.webmedcentral.com/article_view/1173 (accessed 23 May 2017).

Public Health England (2021) NIPE newborn hip screening: screen positive pathway. Available at: www.gov.uk/government/publications/newborn-and-infant-physical-examination-programme-handbook/nipe-newborn-hip-screening-screen-positive-pathway (accessed 25 January 2021).

Rhodes, A. and Aarvold, A. (2022) 'Screening for developmental dysplasia of the hip: current UK practice and controversies'. *Orthopaedics and Trauma*, 36 (6): 317–21.

Tripathy, S., Sen, R., Dhatt, S. and Goyal, T. (2010) 'Legg-Calve-Perthes disease: current concepts'. *WebmedCentral Orthopaedics*, 1 (11). Available at: www.webmedcentral.com/article_view/1173 (accessed 23 May 2017).

Walker, J. (2018) 'Assessing and managing pin sites in patients with external fixation'. *Nursing Times* [online]; 114 (1): 18–21. Available at: www.nursingtimes.net/clinical-archive/tissue-viability/assessing-and-managing-pin-sites-in-patients-with-external-fixation-18-12-2017/.

Young, J.R., Anderson, M.J., O'Connor, C.M., Kazley, J.M., Mantica, A.L. and Dutt, V. (2020) 'Team approach: developmental dysplasia of the hip'. *Journal of Bone and Joint Surgery Reviews*, 8 (9): e20.00030.

CARE OF CHILDREN AND YOUNG PEOPLE WITH HAEMATOLOGICAL PROBLEMS

24

LIZZY HOOLE

THIS CHAPTER COVERS

- Blood cell and bleeding disorders
- Common benign haematological conditions
- Blood transfusions – administration and care
- Care of children and young people with blood disorders and their family

---

REQUIRED KNOWLEDGE

In preparation for this chapter, it would be helpful to understand haematopoiesis (the formation of blood cellular components) and the haematological system.

For a diagram of haematopoiesis, please go to https://commons.wikimedia.org/wiki/File:Hematopoiesis_(human)_diagram_en.svg.

Blood is considered one of the connective tissues in the body, as it consists of cellular components within a fluid matrix called plasma. Blood is the only liquid tissue in the body. It is involved in transportation, regulation and protection and connects the systems of the body together.

Transportation: of oxygen, carbon dioxide and waste products from the tissues to the lungs, and kidneys where these waste products can be removed from the body. Also, in transporting and carrying hormones.

Regulation: of body temperature, pH, and fluid and electrolyte balance.

Protection: by preventing fluid loss through clotting mechanisms and helping to protect the body against microorganisms and diseases.

Table 24.1 outlines the major information about formation and functions of the blood and lymph tissues. The cells within these systems are formed from pluripotent stem cells, originally present in the embryo and capable of forming any type of body cell, which create the two multipotent stem cells from which the range of blood cells are formed.

It is helpful to understand the normal haematology blood ranges in healthy children to know when something is out of range (see Table 24.1 below). Always follow local guidelines for normal blood ranges.

Table 24.1   Normal blood ranges in children

Age	Hb (g/L)	Platelets (x10⁹/l)	WBC (x10⁹/l)	Neutrophils (x10⁹/l)	Lymphocytes (x10⁹/l)
Birth	140-240		10.2-26.0	2.7-14.4	2.0-8.0
2 weeks	134-198		6.0-21.0	1.5-5.4	2.8-9.1
4 weeks	134-198		6.0-21.0	1.5-5.4	2.8-9.1
2-6 months	94-130		5.0-15.0	1.0-5.0	4.0-10.0
6 months-1 year	111-141	150 -400	6.0-17.5	1.0-8.5	4.0-12.0
1-6 years	115-140	(at all ages)	5.0-17.0	1.0-8.5	1.5-9.5
6-12 years	115-140		4.5-14.5	1.0-8.5	1.5-7.0
12-18 years Females	120-160		4.5-13.0	1.5-8.0	1.1-4.5
12-18 years Males	130-170		4.5-13.0	1.5-8.0	1.1-4.5

Information in table above recognised from NBT Southmead:
www.nbt.nhs.uk/sites/default/files/Childrens%20FBC%20Reference%20Ranges.pdf

"Benign haematological conditions vary immensely. Some are very simple to manage. Advice and reassurance to the family and primary care may be all that is needed.
Other conditions are much more complex. They may involve a large number of investigations over a significant period of time. Uncertainty about diagnosis and prognosis can be a key issue for the family that needs holding in this period."

Dr John Moppett, Paediatric Haematology Consultant

INTRODUCTION

Blood helps to maintain homeostasis in the body, therefore any changes to normal blood ranges or functioning of the cells impact health. As highlighted in the opening quote above, some blood disorders are complex, some life-limiting, although through medical advances, many are now manageable and children can lead relatively normal lives. Early detection and intervention are crucial in ensuring morbidities and mortality are avoided, and quality of life maintained.

This chapter includes an overview of the anatomy and physiology of blood and its functions, some of the common blood disorders and bleeding disorders that you may come across in practice and will refer to the genetic and genomic factors associated with a few conditions.

BLOOD ANATOMY AND PHYSIOLOGY

As you can see from Table 24.2, blood is composed of 55% plasma and 45% cells. Red blood cells account for 41% of these cells, while white blood cells and platelets only account for about 4%.

Table 24.2 Blood composition

Component	Function
Haemopoietic stem cells	These cells are pluripotent, meaning they can develop into all types of blood cells, including red and white blood cells, and platelets
Lymphoid progenitor cells: B cells, T cells and natural killer (NK) cells	These white blood cells are involved in acquired or antigen-specific immune response. NK cells are also involved in the innate immune response
Myeloid progenitor cells: neutrophils, eosinophils, basophils, mast cells, monocytes	These white blood cells are responsible for the innate immune response. They release substances to kill invading microorganisms and signal other blood cells to come and help
Dendric cells	These cells guide the immune response by linking innate and adaptive immune responses
Erythrocytes (red blood cells)	These cells contain haemoglobin which carries oxygen around the body
Thrombocytes (platelets)	These cells form clots to stop or prevent bleeding
Plasma (about 55% of blood)	A liquid which carries blood cells around the body, and contains proteins and other vital substances. It helps maintain blood pressure, blood volume, pH balance, and body temperature
Albumin	The protein which makes up half of the plasma content. It helps prevent fluid leaking out of the blood stream and helps vital substances to circulate throughout the body
Clotting factors	Proteins which work together in a series of chemical reactions to stop bleeding and form a blood clot
Immunoglobulins	Known as antibodies, act as a critical part of the immune response, by recognising and binding to particular antigens such as bacteria or viruses

ACTIVITY 24.1: CRITICAL THINKING

Before continuing the chapter, consider the impact to a child or young person's health if they lacked one or more of the components listed in Table 24.2.

BLOOD CELL DISORDERS

Benign blood cell disorders include red and white blood cell and platelet (bleeding) disorders. Pancytopenia is the deficiency of all three of these cellular components. It occurs when there is a problem with the blood-forming stem cells in the bone marrow.

Lack of red blood cells (anaemia) causes fatigue, weakness, dizziness, tachycardia, tachypnoea and pallor. The consequences of long-term anaemia are well documented (Zavaleta and Astete-Robilliard, 2017; World Health Organization, 2023) which are, impaired growth, impaired cognitive and motor development, reduced school performance, reduced quality of life and overall morbidities.

Lack of white blood cells, including neutrophils (neutropenia) puts the child at serious risk of sepsis. Neutropenic sepsis is potentially life-threatening and the assessment and management should include

SEE ALSO
CHAPTER 14

the 'Sepsis Six' screening and action tools which can be found here: www.sepsistrust.org/professional-resources/acute-inpatients-nice/.

Lack of platelets (thrombocytopenia) causes easy and excessive bruising, petechiae (pin prick red/purple spots), purpura (red/purple flat patches similar to bruises), nose bleeds, bleeding gums, blood in urine or stool, unusually heavy periods in older girls, and in extreme cases, internal bleeding.

The assessment of any of these conditions would require:

- Urgent full blood count (FBC) and reticulocytes
- Blood film
- Clotting screen
- A direct Coombs test and immunoglobulins
- A urine dipstick (to assess for non-visible haematuria)
- A full A–E assessment

Each hospital will have clinical guidelines for the assessment and management of children presenting with a potential blood disorder.

If assessing a child with a serious injury or major active bleeding a <C>ABCDE assessment should be carried out, as per the NICE guidelines (NICE, 2016) in order to assess for catastrophic haemorrhage <C> prior to moving on to a structured A–E assessment.

SEE ALSO
CHAPTER 14

SAFEGUARDING STOP POINT

When assessing the child's skin as part of the A-E nursing assessment, any rashes, bruising, or lacerations should be noted. It is also essential to assess bruising in the context of the child's age, developmental stage, known allergies, and exposure. The possibility of non-accidental injury should not be overlooked, and so it is important to assess the child's pattern of injury/illness to ensure ongoing management is appropriate and any relevant treatments are given. Multiple bruises on a non-mobile baby are uncommon and should raise significant concerns about abuse or neglect.

However, large amounts of bruising can also be due to a bleeding disorder. Go to https://patient.info/ and search for immune thrombocytopenia - read the professional article section on immune thrombocytopenia in children for more information.

Common benign haematological conditions

ITP is a condition where the immune system attacks platelets, impacting the body's ability to form clots, resulting in excessive bleeding. ITP is one of the most common acquired bleeding disorders affecting children (Kim and Despotovic, 2021), being more common in girls than boys. The presenting signs and symptoms are as previously described with thrombocytopenia. Treatment should be based on the severity of symptoms and not on platelet count alone. In about 75% of childhood cases the condition is self-resolving within 6 months, requiring no treatment, and the relapse rate is often low. However, in some cases (see Case study 24.1), treatment is required due to the severity of bleeding symptoms, and the condition can become persistent (lasting more than 6 months) or chronic (lasting more than 12 months). It is not often clear what triggers childhood ITP; therefore, continuing active research is vital to further our understanding of the condition.

GO FURTHER

The UK Paediatric ITP registry (https://itp.mdsas.com/?avia_forced_reroute=1) aims to collect data to understand more about childhood cases of ITP, and identify potential causes and treatments.

CASE STUDY 24.1: EVIE

Evie, a 10-year-old girl, presented to the children's emergency department with a 2-week history of bruising, widespread petechial rash and nose bleeds. She had recently suffered with a viral illness. Evie had blood tests performed and was referred to the haematology specialty with a suspected diagnosis of ITP. Her platelets remained severely low, and due to the clinical factors with her presentation she was admitted for intravenous immunoglobulin (IVIg) therapy to raise the platelet levels and prevent further bleeding.

Evie's symptoms improved, she was discharged and reviewed with weekly full blood counts.

Unfortunately, her response to treatment was short-term. She required ongoing management and treatment over the following 12 months; therefore, her condition was considered chronic.

- How would the diagnosis impact Evie and her family?
- What support would Evie and her family require during the initial admission to hospital?
- What teams/professionals would be involved in her ongoing care?

Anaemia is where the number of red blood cells or the levels of haemoglobin are lower than normal. Causes for anaemia include nutrition deficiencies, with iron deficiency anaemia being the most common in children (GOSH, 2016). Iron is an important component of haemoglobin and is found in two forms in several food sources – heme iron commonly found in red meats, chicken and fish, and non-heme iron found in plant-based foods such as grains and vegetables. Therefore, through diet management you can increase the levels of iron in your body, and by consuming foods rich in Vitamin C alongside, you can aid particularly the non-heme iron absorption process (Tan, 2017; Nianyi et al., 2020). Providing support and education to children and families through health promotion techniques are key aspects of the role of a nurse. Empowering parents with nutritional education could significantly prevent iron deficient anaemia in children and could prevent the long-term consequences of anaemia previously mentioned.

Aplastic anaemia is a rare but serious condition where your immune system attacks healthy stem cells in your bone marrow, which therefore stop producing sufficient amounts of new blood cells. This is also termed 'bone marrow failure' and leads to pancytopenia.

Aplastic anaemia can be inherited, meaning it is passed down through the genes from parent to child. Aplastic anaemia is classified as non-severe, severe, or very severe depending on blood cell count. Severe and very-severe aplastic anaemia can be fatal, and stem cell (bone marrow) transplant is the only potential cure; however, a stem cell transplant comes with a risk of serious complications.

Haemoglobinopathies are a group of inherited genetic conditions caused by genetic changes in the structure and production of haemoglobin. Over 1500 genetic changes have been found that result in variants to haemoglobin or thalassaemia (Giardine et al., 2014). According to the World Health Organization (2021), approximately 5% of the world's population are healthy carriers of the genes for haemoglobin disorders, mainly sickle cell disease and thalassaemia.

Sickle cell disease is the most common serious genetic condition affecting people in England, with between 260 and 350 babies born with the condition each year (Public Health England, 2018). It predominantly occurs in people of African, Caribbean, Indian and Middle Eastern ethnicity.

The most common and serious form is called sickle cell anaemia, where red blood cells have an abnormal crescent moon shape, which become rigid and sticky when the haemoglobin is de-oxygenated. The sickle cells can get stuck, blocking capillaries and small vessels, causing painful and serious complications, described as a sickle cell crisis. A sickle cell crisis can be triggered by dehydration, sudden changes in body temperature and infection. The red blood cells in a child with sickle cell disease have a shortened life span, lasting 10–20 days, compared to the normal 120-day lifespan. Severe anaemia is the result and puts the child at risk of infections, strokes and tissue damage. As mentioned by the practitioner below, the management of children with conditions like this should be under a specialist service, providing monitoring, education and nutritional information.

"Many benign haematological conditions are long-term conditions which families and patients need to learn to live with and manage throughout their lives. Throughout this journey families need the support and advice of the whole multi-disciplinary team as their condition affects their growth, development, schooling, and family life."

Dr John Moppett, Paediatric Haematology Consultant

Thalassemia is another genetic condition. Normal haemoglobin contains two alpha and two beta globin chains, each of these chains contains genetic information. The location and extent of a genetic change will determine whether the child has alpha- or beta-thalassemia and will determine the severity of the condition. It is possible to inherit genetic changes to both concurrently. There are approximately 20 babies born with the most common form, beta-thalassemia major, in England each year (Public Health England, 2021). It is most common in individuals of South-East Asian, Mediterranean and Middle Eastern ethnicity.

As mentioned in the practitioner voice above, the management of children with conditions like thalassemia and sickle cell disease should be under a specialist MDT, providing monitoring, physiotherapy, education, and nutritional information.

As we have established, there are several genetically inherited blood cell disorders. Studying the genetic and genomic data using DNA sequencing can significantly impact patient care through improved diagnosis, risk stratification and potential development of novel treatments. Whole genome sequencing is now being offered routinely to child cancer cases, and genomic testing for children with rare diseases (NHS England, 2022). Disease-specific testing is being developed for benign and malignant haematologic conditions (Getawa and Melku, 2022), which can benefit children with unusual presentations and could provide a diagnosis (Zhang et al., 2015). As genomic medicine is mainstreamed into routine practice, it will be increasingly important for nurses to have a comprehensive understanding of its applications in practice. This topic is also covered in Chapter 10.

SEE ALSO
CHAPTER 10

ACTIVITY 24.2: REFLECTIVE PRACTICE

Collaborative working is essential in the care of children with a blood disorder.

Whilst on a placement, spend time with the benign haematology Clinical Nurse Specialist (if possible) and attend a clinic where these children are seen. Reflect on your observations with your practice assessor.

BLEEDING DISORDERS

Bleeding disorders are a group of conditions where there is a problem with the body's ability to form clots. This can be caused by defects in the platelets and/or clotting factors. The body produces several clotting factors, and if any of them are deficient, clotting will be impacted. Clotting factor deficiencies are often inherited. Haemophilia A is caused by a genetic deficiency in clotting factor VIII, and haemophilia B by a genetic deficiency in clotting factor IX. Both conditions are X-linked disorders, which means that the affected gene is found on the 'X' sex chromosome, of which females have two and males have one. These conditions can be passed down in two ways, X-linked dominant and X-linked recessive, and due to the sex chromosome, they are usually inherited from the mother, and affect more boys than girls (Figure 24.1).

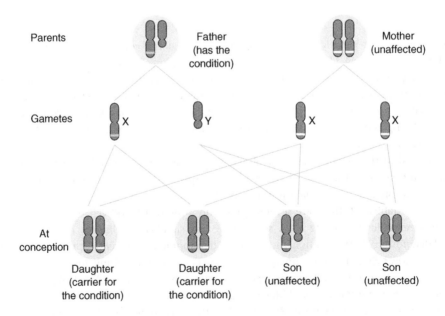

Figure 24.1 X-linked inheritance

https://www.genomicseducation.hee.nhs.uk/genotes/knowledge-hub/x-linked-recessive-inheritance/

Both types of haemophilia have the same symptoms; bruising easily, excessive/prolonged bleeding, bleeding into joints/muscles which can be without obvious cause, causing pain, swelling and long-term damage. Physiotherapy can help to maintain muscle strength and functioning and is an important part of managing the condition. The treatment of haemophilia is by administering a regular intravenous infusions of clotting factor replacement. Over the last decade significant developments have been made through research into new gene therapies, which have been developed for use in adults. Gene therapies offer the chance for a long-term and potentially curative treatment option and could prevent severe bleeds, reduce the need for frequent injections and improve patients' overall quality of life. However, despite continued active research into the efficacy of gene therapies, ongoing data is required to understand the long-term outcomes, and there are currently no licensed gene therapy treatments due to be commissioned by NHS England (Courtney, 2022).

"As a student, looking after these families is a privilege and an honour, they allow us to become part of a journey that they will reflect on for the rest of their life. For that reason, being part of a strong, hardworking team is paramount to the care we provide for these children. Furthermore, understanding their [haematological] condition or diagnosis enables me to deliver holistic patient-centred care to individuals and their families. These patients are with us for a long period of time and naturally, they become part of the ward family."

Amber, nursing student

As you can see from the student voice above, an understanding of haematological conditions is essential to deliver safe and effective care. See Case study 24.2.

CASE STUDY 24.2: JACOB

Jacob was diagnosed with severe haemophilia A when a few months old. Soon after diagnosis he had a port-a-cath inserted and he entered a clinical trial using an extended half-life Pegylated factor given on alternate days. The trial required several monitoring visits which were above routine care and needed to be performed at the Primary Treatment Centre 3 hours from the family's home. By the end of the trial his condition was slightly improved, he had no bleeding issues and very few bruises. He moved on to another treatment administered every 2 weeks, which he remained on, seemed to cope well with and had 6-monthly reviews.

- How do you think this diagnosis impacted Jacob at such a young age?
- Being on a clinical trial required several extra visits. Consider how this impacted the family?
- The treatment at one point was given on alternate days. What education, training and support do you think Jacob's family would need?

Von Willebrand (vW) is the most common inherited bleeding disorder in which children have a deficiency of von Willebrand factor (vWf). There are several types of vW disease, the most common are termed:

Type 1 – mildest and most common. Reduced levels of vWf, bleeding is only a problem if the individual has surgery, dental extraction or suffers an injury. This occurs if one parent has a genetic fault which is passed on.

Type 2 –the vWf does not work efficiently, bleeding can be more frequent and heavier than in type 1. This occurs when one parent has a faulty gene which is passed on.

Type 3 - most rare and severe form. Children have little to no vWf and bleeding is much more common. This occurs when both parents have a faulty gene which is passed on.

As with the previous blood cell disorders we have looked at, patients with haemophilia and vW require management and support from a specialist team, with a collaborative approach. As children are often diagnosed at an early age, they can be under the same team of professionals for most of their childhood, and it is important that transition to adult services is managed in a timely, supportive manner.

Most people with vW disease can lead normal, active lives, and can manage the condition with medicine. It can affect both men and women; however, women are more likely to experience adverse symptoms due to heavy periods and should have monitoring through pregnancy/childbirth. Treatments for vW disease include tranexamic acid, desmopressin, vWf replacement therapy, and contraception measures for menstruating women. In severe cases symptoms similar to haemophilia can occur, such as bleeding in the joints/muscles, and therefore management will be determinant of the person's individual condition.

The chances of inheriting type 1 vW disease can also be affected by blood group; people with blood group O are often more affected than people with blood groups A or B.

Blood groups

The ABO and RhD blood group systems are the most important to understand for clinical practice. Categorising individuals into blood groups is based on the presence or absence of antigens on the surface of their red blood cells as well as the presence of the opposite antibody within the individual's plasma (see Figure 24.2)

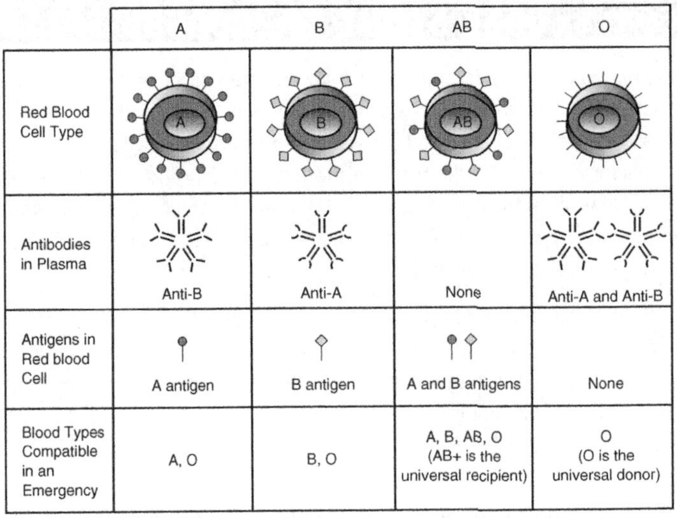

	A	B	AB	O
Red Blood Cell Type				
Antibodies in Plasma	Anti-B	Anti-A	None	Anti-A and Anti-B
Antigens in Red blood Cell	A antigen	B antigen	A and B antigens	None
Blood Types Compatible in an Emergency	A, O	B, O	A, B, AB, O (AB+ is the universal recipient)	O (O is the universal donor)

Figure 24.2 ABO blood groups

https://commons.wikimedia.org/wiki/File:1913_ABO_Blood_Groups.jpg

ABO and Rh

As you can see from Figure 24.2, an individual is categorised into 1 of 4 groups, A, B, AB or O, based on the combination or absence of A or B antigens on their red blood cells. Within the first few months of life, healthy children form ABO antibodies (in the plasma) to the A or B antigens on red blood cells. Individuals with blood group O are sometimes considered 'universal donors' because their red cells have no A or B antigens, and they create all the relevant ABO antibodies, so they can donate blood to any of the other blood groups. However, they can only receive group O blood transfusions.

Each of the blood groups can either be Rh-positive or Rh-negative, and they are commonly termed, for example A positive (A Rh-positive) and A negative (A Rh-negative). The Rh blood group system is comprised by several different antigens, the most important being the D antigen (RhD). Like most blood group antibodies, RhD ('anti-D') antibodies are only created through exposure to the foreign antigen. Individuals only develop antibodies to RhD if a RhD male or female is transfused with RhD-positive red blood cells, or if a RhD-negative female becomes pregnant with a RhD-positive baby.

If a RhD-negative individual who has developed anti-D antibodies through either of the above circumstances, is subsequently transfused with RdD-positive blood, their anti-D antibodies will attack it resulting in a transfusion reaction. Therefore, it is important to avoid giving RhD blood to RhD-negative individuals, except in an extreme emergency. If you have RhD-positive blood, you can receive RhD-positive or negative blood transfusions. See Table 24.3.

Table 24.3 Blood transfusions

Patient's blood group	Blood they can receive
O+	O+ O–
O–	O–
A+	O+ O– A+ A–
A–	O– A–
B+	O+ O– B+ B–
B–	O– B–
AB+	O+ O– A+ A– B+ B– AB+ AB–
AB–	O– A– B– AB–

Information recognised from American Society of Hematology (2023). Available at: www.hematology.org/education/patients/blood-basics/blood-safety-and-matching.
Source: Adapted from www.blood.co.uk/why-give-blood/blood-types/

As plasma contains either A or B, or both A and B antibodies, individuals with AB blood are universal plasma donors, but they can only receive type AB plasma transfusions. Individuals with group O blood can safety receive plasma transfusions from any blood group due to group O not having either A or B antigens. See Table 24.4.

Table 24.4 Plasma transfusions

Patient's blood group	Compatible plasma donor
A	A, AB
B	B, AB
AB	AB
O	O, AB, A, B

Transfusions of blood components may be required for some of the conditions we have discussed in this chapter or following immunosuppressive therapy such as chemotherapy. Nurses must have the appropriate education, training and competencies (as per local policy) in order to check and administer blood products.

GO FURTHER

There are interactive e-learning resources available through LearnBloodTransfusion (www.learnbloodtransfusion.org.uk/), developed by UK Blood Services and recognised by Health Education England, to support healthcare professionals with the safe administration of blood products.

Giving incompatible blood can be fatal; even a very small amount of incompatible blood can result in a significant transfusion reaction triggering a major immune response, and children can die from circulatory collapse. Ideally, people should receive their own precise blood type; however, if this is not possible, a compatible blood type must be given. When a blood transfusion is required, two crossmatch samples should be taken, to confirm the patient's blood group. It is vital that staff are vigilant in checking the patient's name band, confirming patient details with the patient/parent, and ensuring the crossmatch sample tubes are labelled accurately to prevent errors and delays in receipt of a blood product. A crossmatch sample remains valid for 72 hours before a new crossmatch will be required. This is particularly important in bone marrow transplant patients, due to them changing to their donor's blood group.

BLOOD TRANSFUSIONS – ADMINISTRATION AND CARE

Red blood cells transfusions may be required when a child is severely anaemic. For children, the amount is based on weight and haemoglobin levels (usually 15ml/kg). Red blood cells must be stored within a designated blood fridge and the infusion started within 30 minutes and administered within 4 hours of leaving the fridge.

Platelet transfusions may be required if the child has thrombocytopenia. Children can usually be prescribed 10–20ml/kg. Platelets are stored at room temperature on an agitator to prevent clumping. Bags of platelets are yellow/straw coloured, and prior to use the bag should be inspected for discoloration. Platelet transfusions are usually administered over 30 minutes (no quicker), and the unit should be administered within 2 hours of being removed from the agitator; after this they must be discarded. Red blood cells and platelets must be transfused using a dedicated giving set with filter.

Prior to a planned blood transfusion, an assessment should determine if the child is fit to proceed. The assessment should include any previous history of transfusion reactions (in which case a pre-med of chlorphenamine and paracetamol can be administered) and a baseline set of observations including, temperature, pulse, respiratory rate, and blood pressure. If there are any changes to the child's normal parameters, these must be communicated to the medical team. Once the transfusion is started, the child should be monitored with the same observations described above after 15 mins, and then as per local policy (usually hourly throughout the transfusion). Observations should then be repeated at the end of transfusion.

As well as the usual 'double checking', a bedside check with two nurses must be performed for blood product transfusions, as well as re-checking the child details against the blood product bag prior to administration.

Transfusion reactions

If there are any signs of a reaction during any blood product administration, stop the infusion immediately. Reactions could either be haemolytic or hypersensitivity reactions.

Haemolytic reactions can occur if there is an ABO, RhD or other incompatibility. Signs and symptoms include, hypotension, fever, rigors, chills, lower back pain, nausea, vomiting, diarrhoea, chest pain and dizziness. Management of such a reaction includes, an A–E assessment, monitoring of vital signs, administration of high flow oxygen, and administration of hydration and diuretics. The nursing process would need to be followed – Assess, Plan, Implement, Evaluate, Re-Evaluate.

Haemolytic reactions usually occur within the first 5–15 minutes of the transfusion; however, any reactions in the days following a transfusion should be considered as a potential transfusion reaction. To confirm a haemolytic reaction, blood samples would be required from the patient.

Signs and symptoms of an allergic hypersensitivity reaction include, urticaria (hives), facial swelling, wheezing, respiratory distress, nausea, vomiting, diarrhoea, fever, hypotension, shock, loss of consciousness. Reactions with hypersensitivity also usually occur within the first 5–15 minutes of the transfusion, and may initially be mild, often beginning with an itchy rash, but it is essential to stop the infusion and follow an anaphylaxis algorithm or local policies for transfusion reactions.

The medical team should be notified of any reaction and (depending on pre-meds given) paracetamol and chlorphenamine can be administered. If the reaction symptoms reduce, re-commencement of the infusion can be considered at a slower rate. Local policies should be followed regarding storing the empty blood product bag, documenting the reaction, communicating this to relevant teams, and documenting the reaction on the patient's drug chart to flag that pre-meds should be administered prior to future transfusions.

Consent for transfusion of a blood product

Consent must be obtained prior to transfusion of a blood product (unless there are emergency circumstances). When seeking consent, it is important to explain the risks and benefits of the transfusion to the child/parent and document this conversation as well as the type of transfusion required. Information about transfusions and leaflets are available from the National Blood and Transplant Service via: www.nhsbt.nhs.uk/what-we-do/blood-services/blood-transfusion/.

In an emergency, or if the child is critically ill, the blood transfusion should be given as a life-saving treatment, unless there has been prior refusal documented. If consent is not given, this can be overruled and a rapid court order can be obtained (JPAC, 2014).

WHAT'S THE EVIDENCE?

Are there any UK standardised parameters around when to transfuse red blood cells? What evidence can you find around this?

Look at the following:

Local policies for a few geographically spread hospitals in the UK.

NICE (National Institute for Health and Care Excellence) (2022) Blood transfusion. Guideline [NG24]. Available at: www.nice.org.uk/guidance/ng24

NHSBT website to view the RePAST feasibility trial around restrictive vs liberal transfusion strategies in paediatric patients undergoing allogeneic stem cell transplant. Available at: www.nhsbt.nhs.uk/clinical-trials-unit/current-trials-and-studies/repast/

ACTIVITY 24.3: REFLECTIVE PRACTICE

Reflect on your placements so far, list any of haematological blood disorders you have encountered in children you have cared for.

- What assessments and diagnostic tests were carried out?
- What nursing care did the children require?
- Who made up the team providing care?
- Was the child involved in any research/clinical trials?

PROMOTING HEALTH

Health promotion is an important part of the role of a nurse. With the conditions discussed in this chapter, it is essential to involve the child/young person and their family in their care and provide them with education and support in managing their condition. Through medication, nutrition and treatment, children can lead relatively normal lives in many cases, so it is important to empower them to be involved in the whole process and become experts in their condition.

GO FURTHER

There are a variety of ways you can prepare for placements caring for children and young people with haematological conditions, one of which is to understand the condition, as detailed in the advice from this student:

"Some advice I would recommend to other students is to take time to understand the condition or diagnosis and what it entails for that individual, once you have an understanding you can learn how to provide individualised care. Take time to build trust and understand the changes that these patients and families will face, and always show compassion and the desire to help."

Amber, nursing student

CHAPTER SUMMARY

- Blood is vital in carrying oxygen around the body, fighting infection, carrying nutrients and waste products to vital organs, and in repairing damaged tissue
- Blood disorders in children are wide ranging and can greatly impact quality of life

- A collaborative MDT approach is essential for the care and management of the child and their family
- Children having a blood transfusion require specialised care and monitoring

─── BUILD YOUR BIBLIOGRAPHY ───

Weblinks

- Aplastic Anaemia www.youtube.com/watch?v=RBOTrrOBKLO)

FURTHER
READING:
WEBLINKS

REFERENCES

American Society of Haematology (2023) *Blood Safety and Matching*. Available at: www.hematology. org/education/patients/blood-basics/blood-safety-and-matching (accessed 15 February 2023).

Courtney, J (2022) 'First gene therapy treatment for haemophilia to be licensed'. *The Haemophilia Society* [online] 6 July. Available at: https://haemophilia.org.uk/gene-therapy-treatment-for-haemophilia/#:~:text=However%2C%20as%20yet%20there%20are,any%20part%20of%20 the%20UK (accessed 1 September 2022).

Getawa, S. and Melku, M. (2022) 'The application of next generation and whole genome sequencing in the diagnosis of haematological disorders and challenges to apply in routine diagnosis'. *Haematology and Transfusion International Journal*, 10 (2): 24–8. Available at: https:// medcraveonline.com/HTIJ/HTIJ-10-00276.pdf (accessed: 26 August 2022).

Giardine, B., Borg, J., Viennas, E., Pavlidis, C., Moradkhani, K., Joly, P. et al. (2014) Updates of the HbVar database of human hemoglobin variants and thalassemia mutations. *Nucleic Acids Research*, 42 (Database issue): D1063-9. Available at: https://globin.bx.psu.edu/cgi-bin/hbvar/counter (accessed: 1 September 2022).

Great Ormond Street Hospital for Children (GOSH) (2016) Anaemia. Available from: www.gosh.nhs. uk/conditions-and-treatments/general-medical-conditions/anaemia (accessed: 25 August 2022).

JPAC (Joint United Kingdom (UK) Blood Transfusion and Tissue Transplantation Services Professional Advisory Committee) (2014) 12: Management of patients who do not accept transfusion. *Handbook of Transfusion Medicine*, 5th edn. Available at: www.transfusionguidelines.org/transfusion-handbook/12-management-of-patients-who-do-not-accept-transfusion (accessed 21 September 2022).

Kim, T.O and Despotovic, J.M (2021) 'Paediatric immune thrombocytopenia (ITP) treatment'. *Annals of Blood*, 6: doi: 10.21037/aob-20-96. Available at: https://aob.amegroups.com/article/view/6316/ html (accessed: 25 August 2022).

NHS England (2022) *Accelerating genomic medicine in the NHS*. Available at: www.england.nhs.uk/ wp-content/uploads/2022/10/B1627-Accelerating-Genomic-Medicine-October-2022.pdf (accessed: 22 October 2022).

Nianyi, L., Guangjie, Z., Wanling, W., Mengxue, Z., Weiyang, L., Qinfen, C. and Xiaoquin, W. (2020) 'The efficacy and safety of vitamin C for iron supplementation in adult patients with Iron deficiency anaemia'. *JAMA Network Open* [online] 3 (11). (accessed 1 September 2022).

NICE (National Institute for Health and Care Excellence) (2016) Major trauma: assessment and initial management. Nice Guideline 39. Available at: www.nice.org.uk/guidance/ng39 (accessed 24 August 2022).

Public Health England (2018) *Understanding haemoglobinopathies.* Available at: www.gov.uk/government/publications/handbook-for-sickle-cell-and-thalassaemia-screening/understanding-haemoglobinopathies#fn:4 (accessed 1 September 2022).

Public Health England (2021) *Information and choices for women and couples at risk of having a baby with thalassemia major.* Available at: www.gov.uk/government/publications/baby-at-risk-of-having-thalassaemia-description-in-brief/information-and-choices-for-women-and-couples-at-risk-of-having-a-child-with-thalassaemia-major (accessed 1 September 2022).

Tan, V. (2017) *How to increase the absorption of iron from foods.* Healthline. Available at: www.healthline.co/nutrition/increase-iron-absorption (accessed 25 August 2022).

World Health Organization (WHO) (2023) Anaemia. Available at: www.who.int/health-topics/anaemia (accessed: 20 February 2023).

World Health Organization (2021) Sickle cell disease. Available at: www.afro.who.int/health-topics/sickle-cell-disease (accessed 1 September 2022).

Zavaleta, N. and Astete-Robilliard, L. (2017) 'Effect of anaemia on child development: long-term consequences' [in Spanish]. *Revista Peruana de Medicina Experimental Salud Publica*, 34 (4): 716–22. English Abstract available at: https://pubmed.ncbi.nlm.nih.gov/29364424/ (accessed 24 August 2022).

Zhang, J., Walsh, M.F., Wu, G., Edmondson, M.N., Gruber, T.A., Easton, J. et al. (2015) 'Germline mutations in predisposition genes in paediatric cancer'. *New England Journal of Medicine*, 373 (24): 2336–46. Available at: www.ncbi.nlm.nih.gov/pmc/articles/PMC4734119/ (accessed 26 August 2022).

CARE OF CHILDREN AND YOUNG PEOPLE WITH A THERMAL INJURY

25

SHIRIN POMEROY

THIS CHAPTER COVERS

- What is a thermal injury?
- Describing a thermal injury in terms of size and depth
- Treatment options and considerations
- Pain management strategies for the child after thermal injury
- The complexities of caring for children with extensive thermal injuries

---

REQUIRED KNOWLEDGE

It would be helpful to have an understanding of the structure and functions of the skin before you start this chapter.

> "The team approach is imperative to understanding the rehabilitation and emotional, psychological and physiological recovery of burns patients."
>
> **Herndon, 2012, p.13**

INTRODUCTION

Caring for children after thermal injury is both challenging and rewarding. Most people can relate to having had a small burn injury at some point in their life (e.g., from cooking or sunbathing) and afterwards think nothing of it because it heals without any problems. However, a more significant thermal injury can and will impact physically, emotionally and psychologically on the child and the whole family. For some this will have long-term implications.

In recent years, burn care in the UK has acquired a much-improved status as a specialty in its own right. The Burn Care Review (NBCR Group, 2001) paved the way for this, enabling burns to be recognised as a specialised field of healthcare within NHS England. Consequently, the organisation and delivery of burn care across the country is more closely monitored, supported and generally better resourced.

There is international recognition that most thermal injuries in children are preventable (WHO, 2008). The majority result from accidents that occur in the home, with the exploring toddler (aged 12 months to 2 years of age) being the most vulnerable age group. Verey et al. (2014) note that they represent half of all burns admissions in England and Wales. Public awareness of the causes and consequences of burn injury for children and their families is generally poor, hence the ongoing need for injury prevention programmes. Charitable organisations such as the Children's Burns Trust (CBT) (see weblinks) include a prevention remit in their work.

This chapter provides clarity on the definition of a thermal injury, and how treatment is determined after assessment. It is intended that greater knowledge and understanding will be gained of how thermal injury affects child development and all activities of daily living.

WHAT IS A THERMAL INJURY?

A thermal injury is defined as damage to the skin or internal organs caused by the transfer of heat from a direct heat source. There are five generally accepted categories of heat transferring sources: wet heat, dry heat, chemical, electrical and radiation (see Table 25.1) (Bosworth-Bousfield, 2002).

Table 25.1 Different categories of thermal injury with examples

Category	Description	Examples
Wet heat	Liquid-based heat sources (excluding chemicals)	Hot drinks, water, soups, sauces, stews
Dry heat	Non-liquid-based heat sources	Fire, ash, hot objects such as an iron, hob/oven, radiator or hair straighteners
Chemicals	Acids or alkalis	Most household cleaning products are alkaline, including bleach
Electrical	High voltage (>2000v) Low voltage/domestic electricity (240v)	Most electrical burns in children occur from touching or biting exposed cables
Radiation	Radiant heat	Ultraviolet light (sunlight) Hair dryers, fan heaters, radiotherapy burns

Not included in this list are burns caused by exposure to cold. These include frostbite, but also encompass deliberate injuries from aerosol sprays or other cold/chemical sources. These injuries are worthy of mention and are part of the burn care team remit. Usually attributed to risk-taking adolescent behaviour or peer pressure, aerosol spray injuries (a combination of cold and chemical injury) can, if deep, leave permanent scars. Another self-injuring activity currently popular in some schools and amongst adolescent children is the 'ice/salt challenge'. Williams et al. (2013) illustrate a case report of such an injury in a young adult, although local unpublished data within the International Burn Injury Database (iBID, 2010) also shows this in younger teenagers. It is important to identify whether there is a history of bullying or self-harming behaviour associated with these self-inflicted injuries. Any child showing signs of poor emotional, psychological and social well-being (mental health) must be directed to appropriately qualified healthcare professionals so that the right assessment and support can be attained.

The Royal Society for the Prevention of Accidents (RoSPA) (2015) confirms that scalds (wet heat sources) are the most frequent cause of thermal injury in children internationally. Contact burns or flame burns follow thereafter but this depends on how the data are collected and whether outpatient or emergency department figures are included. As a children's nurse it is useful to be aware of what is common, so that safeguarding and health protection questions can be asked when a patient presents with a less common thermal injury.

SAFEGUARDING STOP POINT

The importance of obtaining a detailed history and clinical examination of a child after thermal injury should not be underestimated in the context of safeguarding. While this may not be within the scope of practice for the children's nurse, the recognition of a 'cause for concern' is the responsibility of all members of the burn care team. A recent systematic review by the Royal College of Paediatrics and Child Health (2022) can help in making this judgement call as well as assist clinicians in differentiating between intentional injury and neglect. Some additional information about this can be found in the 'Build your bibliography' section at the end of the chapter.

Describing a thermal injury in terms of size and depth

The extent of a thermal injury is assessed in two ways: the size of the burn in terms of the percentage body surface area affected (the spread of injury), and the depth of injury (how deep through the layers of the skin the damage has occurred) (Chan et al., 2012). It is a combination of both these two assessments, the location of injury with associated inhalation injury and/or other trauma, that determines its significance. A common misconception is that only big burns have a significant impact on the child and family.

Assessing the size of burn injury

The size of injury is measured as a percentage of the total body surface area (%TBSA). There are a variety of tools that can be employed to help in this assessment (see Table 25.2).

Table 25.2 Assessment tools to measure size of burn in children

Tool	Description
Adapted rule of nines (for children) (American College of Surgeons, 1997)	An adult's head and each arm equate to 9% TBSA. An adult's front torso, back torso and each leg are 18% TBSA. A child's head and legs differ, being 18% and 14% (each leg) respectively. As the child grows, the head size lessens, and the legs increase as a percentage of TBSA

(Continued)

Table 25.2   (Continued)

Tool	Description
Rule of palms or 1% rule (Kyle and Wallace, 1951; Rossiter et al., 1996; Berry et al., 2001)	The size of the patient's hand (palmar surface including fingers) equates to 1% TBSA
Lund and Browder chart (Lund and Browder, 1944)	The burn area is drawn on a body map with predetermined size estimations for each body part. Some sizes change with the age of the patient (in years) and are determined from a table on the chart
Serial halving (Allison and Porter, 2004)	Divides the body into a number of halves - front/back, top/bottom, left/right - it is possible to determine whether the injury is ≥50%, ≥25%, ≥12.5% and so on
Mersey burns application (Barnes et al., 2015)	The burn area is drawn directly into a 'smart phone application' (app) body map. The application determines burn size once the age of the patient is entered

ACTIVITY 25.1: REFLECTIVE PRACTICE

Use the Lund and Browder chart to calculate the estimated burn area drawn. Include all coloured areas in your calculation. Consider what the size of burn would be for a child aged under 1 year with one in a child aged 10 years.

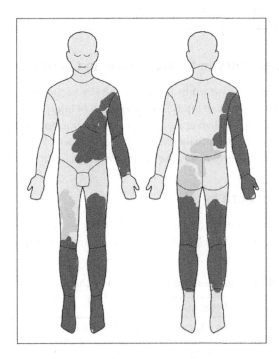

Figure 25.1

Image created from: St Helens and Knowsley Teaching Hospitals NHS Trust (2010-13) *Mersey Burns* http://merseyburns.com

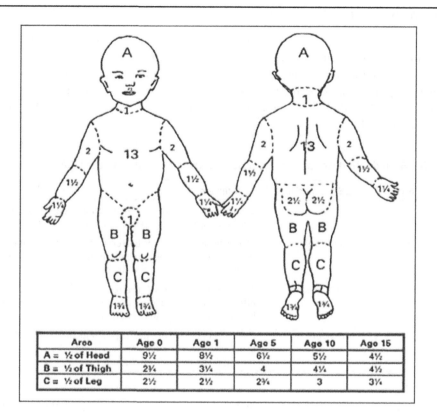

Area	Age 0	Age 1	Age 5	Age 10	Age 15
A = ½ of Head	9½	8½	6½	5½	4½
B = ½ of Thigh	2¾	3¼	4	4¼	4½
C = ½ of Leg	2½	2½	2¾	3	3¼

Figure 25.2 Lund and Browder Chart

From Harwood-Nuss, A., Wolfson, A. and Linden, C. *The Clinical Practice of Emergency Medicine*. Philadelphia: Wolters Kluwer, 2015, with permission

Critical observation of these assessment tools will firstly highlight that they were originally devised for adults and have been modified to fit to children. The literature on burn assessment tools is somewhat mixed, with frequent claims that one tool is more accurate than another. All tools available should be regarded as a helpful aid but with limitations due to inter-rater concordance on their use and interpretation. Giretzlehner et al. (2013) investigated this with a group of just over a hundred clinical staff. Significant discrepancies were found between staff assessments of the same patients. They also found that computer-generated programmes mapping photographic images to 3D-scoring systems were more accurate at burn size calculation. These inaccuracies were also emphasised by Chan et al. (2012) who expressed particular concern for children with increased risk of fluid resuscitation errors if the burn size estimation is correct. The future of burn size estimation may lie in technologically based tools (apps), but an innovative study by Malic et al. (2007) considered the potential for a 'credit card' tool. This has international appeal as all credit cards and most identification badges the world over are made to a standard size of 8.5cm by 5.3cm and equate to 45cm^2. More accurate burn size estimations can potentially be made by mapping the credit card size to the burn area distribution and then calculating this as a proportion of the total body surface area (BSA) of the patient (BSA is calculated using a formula requiring patient weight and height).

Assessing the depth of thermal injury

Assessing the depth of a thermal injury is a complex clinical skill that improves with experience, but still remains a highly subjective task (Serrano et al., 2015). Most clinicians report that the extremes of depth (either very superficial or very deep) are easier to assess, and it is the intermediate or mixed depth injuries that are more difficult. Burn depth classification terminology widely taught and used in the UK, Europe and Australasia differs from that used in the USA, but is more precise (see Table 25.3).

Table 25.3 Burn depth descriptor comparisons between the UK and the USA

Burn depth category	US comparison	Description
Epidermal	1st degree	Epidermis only is affected. Also termed 'superficial burn'. The skin is not broken. The skin looks red
Dermal	2nd degree	Epidermis is denuded or blistered. Also termed 'superficial partial thickness'. The papillary dermis layer is affected. The wound is wet and painful when exposed or touched
	3rd degree	'Deep partial thickness'. The reticular layer of the dermis is affected. The wound looks drier and more leathery. The wound is not as painful due to nerve damage
Full thickness	4th degree	Both layers of skin are destroyed. Subcutaneous tissue and other underlying structures such as muscle, ligaments, or bone may be exposed or charred

Burn depth assessment is generally directed by clinical observation of the wound at the bedside, followed by wound reviews every 1 to 7 days until it is fully healed. The frequency of this review is determined by several factors including: the stage of healing, the clinical condition of the patient and the type of dressing used. Deitch et al. (1983) found that if sufficient re-epithelialisation (healing) is observed over a 2-week period, then the risk of developing hypertrophic scarring and other longer-term complications is deemed minimal. This guiding principle remains current today along with the risk of scarring increasing the longer the wound takes to heal. A more recent interpretation by Cubison et al. (2006) claims that if a burn wound looks like it will heal within 2–3 weeks, then the need for surgical intervention (skin grafting) is less likely or would be much smaller in area. Whilst highly subjective, this approach is often chosen due to a lack of other more objective and reliable methods of burn depth assessment.

The National Institute for Health and Care Excellence (NICE, 2011) recommends as gold standard the use of laser doppler imaging (LDI) to determine the need or avoidance of surgical intervention for intermediate depth wounds. The laser doppler image detects blood flow to the burn injured skin and associated software predicts whether the wound will heal within 14 days, 14–21 days or more than 21 days. At face value the laser doppler seems invaluable to burn care services when used as part of routine burn assessment. Yet the costs of this equipment (initial capital spend, annual servicing and staff training costs) are not insignificant. Other considerations affecting the reliability of the equipment include: taking the image too early or too late, patient movement during the procedure (especially with young children) and interpretation errors of the images obtained. Despite these limitations, Khatib et al. (2014) acknowledge that laser doppler imaging provides a useful contribution to burn depth assessment as an adjunct to clinical observation.

ACTIVITY 25.2: CRITICAL THINKING

The tools illustrated to measure the size of a burn were devised by clinical staff based on the size of patients at the time and all show validation limitations. List what you think the implications are if the burn size is either over- or under-estimated?

Knowledge of the size and depth of injury is necessary for directing initial treatment options of early surgery and fluid management. Fluid management strategies have been subject to much debate in recent years and in children they are a difficult area to research. Go to the 'Build your bibliography' section and read the article which introduces you to this vast topic.

SEE ALSO
CHAPTER 26

WHAT'S THE EVIDENCE?

Often described as dynamic wounds because they can change over time (Jackson, 1953), the size and depth of a thermal injury is influenced by a number of factors, including:

- The promptness and effectiveness of first aid (cooling)
- Judicious fluid management
- Adequacy of pain control
- Sufficient infection control practices to reduce the risk of infection

Deficiencies in any of these can cause the injury to both deepen as well as widen. The Jackson model as described in Yarrow et al. (2009) offers a simple explanation of what is happening at the wound site and within the microcirculation influencing how the injury might evolve over time.

TREATMENT OPTIONS AND CONSIDERATIONS

Irrespective of the size, depth or type of burn injury, a key priority for the burn care team is to achieve wound closure (healing) as promptly as possible with minimal complication. Healing occurs either by secondary intention (on its own with the support of dressings) or with surgery (debridement alone or with skin grafting). On the surface this can seem straightforward, but becomes more complex depending on where the burns are on the body, how long they take to heal and how much they impact on normal activities of daily living. Burns can be described as 'extraordinarily painful' (Stoddard et al., 2002) and this is corroborated by Meyer et al. (2012) who state that all burns will be painful to a greater or lesser extent. The fear and anxiety of pain and painful procedures can be debilitating irrespective of the age of the patient. At times it can be for this reason alone that the child cannot function as normal. It seems pertinent to utilise the activities of daily living as described by Roper et al. (2000) as a guiding principle in the care of burns patients, even for infants and young children who are largely dependent on carers.

SEE ALSO
CHAPTER 3

ACTIVITY 25.3: REFLECTIVE PRACTICE

Use the 12 activities of daily living (ADL) to highlight the potential problems for a child aged 18 months, 5 years and 12 years for the following burn injuries:

- Burns to the face, including eyes, ears, nose and mouth
- Burns to the hands and feet
- Burns to the neck, axilla, elbows, knees and ankles
- Burns to the perineum
- Smoke inhalational injuries

List how you would care for the child and family in light of the above, considering both the physical and psychological needs of both the child and the parents.

SEE ALSO CHAPTER 3, 5 AND 14

Central to burn care is the burn care team. This multidisciplinary team is vitally important in coordinating and delivering treatment/care to children and their families after burn injury, and should not be underestimated. Alongside surgeons and nursing staff, the team might also include general paediatricians, paediatric intensivists, anaesthetics/acute pain services, physiotherapy, occupational therapy, play specialists, clinical psychology, dietetics and microbiology, depending on the severity of injury and the needs of the child and family. Effective interdisciplinary working is crucial to the decision-making process in all 'phases' after burn injury, in conjunction with the child (if able) and family (see Table 25.4).

Table 25.4   Thermal injury recovery phases

Phase	Identified priorities
Emergency (first 1-6 hours)	• Airway, breathing, circulation • Fluid resuscitation • Pain control
Acute (first 5 days)	• Fluid management • Eating/drinking • Wound care/management • Pain and anxiety management • Function and mobility
Rehabilitation (from day 1 until healed)	Needs assessed using a range of assessment tools, including ADL
Long term (from healed date to potentially years later)	As per ADL assessment, and including: • Scar management • School/nursery integration

The role of the children's nurse in burn care is to assess and deliver specific interventions such as wound care, and coordinate holistic treatment/care to support children and their families during initial and intermediate phases of care and after discharge from hospital. It may also be necessary for the nurse to act as the child and family advocate, so that painful procedures are not a source of secondary psychological trauma.

Contemporary burn care espouses two main principles: early debridement and skin grafting of notably deep burns, and 'moist' wound healing. Both practices have shown to improve survival rates, reduce length of hospital stay, and produce better outcomes in terms of reduced scarring and infection rates (D'Cruz et al., 2013). The term 'debridement' is often used to describe anything from simple wound cleansing to surgically cutting away necrotic tissue, and all else in between these extremes. The aim of this process is to remove dead particles from the wound, reduce inflammation and potential sources of infection. For children (in conjunction with good pain/anxiety/symptom control), superficial wound cleansing/debridement is achieved in the bath/shower using gauze swabs to rub/wipe debris away from the wounds. Although there is little evidence to support this, it encourages good hygiene practices through washing the whole body as well as the wound and is common practice nationally (Langschmidt et al., 2014). Particular care is needed to ensure the psychological safety of the child is not overlooked in relation to managing the pain experience, both anticipated and actual pain.

Wound care and dressings and associated psychological preparation and care are essential nursing skills in burns inpatient, outpatient and community settings. These are complex interventions, often involving advanced interpersonal skills and engagement in working collaboratively with parents/carers and children.

To learn more about different types of dressings used in burn care, the Cochrane review 'Dressings for superficial and partial thickness burns' (Wasiak et al., 2013) is a useful starting point.

PAIN MANAGEMENT STRATEGIES FOR CHILDREN AFTER THERMAL INJURY

> "Whilst on placement I participated in the bathing of burns patients. The primary aim of bathing is to reduce infection through removing the necrotic skin. During bathing/wound cleansing some bleeding can occur. The child can also become vocally distressed, hence they are assessed for pain and given analgesia beforehand. Play specialists are usually involved with the procedure providing valuable therapeutic distraction. Parents/carers understandably may become distressed witnessing their child so upset. Procedural preparation is crucial in burn care."
>
> **Matthew, 1st-year children's nursing student**

Effective pain management for the child after thermal injury cannot be over-emphasised. The student's experience above reflects a common example within burns services whereby staff undertake a range of clinical procedures such as wound care, turns/limb positioning, physiotherapy exercises and stretches, all with the potential to exacerbate pain and distress for the child and family. Two key principles in the assessment and management of pain for these patients are that the pain experience evolves over time post-injury and that regular, dynamic assessment is essential to ensure the effectiveness of the pain assessment and management strategies employed. Hospital acute pain services, anaesthetists, hospital play and clinical psychology are key players in helping the children's nurse implement individualised pain management strategies, which also includes post-burn itching.

SEE ALSO CHAPTER 3

Pain management strategies after thermal injury must address all types of pain experienced: background, procedural and breakthrough. Better control is achieved with a combination of both pharmacological and non-pharmacological approaches. Useful summaries of this within burn care can be found in Retrouvey and Shahrokhi (2015) and a more child-centred review by Pardesi and Fuzaylov (2016). Distraction techniques and other forms of non-pharmacological pain management strategies are considered essential armoury within a children's burn care setting, particularly for wound care and dressing changes: television, background music, toys, puppetry, iPad/tablet activities or more sophisticated technological devices such as virtual reality can be employed according to the child's age and stage of development (Miller et al., 2010). The play specialist can be a skilled and welcome ally for the child, especially in the initial and intermediate stages of care management.

WHAT'S THE EVIDENCE?

Recognition that a burn injury can be a stressful and painful experience for the child and family is the first step in supporting physical and psychological recovery. Research in this area is limited and often difficult to individualise because each child and family's experience after a burns/thermal injury is very different. The review article by Bakker et al. (2013) in the 'Build your bibliography' reading section at the end of this chapter provides a useful summary of what is known on this subject.

THE COMPLEXITIES OF CARING FOR CHILDREN WITH EXTENSIVE THERMAL INJURIES

In its simplest form, a comprehensive understanding of this is best achieved in the context of a patient example (see case study 25.1).

CASE STUDY 25.1: RUPERT

Rupert is 4 years old. He was helping his dad build a bonfire to burn rubbish. Something in the bonfire exploded and a fireball occurred. Rupert's clothes caught fire. His dad experienced hand burns as he put the flames out. Rupert has 55% mixed-depth flame burns to his face, torso, arms and hands. Luckily no eye damage or smoke inhalation injury occurred, so his airway and breathing were not of concern after the initial transfer.

- List what supportive measures might help Rupert and family on their journey of recovery after a severe thermal injury.
- Consider what package of care Rupert may require in the community after discharge from hospital.

Employing the 12 activities of daily living (ADLs), the following table maps out the needs, potential risks and likely care plan for this patient from initial injury, through rehabilitation and into the long term (see Table 25.5). This may help guide your thoughts and responses to the above questions.

Table 25.5 Case example, illustrating the complexities of caring for children and young people (CYP) with extensive thermal injuries

Activity	Potential problems/needs	Acute stage	Rehabilitation/long term	Interdisciplinary working
Maintaining a safe environment	• Intravenous/arterial lines, urinary catheter • Risk of falls • Risk of infection from wounds/lines • Pain and medication safety • Psychological safety	Single cubicle for protective isolation Nurse in an appropriate cot/bed Observe and monitor for signs of infection	Proactive line removal when no longer required Support child and family in maintaining physical and psychological safety	Anaesthetists/intensivists Infection prevention and control team Play therapists Clinical psychology services
Communication	• Swelling of face, eyes • Limited vision • Disorientation • Difficulty in speaking • Ability to accurately communicate pain and fear	Nurse upright to reduce swelling Provide reassurance Consider communication aids Developmentally appropriate communication strategies	Support family to encourage the child to communicate own needs Child-centred interventions	Ophthalmologist Hospital play Speech and language therapist Clinical psychology
Breathing	• Poor chest expansion from pain of wounds/bed rest/sedative medications • Risk of fluid retention – wet lungs • Risk of chest infection	Nurse upright for better lung expansion Encourage deep breathing/breathing exercises Observe for signs of chest problems (e.g., breathing changes, increasing oxygen requirement)	Support family to encourage active mobilisation and cardiovascular exercise to prevent long-term chest problems Utilise play and recreation to facilitate normal functions	Physiotherapy Hospital play
Eating and drinking	• Reduced appetite • Increased metabolic demands • Hand injury so unable to self-feed • Risk of reduced gut motility • Fluid losses externally from wounds • Oedema formation due to injury and internal capillary leak	Prescribed supplementary feeding regime via nasogastric or nasojejunal tube Continue to offer oral food/drink Prescribed fluid management regime Maintain a strict fluid balance Observe for signs of fluid overload or dehydration Record-keeping	Support family to normalise and encourage oral diet Enable independent feeding	Intensivists/medical staff Dietician Occupational therapy Hospital play – for example, food play

(Continued)

Table 25.5 (Continued)

Activity	Potential problems/needs	Acute stage	Rehabilitation/long term	Interdisciplinary working
Elimination	• Reduced independence in toileting • Catheterised to enable strict fluid monitoring • Risk of constipation due to immobility and opiate medication • Risk of loose stools from liquid-based feeds • Risk of soiling on wounds	Catheter care Consider aperients to aid bowel motions May require incontinence pads	Support family in enabling independent toileting	Physiotherapy Occupational therapy Hospital play
Washing and dressing	• Significant painful wounds covered in dressings • Unable to wash or wear clothes • High risk of infection	Multiple theatre trips to facilitate wound cleansing Pre- and postop care Observe for 'strike through' on dressings and soiled dressings Support family in following universal infection control procedures	Support family with bathing/showering Support family with wound care and dressings Support family with scar management treatments and reducing contracture formation	Burns surgeons Hospital play Clinical psychology Physiotherapy Occupational therapy Pharmacist
Controlling temperature	• Inflammatory response after injury causes body temperature to rise • Hyper-metabolic state causes body temperature to rise	Nurse in a thermo-neutral environment to maintain body temperature between 37°C–38°C Observe for signs of infection/sepsis Record keeping	Support CYP and family in managing own body temperature	
Mobilisation	• Significant pain on moving and turning • Risk of muscle de-conditioning from prolonged bed rest • Risk of abnormal posturing due to skin tightness	Ensure adequacy of pain assessment using appropriate validated tools Regular appropriate analgesia and non-pharmacological approaches to symptom control Encourage moving and turning on a regular basis Support appropriate positioning when in bed or sitting Follow prescribed splint regime	Support CYP/family in encouraging active stretching and mobilisation	Physiotherapy Occupational therapy Hospital play

Activity	Potential problems/needs	Acute stage	Rehabilitation/long term	Interdisciplinary working
Working and playing	• Reduced concentration ability • Increased fatigue • Risk of developmental/schooling regression • Social deprivation from hospitalisation	Offer play/activities when awake Extra encouragement may be required if low in mood and motivation Ensure adequate rest periods after key stress times (dressing, baths, etc.)	Initiate a daily routine to include play/school activities Support CYP in returning to school	Hospital play Hospital school Clinical psychology
Expressing sexuality	• Fear of scarring and looking different from other boys/girls • For boys: risk of penis deformities • For girls: risk of problems with breast development	Provide realistic expectations for child and family to voice and come to terms with their fears	Support the child and family through puberty	Clinical psychology
Sleeping	• Risk of poor sleep from hospitalisation/pain • Sleep difficulties when weaning off sedative drugs • Risk of flashbacks and nightmares about the injury • Post-traumatic stress disorder potential	Observe and address sleep disturbances as soon as possible May require night time sedation	Encourage the child and family to re-establish a bedtime routine	Hospital play Clinical psychology
Death and dying	• Risk of mortality increases with significant injuries • Post-traumatic stress symptoms at time or later	Support the child and family in voicing their fears of death and dying		Clinical psychology

Traditional burn care practices are gradually being supported, disputed or improved by a greater evidence base and technological advances (particularly within wound assessment and tissue viability). Recovery after thermal injury can be a complex, morbidly painful process with long-term physical and psychological implications even if carefully managed. By employing regular 'activities of daily living', assessments and a team approach, most aspects of burn care can be highlighted and addressed. We should be thankful that children display immense resilience, and with supportive and enabling care from their family alongside healthcare professionals, they can grow to lead able-bodied and meaningful adult lives.

CHAPTER SUMMARY

This chapter has explored:

- Definitions and explanations of thermal injuries and how such injuries may be effectively assessed and managed
- How thermal injuries can affect all activities of daily living across all developmental stages
- Skilled assessment of pain and other symptoms associated with burn care/thermal injury
- The importance of the whole multidisciplinary team in supporting the child and family so that the child can begin to recover after a thermal injury
- The importance of working in partnership with the child and parents/carers in enabling the child to achieve their full potential after a thermal injury

BUILD YOUR BIBLIOGRAPHY

Books

FURTHER
READING

- Herndon, D. (ed.) (2017) *Total Burn Care*, 5th edn. New York: Elsevier.

  This book, with additional online content, is the internationally recognised authority for the burn care community. Although US-centric, it covers every aspect of burn care, is extensively referenced throughout and includes adequate illustrations and images.
- Barret-Nerin, J. and Herndon, D. (2004) *Principles and Practice of Burn Surgery*. New York: Taylor and Francis.

  This book provides a less dense, easier read than *Total Burn Care* although it covers similar subject matter. Focusing on education and training for burn care staff, the various options for the surgical treatment of burns are illustrated.

Journal articles

FURTHER
READING:
ONLINE
JOURNAL
ARTICLES

- Fodor, L., Fodor, A., Ramon, Y., Shoshani, O., Rissin, Y. and Ullmann, Y. (2006) 'Controversies in fluid resuscitation for burn management: Literature review and our experience'. *Injury*, 37: 374–9.

  This article will introduce you to the complex area of fluid management for burn management in children.

- Bakker, A., Maertens, K., Van Son, M. and Van Loey, N. (2013) 'Psychological consequences of pediatric burns from a child and family perspective: a review of the empirical literature'. *Clinical Psychology Review*, 33 (3): 361–71.

  This article highlights the potential psychological consequences of burns for children and their families.

- Wasiak, J., Cleland, H., Campbell, F. and Spinks, A. (2013) 'Dressings for superficial and partial thickness burns'. Cochrane Database of Systematic Reviews. DOI: 10.1002/14651858.CD002106.pub4.

  This article covers different types of dressings used in burns and is a useful starting point.

Weblinks

FURTHER READING: WEBLINKS

- The British Burn Association – founded in 1968, a charity concerned with all aspects of burn care www.britishburnassociation.org/ With its core objectives of burn injury prevention, research, education and standards this website is a primary resource for all members of the burns multidisciplinary team.
- Children's Burns Trust www.cbtrust.org.uk/burn-prevention This is an exemplary resource for children, families and healthcare professionals. A key area of their work is in burn injury prevention – they provide a range of online educational resources and deliver specific awareness campaigns. There is also an opportunity to get involved and support their work.
- Supporting Children with Burns https://supportingchildrenwithburns.co.uk/ An excellent resource for children and families aimed at supporting the emotional and psychological recovery after burn injury.

REFERENCES

Allison, K. and Porter, K. (2004) 'Consensus on the pre-hospital approach to burns patient management'. *Emergency Medicine Journal*, 21 (1): 112–14.

American College of Surgeons (1997) *Advanced Trauma Life Support*, 6th edn. Chicago: American College of Surgeons.

Bakker, A., Maertens, K., Van Son, M. and Van Loey, N. (2013) 'Psychological consequences of pediatric burns from a child and family perspective: a review of the empirical literature'. *Clinical Psychology Review*, 33 (3): 361–71.

Barnes, J., Duffy, A., Hamnett, N., McPhail, J., Seaton, C., Shokrollahi, K., James, M., McArthur, P. and Pritchard Jones, R. (2015) 'The Mersey Burns app: evolving a model of validation'. *Emergency Medicine Journal*, 32: 637–41.

Berry, M., Evison, D. and Roberts, A. (2001) 'The influence of body mass index on burn surface estimated from the area of the hand'. *Burns*, 27: 591–4.

Bosworth-Bousfield, C. (2002) *Burn Trauma: Management and Nursing Care*, 2nd edn. London: Whurr.

Chan, Q., Barzi, F., Cheney, L., Harvey, J. and Holland, A. (2012) 'Burn size estimation in children: still a problem'. *Emergency Medicine Australasia*, 24: 181–6.

Cubison, T., Pape, S. and Parkhouse, N. (2006) 'Evidence for the link between healing time and the development of hypertrophic scars (HTS) in paediatric burns due to scald injury'. *Burns*, 32: 992–9.

D'Cruz, R., Martin, H. and Holland, A. (2013) 'Medical management of paediatric burn injuries: best practice part 2'. *Journal of Paediatrics and Child Health*, 49: 397–404.

Deitch, E., Wheelahan, T., Rose, M., Clothier, J. and Cotter, J. (1983) 'Hypertrophic burn scars: analysis of variables'. *Journal of Trauma*, 23 (10): 895–8.

Giretzlehner, M., Dirnberger, J., Owen, R., Haller, H., Lumenta, D. and Kamolz, L. (2013) 'The determination of total burn surface area: how much difference?' *Burns*, 39: 1107–13.

Herndon, D. (ed.) (2012) *Total Burn Care*, 4th edn. New York: Elsevier.

International Burn Injury Database (iBID) (2010) *iBID Introduction*. Available at: www.ibidb.org/ibid (accessed 24 May 2017).

Jackson, D. (1953) 'The diagnosis of the depth of burning'. *British Journal of Surgery*, 40 (164): 588–96.

Khatib, M., Jabir, S., O'Connor, E.F. and Philp, B. (2014) 'A systematic review of the evolution of laser doppler techniques in burn depth assessment'. *Plastic Surgery International*, 214. Available at: www.hindawi.com/journals/psi/2014/621792 (accessed 24 May 2017).

Kyle, J. and Wallace, A. (1951) 'Fluid replacement in burnt children'. *British Journal of Plastic Surgery*, 3: 194–204.

Langschmidt, J., Caine, P., Wearn, C., Bamford, A., Wilson, Y. and Moiemen, N. (2014) 'Hydrotherapy in burn care: a survey of hydrotherapy practices in the UK and Ireland and literature review'. *Burns*, 40: 860–4.

Lund, C. and Browder, N. (1944) 'The estimation of areas of burns'. *Surgery, Gynecology and Obstetrics*, 79: 352–8.

Malic, C., Karoo, R., Austin, O. and Phipps, A. (2007) 'Resuscitation burn card – a useful tool for burn injury assessment'. *Burns*, 33: 195–9.

Meyer, W., Wiechman, S., Woodson, L., Jaco, M. and Thomas, C. (2012) 'Management of pain and other discomforts in burned patients', in D. Herndon (ed.) *Total Burn Care*, 4th edn. New York: Elsevier.

Miller, K., Rodger, S., Bucolo, S., Greer, R. and Kimble, R. (2010) 'Multi-modal distraction: using technology to combat pain in young children with burn injuries'. *Burns*, 36: 647–58.

National Institute for Health and Clinical Excellence (NICE) (2011) moorLDI2-BI: a laser doppler blood flow imager for burn wound assessment. Medical Technologies Guidance [MTG2]. Available at: www.nice.org.uk/guidance/mtg2 (accessed 24 May 2017).

NBCR (National Network for Burn Care Review) Group (2001) *Committee Report: Standards and Strategy for Burn Care*. Available at: www.britishburnassociation.org/downloads/NBCR2001.pdf (accessed 24 May 2017).

Pardesi, D. and Fuzaylov, G. (2016) 'Pain management in pediatric burn patients: review of recent literature and future direction'. *Journal of Burn Care and Research*, DOI 10.1097/BCR.0000000000000470.

Retrouvey, H. and Shahrokhi, S. (2015) 'Pain and the thermally injured patient – a review of current therapies'. *Journal of Burn Care and Research*, 36: 315–23.

Roper, N., Logan, W. and Tierney, A. (2000) *The Roper–Logan–Tierney Model of Nursing: Based on Activities of Living*. Edinburgh: Elsevier Health Sciences.

Rossiter, N., Chapman, P. and Haywood, I. (1996) 'How big is a hand?' *Burns*, 22: 230–1.

Royal College of Paediatrics and Child Health (RCPCH) (2022) *Child Protection Evidence Systematic Review on Burns*. Available at: https://childprotection.rcpch.ac.uk/child-protection-evidence/burns-systematic-review/ (accessed 9 November 2023).

Royal Society for the Prevention of Accidents (RoSPA) (2015) *Accidents to Children: Scalds and Burns*. Available at: www.rospa.com/home-safety/advice/child-safety/accidents-to-children/#scalds (accessed 24 May 2017).

Serrano, C., Boloix-Tortosa, R., Gómez-Cía, T, and Acha, B. (2015) 'Features identification for automatic Burn classification'. *Burns*, 41: 1883–90.

Stoddard, F., Sheridan, R., Saxe, G., King, B.S., King, B.H., Chedekel, D., Schnitzer, J. and Martyn, J. (2002) 'Treatment of pain in acutely burned children'. *Journal of Burn Care and Rehabilitation*, 23: 135–56.

Verey, F., Lyttle, M., Lawson, Z., Greenwood, R. and Young, A. (2014) 'When do children get burnt?' *Burns*, 40: 1322–8.

Wasiak, J., Cleland, H., Campbell, F. and Spinks, A. (2013) 'Dressings for superficial and partial thickness burns'. *Cochrane Database of Systematic Reviews*. doi: 10.1002/14651858.CD002106.pub4.

Williams, J., Cubbitt, J. and Dickson, W. (2013) 'The challenge of salt and ice'. *Burns*, 39: 1029.

World Health Organization (WHO) (2008) *World Report on Child Injury Prevention*. Available at: http://apps.who.int/iris/bitstream/10665/43851/1/9789241563574_eng.pdf (accessed 24 May 2017).

Yarrow, J., Moiemen, N. and Gulhane, S. (2009) 'Early management of burns in children'. *Paediatrics and Child Health*, 19 (11): 509–16.

CARE OF CHILDREN AND YOUNG PEOPLE WITH FLUID AND ELECTROLYTE IMBALANCE

26

ZOË VEAL AND COLIN VEAL

THIS CHAPTER COVERS

- Homeostasis
- Dehydration
- Gastroenteritis
- Sodium imbalance (hyponatraemia and hypernatraemia)
- Potassium imbalance (hypokalaemia and hyperkalaemia)

REQUIRED KNOWLEDGE

An understanding of the anatomy and physiology of the renal system and homeostasis is recommended before you start this chapter.

> "I don't think it can be emphasised enough that clinical assessment of dehydration can be challenging. The most useful measurement is the degree of weight loss during the illness. I insist that children are reweighed when they re-present to the emergency department with gastroenteritis, as this is by far and away the most accurate way of assessing fluid loss. It is vital to get an actual weight to base fluid calculations on, at the earliest possible opportunity. You don't want to overestimate the weight of a child in diabetic ketoacidosis and prescribe too much fluid, as this puts them at risk of cerebral oedema, etc."
>
> **Nicholas Sargeant, Consultant in Paediatric Emergency Medicine**

INTRODUCTION

This chapter explores fluid and electrolyte imbalance in children, starting with homeostasis and its role in maintaining the body's fluid balance. All children have a daily fluid requirement that can be affected by illness and disease. There are many reasons for fluid and electrolyte imbalance. However, this chapter focuses on the common causes of fluid imbalance and standard treatment as indicated by current guidelines. As a nursing student, you will be involved in caring for children with fluid and electrolyte imbalance and will be tasked with monitoring and recording their fluid input and output.

HOMEOSTASIS

Homeostasis describes the relatively constant internal state of the body within a narrow range of variables, despite changes to the external environment (Brady, 2021). Maintenance of fluid and electrolyte balance is an important aspect of homeostasis and, at its very basic level, means that the body's 'input' of fluid and electrolytes should be roughly equal to the body's 'output'. If the body takes in too much fluid and electrolytes to maintain its homeostatic balance, the excess will need to be eliminated. If too little is taken in, or an excess loss of fluid and electrolytes occurs – for example, through diarrhoea and vomiting – then those fluids and electrolytes will need to be replaced. Maintaining fluid balance and homeostasis is important for all human life, but it is particularly important in infants and young children, as this age group have a higher percentage of water volume in the body compared to older children and adults. This, alongside an immature renal system which cannot concrentrate urine effectively, and an immature immune system which increases susceptibility to gastrointestinal infections, means the risk of rapid fluid loss is greater (Brady, 2019).

Fluid balance

On a daily basis, fluid mainly enters the body via the digestive tract in drink and food, but a small amount of fluid is also obtained through cell metabolism (Jones, 2021). Likewise, fluid is routinely lost through the kidneys (urine), the gastrointestinal tract (faeces), the skin (sweat and diffusion) and the lungs (water vapour). The body maintains homeostasis by regulating the mechanisms through which fluid is routinely lost and this is one reason why humans sweat more and urinate less in hot weather compared to cold.

Normal fluid requirements

The normal volume of fluid required by children on a daily basis is shown in Table 26.1. These are general guidelines and some children may require more or less depending on their disease process, renal function, hormone response and level of consciousness. As a nursing student, you will be actively involved in the recording of fluid input and output and in calculating daily fluid requirements. Daily and hourly fluid requirements are calculated using the formula outlined in Table 26.1.

Table 26.1 Daily and hourly fluid requirement calculation

Daily fluid requirement	Hourly fluid requirement
100ml per kg for the first 10kg	4ml per kg for the first 10kg
50ml per kg for the second 10kg	2ml per kg for the second 10kg
20ml per kg for subsequent kg	1ml per kg for subsequent kg
Example – George is 10 years old and weighs 32 kg. His daily and hourly fluid requirements are calculated as follows	
First 10kg × 100 = 1000ml	First 10kg × 4 = 40ml
Second 10kg × 50 = 500ml	Second 10kg × 2 = 20ml
Subsequent 12kg × 20 = 240ml	Subsequent 12kg × 1 = 12ml
Total daily requirement = 1740ml	**Total hourly requirement = 72ml**

Adapted from Holliday and Segar, 1957

ACTIVITY 26:1 CRITICAL THINKING

You are working with your practice assessor and sharing the care of five patients. Your practice assessor asks you to calculate the daily and hourly fluid requirements for these patients:

- Arthur is 2 years old and weighs 12 kg
- Daisy is 8 years old and weighs 31 kg
- Mohammad is 7 months old and weighs 7.5 kg
- Isabelle is 14 years old and weighs 49 kg
- Elyshia is 5 years old and weighs 18 kg

Daisy and Elyshia are fluid-restricted to an 80% daily fluid allowance. Based on their daily fluid requirements, calculate what 80% would be.

It is also important to know how much fluid is lost. Expected urine output varies, but in general, you should expect to see:

1.5–2ml/kg per hour of urine in neonates and babies
1.5ml/kg per hour in toddlers
1ml/kg per hour in older children and young people.

(Adapted from Batcheler and Dixon, 2012)

For example, 14-year-old Isabelle weighs 49kg, so her kidneys should produce around 49ml of urine each hour, but for Mohammed, weighing 7.5kg, we should expect 15ml of urine produced. As well as urine, vomit and watery faeces would count in fluid output, as well as wound and chest drain losses.

Paediatric fluid balance chart									
Patient Name: Freddie Collins			D.O.B. 7/6/2015			Daily fluid allowance: 1660mls/24hrs			
Patient Number: 25122022						Serum Sodium Results: 140mmols/l			
Date: 9/7/22	INPUT				OUTPUT				BALANCE
Time	Oral fluids	IV fluids	Other	Total In	Urine	Faeces	Vomit	Other	Total Out	
08:00		69mls		69mls	168mls				168mls	-99mls
09:00	250mls	69mls		388mls					168mls	220mls
10:00		69mls		457mls					168mls	289mls
11:00		69mls		526mls	224mls				392mls	134mls
12:00	250mls	Stopped		776mls					392mls	384mls
13:00				776mls		Bowels open			392mls	384mls
14:00	300mls			1076mls	400mls				792mls	284mls
15:00				1076mls					792mls	284mls
16:00	250mls			1326mls	300mls				1092mls	234mls
17:00				1326mls					1092mls	234mls
18:00	300mls			1626mls					1092mls	534mls
19:00				1626mls					1092mls	534mls
Day time total	1350mls	276mls		1626mls	1092mls				1092mls	534mls
20:00										534mls
21:00					250mls				250mls	284mls
22:00									250mls	284mls
23:00									250mls	284mls
24:00:00									250mls	284mls
01:00									250mls	284mls
02:00									250mls	284mls
03:00									250mls	284mls
04:00									250mls	284mls
05:00									250mls	284mls
06:00									250mls	284mls
07:00					260mls				510mls	284mls
Night time total					510mls				510mls	284mls
24 hr total	1350mls	276mls		1626mls	1602mls				1602mls	24mls

Electrolytes

Electrolytes are salts and minerals that conduct electrical impulses around the body to maintain acid–base balance within homeostasis. Found in the blood, they include chemical elements such as sodium and potassium, ions such as chloride and buffers such as bicarbonate. As a nursing student, you will care for children with electrolyte imbalance, as it is frequently seen in conditions such as pyloric stenosis, diabetic ketoacidosis and gastroenteritis. The Report of the Inquiry into Hyponatraemia-related Deaths (2018) contains important findings and should be compulsory reading for all nurses caring for children and young people where there is potential for a fluid or electrolye imbalance.

Normal electrolyte values

Local guidelines mean there is a slight variation in normal values between laboratories. The values given in Table 26.2 are only a guide, so always check the normal value range with the laboratory processing the blood serum level.

Treatment for electrolyte imbalance will depend on which electrolyte is out of balance and by how much. For example, in pyloric stenosis, repeated vomiting and subsequent loss of stomach acid causes low chloride, potassium and sodium concentrations, resulting in the body's acid–base becoming too alkaline. By comparison, diabetic ketoacidosis causes a low bicarbonate, with high potassium, urea and creatinine and a very high glucose concentration, which results in the body's acid base becoming too acidic. In diabetic ketoacidosis, the lack of insulin prevents glucose absorption, which in turn results in fatty acid metabolism and ketone production to provide cellular energy. The kidneys become overloaded by both glucose and ketones and will attempt to excrete them both, causing dehydration and a reduction in bicarbonate, which in turn increases the acidic levels in the body.

SEE ALSO
CHAPTER 4
AND 20

Table 26.2   Normal electrolyte values

Electrolyte	Lower value	Upper value
Sodium (Na+)	136 mmol/l	145 mmol/l
Potassium (K+)	3.5mmol/l	4.5 mmol/l
Chloride (Cl-)	96 mmol/l	106 mmol/l
Calcium (Ca2+)	2.2 mmol/l	2.6 mmol/l
Magnesium (Mg2+)	0.75 mmol/l	1.0 mmol/l
Phosphate (PO43-)	1 mmol/l	1.8 mmol/l
Bicarbonate (HCO3-)	24 mmol/l	30 mmol/l
Urea	3 mmol/l	7 mmol/l
Creatinine	18 micromol/l	70 micromol/l
Glucose	3.9 mmol/l	6.9 mmol/l

ACTIVITY 26.2: CRITICAL THINKING

Return to the earlier section on electrolytes. Make a list of the electrolytes you have come across on placement/in theory. Are you aware of what electrolytes do and why they are so important?

A&P LINK

Drawing on your current knowledge of physiology, spend some time revising the importance of electrolytes in controlling the movement of fluid around the body.

DEHYDRATION

SEE ALSO
CHAPTER 14
AND 29

In children over 1 year of age, around 60% of body weight is made up of water, but in infants, body weight is around 80% water. Clinical dehydration occurs when there is a loss of more than 5% of this water (Miall et al., 2016). Feeling unwell can occur before clinical dehydration is reached. Within the body, fluid is held in two main compartments, intracellular and extracellular, and can be lost from either. Table 26.3 indicates how to assess dehydration in children under the age of 5.

One of the most common causes of dehydration in infants and children is diarrhoea and vomiting, most commonly due to gastroenteritis (Miall et al., 2016), but dehydration can also occur from other causes, such as fluid loss during and after surgery, or fluid maldistribution during sepsis.

Left untreated, dehydration can lead to shock and death (Samuels and Wieteska, 2016), so accurate diagnosis and early assessment is very important, especially in children under 5 years. As Nick, Consultant in Children's Emergency Medicine, stated at the start of this chapter, the clinical assessment of dehydration can be challenging and the most useful measurement is the degree of weight loss during the illness (Lissauer and Carroll, 2022).

Table 26.3 Assessing dehydration in children under 5 years

Increasing severity of dehydration

	No clinically detectable dehydration	Clinical dehydration	Clinical shock
Symptoms (remote and face-to-face assessments)	Appears well	**Red Flag** Appears to be unwell or deteriorating	-
	Alert and responsive	**Red Flag** Altered responsiveness (for example, irritable, lethargic)	Decreased level of consciousness
	Normal urine output	Decreased urine output	-
	Skin colour unchanged	Skin colour unchanged	Pale or mottled skin
	Warm extremities	Warm extremities	Cold extremities
Signs (face-to-face assessments)	Alert and responsive	**Red Flag** Altered responsiveness (for example, irritable, lethargic)	Decreased level of consciousness
	Skin colour unchanged	Skin colour unchanged	Pale or mottled skin
	Warm extremities	Warm extremities	Cold extremities
	Eyes not sunken	**Red Flag** Sunken eyes	-
	Moist mucous membranes (except after a drink)	Dry mucous membranes (except for 'mouth breather')	-
	Normal heart rate	**Red Flag** Tachycardia	Tachycardia
	Normal breathing pattern	**Red Flag** Tachypnoea	Tachypnoea
	Normal peripheral pulses	Normal peripheral pulses	Weak peripheral pulses
	Normal capillary refill time	Normal capillary refill time	Prolonged capillary refill time
	Normal skin turgor	**Red Flag** Reduced skin turgor	-
	Normal blood pressure	Normal blood pressure	Hypotension (decompensated shock)

© NICE [2009] Assesing Dehydration. Available from www.nice.org.uk/guidance/CG84 All rights reserved

SEE ALSO
CHAPTER 27

GASTROENTERITIS

Gastroenteritis is characterised by the sudden onset of diarrhoea and may or may not include vomiting (NICE, 2009). Gastroenteritis is very common and can range from a minor illness to a life-threatening one, as it affects absorption in the gastrointestinal tract, which in turn can lead to dehydration due to fluid loss. The causes of gastroenteritis can be bacterial, viral or parasitic infection (Glasper et al., 2016) and the majority of children are cared for in the community. However, as a nursing student, you will almost certainly care for young children admitted to hospital with dehydration as a result of gastroenteritis.

Treatment and management of gastroenteritis

Initially, infection control measures need to be instigated to prevent cross-contamination. If there is mild to moderate dehydration, then oral rehydration salt (ORS) solutions should be suitable, but if the dehydration is severe, then intravenous fluids will be required. Once rehydration is completed then normal feeding/drinking patterns are recommenced. The use of medications such as antidiarrhoeals, antiemetics or antibiotics are not normally recommended.

Some infections causing gastroenteritis are classed as notifiable diseases under the Public Health (Control of Disease) Act 1984 and Health Protection (Notification) Regulations 2010. This normally only applies to gastroenteritis caused by food poisoning, rather than the more common viral causes such as rotavirus or norovirus. Where the cause is notifiable, a notification form needs to be completed (GOV.UK, 2022).

Where there are no signs of clinical dehydration, current guidelines (see Table 26.4) recommend continuing with breast or formula feeding, encouragement of fluid intake (but not fruit juices or carbonated drinks) and offering ORS solution as supplemental fluid to those whose risk of developing dehydration is high (NICE, 2009).

Table 26.4 Treatment of clinical dehydration and clinical shock based on NICE guidelines

Use of oral rehydration salt (ORS) solution to treat clinical dehydration	Use of intravenous therapy to treat clinical shock
• Use ORS solution to rehydrate children unless intravenous therapy is indicated • Give 50ml/kg for fluid deficit replacement over 4 hours on top of maintenance fluid • Give small amounts of ORS solution frequently • Consider supplementing with usual fluids, including breast/formula milk or water if sufficient amounts of ORS solution are refused • Consider using nasogastric tube if vomiting or an inadequate volume of ORS solution is taken • Use regular clinical assessment to monitor response to therapy	• Use intravenous therapy if shock is suspected or confirmed • Treat with rapid infusion of 20ml/kg of 0.9% saline • Repeat infusion if required and consider consulting paediatric intensive care specialist • If an initial fluid rapid infusion was required for suspected or confirmed shock, then 100ml/kg is recommended on top of the maintenance fluid requirement • Consider other causes of shock rather than dehydration • Monitoring of blood biochemistry should happen from the outset and then be monitored regularly. The composition of the fluid should be altered and infusion rate changed if required

Source: NICE (National Institute for Health and Clinical Excellence) (2009) Diarrhoea and vomiting caused by gastroenteritis in under 5s: diagnosis and management. Guideline CG84. www.nice.org.uk/guidance/cg84

Intravenous therapy

As a nursing student, you may be involved in caring for a patient with an intravenous infusion and keeping a record of the amount infused. It is also important that you are familiar with fluid prescription charts and the standard protocol for rehydration through intravenous therapy, as recommended by NICE (2020) and The Inquiry into Hyponatraemia-related Deaths Report (2018). NICE guidance on intravenous (IV) fluid therapy in children and young people in hospital (NICE, 2020) recommends isotonic crystalloid fluids containing 131–154 mmol/l sodium for routine maintence intravenous fluids. Plasma electrolytes and blood glucose should be measured prior, then checked daily whilst intravenous therapy continues (NICE, 2020). Where fluid restriction is necessary due to fluid retention, the infusion rate should be restricted to between 50-80% of the routine maintenance volume (NICE, 2020). Fluid prescription charts should be signed, dated, timed and written clearly with fluids prescribed in millilitres (ml) per hour. All input and output should be recorded on an hourly basis and a running total kept, with 12-hourly fluid balance subtotals and reassessment of the fluid prescription and hydration status (NICE, 2020). A 24-hour fluid balance should also be calculated, alongside 12-hourly assessment of whether oral fluids can be re-started (NICE, 2020). Training in the principles of intravenous therapy is recommended (NICE, 2017; Report of the Inquiry into Hyponatraemia-related Deaths Report, 2018), and managing the administration of intravenous fluid therapy alongside infusion pumps and devices is now part of the Nursing and Midwifery Council's *Future Nurse: Standards of Proficiency for Registered Nurses* document (NMC, 2018).

After rehydration, the advice is the same as that for preventing dehydration. Breast/formula feeding should be reintroduced and in older children fluid intake should be encouraged, avoiding fruit juice or carbonated drinks. In children who continue to be at risk of dehydration, due to the continuation of diarrhoea and/or vomiting, ORS solution should also be considered (NICE, 2009).

WHAT'S THE EVIDENCE?

Modern nursing care is rooted in an evidence base and, as a nursing student, you should be aware of where to find clinical evidence to provide a rationale for your practice and the care you deliver. Publications produced by the National Institute for Health and Care Excellence (NICE) are one example of evidence-based guidance with a reputation for rigour, independence and objectivity.

Go now to 'Diarrhoea and vomiting caused by gastroenteritis in under 5s: diagnosis and management' (NICE, 2009) and download the full guideline.

- How many articles were reviewed in Chapter 5 'Fluid management', before the recommendations on treating dehydration were made?
- Are you surprised by the detail in this guideline?
- This guidline is now over 10 years old – why has it not been updated?

To help consolidate your learning so far, look at a hypothetical case study based on a common presentation seen in emergency departments. Work your way through the findings presented and answer the questions that follow.

CASE STUDY 26.1: ALBERT

Albert is 18 months old and is brought to the emergency department by his parents, following a 3-day history of diarrhoea and vomiting. Albert's parents noticed his symptoms had become worse in

(Continued)

the last 24 hours. In response to your questions, they inform you that both mum and Albert's 3-year-old sibling have both had an 'upset stomach' recently. Examinations indicate:

A - Self-ventilating in air with saturations >95%
B - Respiratory rate: 45 breaths per minute
C - Heart rate: 140 beats per minute; blood pressure 90/45; capillary refill time 2 secs
D - Albert is irritable
E - Temperature: 37.1°C
F - Reduced skin turgor, dry mucous membranes and his eyes appear sunken

When asked, Albert's mum tells you he hasn't had a wet nappy since yesterday evening.

- Using the assessment of dehydration tool in Table 26.3, how dehydrated is Albert?
- What are your key nursing care priorities for Albert?

SODIUM IMBALANCE (HYPONATRAEMIA AND HYPERNATRAEMIA)

A sodium level of below 136 mmol/l is known as hyponatraemia and can be caused either through sodium loss resulting from diarrhoea, excessive sweating or renal failure, or by an excess of water that causes the body's sodium concentration to become diluted. Hyponatraemia is a serious condition requiring urgent treatment, as a low sodium level can lead to convulsions, caused by the movement of water from the extracellular compartment to the intracellular compartment, increasing brain volume. Treatment is normally through intravenous infusion of an isotonic solution such as 0.9% saline, or 0.9% saline with 5% glucose. Where shock is suspected or confirmed, rapid intravenous infusion is recommended (NICE, 2009).

ACTIVITY 26.3: REFLECTIVE PRACTICE

THE INQUIRY INTO HYPONATRAEMIA-RELATED DEATHS (2018)

This inquiry, which was carried out following the deaths of five children in Northern Ireland, made a total of 96 recommendations. You can read the full report here http://www.ihrdni.org/inquiry-report.htm. The recommendations directly relating to fluid management and hyponatraemia are below:

Recommendation 24: All blood test results should state clearly when the sample was taken, when the test was performed and when the results were communicated and in addition serum sodium results should be recorded on the Fluid Balance Chart.
Recommendation 58: HSC Trusts should ensure that all nurses caring for children have facilitated access to e-learning on paediatric fluid management and hyponatraemia.

Have these recommendations been incorpated into policy in your placement area? Ask your practice assessor/supervisor.

Hypernatraemia is the medical term for a high sodium level, which is defined as being above 145mmol/l. A high sodium level could be caused by dehydration resulting from fluid deprivation or diarrhoea, or through excessive salt intake. Incorrect formula feed preparation or adding salt to solids whilst weaning can cause excessive salt intake, as can deliberate salt poisoning, although this is rare. Hypernatraemic dehydration is very dangerous (Lissauer and Carroll, 2022), because the shift in water from the intracellular compartment to the extracellular compartment means that some of the red flag signs of dehydration, such as sunken eyes and reduced skin turgor, are harder to spot. As water is drawn out of the brain, jittery movements, increased muscle tone, altered consciousness, seizures and cerebral haemorrhage may occur. Treatment involves rehydration using either 0.9% saline, or 0.9% saline with 5% glucose via slow intravenous infusion, typically over 48 hours and reverting to oral rehydration therapy as soon as it is tolerated (NICE, 2009).

In both hyponatraemia and hypernatraemia, sodium levels should be monitored, so you should expect your patient to have their blood taken on a regular basis, as per guidance in 'Intravenous fluid therapy in children and young people in hospital' (NICE, 2020).

POTASSIUM IMBALANCE (HYPOKALAEMIA AND HYPERKALAEMIA)

Potassium imbalance occurs when there is too little (hypokalaemia) or too much (hyperkalaemia) potassium in the bloodstream. It is less common than sodium imbalance, but more serious. Hyperkalaemia (above 5.5mmol/l) is caused by either ineffective elimination of potassium through the renal system or through excessive release of potassium from the cells. Causes of ineffective elimination include renal failure or a sudden reduced urine volume (oliguria) and congenital adrenal hyperplasia. Some medications such as potassium-sparing diuretics, nonsteroidal anti-inflammatory drugs (NSAIDs) and angiotensin-converting enzyme (ACE) inhibitors can also interfere with urinary excretion and may result in raised potassium levels. Excessive release of potassium from cells may occur from tissue necrosis, burn injury or massive haemolysis, during which red blood cells are rapidly broken down and their contents released into the surrounding blood plasma. A high potassium blood result can also be a false positive. This is common in very young children for whom there has been difficulty in obtaining a blood sample. Known as pseudohyperkalaemia, this is the result of laboratory artefact rather than actual potassium imbalance, so where this is suspected, the blood test should be repeated.

Hyperkalaemia is potentially very dangerous as it can cause serious, even fatal, cardiac arrhythmias (Miall et al., 2016). Treatment for hyperkalaemia includes nebulised salbutamol, insulin and glucose infusion to encourage potassium into the cells. Calcium may also be given to protect the myocardium (heart) (Samuels and Wieteska, 2016).

Hypokalaemia (below 3mmol/l) is usually less serious, but still requires treatment as it can lead to muscle weakness, lethargy, gastric ileus and in severe hypokalaemia (below 2.5mmol/l) cardiac arrhythmias. Causes of low potassium include diarrhoea and vomiting, diuretic therapy and an inadequate potassium intake through starvation. As a nursing student, you may care for a young person with anorexia nervosa who has been admitted to hospital with a low potassium level. Depending on the severity of the hypokalaemia, treatment is either via oral potassium supplements (preferred) or an intravenous infusion of potassium (Samuels and Wieteska, 2016).

Because potassium can cause cardiac arrhythmias, children with a potassium imbalance should be nursed under ECG monitoring to observe for any changes to the ECG, and where high dose intravenous infusion of potassium is indicated, close cardiac monitoring is essential (Samuels and Wieteska, 2016). As with a sodium imbalance, you should also expect your patient to have their blood taken frequently to monitor the potassium level.

A summary of sodium and potassium imbalances is presented in Table 26.5.

Table 26.5 Summary of sodium and potassium imbalance

		Caused by	Signs and symptoms
Sodium (Na+)	Hyponatraemia (<136mmol/l)	Diarrhoea Excess sweating Renal failure Excess water = dilute sodium concentration	Convulsions
	Hypernatraemia (>145mmol/l)	Diarrhoea Fluid deprivation Excess salt intake	Jittery movements Increased muscle tone Altered consciousness Cerebral haemorrhage
Potassium (K+)	Hypokalaemia (<3mmol/l)	Diarrhoea and vomiting Diuretic therapy Intake potassium intake through starvation	Muscle weakness Lethargy Gastric ileus In severe hypokalaemia, cardiac arrhythmias
	Hyperkalaemia (>5.5mmol/l)	Excessive release of potassium from the cells through: • Tissue necrosis • Burn injury • Haemolysis Renal failure Congenital adrenal hyperplasia Medications such as: • Potassium-sparing diuretics • Nonsteriodal anti-inflammatory drugs • ACE inhibitors	Nausea and vomiting Dizziness Muscle cramps ECG changes Cardiac arrhythmias which can lead to cardiac arrest

CASE STUDY 26.2: CHELSEA

Chelsea is 9 months old and has been brought to the emergency department by her mother and grandmother. She has jittery movements, decreased consciousness, no history of diarrhoea or vomiting, but her urea and electrolytes show a high sodium level. Chelsea is formula fed and was weaned 3 months ago. Chelsea's grandmother tells you that she makes all of Chelsea's food as 'babies should be encouraged to eat the same food as the rest of the family'.

• What do you think might be the cause of Chelsea's hypernatremia?
• What health promotion may be needed for this family?

SAFEGUARDING STOP POINT

Consider Chelsea's case. Do you identify any cause for concern in the case study?

The grandmother's phrase 'babies should be encouraged to eat the same food as the rest of the family' may indicate the use of food meant for adult consumption and this may place Chelsea at harm.

Read the following news reports into the case of a child who died from accidental salt ingestion. BBC News - http://news.bbc.co.uk/1/hi/uk/404667.stm and The Guardian https://www.theguardian.com/

lifeandstyle/1999/jul/28/familyandrelationships.features101 - What were the factors that contributed to the child's death?

- What weaning advice would you give to parents?

ACTIVITY 26.4: CRITICAL THINKING

Write a plan of care for a child with diarrhoea and vomiting, taking into consideration fluid management and infection control needs. Annotate your care plan with available evidence and discuss this with your practice assessor. Your care plan could be used as evidence towards achieving your learning competencies while in placement.

The ability to manage a child's fluid and electrolyte balance is an important skill in children's nursing, as is the knowledge which underpins the process of homeostasis and acid-base balance in maintaining the body's equilibrium. Children, especially very young children, are at particular risk of dehydration and can become clinically dehydrated very quickly. Caring for a child who is dehydrated is a common occurrence and you will almost certainly come across this during placement.

CHAPTER SUMMARY

In this chapter, you have explored:

- Normal fluid requirements and electrolyte levels for children and young people alongside how to calulate daily fluid requirements and normal urine output for various ages and weights of children
- The importance of early recognition of dehydration and electrolyte imbalance, with a focus on gastroenteritis and how it is treated
- Common causes of sodium imbalance (hyponatraemia and hypernatraemia) and potassium imbalance (hypokalaemia and hyperkalaemia) and their complications.

In addition, you have enhanced your learning through the application of knowledge and understanding using case studies on dehydration and hypernatraemia.

BUILD YOUR BIBLIOGRAPHY

Books

- Glasper, A., Richardson, J. and Randall, D (2021) *A Textbook of Children's and Young People's Nursing*, 3rd edn. London: Elsevier.

  This widely accessible textbook contains information on fluid balance and homeostasis across several of its chapters.

FURTHER READING

- Miall, L., Rudolf, M. and Smith, D. (2016) *Paediatrics at a Glance*, 4th edn. Chichester: Wiley Blackwell.

  Intended as a quick reference, this textbook gives a brief, but thorough, overview of paediatric care, including diarrhoea management, dehydration and electrolyte balance.

Journal articles

FURTHER
READING:
ONLINE
JOURNAL
ARTICLES

- Falszewska, A., Dziechciarz, P. and Szajewska, H. (2014) 'The diagnostic accuracy of Clinical Dehydration Scale in identifying dehydration in children with acute gastroenteritis: a systematic review'. *Clinical Pediatrics*, 53 (12): 1181–8.

  This systematic review explores the data available on the accuracy of the clinical dehydration scale. It is a useful article to test your skills in research analysis.
- Mathieson, L. (2015) 'Vomiting and diarrhoea in children'. *InnovAiT*, 8 (10): 592–8.

  This easy-to-read article provides an overview of vomiting and diarrhoea in children, including common viral causes, clinical assessment, fluid management and complications.
- Mathur, A., Johnston, G. and Clark, L. (2020) Improving intravenous fluid prescribing. *Journal of the Royal College of Physicians of Edinburgh*, 50 (2): 181–7.

  Although this article is written for prescribers, it provides a useful overview of intravenous fluid therapy and best practice in prescription management.

Weblinks

FURTHER
READING:
WEBLINKS

- GOV.UK, *Notifiable Diseases and Causative Organisms: How to Report* www.gov.uk/guidance/notifiable-diseases-and-causative-organisms-how-to-report Reporting certain notifiable infectious diseases aims to help prevent their spread and reduce the risk of epidemic. A list of notifiable diseases requiring report is available on this weblink.
- NICE, *Diarrhoea and Vomiting Caused by Gastroenteritis in Under 5s:* Diagnosis and Management www.nice.org.uk/guidance/cg84 This evidence-based guideline underpins clinical decision-making and care delivery for children under 5 who present with diarrhoea and vomiting.
- Spotting the Sick Child https://spottingthesickchild.com/ The Royal College of Paediatrics and Child Health and the Department of Health, as well as others, support this educational resource. It contains a section on dehydration.
- NICE, *Intravenous fluid therapy in children and young people in Hospital* www.nice.org.uk/guidance/ng29 This evidence-based guideline outlines the general principles for managing intravenous fluids in children and young people under the age of 16 years, and along with its associated quality standard [QS131] aims to improve the safety of intravenous fluid therapy in hospital for children and young people.

REFERENCES

Batcheler, S. and Dixon, M. (2012) 'Care of an infant or child with a cardiac condition or disease', in M. Dixon and D. Crawford (eds), *Paediatric Intensive Care Nursing*. Chichester: Wiley–Blackwell. pp.102–68.

Brady, M. (2019)) 'Homeostasis', in E. Gormley-Fleming and I. Peate (eds), *Fundamentals of Children's Applied Pathophysiology: An Essential Guide for Nursing and Healthcare Students*. Chichester: Wiley–Blackwell. pp.67-81.

Brady, M. (2021) 'Homeostasis', in I. Peate and E. Gormley-Fleming (eds), *Fundamentals of Children's Anatomy and Physiology: A Textbook for Nursing and Healthcare Students*, 2nd edn. Chichester: Wiley–Blackwell. pp.64-88.

Glasper, E.A., McEwing, G. and Richardson, J. (2016) *Oxford Handbook of Children's and Young People's Nursing*, 2nd edn. Oxford: Oxford University Press.

GOV.UK (2022) Notifiable Diseases and Causative Organisms: How to Report. Available at: www.gov.uk/guidance/notifiable-diseases-and-causative-organisms-how-to-report (accessed 27 June 2022).

Holliday, M.A. and Segar, W.E. (1957) 'The maintenance need for water in parenteral fluid therapy'. *Pediatrics*, 19 (5): 823–32.

Jones, N.P. (2021) 'Fluid, electrolyte balance and associated disorders', in I. Peate (ed.), *Fundamentals of Applied Pathophysiology: An Essential Guide for Nursing and Healthcare Students*, 3rd edn. Chichester: Wiley–Blackwell. pp.566–92 (accessed 27 June 2021).

Lissauer, T. and Carroll, W. (2022) *Illustrated Textbook of Paediatrics*, 6th edn. London: Elsevier.

Miall, L., Rudolf, M. and Smith, D. (2016) *Paediatrics at a Glance*, 4th edn. Chichester: Wiley–Blackwell.

NICE (National Institute for Health and Clinical Excellence) (2009) Diarrhoea and vomiting caused by gastroenteritis in under 5s: diagnosis and management. Clinical guideline [CG84]. Available at: www.nice.org.uk/guidance/cg84 (accessed: 27 June 2022).

NICE (National Institute for Health and Care Excellence) (2017) Intravenous fluid therapy in adults in hospital. Clinical guideline [CG174]. Available at: https://www.nice.org.uk/guidance/cg174 (accessed 26 July 2021).

NICE (National Institute for Health and Care Excellence) (2020) Intravenous fluid therapy in children and young people in hospital. NICE guideline [NG29]. Available at: www.nice.org.uk/guidance/ng29 (accessed 26 July 2021).

NMC (Nursing and Midwifery Council) (2018) *Future Nurse: Standards of Proficiency for Registered Nurses*. London: NMC.

Report of the Inquiry into Hyponatraemia-related Deaths (2018) Available at: http://www.ihrdni.org/inquiry-report.htm (accessed: 7 January 2023).

Samuels, M. and Wieteska, S. (2016) *Advanced Paediatric Life Support: A Practical Approach to Emergencies*, 6th edn. Chichester: Wiley–Blackwell.

CARE OF CHILDREN AND YOUNG PEOPLE WITH GASTROINTESTINAL PROBLEMS

27

ZOË VEAL, REBEKAH OVEREND AND DOREEN CRAWFORD

THIS CHAPTER COVERS

- Common gastrointestinal conditions
- Nursing management of gastrointestinal problems
- Nutrition
- Rationale for stoma (ostomy) formation
- Discharge planning and continuing care in the community

REQUIRED KNOWLEDGE

It would be helpful to have an understanding of the anatomy and physiology of the gastrointestinal system before you start this chapter.

> **"**
>
> "You worry that he's getting enough to grow, and that you will be able to manage the tube feeds, then you worry that he won't look like other children of his age because the nasogastric tube is really obvious."
>
> **Ramesh, parent**
>
> **"**

INTRODUCTION

The opening quotation illustrates how a parent can feel when their child requires enteral feeding, for whatever reason. They may feel concern that their child cannot feed 'normally' to grow and develop into a 'healthy' child/adult. They may also be worried their child will be treated differently from others. As a student, you will care for children with a range of gastrointestinal conditions and needs. Some may have acute and short-term conditions that quickly resolve on treatment whereas others may have chronic, lifelong difficulties with eating and digestion, requiring long-term treatment and intervention which impacts on the whole family. A family-focused approach is always essential when delivering child-centred care, and children's nurses are best placed to ensure this happens.

The gastrointestinal system is extensive and complex, consisting primarily of the oesophagus, stomach and small and large intestines, alongside accessory digestive organs: the pancreas, liver and gallbladder. Consequently, there are a number of conditions which can arise, either from a fault during embryological development or via disease process. As a children's nursing student, you may be involved in both the medical and surgical management of gastrointestinal problems, both in hospital and in the community.

COMMON GASTROINTESTINAL CONDITIONS

There are a number of common gastrointestinal conditions that you may come across during your placements. Some, especially those that are congenital/present at birth, require specialist intervention and care from a tertiary children's hospital and are seen less commonly outside of these settings. Others, such as gastroenteritis, are seen more frequently within the community, with children being admitted to hospital only when they become clinically dehydrated.

SEE ALSO
CHAPTER 14

Abdomimal pain

Abdominal pain is very common in children and the pain may be local or generalised. Young children may not be able to locate the exact area of pain within their abdomen and may have their own special words to describe it. Older children with localised pain should be able to point to the source. Older children may hold their tummy; infants may draw up their legs to indicate they have abdominal pain. Abdominal pain can have a surgical, medical or psychological cause.

Causes of abdominal pain

Constipation

Constipation is frequently seen in children and has a number of causes/risk factors:

- A diet low in fibre and not drinking enough fluids
- Unwillingness to use a school or public toilet – 'stool holding'
- Distraction or unwillingness to interrupt activity to use the toilet
- Lack of exercise/impaired mobility
- Fear of pain – previous anal fissure or passing a painful, hard stool in the past can lead to toilet delay/avoidance in the future
- Hirschsprung's disease

Around a third of 4–7-year-olds experience constipation, and many children experience constipation during potty training (Miall et al., 2016). In 2017, NICE updated guidelines on the diagnosis and management of constipation in children. For more information on this guideline, go to the 'Build your bibliography' section at the end of the chapter.

Functional/idiopathic constipation is the most common presentation seen in children and has no known anatomical or physiological cause. When there have been no bowel movements for several days, the faeces becomes hard and compacted in the rectum, making it more difficult and painful to pass. If the bowel becomes very impacted, then soiling can occur as faecal liquid leaks around the faecal mass. This can be mistaken for diarrhoea and can sometimes cause delay in accepting a constipation diagnosis. Treatment for functional constipation is based on a three-pronged approach – disimpaction of the bowel through the use of laxatives, parent and child education and maintenance therapy consisting of improved diet, exercise and regular toileting, and medication (Glasper et al., 2015).

CASE STUDY 27.1: ZAC

You are on placement with the health visitor and you visit Zac, a 4-year-old boy, who according to his mother is a 'picky eater'. Zac has a history of constipation and soiling and is due to start school shortly. His mum has asked for advice.

- What advice would you give Zac's mum to help manage his constipation?
- What advice would you give to Zac's mum regarding school?

Appendicitis/peritonitis

Appendicitis is an infection of the appendix, a small tube-shaped pouch attached to the colon. In many cases a surgeon will use a laparoscopy: precise abdominal incisions allow a small camera and probes to access the abdomen and remove the appendix, meaning children have a shortened recovery. Continual swelling of the appendix due to pus formation can eventually cause perforation of the appendix, releasing bacteria into the peritoneum and causing peritonitis, which can lead to septicaemia. Sudden relief of pain can indicate that perforation has occurred (in the same way that squeezing a spot relieves discomfort). Treatment for perforation is usually surgical removal of the appendix with a laparotomy; a large open incision of the abdominal wall, and nursing care will follow the routine pre- and postoperative care directed by local policy and surgical instruction. Conservative treatment with antibiotics is sometimes used, but its effectiveness as an alternative to surgery remains uncertain.

SEE ALSO
CHAPTER 14,
16 AND 26

Gastroenteritis

This is an extremely common condition in children, which causes diarrhoea and vomiting, often with sudden onset. Common viral causes include norovirus, adenovirus and rotavirus, which are highly infectious. Bacterial causes include *Shigella*, *Escherichia coli*, *Salmonella* and *Campylobacter*. Most cases can be managed successfully at home in the community, but the child may require hospitalisation if symptoms are prolonged and dehydration indicated. Oral rehydration regimes are the primary method for fluid replacement (NICE, 2009).

WHAT'S THE EVIDENCE?

Giving medication to stop vomiting or diarrhoea in gastroenteritis is not normally advised. However, ondansetron – an antiemetic licensed for prescription in children for chemotherapy-induced or post-operative nausea and vomiting – has been shown to be of some benefit in treating gastroenteritis. In studies undertaken outside the UK, more children stopped vomiting when given ondansetron compared to children given a placebo and fewer children needed intravenous therapy or hospitalisation to treat dehydration (NICE, 2014).

- Why might some prescribers be reluctant to prescribe ondansetron to treat gastroenteritis?
- Antiemetic and antidiarrhoeal medication is not normally advised – what might be the reason for this?

Gastritis/peptic ulcer

Gastritis is recognised to be an important cause of abdominal pain in children (Miall et al., 2016). Causes include infection with *Helicobacter pylori*, use of nonsteroidal anti-inflammatory medication, stress and an autoimmune response. Treatment involves symptom management, dietary and lifestyle changes (Knott, 2020).

Other causes of abdominal pain

Abdominal pain can also be caused by mesenteric adenitis, urinary tract infection, Henoch–Schönlein purpura, pyelonephritis, diabetic ketoacidosis and in adolescent girls, gynaecological causes such as ovarian cysts or ectopic pregnancy. Recurrent abdominal pain can also be caused by irritable bowel syndrome, anxiety and problems at home/school causing psychosomatic presentation of pain.

ACTIVITY 27.1: CRITICAL THINKING

A gynaecological cause may be the source of abdominal pain and in addition, the pregnancy status of females should be known before surgery. NICE states that all women of childbearing potential should be asked sensitively about the possibility of pregnancy and a pregnancy test carried out with consent, if there is doubt (NICE, 2016a). This is because there are associated risks with anaesthesia during pregnancy. However, this NICE guideline does not apply to young people under 16 years of age.
Consider the following:

- Should pregnancy checking be routinely carried out on all adolescent females?
- If you do discuss the possibility of pregnancy with your patient, should you document this?
- Should a pregnancy test be carried out without consent?
- What elements of privacy and dignity do you need to consider?
- Does your placement area have a protocol for pregnancy checking in adolescent female patients? Discuss this with your mentor.

Now read the Royal College of Paediatrics and Child Health (RCPCH, 2012) document *Pre-procedure Pregnancy Checking in Under 16s: Guidance for Clinicians*.

Congenital abnormalities of the gastrointestinal system

Gastroschisis/exomphalos (omphalocele)

Often considered to be similar, these are very different in presentation. During development, the intestine lengthens, bulging into the developing umbilical cord. Exomphalos (omphalocele) is the failure of this normal intestinal herniation into the umbilicus to close. Defect size may vary, but can involve the liver, spleen or bladder as well as the intestines. Surgical repair is possible, but the condition is associated with chromosomal abnormalities and other midline defects, so prognosis may be uncertain. In gastroschisis, the intestines are exposed as development of the abdominal wall also fails; consequently there is a risk of peritonitis and thickening of the bowel wall. Treatment is via surgical restoration of the bowel to the abdominal cavity and repair may occur in stages if the lesion is extensive. The infant will require intravenous feeding until the bowel can fulfil normal function. Prognosis is usually good.

SEE ALSO
CHAPTER 16

Oesophageal atresia/tracheo-oesophageal fistula

Tracheo-oesphageal fistula (TOF) is an abnormal passage between the trachea and oesophagus, whereas oesophageal atresia (OA) means the oesophagus ends in a blind pouch. OA can occur in isolation, but this is rare and both defects are usually seen together. Incidence is around 3 in 10000 live births worldwide (Tidy, 2023).

TOF/OA may be suspected antenatally if there is excessive amniotic fluid (polyhydraminos) or the stomach is unclear on ultrasound scan. At birth, if there is swallowing difficulty the midwife may attempt to pass an oragastric tube to check for patency of the oesophagus. Emergency steps are needed to secure the airway and a Repogle tube on low continuous suction is passed into the oesophagus to clear secretions which collect there. This is flushed regularly to maintain patency. Surgical repair is possible, but if the oesophageal gap is large, there may be a period of delay to allow the oesophagus to grow a little. Intravenous nutrition is seldom required, as feeds are usually tolerated through a gastrostomy.

Postoperative complications include stricture (scar tissue) and gastro-oesophageal reflux. TOF/OA is associated with VACTERL syndrome (Miall et al., 2016).

Malrotation/volvulus

Malrotation occurs in 1 in 2500–3000 births and is the failure of the midgut to rotate as it returns to the abdominal cavity during gestation. Although malrotation symptoms can occur at any time, the majority present during the first year of life (Great Ormond Street Hospital, 2019). Volvulus is an associated condition, which results from failure of the small intestine to fix correctly into the abdominal cavity, allowing for twisting and occlusion of the blood supply. For both conditions, bilious vomiting is a key presenting sign, indicating partial or complete bowel obstruction. The presentation of a sick child with a paralytic ileus and obvious abdominal distension is a surgical emergency. Repair is surgical (Ladd's procedure).

Anorectal anomaly/malformation

This is the term given to a range of anal malformations, from anal stenosis where the anal opening is too tight to allow for the passage of stool, to the complete absence of an anal opening and a rectum that ends as a fistula in the vagina (females) or urethra (males). Failure to pass meconium, or the presence of meconium in the urine are presenting signs. Incidence is between 1 in 3500–5000 births and the cause is unknown, although anorectal malformation is often associated other congenital anomalies (Royal Mancester Children's Hospital, 2022). Treatment is always surgical, and in several stages if a temporary colostomy is needed (Great Ormond Street Hospital, 2016). Bowel training or enemas/washouts may be required to help with managing the bowel fully.

Obstructive disorders

Intussusception

Intussusception is the most common form of bowel obstruction in children under the age of 3 years, accounting for 25% of abdominal emergencies in children under 5 years (Willacy, 2022). One part of the bowel telescopes into another part, causing colicky abdominal pain, bile-stained vomiting, pallor, lethargy, irritability, and possible dehydration and shock. A defining feature is the passage of blood and mucus in a 'redcurrant jelly' stool. Depending on the child's clinical condition, treatment is with either an air enema or surgical repair. Untreated intussusception is fatal.

Hirschsprung's disease

The absence of ganglion cells in the colon leads to weak/absent peristalsis – waves of muscular con-tractions along the intestines – meaning faeces cannot pass through normally. The extent of abnormal bowel can vary and symptoms can range from chronic constipation to bowel obstruction, depending on severity. Failure to pass meconium within 48 hours is an important sign (Miall et al., 2016). Repair is surgical to remove or bypass the portion of affected bowel. Occasionally, temporary or permanent colostomy is required.

Adhesions

Adhesions are fibrous bands that occur as a side effect of abdominal surgery, causing twisting and pull-ing, resulting in abdominal pain and bowel obstruction. Adhesions are a surgical emergency.

Problems with the gastric sphincters

Pyloric stenosis

Pyloric stenosis is an idiopathic overgrowth of the pyloric sphincter causing an obstruction to gastric emptying. Peak incidence is at 6 weeks old, is more common in first-born male infants and tends to run in families. The infant presents with projectile vomiting after taking a feed, weight loss and dehydration. Treatment is correction of dehydration and laproscopic incision/dilation of the hypertrophied muscle.

SEE ALSO
CHAPTER 26

Gastro-oesophageal reflux disease (GORD)

This is the passage of gastric contents back into the oesophagus, causing pain and discomfort. Common in babies, especially premature infants and those who have had surgery for TOF. GORD is also seen in older children with cerebral palsy or Down syndrome (Miall et al., 2016).

NICE guidelines currently recommend the following:

- Maintain sleeping position on the back
- Breastfeeding assessment in breastfed infants with marked distress
- Offer smaller, more frequent feeds (maintaining daily amount) in formula-fed infants

- Trial of feed thickener or alginate therapy if the above has been unsuccessful
- Trial of proton pump inhibitors or H$_2$-receptor antagonists recommended only if there is pain and discomfort, and review effectiveness
- Jejunal feeding only if entral feeding is indicated and not tolerated, or if at risk of aspiration pneumonia
- Fundoplication surgery only if medical management has failed or feeding regimes have become impractical (NICE, 2019)

For more information, read the NICE guideline NG1 (see 'Build your bibliography' at the end of the chapter).

Autoimmune disorders

Crohn's disease and ulcerative colitis

Collectively known as inflammatory bowel disease (IBD), Crohn's disease and ulcerative colitis are autoimmune conditions. Crohn's disease can affect any part of the child's gastrointestinal tract from mouth to anus; ulcerative colitis affects the rectum and colon only. The exact cause is unknown but is most likely a combination of genetic, environmental and immunological factors (Crohn's and Colitis UK, 2022). Presentation includes abdominal pain, diarrhoea, rectal bleeding, weight loss and fatigue. Treatment and management depends on severity, but usually involves nutritional support and hydration, corticosteroid and immunosuppressant medication. Wherever possible, surgery is avoided but a resection and anastomosis surgical technique may be required or a resection and formation of a stoma, which may or may not be permanent (Glasper et al., 2016).

There is separate NICE guidance for both Crohn's disease and ulcerative colitis, alongside a NICE quality standard which can be found in the 'Build your bibliography' section.

Coeliac disease

This is a lifelong autoimmune disorder in which the body reacts to gluten, a protein found in wheat, barley and rye. Coeliac disease affects around 1 in 100 people and although it can present in infancy, more commonly it presents in later childhood (Lissauer and Carroll, 2022). Symptoms can range from mild to severe, with faltering growth in extreme cases. Other symptoms include diarrhoea, poor appetite, abdominal distension and lethargy. Diagnosis is via antibody testing and depending on these results, possible intestinal biopsy. Coeliac disease, once confirmed, is managed by a gluten-free diet for life and, if necessary, supplements to treat deficiencies in iron, vitamin B12 or folic acid. There is NICE guidance (NICE, 2015) available to support healthcare decision-making.

Other gastrointestinal problems

Necrotising enterocolitis (NEC)

SEE ALSO
CHAPTER 30

NEC is primarily seen in premature infants where sections of the intestine become necrotic, resulting in potential perforation and peritonitis. The exact cause is unknown. Presentation usually occurs while the infant is still in the neonatal unit and signs may be subtle at first – lethargy, reduced feeding, 'not themselves' and not tolerating handling as well as usual. This may progress to more worrying signs such as apnoea, bradycardia, poor thermoregulation, abdominal distension, vomiting and the appearance of blood in the stools.

Treatment can be either by medical or surgical approaches. The conservative approach of nil by mouth, naso/orogastric tube to empty stomach of contents, intravenous fluids, parenteral nutrition (PN) and antibiotics is usually tried first. If the infant's bowel should perforate, surgery is required to resect the diseased bowel and rejoin (anastomose) the healthy ends. The repair is usually protected by the formation of a temporary stoma.

Lactose intolerance and cow's milk protein allergy

Cow's milk protein allergy (CMPA) is an abnormal reaction by the immune system to proteins found in cow's milk. It affects around 7% of formula-fed and 0.5% of exclusively breast-fed infants, which suggests that exclusive breast-feeding may protect infants from developing CMPA. A range of gastric, respiratory and skin symptoms may be seen, including vomiting, abdominal pain, bloody stools and diarrhoea, hives, eczema, and wheeze (NICE, 2021). Treatment is the elimination of cow's milk from the diet. CMPA is more likely if close family members have asthma, eczema or hayfever. However, prognosis is good with most cases resolving as the child grows (Miall et al., 2016).

Lactose intolerance is the inability to digest lactose due to deficiency in the lactase enzyme (Shah, 2022). Lactose is a type of sugar found in milk and dairy products. Symptoms include flatulence, bloating, abdominal discomfort and diarrhoea, usually occurring within hours of consuming food/drink containing lactose. Infants with lactose intolerance cannot be breastfed – they must have lactose-free formula instead (Shah, 2022). The symptoms are similar to other gastrointestinal disorders and may be confused with CMPA. However, it should be noted that lactose intolerance is *not* the same as a milk or dairy allergy.

Parasite/worm infection

The most common parasite infection is *Giardia lamblia*, which causes diarrhoea, weight loss and abdominal pain. Transmission is via faecal contamination in food/drink or hand-to-mouth contact. Excretion of *Giardia* is intermittent, so collection of three stool samples from different days is advised. Treatment is with tinidazole or metronidazole (Knott, 2022).

Threadworms are common in children. The eggs are laid around the anus, causing itching and are then transferred to fingers when the child scratches. Transmission is via hand-to-mouth contact and because children are very social beings, transmission is particularly easy. Management is via improved hygiene and a single dose of mebendazole. The whole family should be treated at the same time to ensure eradiciation and avoid reinfection (Tidy, 2021).

Roundworm and tapeworms are uncommon in the UK but more serious, and may be seen following a visit overseas. Infection is by the ingestion of contaminated food/water, or from contaminated soil (roundworms) or raw/undercooked meat (tapeworms). Both require medical treatment.

Problems with accessory digestive organs – liver

Neonatal jaundice is very common and usually resolves as the liver enzymes mature during the first week of life. Congenital defects of the liver, such as biliary atresia and choledochal cysts are rare, but result in obstruction of bile flow. Symptoms include jaundice, dark urine, pale stools, abdominal mass, abdominal pain and faltering growth. Early detection of biliary atresia is vital, so infants who remain jaundiced a fortnight after birth should be further investigated (NICE, 2016b), with referral to a specialist centre if biliary atresia is suspected. Surgical treatment to reconstruct or bypass the bile duct is not curative and liver transplantation is usually required by early adulthood.

SEE ALSO
CHAPTER 3, 14
& 26

NURSING MANAGEMENT OF GASTROINTESTINAL PROBLEMS

To a certain extent, the nursing requirement will be dependent on the gastrointestinal problem and whether management is following a medical or surgical route, or being delivered in hospital or at home. However, the type of nursing care you will be expected to deliver is likely to consist of some or all of the following:

- Pain assessment and management
- Assessment of the acutely ill child
- Vital signs observations – temperature, pulse, respiration, blood pressure, oxygen saturations, capillary refill time, level of consciousness (ACVPU) and PEW score
- Management of fluid and electrolyte balance – oral, gastrostomy and/or intravenous fluid intake and urine and gastric output (faeces/vomit/stoma losses), assessment of and treatment for dehydration
- Infection control – management of diarrhoea and vomiting, wound/stoma care
- Nutritional assessment and support via oral, enteral and parenteral routes
- Stool assessment using the Bristol Stool Chart
- Pre- and postoperative care
- Critical Care level 1 and 2 nursing care (Paediatric Critical Care Society, 2021)
- Medication administration
- Parent/child/young person education

SEE ALSO
CHAPTER 4,
16 & 29

As a nursing student, you will be involved in assisting healthcare professionals to carry out diagnostic tests and collecting specimens for examination by biomedical scientists in the pathology, biochemistry and haematology departments. See Table 27.1 for details.

Table 27.1 Common diagnostic tests

Diagnostic test	Purpose
Urinalysis	Rule out urinary tract infection as cause of abdominal pain. Assess dehydration status
Stool culture	Identify causative bacteria/micro-organisms in gastroenteritis/food poisoning
Full blood count (FBC)	Raised white blood cells in appendicitis and urinary tract infection. Anaemia may indicate blood loss, malabsorption, poor iron intake
Urea and electrolytes (U&E)	Assess for electrolyte imbalance and dehydration
C-reactive protein (CRP)	A raised CRP may be seen with infection/inflammatory bowel disease
Blood gas	Identify any acid–base imbalance in the acutely ill child
Abdominal X-ray	Look for dilated bowel loops (intestinal obstruction), abnormal gas pattern (intussusception) or faecal loading (constipation)
Abdominal ultrasound scan	May diagnose appendicitis/intussusception/pyloric stenosis
Barium enema	Used to see the outline of the large intestine
pH study	Diagnosis and severity of GORD
Upper GI contrast study	May be used in GORD, or following bile-stained vomiting to rule out malrotation of gut

Diagnostic test	Purpose
Coeliac antibodies	Test for coeliac disease
Biopsy	A small sample of tissue is taken for examination under a microscope
Endoscopy	Camera investigation of the gastrointestinal tract. Can be either upper GI via the mouth and oesophagus, or lower GI via the rectum

NUTRITION

As a nursing student, an understanding of nutrition and nutritional assessment is important because good nutrition in childhood is vital in maximising growth, development and wellbeing, whereas poor nutrition can cause or complicate childhood ill health.

SAFEGUARDING STOP POINT

Malnutrition is defined as a lack of proper nutrition and can refer to either undernutrition, when a child does not get sufficient nutrients, leading to poor growth and development, or overnutrition, when a child receives more nutrients than are needed, leading to obesity.

There are multiple reasons why a child may be underweight for their age. However, as a children's nurse, it is important to recognise that one cause could be the deliberate withholding of nutrition by the child's parent/carer.

What signs might indicate that a child is being deliberately starved?

When a teacher or a healthcare professional is concerned about a child, it is common for them to speak to the child's parent/carer, but who else should they speak to?

If you think a child is at risk of harm, to whom should you report your concerns?

Enteral and parenteral methods of feeding

Sometimes, the child may be unable to eat and drink normally – they may have had surgery, be unable to swallow properly, or it may be unsafe for them to feed orally. Some conditions dictate that the gastrointestinal tract cannot be used, as there may be mechanical dysfunction, the gut may require 'resting', or the stomach is required to be empty.

"The nasogastric tube was fairly easy to manage but when it turned out he needed a naso-jejunal tube it all got a bit trickier. It's different, we can't insert it ourselves like the NG tube, neither can the CCNs. It goes into the jejunum and takes much longer to put in ... it's very precious, and if it comes out that means a long wait in A&E and then X-rays to check it's where it should be."

Alice, parent

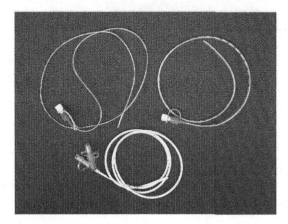

Figure 27.1 Nasogastric tubes

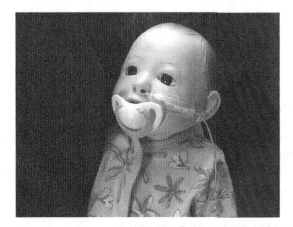

Figure 27.2 Nasogastric tube in position

The decision to move to enteral or parenteral feeding is not taken lightly and the route chosen will depend on the specific needs of each individual child. Knowledge, care and skill are required by the team around the child to ensure safe and effective nutritional support. Enteral feeds may be delivered by bolus or pump-controlled continuous feeding methods, dependent on the route used. For enteral-fed infants, breast milk is the feed of choice, but where breast milk is not available, an infant feeding formula can be used. Children require dietician input and specialist formula feeds to ensure their nutritional needs are fully met. Infants receiving enteral feeding may benefit from non-nutritive sucking of their thumb, fingers or a soother. This reduces length of hospital stay and the transition time from enteral to oral feeding (Foster et al., 2016).

Table 27.2 Types of enteral feeding

Enteral route	How it works
Nasogastric/orogastric tube	A tube inserted into either the nose or mouth, which is then passed into the oesophagus and stomach. Used to aspirate stomach contents or deliver feeds and medication. Tube position must be checked before every use

Enteral route	How it works
Nasojejunal tube	Method of feeding directly into the small bowel, the tube is passed into the nose and through the oesophagus and stomach into the jejunum. Useful in delayed gastric emptying, persistent vomiting or high aspiration risk. Tube position must be checked before every use. Compatibility of medication with the small intestine should be considered, to ensure proper absorption
Gastrostomy/jejunostomy Percutaneous endoscopic gastrostomy/jejunostomy (PEG/PEJ)	Tube inserted through the stomach wall directly into the stomach/jejunem via surgical procedure. Used when long-term feeding is required. Gastrostomy/jejunstomy feeding reduces distress for the child who may not tolerate regular nasogastric/nasojejunal tube insertions. They are also less visible, an important cosmetic and psychological consideration

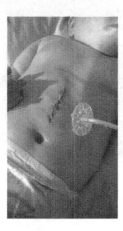

Figure 27.3 Position of gastrostomy

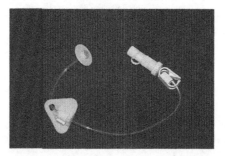

Figure 27.4 Percutaneous endoscopic gastrostomy with internal retention disc and external fixation plate

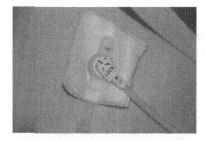

Figure 27.5 Low profile balloon gastrostomy (button) with extension set

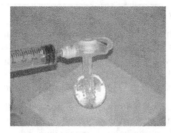

Figure 27.6 Low profile balloon gastrostomy (button) showing inflated balloon

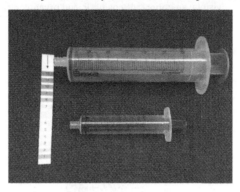

Figure 27.7 Enteral syringes and pH paper

CASE STUDY 27.2: MATTHIS

You are looking after Matthis who is 3 weeks old and was born with gastroschisis. Matthis has a nasogastric tube in place and feeds are slowly being introduced. A feed is due now – when you test the tube for its correct position, you cannot draw back any aspirate.

- What should you do now?

Read the policy on nasogastric feeding for your placement area.

- What does the policy advise?
- How practical is this advice for children in the community who have nasogastric feeds?

Discuss and document your thoughts with your practice assessor.

SEE ALSO
CHAPTER 37

Parenteral nutrition (PN) is the administration of specialised pre-prepared nutrients directly into the bloodstream in children with intestinal failure. It is invasive, requiring intravenous access usually through a central venous access device (CVAD) and carries high risks, so should be used only when there is no alternative method of feeding available. As a nursing student, you may care for children receiving PN, but its administration is regarded as an advanced nursing skill requiring registered nurse involvement and strict adherence to aseptic technique and biochemical monitoring.

Because the risk of sepsis is particularly high in invasive procedures like PN, it is important that you become aware of the early signs of sepsis and know how to act accordingly (NICE, 2017). The UK Sepsis

Trust (http://sepsistrust.org) has produced tools to aid early detection and management in various settings and across various age ranges.

SEE ALSO
CHAPTER 14

STOMA (OSTOMY) MANAGEMENT

When a child is unable to use the normal route of faecal elimination, an ostomy or stoma (opening) may be surgically created through the abdominal wall (see Table 27.3). A stoma may be either temporary or permanent.

Table 27.3 Types of stoma

Type	Location
Colostomy - stoma made from portion of colon	Usually left iliac fossa; typically flat to the abdominal wall
Ileostomy - stoma made from portion of ileum	Usually right iliac fossa; usually sticks out from the abdomen slightly

Where stoma formation is pre-planned, specific multidisciplinary care is required to ensure that the child and family are adequately prepared. Ideally, this involves physical and psychological preparation, familiarisation with the site, appearance, care of the stoma and equipment used such as stoma bags and securing methods. The stoma nurse specialist should be involved as early as possible and the psychological impact of having a stoma should not be ignored.

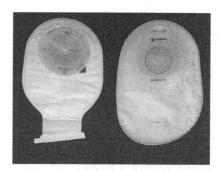

Figure 27.8   Stoma bags - drainable system and closed system

Stoma loss volume and consistency are dependent on the type and location of the stoma, but in general, the higher the intestinal location of the stoma, the greater the volume of losses. Children with a colostomy will have formed or semi-formed losses, whereas children with an ileostomy will have liquid losses and are at risk of sodium depletion due to the volume of losses they experience.

DISCHARGE PLANNING AND CONTINUING CARE IN THE COMMUNITY

Discharge planning should begin on admission to hospital and will be dependent on the reason for admission. The child and family are likely to require information about the condition itself and ongoing care in the community. Some children may have been hospitalised for a long period of time and if this is the first time the family have been able to take their child home, they also need to adjust to being a family, as well as coping with any additional needs their child may have. If the family have received care from a specialist tertiary centre far from home, they may feel anxious about taking their child to their local hospital for continuing care. Brief admission to their local hospital before full discharge home may help to alleviate this and enable the family to build a therapeutic relationship with staff that will continue their child's nursing care.

It is important to ensure parents/carers are trained and competent in all ongoing care needs their child may have. This is important in maintaining the health and safety of the child, both physically and psychologically. As a nursing student, you may be involved in the education and assessment of families, although overall accountability for this lies with the registered nurse. Care in the community for children with long-term conditions is likely to include:

- Wound care (surgical patients)
- Outpatients appointments
- Medication management and administration
- Nutrition management – healthy eating, enteral feeding, parenteral nutrition
- Specialist nursing input – for example, stoma nurse, children's community nurse, enteral feeding nurse
- Open access arrangements to the local children's ward
- Stoma care and prescriptions for stoma equipment
- Feeding tube care and prescriptions for feeds and equipment
- Bloods and other routine monitoring – particularly important for children on parenteral nutrition
- Listening to the concerns of parents and providing emotional as well as practical support

CHAPTER SUMMARY

The ability to understand the gastrointestinal tract and its altered anatomy and functions is an important aspect of children's nursing care. This chapter will have provided you with information about:

- Nursing assessment and management of children with gastrointestinal conditions in hospital and community settings
- Nutritional awareness and the importance of promoting growth and development
- Ostomy/stoma management, education and support
- Proactive discharge planning and care in the community
- The art of listening to and meeting the needs of children and families with gastrointestinal conditions

BUILD YOUR BIBLIOGRAPHY

Books

FURTHER READING

- Dixon, M. and Crawford, D. (eds) (2012) *Paediatric Intensive Care Nursing*. Chichester: Wiley-Blackwell. Chapter 8 on gastrointestinal and endocrine function and Chapter 12 on nutrition and fluid management explore the care needs when gastrointestinal disturbance moves from 'standard' to higher dependency levels of care.

- Bruce, E.A., Williss, J. and Gibson, F. (eds) (2023) *The Great Ormond Street Hospital Manual of Children and Young People's Nursing Practices*, 2nd edn. Chichester: Wiley-Blackwell.

  This practice and procedure based textbook contains an excellent chapter on nutrition and feeding, including procedural guides to enteral and parenteral feeding.
- Peate, I. and Gormley-Fleming, E. (2021) *Fundamentals of Children and Young People's Anatomy and Physiology: A Textbook for Nursing and Healthcare Students*, 2nd edn. Chichester: Wiley-Blackwell.

  This A&P textbook contains a useful chapter on the digestive system and nutrition, along with clinical application sections and other activities.
- Gormley-Fleming, E. and Peate, I. (2019) *Fundamentals of Children's Applied Pathophysiology: An Essential Guide for Nursing and Healthcare Students*. Chicester: Wiley-Blackwell.

  This pathophysiology textbook is the companion text to the antomy and physiology textbook above, and contains a chapter exploring the altered physiology of the gastrointestinal system.

Journal articles

FURTHER READING: ONLINE JOURNAL ARTICLES

- Ismail, N., Ratchford, I., Proudfoot, C. and Gibbs, J. (2011) 'Impact of a nurse-led clinic for chronic constipation in children'. Journal of Child Health Care, 15 (3): 221–9.

  This article on UK-based research demonstrates how a nurse-led clinic was more successful at treating chronic constipation than a general paediatric clinic.
- El-Matary, W. (2011) 'Percutaneous endoscopic gastrojejunostomy tube feeding in children'. Nutrition in Clinical Practice, 26 (1): 78–83.

  This UK-based article explores the use of gastrojejunostomy tube feeding in children for whom PEG feeding is not an option.
- Broekaert, I.J., Falconer, J., Bronsky, J., Gottrand, F., Dall'Oglio, L., Goto, E., Hojsak, I., Hulst, J., Kochavi, B., Papadopoulou, A., Ribes-Koninckx, C., Schaeppi, M., Werlin, S., Wilschanski, M. and Thapar, N. (2019) 'The use of jejunal tube feeding in children: A Position Paper by the Gastroenterology and Nutrition Committees of the European Society for Paediatric Gastroenterology, Hepatology, and Nutrition 2019', *Journal of Pediatric Gastroenterology and Nutrition*, 69 (2): 239-58.

  This position paper provides expert guidance on the indications for the use of jejunal feeding tubes, alongside practical considerations to optimise use and safety.

Weblinks

FURTHER READING: WEBLINKS

- NICE, Constipation in Children and Young People: Diagnosis and Management, Clinical guideline CG99 www.nice.org.uk/guidance/cg99 This guideline outlines the diagnostic criteria and recommended management for constipation in children.
- NICE, Gastro-oesophageal Reflux Disease in Children and Young People: Diagnosis and Management, NICE guideline [NG1] www.nice.org.uk/guidance/ng1 This guideline, updated in 2019, outlines the diagnostic criteria and management of children with gastro-oesophageal reflux disease (GORD).
- NICE, Inflammatory Bowel Disease, Quality standard [QS81] www.nice.org.uk/guidance/qs81 This quality standard, published in 2015, describes the high-priority areas for quality improvement in IBD, detailing diagnosis and management of the condition in adults, children and young people.

REFERENCES

Crohn's and Colitis UK (2022) *Information about Crohn's and Colitis*. Available at: https://crohnsandcolitis.org.uk/info-support/information-about-crohns-and-colitis (accessed 10 September 2022).

Foster, J.P., Psaila, K. and Patterson, T. (2016) 'Non-nutritive sucking for increasing physiologic stability and nutrition in preterm infants'. *Cochrane Database of Systematic Reviews*, 10. doi: 10.1002/14651858.CD001071.pub3.

Great Ormond Street Hospital (2016) *Anorectal Anomaly*. Available at: www.gosh.nhs.uk/conditions-and-treatments/conditions-we-treat/anorectal-anomaly/ (accessed 30 October 2022).

Great Ormond Street Hospital (2019) *Malrotation and Volvulus*. Available at: www.gosh.nhs.uk/conditions-and-treatments/conditions-we-treat/malrotation-and-volvulus/ (accessed 7 November 2022).

Glasper, A., Coad, J. and Richardson, J. (2015) *Children and Young People's Nursing at a Glance*. Chichester: Wiley–Blackwell.

Glasper, E.A., McEwing, G. and Richardson, J. (2016) *Oxford Handbook of Children's and Young People's Nursing*, 2nd edn. Oxford: Oxford University Press.

Knott, L. (2020) *Gastritis*. Available at: https://patient.info/digestive-health/dyspepsia-indigestion/gastritis (accessed 7 November 2022).

Knott, L. (2022) *Giardiasis: Causes, Symptoms and Treatment*. Available at: https://patient.info/doctor/giardiasis#nav-4 (accessed 30 October 2022).

Lissauer, T. and Carroll, W. (2022) *Illustrated Textbook of Paediatrics*, 6th edn. London: Elsevier.

Miall, L., Rudolf, M. and Smith, D. (2016) *Paediatrics at a Glance*, 4th edn. Chichester: Wiley–Blackwell.

NICE (National Institute for Health and Care Excellence) (2009) Diarrhoea and vomiting caused by gastroenteritis in under 5s: diagnosis and management. Clinical guideline [CG84]. Available at: https://www.nice.org.uk/guidance/cg84 (accessed 10 Sept 2022)

NICE (National Institute for Health and Care Excellence (2014) Management of vomiting in children and young people with gastroenteritis: ondansetron. Evidence summary [ESUOM34]. Available at: www.nice.org.uk/advice/esuom34/chapter/Key-points-from-the-evidence (accessed 10 September 2022).

NICE (National Institute for Health and Care Excellence) (2015) Coeliac disease: recognition, assessment and management. NICE guideline [NG20]. Available at: www.nice.org.uk/guidance/ng20 (accessed 10 September 2022).

NICE (National Institute for Health and Care Excellence) (2016a) Routine preoperative tests for elective surgery. NICE guideline [NG45]. Available at: www.nice.org.uk/guidance/ng45 (accessed 10 September 2022).

NICE (National Institute for Health and Care Excellence) (2016b) Jaundice in newborn babies under 28 days. Clinical Guideline [CG98]. Available at: www.nice.org.uk/guidance/cg98 (accessed 30 October 2022)

NICE (National Institute for Health and Care Excellence) (2017) Sepsis: recognition, diagnosis and early management. NICE guideline [NG51]. Available at: www.nice.org.uk/guidance/ng51 (accessed 10 September 2022).

NICE (National Institute for Health and Care Excellence) (2019) Guideline on gastro-oesophageal reflux disease in children and young people: diagnosis and management. NICE guideline [NG1]. Available at: www.nice.org.uk/guidance/ng1 (accessed 30 October 2022).

NICE (National Institute for Health and Care Excellence) (2021) Cow's milk allergy in children: When should I suspect cows' milk allergy? Clinical Knowledge Summary. Available at: https://cks. nice.org.uk/topics/cows-milk-allergy-in-children/diagnosis/diagnosis/ (accessed 30 October 2022).

Paediatric Critical Care Society (2021) *Quality Standards for the Care of Critically Ill or Injured Children*, 6th edn. Available at: https://pccsociety.uk/wp-content/uploads/2021/10/PCCS-Standards-2021. pdf (accessed 10 September 2022).

Royal College of Paediatrics and Child Health (RCPCH) (2012) *Pre-procedure Pregnancy Checking in Under 16s: Guidance for Clinicians*. London: RCPCH.

Royal Manchester Children's Hospital (2022) *Anorectal malformations (ARM)*. Available at: https:// mft.nhs.uk/rmch/services/manchester-centre-for-neonatal-surgery/conditions-we-treat-at-mcns/ anorectal-malformations-arm/ (accessed 30 October 2022).

Shah, S. (2022) *Lactose Intolerance: Causes, Symptoms and Treatment*. Available at: http://patient.info/ doctor/lactose-intolerance-pro (accessed 30 October 2022).

Tidy, C. (2021) *Threadworms*. Available at: https://patient.info/doctor/threadworms-pro#nav-4 (accessed 30 October 2022).

Tidy, C. (2023) *Oesophageal Atresia*. Available at: https://patient.info/doctor/oesophageal-atresia (accessed 16 July 2023).

Willacy, H. (2022) *Intussusception in Children*. Available at: https://patient.info/doctor/ intussusception-in-children (accessed 7 November 2022).

DISCHARGE PLANNING AND TRANSFER FOR CHILDREN AND YOUNG PEOPLE

28

ELIZABETH GILLESPIE AND JAYNE PRICE*

THIS CHAPTER COVERS

- Principles of discharge planning for children and families
- Simple discharge
- Complex discharge
- Transfers
- Transition from children to adult services
- Processes and systems influencing discharge and transfer

> **"** "Then I get the news I'm waiting for: if she does well tonight we get home tomorrow. She does well. In the morning we wait, and wait, for rounds. After lunch, we get to speak to a doctor. It now transpires that we can't go home because she's still on oxygen. If the healthcare team had spoken to me about how we manage our daughter at home, they would have known that she is on oxygen at night at home." **"**
>
> **Mother of a child with complex health needs**

---

*Based on the chapter in the first edition written by Elizabeth Gillespie and Sue Dunlop. We acknowledge and thank Sue Dunlop for her contribution.

INTRODUCTION

Since the Platt Report (Ministry of Health, 1959), it has been accepted that children should only be hospitalised when absolutely necessary, and for the briefest time possible to decrease the level of stress for the child and family (Debelic, 2022).

If children are admitted to hospital, they will require discharge to the community (either home/other organisation) or transfer to another inpatient setting. Although both discharge and transfer are everyday occurrences, these processes can be complex and challenging, leading to risk of fragmentation of care.

The opening quote is a classic example of miscommunication around discharge which led to a prolonged stay and increased parental anxiety. Leyenaar et al. (2017) advise that poor communication during discharge planning can leave parents feeling excluded from the discharge process.

Throughout this chapter we will explore principles of 'getting it right' when you are discharging and transferring children in partnership with the family.

PRINCIPLES OF DISCHARGE PLANNING FOR CHILDREN

Discharge planning is the process that clinicians undertake to ensure safe and effective transition from acute care settings (Holland et al., 2016). Thus, the aim of discharge planning is to reduce the length of hospital stay, unplanned readmission, and to improve the co-ordination of services following the child and family discharge (Gonclaves-Bradley et al., 2016).

Identifying the individual needs of the child and family as early as possible is central to addressing the challenges in the transition ensuring seamless care between hospital and home, including primary and secondary care (Mai et al., 2020). The essential components inherent in discharge planning are examined below.

Assessment

A holistic assessment of the child and family's needs is required in order to identify any support they may require (Foster et al., 2019).

This assessment should commence at an early stage of the admission, incorporating potential complex social and psychological concerns (Brenner et al., 2018). Discharge assessment must involve the family and take in to account their wishes as well as their strengths, resources and the capability of parents/carers to undertake the care of the child (Wellchild, 2021). Consideration of the child's readiness for discharge is required and will include patient safety, and ongoing care requirements and treatment they will require. Assessment also includes identification of the medical supplies and equipment required for the child's ongoing care. (Bowles et al., 2016). This assessment will also identify the potential need for ongoing support from community children's nurses (CCNs), general practitioners (GPs), therapists, and respite services, or increasingly, bespoke packages of care. Once a robust assessment has been carried out a discharge plan can be formulated, keeping the child and family central (Wu et al., 2016). Consideration of these factors will influence health outcomes and potential future readmissions to hospital (Weiss et al., 2020).

ACTIVITY 28.1: REFLECTIVE PRACTICE

Consider the Wellchild 10 principles of complex discharge (see Build Your Bibliography Weblinks). Reflect on how this tool can help clinicians to ensure a safe, timely and effective discharge.

Effective communication and information sharing

Effective communication and knowledge sharing is essential between the child, family and multidisciplinary team (MDT) to ensure a safe and effective discharge (Canary and Wilkins, 2017). Communication that is timely and accurate between multiple providers is key to a seamless transition coupled with an understanding of professional roles and responsibilities at the time of discharge (Manges et al., 2020). Roy et al. (2018) advise that comprehensive discharge information is essential for good communication and continuity of care.

Inadequate discharge communication can delay discharge and have a detrimental effect on outcomes for the child and family (Patel et al., 2022). Parental anxiety, uncertainty, and negative impact on parental confidence can also occur (Lerret et al., 2020). Furthermore, communication issues can result in noncompliance of care, increase adverse drug events and underutilisation of follow-up services (Curran et al., 2020). Effective communication and information sharing is essential within the discharge process and should be tailored for the individual child and family. Frequent repetition may be required to ensure that the child and family understand the information given and written resources should be available (Pladys, 2019). Canary and Wilkins. (2017) suggest communication is both the problem and solution in the discharge process. They advised that to improve the child/family outcomes after discharge healthcare providers need to implement system-wide communication solutions.

Processes to aid communication and knowledge sharing

Using discharge policies, protocols, care pathways, tools and checklists is integral to effective communication often leading to earlier discharge and fewer readmissions (Kucharczuk et al., 2022). Vanmol et al. (2017) advise that it is essential that policies, assessments and discharge protocols are shared across health systems and with the child/family, as this facilitates integration of services across primary and secondary care enabling working across specialist boundaries and closing gaps in care.

Integral to effective communication and knowledge sharing is excellence in record-keeping and documentation. Canary and Wilkins (2017) advise that shared record keeping with all involved professionals is essential for safe effective discharge. When we structure discharge planning, we can reduce readmission, increase family satisfaction and potentially improve quality outcome for children and families.

SEE ALSO
CHAPTER 2

Teaching and education

Teaching and education are essential in providing the child/family with the skill and knowledge to manage their child's care at home. Education regarding the childs's condition and disease trajectory will be central to the education programme developed (Sawin et al., 2017). Furthermore, the family must be enabled to recognise potential changes to the child's health status which may require medical reassessment/intervention (Wilson-Smith et al., 2018).

March (2017) suggests that an individualised child/family centred education programme is integral in ensuring parents and carers are competent/confident to carry out care. Central to this process is ensuring that the parent/carer have adequate time to practise any clinical procedures.

Breneo et al. (2018) advise that nurses have a primary responsibility for discharge teaching. Weiss et al. (2017) further discussed that consideration to the format of the teaching can be more influential than the amount of content.

ACTIVITY 28.2: REFLECTIVE PRACTICE

- Critically reflect on your experience of education for a child's discharge on a clinical placement. Reflect on the content and format of the education provided.
- Read: Kelo, M., Eriksson, E. and Eriksson, I. (2013) 'Perceptions of patient education during hospital visit – described by school-age children with a chronic illness and their parent'. *Scandinavian Journal of Caring Sciences*, 27 (4): 894-904.
- Consider how we can provide best indivdualised child/family education programmes on discharge. Discuss your reflections above with your practice assessor/practice supervisor.
- Reflect on the types of discharge tools/checklists that you have seen used in practice and identify the strengths and drawbacks of each.

ACTIVITY 28.3: CRITICAL THINKING

Refer to *The Code: Professional Standards of Practice and Behaviour for Nurses, Midwives and Nursing Associates* for guidance on documentation and record keeping (NMC, 2018).

- Consider how keeping clear and accurate records is crucial to good discharge planning.

FAMILY-CENTRED CARE AND PARTNERSHIP WORKING

Regan et al. (2018) suggest that family-centred care is a mutually beneficial partnership between the child, family and healthcare providers in the assessing, planning, delivery and evaluation of healthcare tailored to the needs/experiences of the child and family. A family-centred and partnership approach is the cornerstone in the provision of high-quality safe effective discharge care and in ensuring optimal outcomes for the child (Backman and Cho-Young, 2019). Working in partnership with the child and family, sharing information to underpin decision-making will ensure a family-centred continuity of care approach will help to reduce family stress and assist in strengthening the family's coping capacity (Foster et al., 2019). Central to successful partnership working is involving all the professionals and agencies that are required to meet the needs of the individual child and family. Regardless who is inputting their expertise into the care provision, the child and family must remain at the centre of the process. Professionals/agencies that may be involved in the discharge process to the home from hospital may include (not an exhaustive list):

- Consultant pediatrician
- Dietician
- Discharge nurse
- Commuity children's nurse (CCN)
- Health visitor
- Specialist nurse
- School nurse
- Physiotherapists

- Speech and language therapists
- Occupational therapists
- Pharmacy hospital/community
- Social worker
- Education staff
- Voluntary services
- Other carers
- Respite services

SEE ALSO
CHAPTER 1 AND 5

The principles highlighted here are crucial in the planning all types of discharge; we now move on to examine two main types of discharge below.

SIMPLE DISCHARGE

A simple discharge is where the child is discharged home with minimal ongoing care needs that do not require complex planning and delivery by the wider multidisciplinary team. As part of their role in supporting children at home CCNs often provide nursing care for children who require support at home with acute and short-term conditions; this is usually time-limited (Royal College of Nursing, 2020). Going home following a day surgical procedure is an example of a simple discharge.

Read the following example and undertake Activity 28.4.

"My operation had finished and it was time to go home. My mum and I went into a room with one of the nurses. The nurse was smiling at me and was telling us about different medicines that can help ease the pain and what times to take them at. She was kind and made sure everything was OK. Talking about it definitely made me feel a lot better. She also told me to take baths regularly. She said that they might hurt at first, but then I would get used to it. There was a lot to remember because we didn't write any instructions down and we never got a handout. I was given my medicine and it was time to go home. I was happy to be going back home because I knew that I had everything that I needed to help me and also my mum to look after me. I was a wee bit worried because it was sore to move around and go different places. Before leaving, we were told if I got very sore or any had difficulties, I should come back to the A&E department. I was a bit upset and worried about it when I was told that, but my mum gave me a hug and said that everything would be OK. The nurse said she was sad to see me upset but told me that my mum would take very good care of me."

Ross, child

ACTIVITY 28.4: CRITICAL THINKING

Think critically regarding how the communication needs of the child could have been met more effectively.

- Identify three things that the child found positive about the discharge.
- Explore what could have been done differently to ensure the discharge was more effective.
- Consider the main take home messages for your practice.

COMPLEX DISCHARGE

Increasing numbers of children are discharged home with long-term illness, complex or exceptional healthcare needs (Carter et al., 2016). While advances in treatment, medical technology and pharmacology have been progressive for this cohort of children, health systems in which these children are discharged have been static. Children with complex needs experience frequent transitions to home and within healthcare settings, often presenting extensive challenges to the child, family (Curran et al., 2017) and professional (Bleazard, 2020). This cohort of children frequently experience fragmented care which has the potential to increase adverse effect, compromise care quality and increase usage of healthcare resources and costs. Ronan et al. (2020) state that repeated and unplanned hospital admissions are significantly higher for this group of children. Effective multi-agency planning and agreements, robust governance and risk management, accessible accommodation and well-functioning acute/community relationships are core. Barone et al. (2020) advise that critical to effective complex discharge planning is the need for the professionals to understand how ongoing medical/care needs are translated into the home. They discuss that this lack of professional knowledge can lead to gaps in care, medical errors and problems with medical technology at home.

The role of the discharge liaison nurse, care coordinator key worker or specialist nurse can provide a crucial link between these child, family and other services (Ramshaw, 2020).

WHAT'S THE EVIDENCE?

Read the systematic review by Ronan et al. (2020).

- Identify the emotional experiences of parents when their child with complex needs is discharged to home from hospital.
- What does the review highlight regarding the role of the children's nurse in the discharge process?
- What are the three main learning points that you take from this systematic review for your practice?

Brenner et al. (2018) reviewed the literature identifying concerns of parents who had become the primary caregiver when their child was discharged home and advised that parents felt frustrated by the length of time taken by the discharge process. Parents were also fearful of the levels of competence in community services and worried about how they were going to cope in the future. Within the findings, parents did indicate the value of a staged process to going home; they collectively indicated feeling overwhelmed when they were eventually discharged from hospital. Parents stated that they were often 'petrified' or 'terrified' in their initial days at home despite their perceived clinical readiness and sense of empowerment while in the hospital.

Leyenarr et al. (2017), in their study of families who have a child with complex health needs, voiced that the family's priority on discharge were the reestablishment of home routines and a desire for normalisation; for this to occur, support from professionals was essential. To increase positive care outcomes for this cohort of children and their families it is critical that practitioners understand parents' experiences and needs during transition from hospital to home. Ronan et al. (2020) in their systematic literature review discussed the use of step down services for a phased discharge for some children with very complex technological needs and their families. This enabled parents taking increased responsibility for care as the process rolled out.

Step Down Care

In recent years, a number of children's hospices and other organisations have expanded the services they offer by providing step down care to technology-dependent children who experience a protracted discharge from hospital to home. Price et al. (2018) defined step down care as: 'a term used to reflect the transition from a highly medicalised hospital environment with prompt access to a multi-professional team of doctors, nurses and allied health professionals, to the more home like hospice environment where care is delivered by a nurse led team in a closer manner to the way care will be delivered at home.'

WHAT'S THE EVIDENCE?

Examine the three forms of evidence below and answer the questions based on what you have discovered collectively.

Watch this film clip and identify the main elements of step down care offered: https://www.the-childrenstrust.org.uk/our-services/step-down-care

Read this research paper: Price., J., McCloskey, S. and Brazil, K. (2018) 'The role of hospice in the transition from hospital to home for technology-dependent children – a qualitative study'. *Journal of Clinical Nursing*, 27 (1-2): 396–406. doi: 10.1111/jocn.13941.

Read case study 28.1.

CASE STUDY 28.1: CAROLINE

I can't wait to get home. This is a recurrent thought from the moment we are on route to hospital, never mind the weeks that my daughter is an inpatient. Then I get the news I'm waiting for: if she does well tonight we get home tomorrow. She does well. In the morning we wait, and wait, for rounds. After lunch, we get to speak to a doctor. It now transpires that we can't go home because she's still on oxygen. She will require a drizzle of oxygen for about a month after this infection. It's how she rolls. The healthcare staff would have known that if they had spoken to me. We have oxygen at home and portable oxygen for car journeys.

After a long discussion it is agreed that we go to our local district general hospital. We stay overnight at the local hospital and they agree we can go home the next morning. Overall this is a much smoother final discharge for us. Yes, we are going home on a drizzle of oxygen. Yes, we have supplies of medicines which we require for home. Yes, I'm confident that we are making the correct and safe choice for my daughter.

How could discharge have been more streamlined? This is the mother's view:

- *Anticipate discharge:* you know we will need supplies of regular medication for discharge so order them up at least 24 hours in advance so that they are ready for discharge.
- *Manage my expectations:* give me a clear and concise plan of what is going to happen and when.
- *Ask me questions:* if you had spoken to me at all about how we manage my daughter at home you would have known that she is on oxygen at night, but that she habitually requires a 'drizzle' of oxygen (low-flow oxygen) in the daytime for weeks after a bad respiratory virus.
- *I know my daughter:* please listen to what I have to say about her day-to-day care.
- *Continuity is important:* make sure each health professional has the same opinion before speaking with parents/child.
- *A multidisciplinary (MDT) meeting is important:* it would have been easier to assess my daughter's health progress if she wasn't admitted as an unknown entity; don't discharge her like one either.
- *It is important to be honest and open with parent/child:* after a long period of having my daughter as an inpatient I am getting less sleep, feeling more exhausted, more worried and less tolerant. Do me the courtesy of paying attention to the little things.

- *Update relevant professionals of changes to care needs*: one recurrent problem that we have is that my daughter's medicines change by weight or by condition. If you are discharging a patient with complex care needs it would help to give the patient/parent an updated medicine/dosage list detailing changes to hand in to their GP on discharge.

After reading this mother's account and the systematic literature review by Ronan et al. (2020) – consider:

- What could the staff have done to better facilitate her daughter's discharge?
- What ways can the multidisciplinary teams work in partnership with the mother on the detail of the discharge plan?
- What aspects of the discharge process could have been anticipated and arranged prior to the day of discharge?

TRANSFERS

Some children may be transferred to other wards within the same hospital or to other hospitals. An inter-hospital transfer (IHT) may be required when the child requires diagnostic or therapeutic facilities that are not available at the current hospital. IHT may, for example, take place from an emergency department to a regional paediatric intensive care unit (PICU). Occasionally, a child may require an IHT if a bed is not available locally. IHT of children is a process requiring the same discharge planning principles outlined above.

Transition from children's services to adult service

An increasing number of children with complex health needs are now surviving into adulthood and require transition from children's services to adult services. NICE (2016) defines transition as a purposeful and planned process of supporting young people to move from children's to adults' services. Occurring usually in the teenage years, such a move can present many challenges for the young person, their family and healthcare professionals in both child and adult services (Truesdale and Brown, 2017). Campbell et al. (2016) found that the transition process to adult services can be a negative experience for young adults and their families and an ineffective transition process has the potential to have a detrimental effect on health and life outcomes for the young adult (Kerr et al., 2017). A family-centred approach and partnership working with all parties is integral, with continuous robust support for the young person and family throughout the journey. To ensure a smooth transition a clearly identified lead person, a transition coordinator, is essential (White and Cooley, 2018).

ACTIVITY 28.5: CRITICAL THINKING

Read the article below and then complete the Activity.

- Kerr, H., Price, J., Nicholl, H. and O'Halloran, P. (2017) 'Transition from children's to adult services for young adults with life-limiting conditions: a realist review of the literature'. *International Journal of Nursing Studies*, 78: 1-27. Doi:10.1016/j.ijnurstu.2017.06.013.

SEE ALSO
CHAPTER 5

(Continued)

Consider why children need to transition from children's to adult services.

- Reflect on the positive aspects of transfer to adult services, and the challenges which transition may present both to the child and family and the practitioners involved in the transition process.
- Reflect on the reported experiences of teenagers moving into adult-focused services.
- Think about what children's services do to improve transfer and subsequent experiences for teenagers.

Access the Ready, Steady, Go programme at www.readysteadygo.net/

- Consider how the Ready, Steady, Go programme could be implemented in the transition of children to adult health services.

SAFEGUARDING STOP POINT

SEE ALSO
CHAPTER 9

All organisations involved in caring for children have safeguarding policies to ensure children are protected from harm (NSPCC, 2016). Where there are concerns about possible child protection issues, there must be a multi-agency action plan agreed and recorded before the child is transferred or discharged, and the safety of the transfer or discharge must be agreed between children's social care and the child's consultant. All professionals involved with the child need to consider what future support may be required and who else needs to be informed of the situation. Consideration always needs to be given to the sharing of information and confidentiality (Parkin, 2016).

PROCESSES AND SYSTEMS

Health services and Trusts are large, complex systems, and within such systems children and families depend on high-quality evidence-based care to be planned and provided to meet their many needs (World Health Organization, 2020). When discussing the discharge of older people, a health ombudsman (Mellor, 2016) recognised that there are structural and systematic barriers to effective discharge planning, which have massive human costs. Structural and systematic barriers also exist when discharging/transferring children and their families. We as children's nurses need to ensure that we work within existing polices and processes, but also that we look at different ways of working. At all times the voice of the child and family should be central to care.

Overall, then, discharge planning and transitional care need to be viewed as a dynamic, continuous, unified process, and not as a single clinical event when the child and family leave hospital. Planning therefore begins on admission, or in elective cases, before admission and continues as a set of care processes throughout the inpatient period (Vaish et al., 2019). As such, this enables the development of a robust discharge plan which ensures more opportunities for child and family engagement in planning and decision-making as well as opportunities to prepare and educate them for discharge (Hua et al., 2021). It also enables efficient coordination of services through communication with the healthcare team and community service providers.

CHAPTER SUMMARY

- Effective discharge planning improves quality of care for the child, enables continuity of care, improved compliance and ensures good patient outcomes, often preventing readmission
- Discharge planning is a dynamic ongoing process which should begin as early as possible before or during admission to hospital
- Planning, preparation and communication are vital when transferring and discharging children. Effective team working and communication are vital to the success of discharge planning and transfer
- The child and family must be actively engaged and welcomed as partners in the discharge process, goal-planning and decision-making

BUILD YOUR BIBLIOGRAPHY

Books

- Lees, L. (2012) *Timely Discharge from Hospital*. Keswick: M&K Publishing.

  A book designed to explore multidisciplinary and multi-agency perspectives of discharge planning.
- National Leadership and Innovation Agency for Healthcare (2008) *Passing the Baton: A Practical Guide to Effective Discharge Planning*. Cardiff: NLIAH.

  This book is aimed at practitioners working in acute, community, intermediate and ambulatory care settings; all areas of practice are featured. Each section is arranged in themes but written to stand alone, allowing the reader to dip in and out. The book is further enhanced by a comprehensive selection of case studies.
- Thurston, C. (2013) 'Transferring to adult services for young people with long-term conditions', in C. Thurston (ed.) *Essential Care for Children and Young People: Theory, Policy and Practice*. New York: Routledge.

  This chapter explores the transition from young person to adult and examines the development approach to encouraging independence. It highlights relevant theories and examines the implication for policy and practice. The chapter discusses the changing context of young people's lives and the services they may require, advising that this means that health professionals should develop their capacity to undertake assessments and interpretation in a wide variety of settings. The chapter will also assist practitioners in understanding their role in the context of their statutory duties, agency requirements and the needs and wishes of the young person.

FURTHER READING

Journal articles

- Anderson, N. and Narvey, M. (2022) 'Discharge planning of the preterm infant'. *Paediatrics & Child Health*, 27 (2): 129.

  This article provides guidance for the safe discharge of infants born before 37 weeks. Citing that the discharge process should start at the time of admission to NICU, and with a plan for assessing physiological markers including thermoregulation and control of breath. It explores the family unit as a crucial part of the care team and discusses that their involvement in the NICU will promote confidence, decrease anxiety, increase resilience and help ensure a safe discharge environment.

FURTHER READING: ONLINE JOURNAL ARTICLES

- Ingram, J.C., Powell, J.E., Blair, P.S., Pontin, D., Redshaw, M., Manns, S., Beasant, L., Burden, H., Johnson, D., Rose, C. and Fleming, P.J. (2016) 'Does family-centered neonatal discharge planning reduce healthcare usage? A before and after study in South West England'. *BMJ Open.* 6: e010752.

  This study measures the impact of a neonatal family-centred care intervention on parental self-efficacy on use of emergency department (ED) post discharge for moderately preterm infants. Using health economic data collection, the study found that lack of time for implementing the Train-to-Home intervention meant that some staff were not confident in using the family-centred approach to discharge planning.

- Shillington, J. and McNeil, D. (2021) 'Transition from the Neonatal Intensive Care Unit to home: A concept analysis'. *Advances in Neonatal Care*, 21 (5): 399-406.

  This article highlights the complex and challenging process of transistion from the NICU to home. It discusses that this complex and challenging process requires increased attention by healthcare providers and researchers to promote a successful transitional experience for families in the NICU. It suggests that transition is a central concept of the nursing discipline, as nurses care for people during a time of transition between health and illness. Appreciating the concept of transition regarding nursing phenomena will help lessen patient vulnerability and disparity in the future.

Weblinks

FURTHER
READING:
WEBLINKS

- What? Why? Children in Hospital, *Preparing for Hospital* www.whatwhychildreninhospital.org.uk Prepares children, parents and carers for a positive hospital experience by sharing age-appropriate videos and information.
- Children with Exceptional Healthcare Needs Network www.cen.scot.nhs.uk The National Managed Clinical Network for Children with Exceptional Healthcare Needs (CEN) started in March 2009, with the aim of strengthening specialist services for children with complex and exceptional healthcare needs in Scotland. Parents/carers, voluntary sector organisations and professionals are invited to join the network and attend working group meetings and events. The website provides a good source of information for professionals and carers.
- Great Ormond Street Hospital for Children www.gosh.nhs.uk
- Wellchild 10 principles of complex discharge www.wellchild.org.uk/for-professionals/ research-resources/10-principles-for-complex-discharge

REFERENCES

Backman, C. and Cho-Young, D. (2019) 'Engaging patients and informal carers to improve safety and facilitate person and family-centered care during transitions from hospital to home – a qualitative descriptive study'. *Patient Preferences and Adherence*, 13: 617–26.

Barone, S., Boss, R., Rainsanen, J., Shepard, J. and Donohue, S. (2020) 'Our life at home: photos from families inform discharge planning for medically complex children'. *Birth*, 47 (3): 278–89.

Bleazard, M. (2020) 'Compassion fatigue in nurses caring for medically complex children'. *Journal of Hospice and Palliative Nursing*, 22 (6): 473–47.

Bowles, J., Jnah, A.J., Newberry, D.M., Hubbard, C.A. and Roberston, T. (2016) 'Infants with technology dependence: facilitating the road to home'. *Advances in Neonatal Care*, 16 (6): 424–9.

Breneo, S., Hatty A., Bishop, A. and Curran, J. (2018) 'Nurse-led discharge in pediatric care: a scoping review'. *Journal of Pediatric Nursing*, 41: 60–68.

Brenner, M., Kidston, C., Hilliard, C., Coyne, I., Eustace-Cook, J., Doyle, C. et al. (2018) 'Children's complex care needs: a systematic concept analysis of multidisciplinary language'. *European Journal of Pediatrics,* 177: 1641–52.

Campbell, F., Biggs, K., Aldiss, S.K., O'Neill, P.M., Clowes, M., McDonagh, J. et al. (2016) 'Transition of care for adolescents from paediatric services to adult health services'. *Cochrane Database of Systematic Reviews,* Issue 4. Art. No.: CD009794.

Canary, H.E. and Wilkins, V. (2017) 'Beyond hospital discharge mechanics: managing the discharge paradox and bridging the care chasm'. *Qualitative Health Research,* 27 (8): 1225–35.

Carter, B., Bray, L., Sanders, C., van Miert, C., Hunt, A. and Moore, A. (2016) 'Knowing the places of care: how nurses facilitate transition of children with complex health care needs from hospital to home'. *Comprehensive Child and Adolescent Nursing,* 39 (2).

Curran, J., Breneo, S. and Vine, J. (2020) 'Improving transition in care for children with complex and medically fragile needs: a mixed methods study'. *BMC Pediatrics,* 20 (1): 219.

Debelic, I., Mikolcic, A., Tihomirovic, J., Baric, I., Lendic, Ð., Niksic, Z., Sencaj, B. and Lovric, R. (2022) 'Stressful experiences of parents in the paediatric intensive care unit: searching for the most intensive PICU stressors'. *International Journal of Environmental Research and Public Health,* 19 (18): 11450.

Foster, K., Mitchell, R., Young, M., Van, C. and Curtis, K. (2019) 'Parent experiences and psychosocial support needs 6 months following paediatric critical injury: a qualitative study'. *Injury,* 50 (5): 1082–8.

Gonçalves-Bradley, D., Lannin, N., Clemson, N., Cameron, I. and Shepperd, S. (2016) 'Discharge planning from hospital' (Review). *Cochrane Database of Systematic Reviews,* 2016 (1): CD000313.

Holland, D., Vanderboom, C., Delgado, A., Weiss, M. and Monsen, K. (2016) 'Describing pediatric hospital discharge planning care processes using the Omaha System'. *Applied Nursing Research,* 30: 24–28.

Hua, W., Wang, L., Simoni, J.M., Yuwen, W. and Jiang, L. (2021) 'Understanding preparation for preterm infant discharge from parents' and healthcare providers' perspectives: challenges and opportunities'. *Journal of Advanced Nursing,* 77 (3): 1379–90.

Kerr, H., Price, J., Nicholl, H. and O'Halloran, P. (2017) 'Transition from children's to adult services for young adults with life-limiting conditions: a realist review of the literature'. *International Journal of Nursing Studies,* 76: 1–27.

Kucharczuk, C., Lightheart, E., Koden, A., Haynes, C., Rabatin, S., Burke, J. et al. (2022) 'Standardized discharge planning tool leads to earlier discharges and fewer readmissions'. *Journal of Nursing Care Quality,* 37 (1): 54–60.

Lerret, S., Joshson, M., Polfuss, N.L., Weiss, M., Gralton, K., Klingbeil, C. et al. (2020) 'Using and engaging parents in education of discharge (eped) iPad applications to improve patient discharge experience'. *Journal of Paediatric Nursing,* 52: 41–8.

Leyenaar, J., Rizzo, P., Khodyakov, D., Leslie, L., Lindenauer, P. and Mangione-Smith, R. (2017) 'Importance and feasibility of transitional care for children with medical complexity: results of a multi stakeholder Delphi process'. *Academic Paediatrics,* 18 (1): 94–101.

Mai, K., Davis, R., Hamilton, S., Robertson-J, C., Calaman, S. and Turchi, R. (2020) 'Identifying caregiver needs for children with a tracheostomy living at home'. *Clinical Pediatrics,* 59 (13): 1169–81.

Manges, K., Groves, P., Farag, A., Peterson, R., Harton, J. and Ryan, S. (2020) 'A mixed methods study examining teamwork shared mental models of interprofessional teams during hospital discharge'. *BMJ Quality and Safety,* 29 (6): 499–508.

March, S. (2017) 'Parents' perceptions during the transition to home for their child with a congenital heart defect: how can we support families of children with hypoplastic left heart syndrome?' *Journal for Specialists in Pediatric Nursing,* 22 (3). doi: 10.1111/jspn.12185.

Mellor, J. (2016) *A Report of Investigation into Unsafe Discharge from Hospital.* Parliamentary and Health Service Ombudsman. Available at: www.ombudsman.org.uk/sites/default/files/page/A%20 report%20of%20investigations%20into%20unsafe%20discharge%20from%20hospital.pdf (accessed 26 May 2017).

Ministry of Health (1959) *The Welfare of Children in Hospital.* The Platt Report. London: Her Majesty's Stationery Office.

National Institute for Health and Care Excellence (NICE) (2016) Transition from children's to adults' services for young people using health or social care services. NICE guideline [NG43]. Available at: www.nice.org.uk/guidance/ng43 (accessed 19 June 2023).

NSPCC (National Society for the Prevention of Cruelty to Children) (2016) *Child Protection in the UK.* Available at: www.nspcc.org.uk/preventing-abuse/child-protection-system (accessed 26 May 2017).

Nursing and Midwifery Council (NMC) (2018) *The Code: Professional Standards of Practice and Behaviour for Nurses, Midwives and Nursing Associates.* London: NMC. Available at: www.nmc.org. uk/standards/code/.

Parkin, E. (2016) *Patient Health Records and Confidentiality.* House of Commons Library. Briefing paper 07103. 25 April.

Patel, H., Yirdaw, E., Yu, A., Slater, L., Perica, K., Read, G., Amaro, C. and Jones, C. (2022) 'Improving early discharge using a team-based structure for discharge multidisciplinary rounds'. *Professional Case Management,* 24 (2): 83–9.

Pladys, P., Zaoui, C., Girard, L., Mons, F. Reynaud, A. and Casper, C. (2019) 'French neonatal society position paper stresses the importance of an early family centred approach to discharging preterm infants from hospital'. *Acta Scandinavica Paediatrics,* 109 (7): 1302–9.

Price, J., McCloskey, S. and Brazil, K. (2018) 'The role of hospice in the transition from hospital to home for technology-dependent children. A qualitative study'. *Journal of Clinical Nursing,* 27 (1-2): 396–406.

Ramshaw, S. (2020) 'Healthcare professionals' perceptions and experiences regarding what works well in the discharge of children with medical complexity: a qualitative service evaluation'. *Archives of Disease in Childhood,* 2020-10, 105 (Suppl 1). Available at: https://adc.bmj.com/content/105/ Suppl_1/A123.1.

Regan, K., Curtin, C. and Vorderer, M.A. (2018) 'Paradigm shifts in inpatient psychiatric care of children: approaching child- and family centred care'. *Journal of Child and Adolescent Psychiatric Nursing,* 30 (4): 186–94.

Ronan, S., Brown, M. and Marsh, L. (2020) 'Parents experience of transition from hospital to home of a child with complex health needs: a systematic literature review'. *Journal of Clinical Nursing,* 29 (17–18): 3222–35.

Roy, C., Langschymidt, J. and. Starritt, N. (2018) 'Improving documentation and information-giving in tonsillectomy discharges at a paediatric centre'. *International Journal of Surgery,* 55: S54–S55.

Royal College of Nursing (RCN) (2020) *Futureproofing Community Children's Nursing.* RCN guidance. London: RCN.

Sawin, K., Weiss, M., Johnson, N.L., Gralton, K. and Malin, S. (2017) 'Development of a self-managed theory guided discharge intervention for parents of hospitalised children'. *Journal of Nursing Scholarship,* 49 (2): 202–13.

Truesdale, M. and Brown, M. (2017) *People with Learning Disabilities in Scotland: 2017 Health Needs Assessment Update Report.* Glasgow: NHS Health Scotland.

Vaish, S., Power, G., Fagan, C., Fitzgerald, E. and Ryan, S. (2019) 'A pilot quality improvement (QI) initiative to improve discharge planning process for patients with complex care needs at Temple Street Children's Hospital (TSCHU) Dublin'. *Archives of Disease in Childhood,* 104 (Suppl 3), p.A242.

Vanmol, M., Nijkamp, M., Markam, C. and Ista, E. (2017) 'Using intervention mapping approach to develop a discharge protocol for intensive care patients'. *BMC Health Services Research,* 17 (1): 837.

Weiss, M., Squin, J., Gralton, K., Johnson, N., Kingbell, C., Lerret, S. et al. (2017) 'Discharge teaching readiness for discharge and post discharge outcomes in parents of hospitalised children'. *Journal of Paediatric Nursing*, 34: 58–64.

Weiss, M., Lerret, S., Sawin, K. and Schiffman, R. (2020) 'Parent readiness for hospital discharge scale: psychometrics and association with postdischarge outcomes'. *Journal of Pediatric Health Care*, 34 (1): 30–7.

Wellchild (2021) 10 Principles for Complex Discharge Guidance and Toolkit. Available at: www.wellchild.org.uk/.../10-principles-for-complex-discharge (accessed 19 June 2023).

White, P.H. and Cooley, W.C. (2018) 'Transitions Clinical Report Authorizing Group, American Academy of Pediatrics, American Academy of Family Physicians and American College of Physicians. Supporting the health care transitions from adolescence to adulthood in the medical home'. *Pediatrics*, 142 (5): e20182587.

Wilson Smith, M.G., Sachse, M. and Perry, M.T. (2018) 'Road to Home Program: a performance improvement initiative to increase family and nurse satisfaction with the discharge education process for newly diagnosed pediatric oncology patients'. *Journal of Pediatric Oncology Nursing*, 35 (5): 368–74.

Wu, S., Tyler, A., Logsdon, T., Holmes, N., Balkian, A., Brittan, M. et al. (2016) 'A quality improvement collaborative to improve the discharge process for hospitalized children'. *Pediatrics*, 138 (2): e201435604. Doi: 10.1542/peds.2014-3604.

PART 4 CARING FOR CHILDREN AND YOUNG PEOPLE WITH COMPLEX AND HIGH DEPENDENCY NEEDS

CARE OF HIGHLY DEPENDENT AND CRITICALLY ILL CHILDREN AND YOUNG PEOPLE

29

USHA CHANDRAN AND FIONA LYNCH

THIS CHAPTER COVERS

- An introduction to the paediatric critical care unit (PCCU)
- Assessing and caring for critically ill children
- Holistic and child/family-centred care
- PCC outcomes

" "As a parent my world was tipped upside down completely, unexpectedly and suddenly, with the life of the most precious thing in the world to me hanging in the balance. I was helpless, scared, and shell-shocked. The nurses were our advocates, support, voice of reason, teachers, interpreters, substitute parents, in addition to providing expert medical care to our child. They made us laugh, listened when we were worried, looked after us when we cried. The people we relied on 24 hours a day, who I still think of so incredibly fondly."

Leah, parent of 18-month-old girl with multi-organ failure "

" "I initially dreaded coming to the PCCU. I imagined myself irrelevant and unable to do anything. On the contrary, the staff are always so well organised and prepared. The nurses have taught me so many things and I'm so happy. I now feel ready to take on life as a qualified nurse. I've learnt skills here and gained knowledge at three times the rate I have elsewhere. Consider yourself lucky if you're placed in the PCCU. There are many learning opportunities that await you."

Zakinah, 3rd-year children's nursing student "

INTRODUCTION

In this chapter we will look at how PCCUs in the UK are organised and structured and describe how to systematically assess and manage critically ill children. This will include the common types of interventions on a critical care unit and highlight the principles for delivering safe and high-quality critical care. Teamwork and holistic care of the child and family-centred care are key principles.

To understand this chapter, you need a good grasp of the anatomy and physiology of the major organ systems of children. This is because critical care is to do with supporting and/or managing failing organs and so it is important to know normal functions before we can appreciate its dysfunction and management – the hallmark of critical care practice. A good resource for revising these is: *Fundamentals of Children and Young People's Anatomy and Physiology: A Textbook for Nursing and Healthcare Students*, 2nd edition (Peate and Gormley-Fleming, 2021).

AN INTRODUCTION TO THE PAEDIATRIC CRITICAL CARE UNIT (PCCU)

The Paediatric Critical Care Society describe paediatric critical care (PCC) as the care of children who need an advanced level of observation, monitoring or intervention which cannot be safely delivered in general wards (PCCS, 2021). The different levels of PCC interventions are also defined clearly in this document (PCCS, 2021). Additionally, the Royal College of Paediatrics and Child Health (RCPCH, 2014), sets standards for PCC outside of the paediatric intensive care unit (PICU) describing situations where critical care may be offered outside of the critical care unit depending on patient complexity. For instance, levels 1 and 2 PCC can be delivered in dedicated high-dependency areas (HDU) whereas level 3 PCC can only be delivered in an ICU environment (RCPCH, 2014). Highly dedicated/specialised units provide specialist services such as burns, liver and cardiac surgery. Patients with PIM-TS (also known as MIS-C), a hyperinflammatory condition associated with a SARS-CoV-2 (COVID-19) infection that some children developed, would be referred to a cardiac centre if the heart was involved (Sperotto et al., 2021). Do have a look at these two documents if you would like to know more about how PCCUs are structured and set up.

Table 29.1 Essential bedside equipment

System	Equipment	Comments
Airway	Wall suction	Must be accessible and functional in an emergency or arrest. Portable suction is required for transfers
	Wide-bore rigid suction catheter (Yankauer)	Essential for clearing the airway and for all intubation/extubation and transfers
	Guedel airways	Maintains a patent airway
	Soft suction catheters	For clearing nasopharyngeal and artificial airways. For artificial airways, suction catheters are twice the size of the endotracheal (ETT) or tracheostomy tube. For example, for size 4 ETT, you will need size 8 FG suction catheters
Breathing	Self-inflating Ambu bag and face mask	Not dependent on gas flow. Mandatory on all transfers
	Ayers T-piece, Mapleson circuit or similar hand-ventilation circuit and face-mask	Requires gas flow to inflate. Most preferred mode of hand/manual ventilation. Essential for intubation/extubation procedures
	¾ or full oxygen cylinder	In case piped oxygen fails
	Pulse oximetry (SpO2)	Monitors oxygenation
	End-tidal CO2 sensor	Monitors carbon dioxide (CO_2) clearance
	Stethoscope	Auscultate breath sounds (BS)

System	Equipment	Comments
Circulation	ECG monitoring	Monitors heart rate (HR) and rhythm. If patient is paced, pacing spikes must be visible on monitor
	Invasive or non-invasive blood pressure (BP)	Invasive BP must show a reliable waveform on monitor
Disability	Drugs/infusions	Must be checked and verified as correct
Exposure	Health and safety	Adheres to policies and procedures
		Clean and clutter-free environment

Nursing practice

This begins with the handover report of the child. It includes patient demographics, past medical and presenting history, family structures, treatment to date and safeguarding issues. An initial 'eye-balling' observation during the handover provides much information about the child (and family, if present) almost immediately. The information you obtain during this time is then substantiated by other reports, communication, observations, vital signs and other data.

A structured approach (e.g., ABCDE – airway, breathing, circulation, disability and exposure) is used to communicate clinical data, patient problems, needs and treatment goals during the handover. Following this, the child's bedspace area is checked to ensure it is safe and appropriate for the child (see Table 29.1 which suggests equipment required). These tasks are only superseded if an unexpected event occurs that places the child at immediate risk, for example the desaturating child, cardiorespiratory arrest, or the child at risk of harming him/herself. During such events, patient priority takes precedence over checking of the bedspace and the reason for always ensuring that the bedspace area is set-up and ready for emergency management.

CASE STUDY 29.1: BILLY

Billy is a 2-year-old boy with toxic shock secondary to chicken pox. He has been very unwell in his local hospital and a referral has been made to the PCC transport service for ongoing advice and transfer to a level 3 PCCU. He has been intubated and ventilated, volume (fluid) resuscitated and commenced on vasoactive drugs to support his BP.

What do you think Billy, his family and the transport team will require on arrival to the PCCU?

Useful information on PCC transport principles and process, clinical management of different conditions and information on parental advice can be found can be linked to 'transport of critically ill infants and children' chapter 13 in *Children in Intensive care – A survival guide* by Davies, J.H. and McDougall, M. (2018) 3rd edition, Elsevier.

PCC monitoring

All PCC children will have basic essential monitoring that includes ECG (electrocardiogram) monitoring, blood pressure (BP), respiratory rate (RR), temperature, oxygen saturation (SpO_2) and pulse rate (PR). Special or intensive monitoring is one of the reasons for admission to a critical care unit. However, you must never rely solely on monitoring without first checking the child. For instance, in pulseless electrical activity – a type of cardiac arrest with normal electrical activity but no cardiac output (CO) or perfusion – the ECG trace can show a normal cardiac rhythm and heart rate (HR), yet the child is in cardiac arrest.

Intubated patients will have end-tidal CO_2 ($EtCO_2$) monitoring. Intubation is the process by which a tube is inserted into the trachea to support the airway. Although there are a number of ways to determine that the trachea has been properly intubated such as chest X-ray and auscultation for breath sounds, $EtCO_2$ is one of the most effective means of providing information on endo-tracheal intubation. $EtCO_2$ provides information on how effectively the child is ventilating and acts as a safety device for intubated patients as the waveform will change should the endotracheal or tracheostomy tube become displaced.

$EtCO_2$ is a non-invasive sensor applied to the child's ventilator circuit to detect exhaled CO_2. The loss of the $EtCO_2$ trace on the monitor is a reliable indicator of a dislodged or misplaced airway tube. This is because for $EtCO_2$ to be detected the artificial airway (ETT or tracheostomy) must be positioned correctly in the airway. Basic monitoring also includes physical assessment parameters such as capillary or venous blood gas analysis.

ACTIVITY 29.1: CRITICAL THINKING

When you look after a child with ECG monitoring, you must recognise the normal ECG pattern and what it means. To support this learning, look up the normal PQRST ECG pattern and explain its link to cardiac contraction (systole) and relaxation (diastole). Describe in simple terms what the PR interval and ST segment mean. Watch the video at https://www.youtube.com/watch?v=RYZ4daFwMa8 to enhance your understanding.

Advanced monitoring supports more complex decision-making and includes, for example, invasive continuous arterial blood pressure (ABP) and/or invasive central venous pressure (CVP) monitoring. ABP requires arterial cannulation (commonly referred to as an arterial (art) line). These are used for continuous blood pressure monitoring, blood sampling and is the gold standard for arterial blood gas (ABG) analysis. Not all sick children will require this type of monitoring, but many sick children do.

Invasive lines such as arterial lines require special care and management only possible in the critical care environment and is one of the reasons for a PCCU admission. An arterial line that becomes disconnected for instance can cause the child to exsanguinate. For this reason, arterial lines must be visible and are clearly labelled. An erroneously infused drug or fluid into an arterial line can result in serious consequences, e.g., loss of limb or even be fatal (NPSA, 2008). Blood pressures through an arterial line should be compared with a non-invasive BP device to determine its accuracy at the start of the shift.

A cannula inserted into a large central vein is known as as central line. This line can be used to measure central venous pressure (CVP) to monitor right heart preload (end-diastolic pressure) which can be a surrogate marker for circulating volume. The spare lumens on this line can be used for infusing viscous, high concentration, toxic or vasoactive drugs – for example, total parenteral nutrition, high-dose chemotherapy, adrenaline (epinephrine) and noradrenaline (norepinephrine). All these invasive lines must be checked, labelled and handled carefully. Check perfusion distal to the limb for femoral lines as blood flow can be compromised by these lines and children can also develop deep vein thrombi.

In special cases, such as traumatic brain injury or cardiac arrest, a child's temperature may be tightly regulated and controlled using specialised invasive thermometry (e.g., oesophageal or rectal probe) and/or a cooling blanket. This is known as targeted temperature management (TTM) protocol and aims to protect the child's brain through cooling mechanisms and/or maintenance of a targeted temperature (Kochanek et al., 2019; Resuscitation Council UK, 2021). These interventions are usually only provided in a level 3 PCCU. Other invasive lines are more specialised. For instance, cardiac patients may have left atrial (LA) lines.

Some of the more standard critical care monitoring tools are listed below:

- Three-lead ECG
- RR, SpO_2 and PR
- Temperature
- $EtCO_2$
- Non-invasive or invasive arterial BP
- Central venous pressure (CVP)

Patient alarms

Setting alarms is an important task as alarms alert you to any problems. It can be frightening for both children and families if they are unsure what this means. High and low monitoring alarms are set to the child's age, weight and/or condition and predetermined goals. Although artefacts cause false alarms, all alarms must be attended to promptly. Unattended alarms compromise patient safety and contribute to sensory overload, alarm fatigue and child/family stress.

ACTIVITY 29.2: REFLECTIVE PRACTICE

Reflect on a time when you were either in a noisy, chaotic and confusing environment or even in your first placement when you were unsure of what to expect. How did you feel? This experience will be significantly worse for critically ill children and their families who have little control over their own environment on the PCCU.

ASSESSMENT AND CARE OF CRITICALLY ILL CHILDREN

A structured approach is the most comprehensive way for assessing and managing critically ill children. This chapter illustrates two models – ABCDE and a top-to-toe/front-to-back model. We will start with the most common model – ABCDE – which stands for: airway, breathing, circulation, disability and exposure.

Airway

If the child in the HDU has the ability to talk, babble or cry, the airway is patent. Drooling, gurgling or snoring and stridor are signs of airway problems. Noisy breathing that quietens, or muffled and hoarse speech signals an airway emergency. Loss of airway reflexes, a weak cough or the inability to cough requires urgent airway protection. You should not be able to hear any vocalisation in a properly positioned endotracheal tube or tracheostomy tube. If you can hear sounds from such a child, then a leak around the tube is present and should be escalated to senior staff. Vocalisation can be a normal event for a child with a tracheostomy. You should always check if this is the case with senior staff.

For intubated children, assessment, and management of the endotracheal tube (ETT) or tracheostomy is essential. The artificial airway must remain patent, stable and secure.

Breathing (respiratory)

Assessment of the child's respiratory state, breathing pattern and work of breathing (WOB) is next. This consists of observing the child's RR, SpO_2, HR, colour and use of accessory muscles. Increased WOB is characterised by the use of accessory muscles (e.g., recession, nasal flaring, grunting, head-bobbing) and can indicate the need for additional respiratory support, e.g., high-flow nasal cannula oxygen therapy, invasive or non-invasive ventilation. Not tolerating being handled, agitation and irritability are also signs of airway compromise. In the infant with bronchiolitis, for instance, high-flow nasal cannula oxygen or NIV has shown some benefit (Fainardi et al., 2021). A new or rising trend in supplementary oxygen confirms the need for review.

Cyanosis, a late sign, and the child who is too breathless to speak, eat or drink, is in a life-threatening state. Gasping, cyanosis, bradypnoea/apnoea and fatigue/exhaustion all herald impending collapse. These symptoms must be escalated immediately.

Observing the breathing pattern and how the chest/abdomen moves and expands is an important part of the respiratory assessment. As different pathologies cause different patterns of breathing, it is important to observe and report these early. For instance, upper airway obstruction causes paradoxical (see-saw) breathing. A pneumothorax, pleural effusions, or mucus plugs may cause unequal chest wall expansion and could require chest drains and airway clearance manoeuvres. Metabolic acidosis causes comfortable tachypnea but requires correction of the metabolic acidosis. Children with head injuries with irregular breathing patterns may be developing raised intracranial pressure (RICP) – a life-threatening condition which may require urgent management and/or scan.

Secretion management is a simple strategy for supporting airway and breathing difficulties. Secretions/sputum must be assessed properly as different types may indicate different problems. For example, green sputum indicates infection, pluggy, thick copious secretions are seen in asthma. Regular physiotherapy, good humidification of gases, nebulisation and mucolytics can be prescribed to support respiratory problems. Severe cases may require specialist input – for example, bronchoscopy and/or broncho-alveolar lavage or even chest drains.

An essential part of bedside respiratory assessment is the auscultation of breath sounds (BS). Normal BS are clear from the apex to the bases.

You may be able to auscultate a variety of different breath sounds. For instance, coarse crackles are a feature of retained secretions and you may be able to palpate/feel this by placing your hand on the child's chest. Fine crackles at lung bases suggest pulmonary oedema. A positive fluid balance and hepatomegaly in a young child may confirm this finding. Wheeze is an intrathoracic sound from narrowed airways. Practise this skill in your placement and if you hear adventitious sounds make a note of where you hear them and what they sound like. Note whether you hear them during inspiration, expiration or both and other symptoms that may be associated with it.

DOPE(S) is a mnemonic to identify clinical emergencies causing hypoxia or desaturations in a child with an artificial airway. DOPES stands for:

- **D**isplaced or dislodged ETT or tracheostomy
- **O**bstruction: any causes of tube obstruction (e.g., secretions, kink in ETT)
- **P**neumothorax (ventilated patients, patients with fragile lungs or insertion of neck lines may cause this)
- **E**quipment failure or problem (e.g., malfunctioning ventilator, disconnection)
- **S**tomach (if too full of air or fluid will splint the diaphragm, hindering lung expansion and ventilation)

Loose ETT or tracheostomy tapes must be resecured without delay. This is a two-person procedure that requires access to an airway expert in case reintubation is required. For secure tubes, note the tube position (oral/nasal/tracheostomy), type and size of tube, whether it is cuffed or uncuffed and the volume of air in the cuff (if inflated). Cuff pressure should be checked with a cuff manometer every shift. High cuff pressure and mobile tubes cause tracheal damage and airway swelling. Blocked tubes are an airway emergency.

Mechanically ventilated patients can continue to breathe comfortably and synchronously on the ventilator. Synchrony means the ventilator is synchronising the patient's efforts and is comfortable for the patient. Asynchrony means that the patient is not comfortable and is 'fighting' the ventilator. Asynchrony requires management. Parents become upset when they observe their child not synchronising with the ventilator and appearing uncomfortable. Apart from ventilator modes and/or settings, retained secretions, suboptimal sedation, pain and discomfort (e.g., from a full bladder) are some causes of asynchrony.

Airway obstruction can cause problems and must be managed. Airway clearance strategies – which may include preoxygenation and manually ventilating the child, saline instillation, chest physiotherapy and suction – are all part of this intervention. Unnecessary or routine airway clearance procedures are counterproductive, even dangerous (Strickland et al., 2013). Evidence-based guidelines (Tume and Copnell, 2015) and the endotracheal suction assessment tool are valuable strategies for supporting this practice (Davis et al., 2017). You can learn more about airway clearance manoeuvres in placement by teaming up with physiotherapists who are experts in this field.

ACTIVITY 29.3: TEAM WORKING

An intubated baby has copious, tenacious and thick secretions and his oxygen saturations fall to 87%. Following a systematic assessment, his nurse identifies ETT secretions to be the problem and prepares to perform an airway clearance maneouvre.

- Which members of the multidisciplinary team (MDT) should, or could, be involved in this baby and family's care during this episode of desaturation?

"Spend some time alongside other members of the multidisciplinary team, for example dieticians, physiotherapists and pharmacists. Talk to parents and patients. Ask them about their experience and try to see what it would be like if you were in their shoes."

Staff nurse

Although advanced interventions such as mechanical ventilation (MV) and non-invasive ventilation may be required, one simple intervention for optimising airway and breathing is positioning. Effectively positioning the child facilitates not only airway opening but also optimises lung expansion, ventilation–perfusion (VQ) matching and gas exchange (Johnson and Meyenburg, 2009). Children in HDU with the ability to position themselves adequately will normally do this independently (e.g., tripod position). Dependent patients require assisted therapeutic positioning. For instance, in unilateral lung disease, dependent patients are positioned with the 'good' lung up (Davis et al., 1985). In bilateral lung disease, prone positioning may be beneficial (Wells et al., 2005).

Prone positioning is a special ventilatory position that became popular during the COVID-19 pandemic (Venus et al., 2020). Proning displaces the child's abdominal and thoracic structures to make more space for the lungs to expand, recruits atelectatic lungs and promotes VQ matching and gas exchange (Messerole et al., 2002). Always perform a risk assessment considering contraindications and local moving and handling policies prior to these procedures.

It is important to ensure that parents recognise proning as a special ventilatory mode – safe only on the PCCU where there is continuous monitoring. There is a recognised risk of sudden infant death syndrome in babies who are placed prone at home (Lullaby Trust, 2013).

Circulation

Circulatory/cardiovascular (CVS) assessment is the next stage of the structured assessment approach. It is about assessing and managing circulation and perfusion. Adequate perfusion is needed for organ survival. Capillary refill time (CRT), skin warmth, colour (flushed, pale or cyanotic or mottled) and toe-to-core temperature gradients are non-invasive means of assessing perfusion. These provide valuable information on how the heart is functioning, on cardiac output (CO) and circulating volumes. It can help to differentiate compensating children from decompensating children. A bounding pulse, flash CRT and flushed appearance in septic shock, for instance, shows a compensating patient with a high CO and increased stroke volume (SV) (i.e., vasodilated patients). A low volume, thready pulse, prolonged CRT and mottled and cool skin are features of low CO, vasoconstriction and hypoperfusion. These children may appear pale or cyanosed and diaphoretic (i.e., decompensated, also known as cold shock). Both types of children can deteriorate into circulatory failure and collapse. Not all children will go through both phases. In children, the compensated phase might be short-lived. Cold shock is the more likely scenario in young children.

HR and rhythm assessment is an important assessment parameter. It influences CO, stroke volume (SV) and organ perfusion. Children under the age of 2 are particularly HR-dependent for increasing their CO as they cannot improve their SV to any great extent – hence early tachycardia in this group. However, very rapid HR (in excess of 200 beats/minute in young children) and serious arrhythmias (e.g., supraventricular tachycardia) will compromise CO in all age groups (Hazinski, 2013).

Mean BP (MAP) is another critical care haemodynamic parameter in PCC. It requires skilled monitoring and observation as MAP is all about organ perfusion and perfusion pressure. Poor perfusion pressures (i.e., MAP) can lead to organ failure and death. If one organ fails, this is termed single-organ failure. If more than one organ fails, then the child is in multi-organ failure. Maintaining a good CO and perfusion pressure minimises the risk of organ failure, PCC complications and/or death.

Lack of perfusion can be life-changing. Lack of perfusion to limbs and limb digits compromises the viability of that limb/digit and may lead to amputations. This is a life-changing event for the child. If there is inadequate perfusion to the heart, myocardial dysfunction and life-threatening arrhythmias can occur. In traumatic brain injury, an adequate cerebral perfusion pressure is required to prevent secondary brain injury, swelling, herniation and brain-stem death. Common strategies for maintaining MAP in these children who are no longer fluid responsive is to use vasopressor drugs. In severe cases, specialised mechanical support may be required, such as extra corporeal life support (ECLS, or extracorporeal membrane oxygenation, ECMO). Units that provide these highly specialised interventions are defined as Advanced 5 PCCU (PCCS, 2021) and this is the highest level of care any PCCU can provide.

Lactate, which can be obtained through a blood gas, is a useful marker of poor CO and perfusion. As lactate is a by-product of anaerobic metabolism, poor CO will cause a rise in lactate. A rising lactate (normal <2mmol/l) is associated with increased mortality (Wheeler, 2013). Some caution is required in interpreting this result in liver disease as lactate is cleared by the liver. Initial management of deranged lactate levels is fluid resuscitation and/or vasoactive drugs to optimise CO. Blood transfusions and oxygen therapy may be required to improve the oxygen content of the blood for aerobic metabolism (Wheeler, 2013).

One early marker of hypoperfusion is acute kidney injury (AKI). AKI results in poor urine output, deranged kidney function and acid–base imbalance. Early AKI can be detected at the bedside by closely monitoring urine output and fluid balances. Mild AKI may respond to volume resuscitation and vasopressors to improve CO and perfusion pressure to this organ, and may reverse AKI. Severe AKI requires renal replacement therapy (RRT) in the form of peritoneal dialysis or continuous RRT.

Pulse pressure – the difference between systolic and diastolic BP – is another important early marker of deterioration in PCC. In dehydration, reduced pulse pressure is detected long before a drop in BP and hypotension. Unlike adults, hypotension is a late and pre-terminal finding in children and the pulse pressure provides valuable information prior to this pre-terminal event.

CVP (sometimes referred to as right atrial pressure) (as opposed to left atrial pressure/LAP) measures right heart (atrial) filling pressures and circulating volume. It provides information on how well children are responding to fluid resuscitation and other interventions that aim to improve CO. Children who respond to fluid resuscitation will sustain a higher CVP. High CVP (but not necessarily high LAP) is seen in overloaded children and children in right-heart failure. Hepatomegaly, basal lung crackles and a positive fluid balance chart will also support the diagnosis of fluid overload. Low CVP is associated with dehydration, hypovolaemia and low circulating volume (Darovic, 2002). A prolonged CRT, cool skin or poor skin turgor and a sunken fontanelle in the young child will also support this finding although in certain conditions (e.g., diabetic ketoacidosis) these classical signs may not be evident. Patient history and presentation are important when interpreting these findings.

Disability

The assessment of disability focuses on neurological state and arousal, drugs impacting on neurology and blood glucose monitoring. Neurological assessments comprise the assessment of mental state and/or behaviour, Glasgow Coma Scale, tone/flaccidity, and pupils assessment to check pupils are equal and reactiong to light (PEARL). For children with epidural analgesia, spinal drains and/or other neurological conditions or surgical interventions involving the brain and/or spine, sensation and motor function are also assessed. Young babies will very quickly present with poor tone and floppiness if unwell. In hypoxia, hypercapnia or other forms of encephalopathy, agitation, confusion, drowsiness, seizure activity or coma may be the presenting features. Any drug that affects the neurological state or assessment must be reviewed.

Pupil assessment is an important part of neurological assessment. Fixed dilated and/or unequal pupils and a bulging or tensed fontanelle in infants is a sign of RICP. Evidence-based 'neuro-protective' strategies (e.g., normothermia, normocapnia, adequate MAP and normoglycaemia) are life-saving strategies (Kochanek et al., 2019). In the sedated or opioid-managed child, sluggish or pin-point pupils can be a sign of over-sedation.

Pain and sedation are a part of neurological assessments and a PCC priority as sedated children may still be able to experience pain. Various pain tools are used to assess pain in PCC (RCN, 2009) and the COMFORT scale is commonly used to assess comfort and sedation in MV children (Ambuel et al., 1992; Harris et al., 2016). Suboptimal pain and sedation management are detrimental and compromise patient safety but too much sedation in MV patients will prevent patients from weaning their ventilation, induce withdrawal symptoms and prolong their stay in the PCCU (Grant et al., 2013). Delirium, a distressing event for both children and families, is now an important part of neurological assessment for recovering PCC children.

Exposure

Children must be exposed (preserving their dignity and warmth as much as possible) to assess them fully. Abdominal assessment, assessment of pressure areas, lines and wound sites, tubes or drains, and the assessment of patients' limbs for any abnormality require proper exposure.

Abdominal assessment consists of observing the abdomen for any abnormality (e.g., distension, discoloration or shape). In critical illness, hypoperfusion to abdominal organs can result in deranged function, ischaemia, necrosis, bleeding and/or perforation. The bowel, liver and other gastrointestinal organs can become involved. Many of these complications may result in abdominal discomfort, abdominal discoloration and/or distension. As a distended abdomen reduces chest wall compliance and complicates mechanical ventilation and weaning, you may be required to monitor distension by measuring abdominal girth. Auscultating for bowel sounds is part of the abdominal assessment and a core PCC nursing skill. Learn to auscultate bowel sounds in your placement.

Top-to-toe/front-to-back assessment

Hygiene and other personal and health needs are thoroughly assessed using the above approach. Meeting PCC patients' personal hygiene needs is a nursing priority not only for infection control purposes, but it is also integral to patient dignity and welfare. It normalises the critical care process for children and provides opportunities for families to participate in the child's care. This is an area where you can participate more fully with support.

Assess all areas of the child's skin and mucous membranes. Observe for any abnormality, pressure damage and/or tissue oedema. In babies and young children, the occipital area is very much at risk for pressure damage and in all critically ill children the ears, ETT and other pressure points are vulnerable. In sedated patients with poor blinking reflexes, the children's eyes should remain moist and closed to prevent complications such as corneal keratitis and other eye infections. One of the first signs of keratitis is pink-tinged eyes.

Tissue oedema is a common PCC complication. One of the causes of this complication is hypoalbuminaemia and increased vessel permeability which can be exacerbated by critical illness and MV. Tissue oedema is not only a potential risk factor for pressure ulcer formation, but it can also impede chest wall compliance and interfere with ventilation and weaning. It causes oozing/leaking at line, tube and punctures sites, prevents dressings from adhering to skin and is a potential contributor for infection and poor wound healing. It also causes parents much distress if their child's normal appearance changes. Reassure families that you will report these problems to senior staff who may explain the causes and its management which could include fluid restriction and drugs (diuretics).

Comprehensive assessment includes a thorough assessment of the child's limbs and other areas. Here, observe the child's limbs for any abnormality or deformity (e.g., swelling from IV lines) and perfusion. Assess colour, warmth, capillary refill, motor, and sensory function. For children who have had surgical grafts or flaps, you may be required to perform a hand-held Doppler assessment of peripheral pulses. Promptly report swelling, inflammation, tenderness, or pain as femoral and other lines can cause complications (e.g., thrombus, infiltration or extravasation of drugs and fluids). Remove thromboembolic stockings (if applicable) and check calves, heels, and feet. Signs of calf inflammation, swelling, warmth or erythema may be the early signs of deep vein thrombosis. Demarcation, discoloration, and coolness may be signs of hypoperfusion, and rashes have various causes, some of which may be ominous (e.g., petechial rash in meningococcal infection).

Disseminated intravascular coagulopathy (DIC) is a complication that some critically ill children develop. DIC is caused by factors that trigger a dysfunctional clotting system (e.g., sepsis, cancer or liver dysfunction). In septic shock, endothelial injury and microvascular damage activates the clotting system. This results in thrombus formation in small vessels, thrombocytopenia, and depletion of clotting factors.

The depletion of platelets and clotting factors and the activation of fibrinolysis place patients at risk of bleeding and haemorrhage, some of it severe, hence the acronym DIC: 'death is coming' (Moore et al., 2010). Thus, thorough and comprehensive assessment for signs of bleeding at line, tube and puncture sites and observing for signs of covert or internal bleeding are important features of PCC assessment.

COVID-19 (SARS-CoV-2) is also associated with clotting problems such as hypercoagulopathy. Whilst not many children have been critically ill with COVID-19, those who do contract the disease may experience these problems.

CASE STUDY 29.2: PEARL

Fifteen-year-old Pearl, an oncology patient, is septic and has received 40ml/kg volume resuscitation and antibiotics on the ward according to sepsis guidelines (NICE, 2017). Pearl was unresponsive to this treatment so she was transferred to PICU for ongoing management. On PICU, Pearl received another 20ml/kg of fluid to support her blood pressure and normalise tachycardia (Weiss et al., 2020).

Here are Pearl's assessment details:

Airway: Patent, weak cough

Breathing: RR: 47 breaths/minute; saturations: 98% on 15 litres oxygen via non-rebreathe bag. Comfortable but shallow, rapid breathing. BS: resonant, clear to lung bases. ABG: metabolic acidosis

Circulation: HR: 157 beats/minute. Radial pulse regular, high volume, bounding; ECG: sinus tachycardia; BP is hypotensive – 89/30 (mean: 50mmHg). Temperature: 39°C. Shivering (rigors). CRT: flash; hot to touch, dry skin, pink, flushed appearance. Urine output: oliguria. Lactate 4mmol/l (high)

Disability: GCS: Responding to questions. $E_4V_5M_6$ (15/15), PERL size 4mm, moving all limbs, blood glucose: 4.0mmol/l, denies pain. Not agitated. Looks lethargic/exhausted

Exposure: No rashes. Hickman line site appears inflamed

Problem: Warm shock

Potential problem: Decompensated shock and organ failure

Goal: Pearl will respond to treatment and recover from this deterioration

What actions can we take to help Pearl's parents cope with this crisis?

PCC management

The journey for children like Pearl can be painful, traumatic, and unpredictable. These children may have advanced and/or specialised monitoring and all children with sepsis will have the source of infection aggressively treated (e.g., antibiotics and removal of invasive lines, if line sepsis). Most ventilated patients will have an indwelling urethral catheter to monitor their urine output, kidney function and fluid balances. A central line may be inserted for high-volume fluid resuscitation, infusing vasoactive drugs and CVP measurement. An arterial line is useful for regular blood sampling, ABG and continuous BP monitoring.

Unstable or severely deteriorating children are always electively intubated and sedated to support their respiratory and cardiovascular status. Intubation and ventilation allow for additional sedation to be given to enable tolerance of invasive procedures and painful interventions. It also induces a necessary sense of amnesia for unpleasant events. Deep sedation is beneficial as it reduces the metabolic rate, but it also compromises the patient's ability to protect their airway and depresses respiratory function – hence the need for airway support. Some children (e.g., oncology or asthmatic patients) are very high-risk intubations as they can decompensate very quickly and the team must be prepared for this.

HOLISTIC AND CHILD/FAMILY-CENTRED CARE

All PCC interventions are underpinned by a holistic and child-/family-centred care (FCC) approach (Hakio et al., 2015). This approach facilitates child/parental involvement and empowerment. Reassurance, communication, meeting parents' basic needs and their need for information is all part of FCC (Latour, 2011). Looking for opportunities to involve parents, such as teaching them how to provide eye and mouth care for their ventilated child, changing a nappy on the child with an indwelling catheter or other invasive lines, assisting with bed-bathing or repositioning the intubated child plus comforting the critically ill child, are supportive of the parental role and empowering (McGraw et al., 2012).

Negotiation is a key concept in child/FCC (Tume and Latour, 2015). On the PCCU, negotiate to maintain as much of the child's normal routines as possible. Find out about the child's likes and dislikes and remember that beneath all lines, tubes and technology is a child who is unique, an individual and someone's child. Despite being in a busy and technological environment, aim to promote normality and dignity, a child-friendly atmosphere and psychological/emotional security. Facilitating a normal circadian rhythm and providing protected rest periods during the day, increasing natural light, decreasing artificial light may all help. Bear in mind that families also provide the emotional love and bond for the child, so create opportunities for open visiting and minimise family waiting times. Importantly, form therapeutic partnerships with families and critically ill children and within professional boundaries do all you can to facilitate a sense of control for children and their families (NMC, 2018). In some cases, however, parents may be too distressed or not have the ability to engage. This requires referral to a family counsellor, psychologist or faith chaplain of their choice with their consent. Safeguarding issues may materialise. As stress and distress can be an ongoing event, even following PCCU discharge, follow-up care in the community may be required.

Parents' views of helpful nurse behaviours (Harbaugh et al. (2004) include:

- Nurturing and protective
- Allowing access and proximity to their child
- Openly being affectionate and caring
- Reducing stress and uncertainty
- Including parents in care
- Appreciating the individuality of their child
- Conducting care in a competent, coordinated manner
- Providing accurate information and reassurance

Parents' views of unhelpful nurse behaviours (Harbaugh et al., 2004; Brooten et al., 2012) include:

- Separation from child
- Exclusion from their child's care
- Poor communication of child's progress
- Nursing care without affection
- Nursing care without protection
- Conflict between staff and parents
- Inexperienced staff

ACTIVITY 29.4: REFLECTIVE PRACTICE

Give examples of your own behaviours that children and their families may have found helpful. List the actions and behaviours that may have been perceived as negative.

"Our nurses were amazing from the time we arrived, when we knew the least but needed them the most. I say our nurses as they were there for the whole family. We needed to trust that they cared as much as we did about the survival of our child. We physically could not be there 24 hours a day, and our nurses told us not to be, but the assurance and confidence of our nurses allowed us to rest, trusting that our child would be looked after. There were so many people involved in the care that came and went but the nurses were our constant. I would ensure I was there for every shift change so I would know who was looking after our child so I could then relax. I felt a bond with those nurses we had more than once."

Leah, parent of 18-month-old girl with multi-organ failure

SAFEGUARDING STOP POINT

Always clarify safeguarding issues during handover and as the situation changes on the PCCU. You must be aware of how actively parents and other visitors are allowed to participate in care, with or without supervision, and who is visiting your patient and if there are any restrictions to this.

WHAT'S THE EVIDENCE?

Some critically ill children and their families experience post-traumatic stress disorder (PTSD) following a PCCU admission and require follow-up care on discharge from the PCCU. Read Colville and Pierce's (2012) article 'Patterns of post-traumatic stress symptoms after paediatric intensive care'.

- What are the potential causes of PTSD for critically ill children and their parents?

PCC OUTCOMES

Many children and their families look forward to leaving the PCCU. For a few, the prospect of leaving can be daunting (Keogh, 2001). Being able to visit the ward and meet ward staff beforehand is an ideal strategy for reassuring children and their families. Where this is not possible, effective communication, reassurance and sensitive 'deintensifying' or 'de-escalating' monitoring may be the only option. Some units will have an outreach team or discharge nurse to support discharge and a minority of patients will be prepared for home/community care (e.g., those with life-limiting, long-term or rehabilitation/complex needs). This process requires the involvement and coordination of many hospital and community teams.

SEE ALSO
CHAPTER
28

CASE STUDY 29.3: HASAN

Hasan, a 2-month-old baby who was intubated and ventilated for bronchiolitis leading to respiratory failure, has been recently extubated (removal of ETT) and transitioned to high dependency unit (HDU) care. Hasan's assessment is highlighted below:

Observation: Lying comfortably on his back, breathing spontaneously and watching and interacting with his mum

Airway/Breathing: *Inspection*: Naris clear and patent, no excessive secretions, in room air saturating at 97%, RR: 42 breaths/min. No excessive WOB. No stridor or other signs of airway obstruction or swelling – a risk factor for recently extubated young children. Hasan's breathing is synchronous and there is bilateral chest wall expansion (equal). He has a strong, intermittent and non-problematic cough. His colour is normal for his ethnicity

Palpation: No evidence of retained secretions on chest

Auscultation: Bilateral breath sounds clear to bases. No crackles or wheeze

Circulation: Stable. HR: 115 beats/min, sinus rhythm, afebrile, CRT <2 seconds, normotensive, warm and well-perfused, urine output: 1.5ml/kg/hr

Disability: All sedation discontinued; no signs of withdrawal. $E_4V_5M_5$ (14/15), appropriate for age, fixing and following, moving all limbs normally and has normal tone. PEARL 3mm. Blood glucose: 4mmol/L

Exposure: Hasan has an intravenous cannula on the right hand which is infusing maintenance fluids at a normal rate. A spigotted nasogastric tube is in situ. He has a urethral catheter which can be removed

Problem/need: Hasan and his family need to feel prepared for ward discharge

Potential problem: Hasan is recently extubated and may deteriorate to the extent of needing reintubation or respiratory support. His family may feel anxious about his discharge

Goal: Hasan will continue his recovery. Hasan and his parents will feel fully prepared for his discharge

How can we prepare Hasan and his parents for discharge?

Sadly, for some patients and their family, end-of-life care is a reality. Discussion around palliation, futility of care, the need to limit or withdraw treatment (we never withdraw care) and organ donation is distressing, not least for the families involved (Griffiths and Danburry, 2015). Involving the palliative care team during this time is essential (Truog et al., 2006), and the RCPCH (Larcher et al., 2015) provide guidelines generally for the medico-legal issues surrounding treatment and treatment withdrawal. Managing death in a hospice or at home may be more comforting for families and dignified for the child but requires intense preparation. These issues must be sensitively raised and handled with children and their families as appropriate. Many roles and responsibilities are associated with supporting children and families in this phase of their lives (Michelson et al., 2013) and moral distress can be unbearable (Mu et al., 2019).

SEE ALSO
CHAPTER 33

"Do some reading before your placement so you are not so overwhelmed. Show you are interested and willing to learn. Ask the nurses if you can do things. They let you do a lot which helps you learn new skills."

Francesca, 3rd-year children's nursing student

CHAPTER SUMMARY

- Skillful ongoing structured assessment/monitoring is crucial when caring for the critically ill child
- Holistic child/family centred care is key within the technological environment
- Interventions/care management impact patient outcomes and family experiences

BUILD YOUR BIBLIOGRAPHY

Books

- Crawford, D. and McNee, P. (2012) Chapter 16: 'Care of the family', in M. Dixon and D. Crawford (eds), *Paediatric Intensive Care Nursing*. Chichester: Wiley-Blackwell.

  This chapter provides you with a comprehensive and detailed view of the strategies nurses can use to facilitate FCC.

- Davies, J.H. and Hassell, L.L. (2018) Chapter 12: 'Handy hints for various conditions', in J.H. Davies and L.L. Hassell, *Children in Intensive Care: A Survival Guide*, 3rd edn. London: Elsevier Churchill-Livingstone.

  This chapter provides a quick reference for the management of common conditions. Critical care is a complex area of nursing where not only do you come across many different conditions and injuries, but its management can be difficult to understand.

- Dixon, M. and Teasdale, D. (2012) Chapter 3: 'Physiological monitoring of infants and children in the intensive care unit', in M. Dixon and D. Crawford (eds), *Paediatric Intensive Care Nursing*. Chichester: Wiley-Blackwell.

  This chapter describes PCCU monitoring. One of the core experiences you will come across in your placement is the range of monitoring systems available in the critical care setting.

FURTHER
READING

Journal articles

- Colville, G., Kerry, S. and Pierce, C. (2008) 'Children's factual and delusional memories of intensive care'. *American Journal of Respiratory and Critical Care Medicine*, 77: 976-82.

  It is important to appreciate that critically ill children's true experiences may differ from the assumptions we make about what they may or may not remember about their critical care

FURTHER
READING:
ONLINE
JOURNAL
ARTICLES

admission and management and continuing support following discharge. This paper explores how accurately children's perceptions reflect their critical care experiences and the support they may or may not require recovering.

- Carnevale, F.A., Benedetti, M., Bonaldi, A., Bravi, E., Trabucco, G. and Biban, P. (2011) 'Understanding the private worlds of physicians, nurses and parents: a study of life-sustaining treatment decisions in Italian paediatric critical care'. *Journal of Child Health Care*, 15 (4): 334-49.

We may never know the true impact that critical illness has on all those who are closely involved in this process. This important study provides some insights into the emotional and psychological costs of caring for or being a parent of a critically ill child.

- LaFond, C.M., Van Hulle Vincent, C., Corte, C., Hersheberger, P.E., Johnson, A., Park, C.G. and Wilkie, D.J. (2015) 'PCCU nurses pain assessments and intervention choices for virtual human and written vignettes'. *Journal Pediatric Nursing*, 30 (4): 580-90.

It is morally, ethically and professionally important to ensure that pain is effectively and adequately managed in any setting, including on PCCUs where assumptions may be made about children's pain experiences. This article provides important insights into how pain may be viewed, assessed or managed in this medicalised setting.

Weblinks

FURTHER
READING:
WEBLINKS

- Children's Hospitals and Clinics of Minnesota youtube.com/watch?v=X49hzjE9cLs PCCUs can be somewhat threatening in appearance to a novice. This video gives you an insight into how a PCCU may appear and help you to identify some of its structures before you commence your placement.
- The Guardian, 'Children's lives in the balance at NHS paediatric intensive care unit' youtube.com/watch?v=picfVuZr93s Family-centred care (FCC) is an integral part of critical care nursing. This video will provide you with some strategies on how FCC may be facilitated in the critical care environment.
- https://georgespicu.org.uk/wp-content/uploads/2017/01/Psychology-Road-to-recovery-Guide-for-Families.pdf Many children and their families continue to be traumatised by the critical care experience even following their discharge from the PICU. This video by Colville and Atkins, describes some of these families' anxieties and fears and provides you with an insight into their psychological and emotional wellbeing.

REFERENCES

Ambuel, B., Hamlett, K.W., Marx, C.M. and Blumer, J.L. (1992) 'Assessing distress in paediatric intensive care environments, the COMFORT scale'. *Journal of Pediatric Psychology*, 17 (1): 95–109.

Brooten, D., Youngblut, J.M., Seagrave, L., Caicedo, C., Hawthorne, D., Hidalgo, I. and Roche, R. (2012) 'Parent's perceptions of health care providers actions around child ICU death, what helped, what did not'. *American Journal of Hospice and Palliative Medicine*, 30 (1): 40–9.

Colville, G. and Pierce, C. (2012) 'Patterns of post-traumatic stress symptoms after paediatric intensive care'. *Intensive Care Medicine*, 38: 1523–31.

Darovic, G.O. (2002) *Haemodynamic Monitoring, Invasive and Non-invasive Clinical Applications*. London: WB Saunders.

Davis, H., Kitchman, R., Gordon, I. and Helms, P. (1985) 'Regional ventilation in infancy, reversal of adult pattern'. *New England Journal of Medicine*, 313: 1625–8.

Davis, K., Bulsara, M.K., Ramelet, A.S. and Monterosso, L. (2017) 'Audit of endotracheal tube suction in a pediatric intensive care unit'. *Clinical Nursing Research*, 26 (1): 68–81.

Fainardi, V., Abelli, L., Muscarà, M., Pisi, G., Principi, N. and Esposito, S. (2021) 'Update on the role of high-flow nasal cannula in infants with bronchiolitis'. *Children*, 8 (2): 66. https://doi.org/10.3390/children8020066

Grant, M.J.C., Balas, M.C., Curley, M.A.Q. and RESTORE investigation team (2013) 'Defining sedation-related adverse events in the PICU'. *Heart and Lung*, 42 (3): 171–6.

Griffiths, S. and Danburry, C. (2015) 'Medico-legal issues for intensivists caring for children in a district general hospital'. *Journal of the Intensive Care Society*, 16 (2): 137–41.

Hakio, H., Rantanen, A., Astedt-Kurki, P. and Suominen, T. (2015) 'Parents' experiences of family functioning, health and social support provided by nurses – a pilot study in paediatric intensive care'. *Intensive and Critical Nursing*, 31: 29–37.

Harbaugh, B.L., Tomlinson, P.S. and Kirschbaum, M. (2004) 'Parents' perceptions of nurses' caregiving behaviours in the pediatric intensive care unit'. *Issues in Comprehensive Pediatric Nursing*, 27 (3): 163–78.

Harris, J., Ramelet, A-S., van Dijk, M., Pokorna, P., Wielenga, J., Tume, L., Tibboel, D. and Ista, E. (2016) 'Clinical recommendations for pain, sedation, withdrawal and delirium assessment in critically ill infants and children: an ESPNIC position statement for healthcare professionals'. *Intensive Care Medicine*, 42: 972–86.

Hazinski, M.F. (2013) *Nursing Care of the Critically Ill Child*, 3rd edn. St Louis, MO: Mosby.

Johnson, K.L. and Meyenburg, T. (2009) 'Physiological rationale and current evidence for therapeutic positioning of critically ill patients'. *AACN Advanced Critical Care*, 20 (3): 228–40.

Keogh, S. (2001) 'Parents' experiences of the transfer of their child from the PICU to the ward: a phenomenological study'. *Nursing in Critical Care*, 6 (1): 7–13.

Kochanek, P.M., Tasker, R.C., Bell, M.J., Adelson, P.D., Carney, N., Vavilala, M.S. et al. (2019) 'Management of pediatric severe traumatic brain injury: 2019 consensus and guidelines-based algorithm for first and second tier therapies'. *Pediatric Critical Care Medicine*, 20 (3): 269–79. Doi: 10.1097/PCC.0000000000001737.

Larcher, V., Craig, F., Bhogal, K., Wilkinson, K. and Brierley, J. (2015) 'Making decisions to limit treatment in life-limiting and life-threatening conditions in children: a framework for practice'. *Archives of Disease in Childhood*, 100 (Suppl. 2): s1–26.

Latour, J.M. (2011) *Empowerment of Parents in the Intensive Care: A journey discovering parents' experiences and satisfaction of care.* Rotterdam: Erasmus Universiteit Rotterdam.

Lullaby Trust (2013) *Sudden Infant Death Syndrome: A Guide for Professionals.* London: The Lullaby Trust.

McGraw, S.A., Truog, R.D., Solomon, M.Z., Cohen-Bearak, M.P.H., Sellers, D.E. and Meyer, E.C. (2012) '"I was able to still be her mom": parenting at end of life in the PICU'. *Pediatric Critical Care Medicine*, 13 (6): e350–6.

Messerole, E., Peine, P., Wittkopp, S., Marini, J.J. and Albert, R.K. (2002) 'Clinical commentary: the pragmatics of prone positioning'. *American Journal Respiratory Critical Care Medicine*, 165: 1359.

Michelson, K.N., Patel, R., Haber-Barker, N., Emanuel, L. and Frader, J. (2013) 'End-of-life care decisions in the PICU: roles professionals play'. *Pediatric Critical Care Medicine*, 14 (1): e34-44. Doi:10.1097/PCC.0b013e31826e7408.

Moore, G., Knight, G. and Blann, A. (2010) *Haematology, Fundamentals of Biomedical Science.* Oxford: Oxford University Press.

Mu, P.F., Tseng, Y.M., Wang, C.C., Chen, Y.J., Huang, S.H., Hsu, T.F. and Florczak, K.L. (2019) 'Nurses' experiences in end-of-life care in the PICU: a qualitative systematic review'. *Nursing Science Quarterly*, 32 (1): 12–22.

NICE (National Institute for Health and Care Excellence) (2017) Sepsis: recognition, diagnosis and early recognition. NICE guideline [NG51]. Available at: www.nice.org.uk/guidance/ng51 (accessed 20 June 2023).

NPSA (National Patient Safety Agency) (2008) *Problems with Infusions and Sampling from Arterial Lines*. Rapid Response Report, NPSA/2008RRRS006, From Reporting to Learning. National Patient Safety Agency.

Nursing and Midwifery Council (2018) *The Code: Professional Standards of Practice and Behaviour for Nurses and Midwives*. London: NMC. Available at: www.nmc.org.uk/standards/code/.

PCCS (Pediatric Critical Care Society) (2021) *Quality Standards for the Care of Critically Ill or Injured Children*, 6th edn. Available at: https://pccsociety.uk/about-pccs/pics-standards/ (accessed 20 June 2023).

Peate, I. and Gormley-Fleming, E. (eds) (2021) *Fundamentals of Children and Young People's Anatomy and Physiology: A Textbook for Nursing and Healthcare Students*, 2nd edn. Chichester: Wiley–Blackwell.

Resuscitation Council UK (2021) *Paediatric Advanced Life Support Guidelines*. Available at: www.resus.org.uk/library/2021-resuscitation-guidelines/paediatric-advanced-life-support-guidelines (accessed 20 June 2023).

Royal College of Nursing (RCN) (2009) *The Recognition and Assessment of Acute Pain in Children*. Clinical Practice Guidelines, update of full guideline. London: RCN.

Royal College of Paediatrics and Child Health (RCPCH) (2014) *High Dependency Care for Children: Time to Move: A Focus on the Critically Ill Child Pathway beyond the Intensive Care Unit. A Set of Recommendations to Improve the Care of the Critically Ill Child*. London: RCPCH.

Sperotto, F., Friedman, K.G., Son, M.B.F., Van der Pluym, C.J., Newburger, J.W. and Dionne, A. (2021) 'Cardiac manifestations in SARS-CoV-2-associated multisystem inflammatory syndrome in children: a comprehensive review and proposed clinical approach'. *European Journal of Pediatrics*, 180 (2): 307–22.

Strickland, S.L., Rubin, B.K., Dreschu, D.H., O'Malley, C.A., Volskot, A., Branson, R.D. and Hess, D.R (2013) 'AARG clinical practice guidelines: effectiveness of non-pharmacological airway clearance therapies in hospital patients'. *Respiratory Care*, 58 (1): 2187–93.

Truog, R.D., Meyer, E.C. and Burns, J.P. (2006) 'Toward interventions to improve end-of-life care in the pediatric intensive care unit'. *Critical Care Medicine*, 34 (11 Suppl): S373–9.

Tume, L.N. and Copnell, B. (2015) 'Endotracheal suctioning of the critically ill child'. *Journal of Pediatric Intensive Care*, 4 (2): 56–63.

Tume, L.N. and Latour, J.M. (2015) 'Family involvement in PICU rounds: reality or rhetoric?' *Paediatric Critical Care Medicine*, 16 (9): 875–6.

Venus, K., Munshi, L. and Fralick, M. (2020) 'Prone positioning for patients with hypoxic respiratory failure related to COVID-19'. *Canadian Medical Association Journal*, 23 (192): E1532-7.

Weiss, S., Peters, M.J., Waleed, A., Agus, M., Flori, H., Inwald, D. et al. (2020) 'Executive Summary: Surviving Sepsis Campaign international guidelines for the management of septic shock and sepsis-associated organ dysfunction in children'. *Pediatric Critical Care Medicine*, 21 (2); 186–95.

Wells, D., Gillies, D. and Fitzgerald, D. (2005) 'Positioning for acute respiratory distress in hospitalized infants and children'. *Cochrane Database of Systematic Reviews*, 2005 (2): CD003645. doi: 10.1002/14651858.

Wheeler, D.S. (2013) '*Critical care of the pediatric patient*'. An Issue of *Pediatric Clinics* 60(3). Epub June 2013. Elsevier.

CARE OF THE NEONATE

KATHLEEN MANGAHIS AND CATHARINE GROB*

THIS CHAPTER COVERS

- Organisation and provision of neonatal care
- The term, preterm and growth-restricted baby
- Environmental challenges to the infant
- Environmental stressors for the baby
- Environmental challenges to the family
- Decision-making and ethics in neonatal care

"The unexpected birth of my daughter at 28 weeks gestational age gave me a unique entry into the world of neonatal care. I had lived in this world as a nurse caring for babies and their families. Now I was to experience this as the recipient. During the next 12 weeks we occupied an environment that provided many noxious stimuli: light, noise, multiple caregivers, occasional lack of understanding and insensitivity. The sense of loss of being unable to parent my daughter was overwhelming. The dependency on others, the unknown road ahead, the setbacks, the holding onto hope, the pain and discomfort – these were some of the experiences lived through on a daily basis. Setbacks knocked both hope and optimism. Parenting through this journey was conducted in a very public environment and always in the presence of others. The very environment that ensured her survival had also deprived me of privacy with my daughter. Developing friendship with other parents in the same situation was a source of support and joy. Throughout the journey staff unfailingly provided expertise, care, support, love to my daughter and to me. It is difficult to adequately articulate my gratitude and impossible to quantify it."

Kate, parent

---

*Based on the chapter in the first edition written by Elisabeth Podsiadly and Mary Goggin.

INTRODUCTION

Neonatology is the care given to a baby in its first 4 weeks of life and addresses the needs of infants born too soon (premature), too small (growth-restricted) and ill. Care needs will vary depending upon the degree of prematurity and the condition of the infant and will identify what type of neonatal unit should provide infant and family care. Admission to a neonatal unit can be life-saving, but also exposes the vulnerable infant to an inappropriate environment for neurodevelopment during a critical time and can therefore have a lifelong impact on neurobehavioural outcomes. This chapter explores the current provision of neonatal care to demonstrate its uniqueness in relation to other areas of child health and provide the setting for a comparison of the characteristics, problems/conditions and care of the term, preterm and growth-restricted baby. The chapter then considers the environmental challenges experienced by both the infant and family admitted to the neonatal unit with a focus on family-centred care to enable you to support a parent like Kate, the voice that introduced the chapter.

ORGANISATION AND PROVISION OF NEONATAL CARE

Providing care to infants and families in a neonatal unit requires you to have an understanding of how care is organised nationally and locally by network.

Not all neonatal units are the same. The British Association of Perinatal Medicine (BAPM) represents neonatal healthcare professionals and is responsible for defining the levels/designation and categories of care that can be provided by neonatal units – the higher the level (1 to 3), the greater the complexity of care offered. Four categories of neonatal care have been identified (BAPM, 2011). These are, increasing in the order of care complexity: transitional care, special care, high dependency and intensive care. Since 2003, England has structured its neonatal care locally into managed clinical networks or organisational delivery unit networks. Scotland, Wales and Northern Ireland have followed suit. Such networks develop expertise in a small number of neonatal units which deliver all levels of care in order to improve infant morbidity and mortality. Not all units will provide all levels of care. Who provides what levels of care is negotiated and agreed within each network. A network will consist of special care units (SCUs), local neonatal units (LNUs) and usually one or two lead neonatal intensive care units (NICUs).

Ideally, infants requiring a higher level of care are delivered at the lead NICU. Transfer before delivery is known as an in-utero transfer. Some networks have arrangements whereby all mothers likely to deliver on or before, for example 26 weeks, do so in the maternity unit attached to the lead NICU. If an infant delivers before an in-utero transfer can be arranged, then the baby will be transported (ex-utero) to the network NICU for a higher level of care provided by a specialist team.

ACTIVITY 30.1: REFLECTIVE PRACTICE

Explore the provision of neonatal care in the hospitals affiliated with your university by using the 'Network Information' on the BAPM website (www.bapm.org/pages/19-neonatal-networks).

- What levels of care are available in your local network?
- How far would parents have to travel from an SCU or LNU to receive neonatal intensive care?
- What might be the emotional, social and financial impact on the family involved in a transfer for a higher level of care?

Neonatal and family care is mainly provided by neonatal nurses and paediatric doctors trained or undergoing training in the care of neonates. Nurses could be child or adult trained and, depending on where in the UK you are working, midwives. Neonatal nurses, who have undertaken further post-registration training and are identified as qualified in specialty (QIS), deliver and oversee all levels of care. Lower levels of care can be provided by nurses (not QIS), nursery nurses and/or healthcare assistants under supervision of a QIS nurse. Many neonatal units now have advanced neonatal nurse practitioners who often work as part of the medical team. Additional healthcare professionals contributing to neonatal care include pharmacists, physiotherapists, speech and language therapists, counsellors, family support nurses and paediatric surgeons, to name a few. Like many areas of nursing, neonatal units are experiencing staff shortages, particularly of staff that are QIS and are keen to recruit to 'grow their own' from both adult and child field-specific graduates.

WHAT'S THE EVIDENCE?

The annual National Neonatal Audit Programme (NNAP) was established in 2006 and it aims to assess whether babies admitted to neonatal units in England, Scotland and Wales receive consistent high-quality care. The report covers key outcomes of neonatal care and measures of optimal perinatal care, maternal breastmilk feeding, measures of parental partnership, neonatal nurse staffing, and other important care processes (RCPCH, 2022).

In the 2021 report, it found that just 78.6% of shifts are numerically staffed according to national guidelines. It also showed that only about 47% of nursing shifts have sufficient QIS staff care for the babies in NICU. You can read the report at www.rcpch.ac.uk/resources/national-neonatal-audit-programme-summary-report-2021-data.

Compare the research findings with a neonatal unit affiliated with your university by organising a visit to speak with a neonatal nurse manager or a neonatal tutor/practice educator to discuss the following about medical and nursing staffing levels.

- Is the unit fully staffed?
- If not, which grades are they short of? What are the reasons for this?
- How is this affecting the unit's provision of care to infants and families?

THE TERM, PRETERM AND GROWTH-RESTRICTED BABY

This overview presents a systems approach (rather than a nursing framework) to reflect the shared assessment approach used by the multidisciplinary (MDT) healthcare team in many neonatal units. The overview is followed by a diagrammatic representation of the interrelationships between neonatal systems to help you deliver holistic care (Figures 30.1–30.5).

The following tables (30.1–30.3) provide a concise introduction to the problem experienced by the preterm, intrauterine growth-restricted and term infant requiring admission to the neonatal unit. The tables identify the system, problem, assessment and nursing action. Prior to assessment it is essential to understand the antenatal, intrapartum and resuscitation history to enable accurate assessment in context. Documentation of nursing observations and interventions must be completed in a timely manner.

Characteristics and problems associated with the small for gestational age infants (<10th centile on weight chart)

Small for gestational age (SGA) infants may be divided into two subgroups: small but appropriately and symmetrically grown (constitutionally small) and SGA due to growth restriction (IUGR). These infants present with asymmetrical growth.

Table 30.1 Overview: Characteristics and problems associated with the preterm infant (<37 weeks gestational age)

System	Characteristics and problems	Assessment skills	Nursing action
Neurological	Immature/fragile walls of cerebral blood vessels	Positioning	Appropriate position: head aligned with the body
	Less able to tolerate an asphyxia insult: risk of intraventricular haemorrhage (IVH) and periventricular leukomalacia	Oxygen saturation appropriate to gestational age and oxygen requirement	Nesting to maintain head aligned with body
		Method of feeding	Physical boundaries
	Absent/immature suck swallow reflex	Susceptible to changing pressure	Alternate positioning: supine, right lateral, left lateral
	Immature visual system: potential for the development of retinopathy of prematurity (ROP)		Avoid prone position in the first week of life as head cannot be aligned with body
	Small muscle mass: inability to adopt flexed position conducive to development		
	Poor muscle tone		
Respiratory	Immature lungs	Stages of lung development	Assist with the administration of surfactant
	Lack of surfactant	Effect of lack of surfactant	Monitor effects of surfactant
	Apnoea of prematurity		Monitor O_2 saturation levels
	Transient tachypnoea of the newborn (TTN)	Pattern of breathing	Adjust oxygen requirements in response to effects of surfactant
	Pneumonia	Assess need for degree of respiratory support	Check blood gas in response to changes in ventilation: oxygen requirement, rising CO_2
	Chronic lung disease (CLD)	Presence of apnoea and/or bradycardia	
	Signs of respiratory distress include the following: tachypnoea, nasal flaring, recession, grunting, asynchronous chest movement, cyanosis and apnoea		Monitor respiratory function: colour, respiratory rate, work of breathing
Cardiovascular	Patent ductus arteriosus (PDA) with associated risk of Intraventricular Haemmorhage (IVH)	Monitoring to include: observe colour	Observe central and peripheral colour
	Low blood pressure (BP)	SaO_2 level and variations	Continuous monitoring of oxygen saturation levels, respiratory and heart rate
	Poorly oxygenated tissues: acidosis	skin temperature	Note variations in oxygen saturation and bradycardia
	Bradycardia (<100)/tachycardia (>180)	capillary refill time (CRT)	Pre and post ductal saturation measurement.
		heart rate (HR)	
		note presence or absence of PDA	Take regular temperature measurements
		measure BP	Use appropriate BP cuff and monitor blood pressure- consider 4 limb BP measurement

System	Characteristics and problems	Assessment skills	Nursing action
Digestive	Immature gut motility limiting enteral intake	Pass oro/nasogastric tube (O/NGT)	Feed with colostrum initially then breast milk
	Risk of necrotising enterocolitis (NEC)	Check and monitor O/NGT; aspirate for volume, colour and pH	Trophic feeds
	Limited enzyme activity		Initiate small volume (once breastmilk is available)
	Intermittent uncoordinated peristalsis	Monitor tolerance	Increase as tolerated
		Increase milk feeds slowly	
		Observe abdomen for signs of distension/ loopy bowels	
Excretory	Feed intolerance due to immature gut motility	Observe abdomen for signs of distension, colour and presence of loopy bowels	Document status of abdomen
	Renal immaturity: inability to concentrate urine, inability to excrete acid load with low bicarbonate threshold resulting in metabolic acidosis		Weigh nappies and measure urinary output (2-4mls/kg/hour)
		Monitor urinary output	Test urine using clinistix reagent strips
			Document findings
Metabolic	Hypoglycaemia	Assess glucose levels	Monitor glucose levels
	Lack of glycogen stores	Issue that may increase energy consumption (e.g., infection, procedures, pain, respiratory distress, activity, handling, work of breathing)	Provide adequate glucose intake; i.e., breast milk, IV fluids, TPN
	Immature gluconeogenic pathway		Minimal handling to conserve infant energy
	Jaundice: high cell mass		Monitor SBR levels
	Immature liver: inadequate enzyme activity/immature enzymes		Plot levels on the appropriate treatment threshold graphs and initiate treatment when indicated (NICE CG 98, 2016)
		Assess serum bilirubin (SBR)	
Skin	Immature skin	Daily assessment of skin	Nurse in incubator
	Iatrogenic injury	Soft bedding to prevent pressure injury	Humidified environment (80-100%)
	Transepidermal water loss		Avoid use/minimise tape on infant's skin and where unavoidable use specialist tape (e.g., Siltape®) to secure dressings
		Check position of ears if infant wearing hat	Use Apeel® to remove tape from immature skin
			Avoid the use of ECG electrodes on extremely immature skin (<26 weeks gestation)
			Nurse the very immature infant on 100% cotton or sateen sheets
Skeletal	Immature and soft bone	Assess position	Promote bone mineralisation
	Risk of metabolic bone disease		Administer vitamins and phosphate supplements as prescribed
	Exacerbation of respiratory distress		Use nests/rolls to support baby's position
			Ensure baby is in flexed position
			Position to help baby establish midline, hand to hand, and hand to mouth

(Continued)

Table 30.1 (Continued)

System	Characteristics and problems	Assessment skills	Nursing action
Immunity	Relatively immature immune system (immunity transferred by mother in last trimester) Skin integrity breached by IV cannula/central lines	Documentation Prevent Assess for signs of infection and extravasation	Strict handwashing Universal precautions Weekly screening (as per local policy) Review stop date for antibiotics Hourly documentation of lines, sites and pump pressures Access 'plastics' team in the event of an extravasation injury Awareness of extravasation protocol Aseptic technique when accessing vascular devices.

Infants who are SGA and are small but appropriately and symmetrically grown (constitutionally small) experience an insult in the first trimester, during embryogenesis. This results in a failure of growth which is sustained throughout pregnancy. The infant is undersized with fewer cells, but these cells grow normally. Causes include intrauterine infection, genetic abnormalities, smoking and alcohol. All can affect long-term prognosis.

Infants who are SGA due to growth restriction (IUGR) and who present with asymmetrical growth often experience an insult in the second to third trimester due to a lack of nutrition (starved). This results in slow/failure in weight gain, while head circumference is not affected. There is little subcutaneous fat, the skin may appear loose and thin, the muscle mass is greatly decreased, notably on the buttocks and thighs. The infant often has a wide-eyed anxious appearance. These infants can experience many potential problems (Table 30.2).

Term babies are admitted to the neonatal unit due to congenital abnormalities, antepartum/intrapartum events, maternal and environmental pregnancy-related issues. A summary of conditions can be found in Table 30.3.

Table 30.2 Potential problems of the small for gestational age (SGA) infant due to growth restriction

Problems	Effect	Assessment	Nursing action
Perinatal asphyxia	Reduced oxygen is poorly tolerated and the impact may not be seen until later in life	Observation of vital signs, skin colour and capillary refill time (CRT) Appropriate positioning of saturation probe Observation of skin and frequent position change	Maintain oxygen saturation levels within the desired values for gestational age
Hypoglycaemia	Reduced energy to the brain and body tissues Apnoea and bradycardia	Assess glucose level Assess response to handling Assess physiological signs and behaviour that may increase energy expenditure	Ensure delivery of prescribed nutrition Monitor nutritional intake: 10% dextrose, TPN, enteral feeds Tolerance to enteral feeds Monitor glucose levels and document Initiate hypoglycaemia policy

Problems	Effect	Assessment	Nursing action
Polycythaemia	Viscous circulation resulting in poor oxygenation to the tissues Low oxygen saturation levels Renal thrombi Blood in urine	Colour Temperature Peripheral temperature Blood gas SBR Hb/Haematocrit level	Monitor and document oxygen levels Test urine for the presence of blood Monitor SBR levels Plot levels on the appropriate treatment threshold graphs and initiate treatment when indicated (NICE, 2016)
Thermal instability	Large surface area and small body mass increases risk of hypothermia, acidosis, hypoglycaemia and poor growth	Colour and temperature of peripherals Core temperature Assess temperature control Weight gain	Monitor closely to exclude other causes, i.e., infection Nurse infant in an incubator and maintain a neutral thermal environment to minimise energy and oxygen consumption Transfer to cot when infant is maintaining own temperature and achieving growth Ease the transition to cot by the initial use of heated mattress Monitor temperature and weight gain (aim for 15-25g/kg/day)

Table 30.3 Conditions of term babies requiring admission to the neonatal unit

Condition	Effect	Assessment	Nursing action
Congenital abnormalities			

Congenital diaphragmatic hernia (CDH)	Perforation of the diaphragm results in the abdominal organs (e.g., the stomach, liver, spleen, intestines) entering the chest cavity, causing compression of developing lungs
	
	May occur on left or right (most severe due to larger right lung)
	
	Difficult to achieve lung expansion due to pressure from organs in chest
	
	Air in the stomach may exacerbate the situation by reducing available space for lung expansion
	
	Resuscitation: infant is intubated; do *not* bag and mask
	
	Inflation breaths are given once infant intubated
		Colour
		
		Chest movement
		
		Heart rate
		
		Dextrocardia
			Stabilisation/preop care:
			
			pass O/NGT (size 8Fr) and aspirate stomach contents, maintain on free drainage
			
			no hand bagging
			
			Provide supportive care:
			
			   intubation and ventilation
			
			   paralysis and sedation
			
			   inotropic support
			
			   pain/discomfort management
			
			   IV fluids/TPN
			
			Blood gas monitoring
			
			Check glucose levels regularly
			
			Bilirubin measurement
			
			Monitor urinary output (2-4ml/kg/hour)

(Continued)

Table 30.3 (Continued)

Tracheoesophageal atresia/fistula	The upper part of the oesophagus ends in a blind pouch and does not connect to the lower oesophagus Swallowed saliva gathers in the upper pouch and if untreated may be aspirated If the baby feeds, milk fills the pouch overflowing increasing the risk of aspiration The oesophagus must grow to enable anastomosis of the upper and lower pouch; this may take many weeks Baby must remain hospitalised during this period of growth Nutrition is provided via a gastrostomy	Assess colour Presence of mucous at mouth Access success in passing O/NGT, if resistance felt stop procedure	Protecting the lungs by preventing aspiration of pouch contents is *essential* Pass an 8Fr. Replogle tube into the pouch end, attach the end of the tube to a continuous low suction (5Kpa – may vary depending on the size of baby and thickness of secretions) Flush the Replogle tube every 15 minutes with 0.5ml of NaCl 0.9% to prevent blockage of tube, documenting all flushes Monitor viscosity of mucous; if thick a larger flush may be required (1ml) Observe closely during flushing and ensure volume of flush is returned Prevent oral aversion by providing non-nutritive sucking

Antepartum/intrapartum events

Perinatal asphyxia due to: antepartum or intrapartum haemorrhage	Lack of oxygen delivered to the tissues results in: brain deprived of oxygen raised CO_2, raised lactic acid (>2mmol/l) low glucose level (<2.5mmol/l)	Colour Tone Activity Chest movement Respiratory rate	Assist with resuscitation: dry infant, consider passive cooling maintain clear airway provide inflation breaths
foetal distress due to prolonged labour	abnormal brain activity possible seizures	Oxygenation status Glucose level Blood gas	measure O_2 saturation levels check blood gas and glucose level Once stabilised transfer infant to the NNU Initiate appropriate monitoring Provide respiratory support Provide nutritional support: IV fluids (10% dextrose initially) Commence cooling if infant meets the criteria Keep parents informed

Shoulder dystocia	Baby's head is delivered, but one shoulder becomes stuck behind the mother's pubic bone, delaying the birth of the baby's body	Colour	Support shoulder and arm
		Tone	Provide comfort measures
		Activity	Provide analgesia for pain
	Prolonged labour	Chest movement	Careful dressing of the infant to prevent discomfort
	Brachial plexus injury (BPI) which may cause loss of movement to the arm	Respiratory rate	
		Oxygenation status	Support and keep parents informed
	Most common injury is Erb's palsy, usually temporary and movement returns within hours or days	Tone, position and movement of affected limb	
	Sometimes infants can suffer brain damage if they do not get enough oxygen due to delayed delivery		
Fractured clavicle	Sometimes shoulder dystocia can cause other injuries including fracture of the infant's arm or shoulder	Use appropriate pain tool to assess level of pain/discomfort	Provide comfort measures
			Administer analgesia as required
	In the majority of cases these heal well		Reduce discomfort by carefully dressing and positioning
			Use figure-of-8 support if indicated
			Support parents
Cardiac: acyanotic heart problems patent ductus arteriosus (PDA) atrial septal defect (ASD) ventricular septal defect (VSD)	PDA results in increased pulmonary blood flow from the aorta across the ductus arteriosus into the pulmonary artery; this results in increased blood flow to the lungs (left to right shunt)	Assessment is focused on cardiac output: observe central and peripheral colour assess CRT oxygenation saturation levels blood pressure	Maintain adequate gas exchange
			Monitor oxygen requirement
			Maintain saturation levels within the desired values (based on gestational age and oxygen dependency)
	Reduced systemic blood flow		Support parents
	Increased oxygen requirement		
	ASD less significant (atria are filling chambers) than VSD (ventricles are pumping chambers); mixing of arterial and venous blood more significant by lowering oxygen to the systemic circulation		
Cardiac: Cyanotic heart problems e.g., tetralogy of Fallot	Cyanosis	Colour	Respiratory support as required
	Respiratory distress	Femoral pulses	SaO_2 levels are prescribed
	Acidosis	Four limb blood pressure	Administer prostaglandin E1
			Monitor for apnoea
			Prepare infant and parents for transfer to the cardiac centre

(Continued)

Table 30.3 (Continued)

Environmental and pregnancy-related events

Maternal diabetes which can be: insulin dependent gestational diabetes type II diabetes	The foetus receives a higher than normal level of glucose from the maternal blood (via the umbilical vein) Foetal insulin axis is independent of the mother Infant produces a corresponding level of insulin to metabolise the glucose In the postpartum period the infant experiences a period of adaptation and is dependent on an exogenous supply of glucose while at the same time continues to produce high levels of insulin The effect is hypoglycaemia blood glucose level <2.5mmol/l, which if uncorrected may cause irreversible brain damage Increased risk of respiratory distress syndrome (RDS), congenital abnormality, polycythaemia, hypocalcaemia and jaundice	Colour Tone Activity Heart rate Respiratory rate Glucose level	Check and monitor glucose levels at regular intervals to prevent hypoglycaemia Initiate hypoglycaemia policy Provide a suitable glucose supply Administer IV fluids (10% dextrose) Support mother to breastfeed or provide formula Cautious weaning of IV fluids to ensure maintenance of safe glucose levels Measure blood gas and bilirubin levels

Maternal substance abuse

Neonatal abstinence syndrome most commonly due to: alcohol cocaine heroin cannabis	Withdrawal symptoms can affect all systems and signs and symptoms may include: irritability unsettled high-pitched cry difficult to console and settle hyperactive higher than normal demand for energy high temperature sneezing seizures	Observe the baby at rest and post feed Note all activity at rest and when awake Frequency of feeds Vital signs	Appropriate environment: quiet part of the nursery with reduced lighting Loose clothing Comfort measures Nutritional support: baby may demand frequent feeds Complete withdrawal chart and monitor score Administer morphine as prescribed to manage symptoms Support parents and family Consider safeguarding issues MDT approach to discharge planning

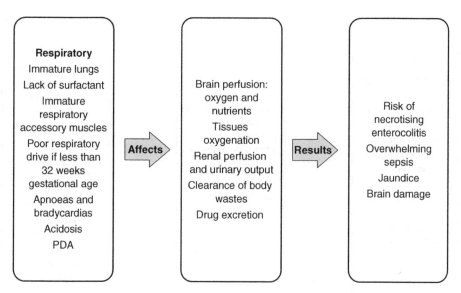

Figure 30.1 How a problem arising in the respiratory system can affect other systems

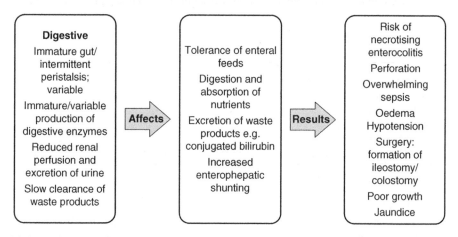

Figure 30.2 How a problem arising in the digestive system can affect other systems

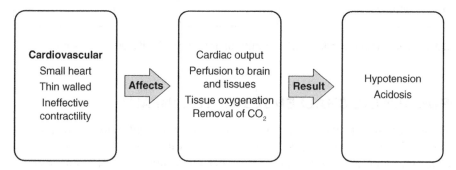

Figure 30.3 How a problem arising in the cardiovascular system affects oxygenation to the brain, tissues and removal of waste products

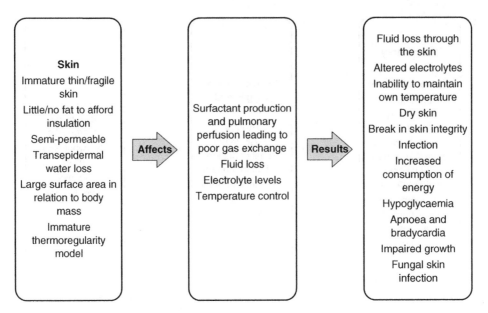

Figure 30.4 How immature skin affects temperature control, fluid loss, infection and energy consumption

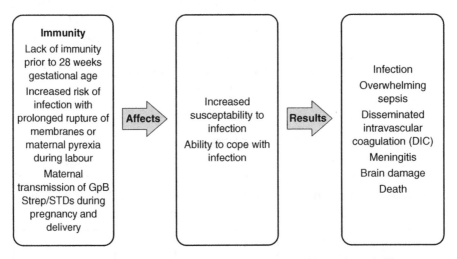

Figure 30.5 The impact of a lack of immunity on infant morbidity and mortality

ENVIRONMENTAL CHALLENGES TO THE INFANT

The neonatal environment compared to the intrauterine environment is hostile and provides the preterm and sick neonate with challenges. These challenges create risks and if not managed can impact on the infant and family journey through the neonatal unit by undermining treatment and increasing morbidity and mortality. These risks include infection and the influences of light and noise, and pain resulting from disease state and care interventions required to manage their condition.

Neonatal infection

Despite advances in neonatal care, neonatal infection remains a significant cause of neonatal morbidity and mortality, particularly for the IUGR and preterm infant whose host defences are poor (Bedford-Russell, 2015). The presentation of infection in the neonate is generalised or often expressed as non-specific (see Table 30.4). As a result, we have difficulty diagnosing sepsis early. Treatment is based on a total reliance of killing the identified organism by using appropriate antibiotics (Bedford-Russell, 2015). The consequences of neonatal infection can include meningitis, septicaemia, septic shock, disseminated intravascular coagulation (DIC), poor developmental and neurological outcome and death (see Figure 30.5).

Table 30.4 Signs of infection

System	Signs
Neurological	Irritability, listlessness/lethargy, poor suck, unresponsive, high-pitched cry, jitteriness, full or bulging fontanelle, tense fontanelle, episthotonos, hypo/hypertonic seizure activity, unstable temperature
Cardiovascular	Tachycardia, pale, mottled poor cutaneous circulation, capillary refill >3 seconds, cyanosis, irregular heartbeat, hypotension
Respiratory	Tachypnoea, apnoea, nasal flaring, recession grunting, cyanosis, irregular respirations, desaturation, increasing FiO_2
Gastrointestinal	Vomiting, diarrhoea, abdominal distension, poor weight gain, 'not interested in feeding'
Hepatic	Jaundice, altered coagulation, hypo/hyperglycaemia
Integumentary	Petechia, rash, heat and redness in an infected area
Immunological	Neutropenia, neutrophilia, thrombocytopenia, raised C-reactive protein (CRP)
Own learning Tacit or intuitive	'Just not right'; 'Handled better yesterday'; 'not him/herself'

Table 30.5 Comparison of early and late onset infection

	Early onset infection	Late onset infection
Onset	<72 hours	>72 hours
Source	Mother's genital tract	Postnatal environment Mother's genital tract
Organism	Group B streptococcus Listeriosis *Stapylococcus aureus* *Haemophilus*	*Escherichia coli* *Pseudomonas* *Klebsiella* Group B streptococcus *Enterobacter* *Staphylococcus aureus* Coagulase-negative staphylococi
Disease presentation	Fulminant Multisystem	Insidious Focal Pneumonia frequent Meningitis frequent

Three groups of infection have been identified: transplacental or congenital infections (e.g., toxoplasmosis, hepatitis, parvovirus, rubella, cytomegalovirus and herpes), intrapartum or early onset infections, and finally postpartum or late onset infections. See Table 30.5 for a comparison of early and late onset infection.

Nursing care is supportive. The key intervention in reducing nosocomial or late onset infection sepsis is to ensure all who interact with the infant adhere to the neonatal unit hand-washing policy in order to prevent cross-infection. Nurses need to lead by example and ensure that all who interact with infants follow unit guidelines. Parents taught how to correctly hand wash on their first visit generally go on to demonstrate good technique, ensuring all those who come into contact with their infant comply with unit policy.

ENVIRONMENTAL STRESSORS FOR THE BABY

The uterine environment is temperature-consistent and dark, and as the foetus matures it provides a supportive positional environment with natural maternal noises and a muffled outside world. This environment ensures appropriate infant growth and development. When an infant is born prematurely or ill, the safe and nurturing environment is replaced by the neonatal unit which can be deemed hostile and not developmentally friendly. Increased survival and decreasing gestational age results in an infant less able to cope with the stresses of the neonatal environment, which include light, noise and pain.

Light

Circadian rhythms or how we respond to day and night are essential to wellbeing. They determine a range of biological activities including brainwave activity, hormone production, cell regeneration, sleep and feeding patterns (Robert, 2010). Foetal circadian rhythms are regulated by the mother, but lost if born early (Haumont, 2012). Preterm eyes open more frequently and their thin lids are easily penetrated by the bright light of the neonatal environment (Robinson and Fielder, 1992). The bright and harsh lighting of this environment can lead to behavioural disorganisation, physiological instability, potentially ROP (retinopathy of prematurity) and disruption/deprivation of much-needed sleep (Haumont, 2012). Lighting in nurseries should be as natural as possible and adjustable, with directable procedural light available when needed. Many units now employ the use of cot covers and ensure periods when nursery lighting is dimmed if not off. These periods known as 'quiet time' or 'quiet hour' also address the other environmental stressor, noise.

Noise

Neonatal units provide 24-hour care and potentially 24 hours of varied but continuous noise. Unlike staff and parents, the infants cannot escape the sounds of the unit environment and are entirely dependent on us to regulate the levels of noise generated by equipment, care-giving and talking. Intense and sustained noise may lead to physiological and behavioural instability, hearing deficits, long-term neurodevelopmental outcomes and delayed language acquisition (Wachman and Lahav, 2011; Venkataraman et al., 2018). The nurse plays a key role in moderating noise levels in response to infant behavioural cues. Kuhl and Melzoff (1984) suggest that noise in the NICU may be a contributing factor in delayed parent–infant interaction as it masks meaningful sounds.

Neonatal pain

Neonates feel acute and chronic pain. The causes may be related to procedural activities, handling/care and of course illness itself. The infant's responses to pain are also influenced by gestational age, previous experience of pain and sleep state (Anand, 2015). Pain results in immediate physiological and behavioural instability (and if left untreated, may lead to long-term neurological damage, developmental delays and behavioural problems resulting in learning difficulties (Mitchell and Boss, 2002; Campbell-Yeo, Eriksson and Benoit, 2022)).

Pain assessment is central to good neonatal care (Anand, 2015). A large number of multidimensional pain assessment tools, for procedural and acute pain, are available to practice. These assess specific physiological and behavioural responses, but are also dependent on the caregivers' subjective assessment (Anand, 2015). Pain relief is dependent on using the correct tool and staff appropriately trained in its use.

SEE ALSO
CHAPTER 3

Pharmacological and non-pharmacological interventions, together or alone, can be used to prevent, reduce or eliminate neonatal pain. Opiates, like morphine, continue to be the drug of choice for many ventilated or surgical neonates with moderate to severe pain. The use of opiates still creates anxiety about their short- and long-term side effects (Kariholu et al., 2014). Oral sucrose is frequently used to manage single-event procedural pain. In addition to modulating the neonatal environment by reducing light and noise, a range of non-pharmacological interventions can be used to alleviate pain during procedures, encourage behavioural organisation and general comfort. These measures give parents an active role and include non-nutritive sucking, breastfeeding, swaddling, facilitated tucking, kangaroo care and touch by means of containment holding.

ACTIVITY 30.2: REFLECTIVE PRACTICE

A neonatal nurse has assumed the voice of a preterm baby in order to help parents understand the different needs of their preterm infant. The advice offered is not only relevant to parents but will provide you with insight into the preterm infant's developmental needs in light of the environmental stressors just discussed.

Confessions of a Preemie- How Am I Different From a Full Term Baby? (www.peekabooicu.com/crib-notes/confessions-of-a-preemie/)

Once read, formulate a framework of care to meet the developmental needs of the pre-term infant.

ENVIRONMENTAL CHALLENGES TO THE FAMILY

The following section will explore, by means of a case study, the environmental challenges that are experienced by parents and the family. A series of questions relating to the case study will be asked to enable you to gain an understanding of the family experience and journey and identify appropriate supportive strategies.

CASE STUDY 30.1: THE HUNTER FAMILY

Louise, Ian and Ted (aged 18 months) were on holiday in Lanzarote. On their last day there, Louise, 24+5 weeks pregnant, went into premature labour. The family were transferred to Las Palmas, where Louise delivered Hugh. He weighed 660 grams, required ventilation, suffered an intraventricular haemorrhage

(Continued)

and at 4 weeks required ligation of his patent ductus arteriosus. Hugh then developed necrotising enterocolitis (NEC), which was medically managed. His condition deteriorated and Hugh was baptised.

Hugh, 8 weeks old, was transferred to the UK for ongoing intensive care. Unfortunately, his local network NICU was closed to admissions, so Hugh transferred to a NICU outside the network for a few days, where Louise had her first cuddle with him.

Hugh's progress was slow. He made small steps forward and many large strides back. On arrival to his local NICU, complications from his original episode of NEC resulted in further bowel surgery. After 3 months Hugh was transferred to special care and appeared to be on the road to home. Due to further bowel complications and sepsis, Hugh moved back and forth between IC/HD and SC. On his third attempt he managed to stay in special care and make the required progress in feeding and growing to be considered for discharge. On day 246 Hugh was discharged home.

To celebrate Hugh's first birthday and as a thank you, Ian posted a video, which captures Hugh's and his family's journey. Explore the feelings and needs of Louise, Ian and Ted on Hugh's various admissions and transfers to receive the appropriate level of care, by answering the following questions:

- What feelings might Louise and Ian be experiencing as a result of Hugh's unexpected arrival and subsequent admission to the neonatal unit in Las Palmas?
- What feelings and issues may arise for Louise and Ian when Hugh is re-patriated to the UK, and then as he moves between nurseries as his condition improves and deteriorates?

An unanticipated early end to a normal pregnancy has resulted in Louise and Ian having to reappraise their expectations and adjust to a new reality. All babies born <26 weeks' gestation should be cared for in a NICU. Once the baby is in the recovery stage a lower level of care is required. This can be delivered by transferring the baby within the unit to a special care nursery or transferring the baby to another hospital to deliver that lower level of care. Both transfers result in leaving a familiar environment and can result in a range of different emotions.

Supportive care offered to the family is informed by research which provides an understanding of the parent's reality. The whole experience of having a premature or sick baby can have a long-term psychological impact to the parents due to the anxieties and emotional distress they have experienced throughout their child's journey (Shaw et al., 2013). There is now growing evidence of the emergence of post-traumatic stress disorder (PTSD) and high levels of depression among parents and this could persist for years (Shaw et al., 2013; Winter et al., 2018). A key role of the neonatal nurse is to help minimise the impact of baby–family separation and role loss, and to promote parental adaptation. This role also includes sign posting the parents and referral to psychological and mental health services, especially during difficult times (Dickinson et al., 2022).

ACTIVITY 30.3: REFLECTIVE PRACTICE

- Considering the case study of the Hunter family, what strategies can you employ to help the parent deal with their feelings?
- When and how would you promote parent–infant attachment?

"Family-centred care is at the heart of neonatal practice; every care is taken to involve the whole family in the care of their baby ... siblings are not ignored – they are encouraged to draw their new brother or sister pictures or bring in toys."

Sacha, 3rd-year children's nursing student

SEE ALSO
CHAPTER 1

ACTIVITY 30.4: REFLECTIVE PRACTICE

- What might be the impact of the neonatal environment on family-centred care?
- What strategies would you employ to involve the whole family in the care of their baby?

Health promotion commences on the admission of the baby and family to the unit and continues throughout to discharge. Handwashing, the first skill taught to the parents, is essential to infant well-being. Mothers require support to initiate and maintain breastfeeding. The feeding of expressed breast milk not only provides a milk best tolerated but the non-nutritional benefits play an important role in preventing conditions such as NEC. Health promotion materials should be widely available in a range of languages and should include guidance on newborn screening and the prevention of sudden infant death syndrome (SIDS).

ACTIVITY 30.5: REFLECTIVE PRACTICE

- How can you support Louise to initiate and maintain her lactation? You might find it helpful to watch the video *From Bump to Breastfeeding* via www.bestbeginnings.org.uk/from-bump-to-breastfeeding
- What routine newborn screening takes place in the UK?
- What are the implications for screening an infant admitted to a neonatal unit? Access the screening website for health professionals.
- What advice should be offered to Louise and Ian on how to prevent SIDS while Hugh is on the unit and in preparation for discharge? Access the Lullaby Trust website.

SAFEGUARDING STOP POINT

Safeguarding in a neonatal unit is less obvious than other areas where parents assume full responsibility and care for their children. All neonates are vulnerable and their needs must be considered and infant/family support provided throughout their journey to identify and mitigate problematic issues at the earliest opportunity. Clear-cut safeguarding situations include known maternal substance abuse and domestic violence.

- What early warning signs might alert you in parent behaviour/actions that there may be a safeguarding issue?

SEE ALSO
CHAPTER 28

Preparing parents for discharge commences on admission. Discharge planning is essential to ensure parents can make a seamless transition from hospital to community.

ACTIVITY 30.6: REFLECTIVE PRACTICE

- What feelings might Louise and Ian have while preparing for and at the discharge of Hugh from the neonatal unit?
- What parentcraft and support are required to help make a smooth transition home?

DECISION-MAKING AND ETHICS IN NEONATAL CARE

Decision-making at the beginning of life has become more nuanced with ongoing advances in technology, treatment and the shared expertise of skilled neonatal intensive practitioners/nurse specialists. There has been a significant increase in the survival rates of extremely premature babies born between 22 and 23 weeks over the last decade (Bell et al., 2022). These babies are on the very edge of viability, which brings the abortion limit set at 24 weeks in England into question. They also survive at a cost, whether that is through expensive innovative treatments, neurological deficits/other impairments or impact on the family as a whole. Ethical considerations surrounding the resuscitation and continued care of premature infants or infants with life-limiting conditions continues to be debated.

A neonatal nurse may need to act as an advocate and in the best interests of the baby and this may be at odds with the parents' wishes. Wilkinson and Savulescu (2017) argue that there should be a limit to the decision-making that parents have, especially with regard to experimental treatments that may or may not carry a significant risk of serious harm to the baby. In caring for neonates that raise ethical issues, it is vital that the neonatal nurse is able to put personal views aside. This is often easier said than done.

ACTIVITY 30.7: REFLECTIVE PRACTICE

- How would you ensure that parents are involved in decision-making?
- Who needs to be involved and how would the decision/prognosis be delivered?

—————— CHAPTER SUMMARY ——————

In this chapter we have looked at the care of a neonate. Key messages include:

- Neonatal care and service provision continues to evolve in order to optimise neonatal outcomes
- Neonatal nursing offers a challenging and rewarding career pathway. Quality care is ensured by ongoing professional development to achieve QIS status
- Delivery of appropriate and optimal care requires an understanding of the similarities and differences between infants born preterm, small for gestational age or with problems at term and knowledge of the interrelationships between the infant's body systems
- Neonatal care should be baby-centred, with parents the key caregivers working in partnership with and supported by the healthcare team

———— BUILD YOUR BIBLIOGRAPHY ————

Books

FURTHER
READING

- Petty, J. (2015) *Bedside Guide for Neonatal Care: Learning Tools to Support Practice*. London: Palgrave.

  A useful bedside resource providing the student/novice neonatal nurse with the tools needed to support practice.
- Bliss (2011) *The Bliss Baby Charter Standards*, 2nd edn. London: Bliss Publications.

  A practical guide to help neonatal units provide the best possible family-centred care for premature and sick babies.

Journal articles

FURTHER
READING:
ONLINE
JOURNAL
ARTICLES

- Rossman, B., Kratovil, A.L., Greene, M.M., Engstrom, J.L. and Meier, P.P. (2013) '"I have faith in my milk": the meaning of milk for mothers of very low birth weight infants hospitalized in the neonatal intensive care unit'. *Journal of Human Lactation*, 29 (3): 359-65.

  Mothers of preterm infants are actively encouraged to express breast milk predominantly for its therapeutic or non-nutritional benefits; this article explores the mother's perspective of the importance of her milk to her infant's well-being.
- Strandås, M. and Fredrikson, S-T.D. (2015) 'Ethical challenges in neonatal nursing'. *Nursing Ethics*, 22 (8): 901-12.

  Advancements in neonatal technology and pharmacology combined with our understanding of neonatal pathophysiology have led to the survival of neonates at the edges of viability. Neonatal care provides many ethical dilemmas. This research article is useful as it provides insight into the ethical challenges that can face neonatal nurses in their daily work, rather than the obvious life and death decisions associated with neonatal care.
- Stuart, M. and Melling, S. (2014) 'Understanding nurses' and parents' perceptions of family-centred care'. *Nursing Children and Young People*, 26 (7): 16-20.

  Family-centred care is an essential component of neonatal care. Therefore, in order to work effectively together and facilitate optimal parental partnership, it is essential that you explore parental and nursing perceptions of the concept.
- Trajkovski, S., Schmied, V., Vickers, M. and Jackson, D. (2015) 'Using appreciative inquiry to bring neonatal nurses and parents together to enhance family-centred care: a collaborative workshop'. *Journal of Child Health*, 9: 239-53.

  This article is useful as it considers strategies that can be used to enhance the delivery of family-centred care in the neonatal unit.

Weblinks

FURTHER
READING:
WEBLINKS

- NHS and Department of Health, Toolkit for High-quality Neonatal Services http://webarchive.nationalarchives.gov.uk/20130107105ents/digitalasset/dh_108435.pdf The Toolkit, originally developed for England, now identifies the structure and principles needed to deliver neonatal care across the four countries of the UK.
- Royal College of Nursing, *Career, Education and Competence Framework for Neonatal Nursing in the UK* www.rcn.org.uk/-/media/royal-college-of-nursing/documents/publications/2015/january/pub-004641.pdf A useful document to enable you to explore the possible career opportunities in neonatal nursing.

- Best Beginnings, *From Bump to Breastfeeding* www.bestbeginnings.org.uk/from-bump-to-breastfeeding A set of films following the journey of mothers wishing to breastfeed their babies, providing detailed information on how to breastfeed successfully.
- Best Beginnings, *Small Wonders* www.bestbeginnings.org.uk/small-wonders A set of 12 short films following 14 families through their neonatal unit journey.

REFERENCES

Anand, K. (2015) 'Pain assessment in preterm neonates'. *Pediatrics*, 119 (3): 605–7.

Bedford Russell, A. (2015) 'Neonatal sepsis'. *Paediatrics and Child Health*, 25 (6): 271–5.

British Association of Perinatal Medicine (BAPM) (2011) *Categories of Care*, 3rd edn. London: BAPM.

Bell, E., Hintz, S., Hansen, N. et al. (2022) 'Mortality in-hospital morbidity, care practices, and 2-year outcomes for extremely preterm infants in the US (2013–2018)'. *JAMA*, 27(3): 248–63.

Campbell-Yeo, M., Eriksson, M. and Benoit, B. (2022) 'Assessment and management of pain in preterm infants: a practice update'. *Children*, 9 (2): 244.

Dickinson, C., Vangaveti, V. and Browne, A. (2022) 'Psychological impact of neonatal intensive care unit admissions on parents: a regional perspective'. *Australian Journal of Rural Health*, 30 (3): 373–84.

Haumont, D. (2012) 'Environment and early development care', in G. Buonnocore, R. Bracci and M. Weindling (eds), *Neonatology: A Practical Approach to Neonatal Disease*. Milan: Spinger-Verlag.

Kariholu, U., Banerjee, J., Selkirk, L., Warren, I., Chow, P. and Godambe, S. (2014) 'Managing neonatal pain while rationalizing the use of morphine using a structured systematic approach'. *Infant*, 10 (1): 30–4.

Kuhl, P.K. and Meltzoff, A.N. (1984) 'The intermodal representation of speech in infants'. *Infant Behavior and Development*, 7 (3): 361–81.

Mitchell, A. and Boss, B. (2002) 'Adverse effects of pain on the nervous systems of newborns and young children: a review of the literature'. *Journal of Neuroscience Nursing*, 34 (5): 228–36.

NICE (National Institute of Health and Care Excellence) (2016) Jaundice in newborn babies under 28 days. Clinical guideline [CG98]. Available at: www.nice.org.uk/guidance/cg98 (accessed 29 May 2017).

Robert, J. (2010) *Circadian Rhythm and Human Health*. Available at: www.photobiology.info/Roberts-CR.html (accessed 29 May 2017).

Robinson, J. and Fielder, A.R. (1992) 'Light and the neonatal eye'. *Behavioural Brain Research*, 49 (1): 51–5.

Royal College of Paediatrics and Child Health (RCPCH) (2022) About the National Neonatal Audit Programme (NNAP). Available at: www.rcpch.ac.uk/work-we-do-/quality-imorovement-patient-safety/neonatal-audit-programme-nnap/about#about.

Shaw, R.J., Bernard, R.S., Storfer-Isser, A., Rhine, W. and Horwitz, S.M. (2013) 'Parental coping in the neonatal intensive care unit'. *Journal of Clinical Psychology in Medical Settings*, 20: 135–42.

Venkataram, R., Kamaluddeen, M., Amin, H. and Lodha, A. (2018) 'Is less noise, light and parental/caregiver stress in the neonatal intensive care unit better for neonates?'. *Indian Pediatrics*, 55 (1): 17–21.

Wachman, E.M. and Lahav, A. (2011) 'The effects of noise on preterm infants in the NICU'. *Archives of Disease in Childhood Foetal and Neonatal Edition*, 96 (4): F305–F309.

Wilkinson D., and Savulescu J. (2017) 'Hard lessons: learning from Charlie Gard case'. *Journal of Medical Ethics*. Available at: https://jme.bmj.com/content/44/7/438.

Winter, L., Coldiz, P.B., Sanders, M.R., Boyd, R.N., Pritchard, M., Gray, P.H., Whittingham, K., Forrest, K., Leeks, R., Webb, L., Marquart, L., Taylor, K. and Macey, J. (2018) 'Depression, posttraumatic stress and relationship distress in parents of very preterm infants'. *Archives of Women's Mental Health*, 21 (4): 445–51.

CARE OF CHILDREN AND YOUNG PEOPLE WITH A MALIGNANT CONDITION

31

JAYNE PRICE AND SUZANNE COULSON

--- **THIS CHAPTER COVERS** ---

- Childhood cancer types
- Presentation of childhood cancer
- Psychosocial impact of childhood cancer
- Treatment of childhood cancer
- Team working in childhood cancer care

> "We had to be strong at the time it was happening and just get on with it. The kindness of the hospital staff was really important to help us get through it. Until you've gone through something like this yourself it's really hard to understand how horrific your child being diagnosed with cancer really is."
>
> **Aimee, parent**

Please note this chapter focuses on cancer in children and young people (YP). Childhood cancer is a collective term to include both child and young person. Anything specific to YP will be highlighted as such.

INTRODUCTION

Cancer is a group of diseases in which cells grow uncontrollably and can spread from the originating site to another part of the body. Approximately 1900 children in the United Kingdom (UK) are diagnosed with a childhood cancer each year (Children with Cancer UK, 2021).

Whilst great improvement in survival of children/YP with cancer have been noted in recent years and cure rates are much higher than for most adult cancers, receiving such a diagnosis plunges children and families into a state of disarray and disruption, given that the term cancer is often synonymous with death. More than 8 out of 10 children (all childhood cancers combined) in England survive for 5 years or over, more than doubled from the 1960s (Children's Cancer Leukaemia Group, 2022). Improvements in outcomes for children/YP with cancer have been attributed to clinical trials and collaborative working regarding treatment protocols. Improvements in supportive care are also evident, enhanced through some key publications. Over the past decades enhancements in care and service development have been implemented; NICE (2005) produced guidance on the healthcare children with cancer should receive followed by Quality Standards (NICE, 2014). Further, Children's Cancer Measures (2013) provide a benchmark for services throughout the UKs, further updated in 2021 with Service Specifications for the provision of cancer services for children aged 0–15 years in England (NHS England, 2021). Cancer is classed as a 'life threatening' condition in that curative treatment is feasible but not guaranteed. While treatment is given from a Children's Cancer and Leukaemia Group (CCLG) treatment centre, supportive care is sometimes provided in shared care centres (hospitals closer to the child's home).

The parent voice cited at the beginning of this chapter indicates that despite increased survival rates the impact of childhood cancer is wide-ranging, meaning children and families require intense care throughout treatment as well as ongoing support for years afterwards. This chapter will unravel the needs of children and families whilst highlighting the nurse's role during diagnosis, treatment and beyond.

CHILDHOOD CANCER

Cancers in children and YP often result from DNA changes in cells, that take place very early in life, unlike adult cancers, which often have links to environmental or lifestyle factors. While causes of childhood cancer are generally unknown, certain genetic and familial traits are thought to influence the development of some cancers.

Childhood cancer generally falls into these groupings:

- Haematological malignancies – arising in blood-forming tissue (leukaemia and lymphoma)
- Solid tumours – arising from tissue or organ (sarcoma, blastoma, germ cell)

Haematological malignancies can spread out with the blood and lymph system into the cerebrospinal fluid (CSF) or occasionally cause skin lesions. Solid tumours may be confined to the primary site or may have local or distant metastatic spread. While metastatic disease can be cured, it is more challenging, and longer, more intense treatment is required.

Common childhood cancers

Leukaemia is the commonest form of childhood cancer, with approximately 400 new cases diagnosed each year within the UK. Leukaemia is the uncontrolled proliferation of immature blood cells (blasts) following an abnormality occurring during development in either the lymphoid or myeloid blood cell line. Acute lymphoblastic leukaemia (ALL) accounts for 80–85% of diagnoses, and while it occurs at any age it is most common in children under 5 years (National Cancer and Analysis Service, 2021). Most of the remaining 15–20% of children present with acute myeloid leukaemia (AML). Chronic leukaemia is very rare in childhood. Of children diagnosed with acute lymphoblastic leukaemia, 88% will live beyond 5 years of their diagnosis (Children with Cancer UK, 2021).

Brain tumours are the second most common childhood cancer and commonest solid tumour. They are usually named after the type of cells and area of the central nervous system (CNS) in which they develop. Most CNS tumours start in glial cells, the supporting cells of the brain. These tumours are known as gliomas and include astrocytomas, ependymomas and oligodendrogliomas. Another group arise from embryonal cells and include medulloblastomas and PNETs (primitive neuro-ectodermal tumours).

Other childhood cancers

A number of malignancies are seen almost exclusively in young children, others more often in the older child or young person and some in both children and young people – though treatment and prognosis can be quite different (Table 31.1).

Table 31.1 Other types of childhood cancer

Type of cancer and age group	Common types	Organ or tissue of origin
Sarcomas – arising in bone and soft tissue All ages but especially older children/ teenagers	Osteosarcoma	Bone, often the long bones
	Ewing's sarcoma and peripheral primitive neuroectodermal tumour (PPNET)	Bone or soft tissue
	Rhabdomyosarcoma	Primitive muscle cells, occurring in soft tissue almost anywhere in the body
Embryonal tumours (blastomas) – arising in immature embryonal tissue Mainly pre-school children	Neuroblastoma	Sympathetic nervous system pathway, often developing in the adrenal glands
	Retinoblastoma	Retina, small number of cases are bilateral
	Nephroblastoma (Wilm's tumour)	Kidney, small number of cases are bilateral
	Hepatoblastoma	Liver
Germ cell tumours	Germ cell tumours (GCT)	Immature tissue destined to become the ovaries or testes; include yolk-sac tumours, germinomas, embryonal carcinomas, teratomas and immature teratomas
Lymphoma	Non-Hodgkin's lymphoma	B or T lymphocytes – lymphoblastic, Burkitts and anaplastic large cell lymphoma
	Hodgkin's disease	Lymphatic system, distinguished by presence of Reed Steinberg cells
Rare tumours Occasionally in children – more common in adults	Carcinoma	Lining tissue (epithelial tissue) – possible sites include adrenal gland, nasopharynx, thyroid gland
	Melanoma	Arising in melanocytes, usually skin

PRESENTATION

Children and YP can present with a wide variety of symptoms depending on the condition and position of the tumour, its size and the impact on tissues and organs close by. Reaching a diagnosis can be protracted. Symptoms can seem vague and in isolation may appear like regular childhood illnesses (see Figure 31.1).

Diagnostic aids to support professionals less familiar with childhood cancer have been developed and include:

- Headsmart – www.headsmart.org.uk

and

The Grace Kelly Childhood Cancer Trust, Regional Red Flags for Clinicians – www.gkcct.org/regional-red-flags-clinicians

Diagnostic tests aim to:

- Achieve an accurate diagnosis and establish the extent of disease
- Assess the child/YP's general health status

Investigations are guided by the type of cancer suspected. For commonly used tests, see Table 31.2.

Identifying risk factors is an important area enabling treatment protocols to be tailored more specifically, for example, for CYP with genetic factors present that can influence overall prognosis (Bailey and Skinner, 2010).

Continued, Unexplained weight loss

Headaches, often with early morning vomiting

Increased swelling or persistent pain in bones, joints, back, or legs

Lump or mass, especially in the abdomen, neck, chest, pelvis, or armpits

Development of excessive bruising, bleeding, or rash

Constant infections

A whitish colour behind the pupil

Nausea which persists or vomiting without nausea

Constant tiredness or noticeable paleness

Eye or vision changes which occur suddenly and persist

Recurrent or persistent fevers of unknown origin

Figure 31.1 Symptoms of childhood cancer (not exhaustive and relate to type of cancer)

Source: Ped-Onc Resource Center (2015) Signs of Childhood Cancer. Reproduced with permission.

Table 31.2 Diagnostic investigations (not exhaustive)

Investigation	Definition	Reason for investigation
Blood test (Full blood count [FBC]) and biochemistry	Peripheral blood sample	Presence of leukaemic (blast) cells
		Normal blood cell levels
		Biochemistry picture for renal and liver function
Bone marrow aspirate and trephine	Sample of bone marrow cells (aspirate) and segment of bone marrow (trephine) from hipbone. Performed under general anaesthetic	Presence, extent and type of leukaemia
		Presence of metastatic disease – solid tumours
		Also performed during treatment to monitor response
Lumbar puncture (LP)	Aspiration of cerebrospinal fluid (CSF) Performed under general anaesthetic	Establish if cancer cells have infiltrated the CSF in leukaemia or lymphoma
		Cytotoxic chemotherapy drugs can be given intrathecally during the LP
Ultrasound scan (U/S)	A non-invasive scan utilising high frequency sound waves to capture images inside the body, showing structure and movement of internal organs	Presence of a solid tumour or metastases
		Presence of testicular involvement in leukaemia
Chest X-ray	Ionising radiation used to take images of chest area	Presence of mediastinal mass, infiltrated lymph nodes (leukaemia or lymphoma) or tumour – primary or metastatic
CT (computerised tomography) scan	A CT scan using X-rays takes a series of images, providing a three-dimensional picture of organs inside the body. Provides more detail of internal organs, bones, soft tissues and blood vessels than ordinary X-rays	Presence, position and extent of primary tumour and existence of metastatic disease
MRI (magnetic resonance imaging) scan	Similar to CT but instead of X-rays MRI uses magnetism to build up a detailed picture of areas of the body. MRI is non-invasive but the machine noise can be frightening. A sedative or general anaesthetic may be used if the child is unable to lie still	Presence, position and extent of primary tumour, and existence of metastatic disease
Biopsy	Needle biopsy – a needle inserted through the skin into the tumour to remove a small part for examination. May be performed under local anaesthetic. Open biopsy – under general anaesthetic an incision is made and a piece of tumour removed for examination	To identify the tumour type
Bone scan	A small amount of radioactive substance is injected into a vein and subsequently absorbed by the bones. Diseased bone is highlighted as it absorbs more than healthy bone	If a bone tumour is suspected or if a primary tumour may have spread to bones

"When we first found out Jack had bone cancer I felt very guilty, thinking it was something I missed or did wrong."

Astrid, parent

CASE STUDY 31.1: BELLE (1)

Belle is 5 years old. Her mum had taken her to the GP repeatedly over the past 6 months. Initially Belle had a lingering ear infection, even after antibiotics. Mum then reported Belle being 'off form', with a poor appetite. She subsequently required further antibiotics for a sore throat. Mum felt the GP saw her as a paranoid mother. A few weeks later Belle experienced a nosebleed which settled spontaneously. Dad then noticed bruises on Belle's leg, but she explained she fell at school. Then Belle fell off her bike, complained of a painful wrist and her nose bled heavily again. Mum took Belle to the emergency department but felt under suspicion when the doctor, then the nurse, asked about the bruising. During a detailed history it was noted she was pale. Belle had her wrist X-rayed. An FBC was taken; her haemoglobin was low (anaemia), platelets were low (thrombocytopenia) and white cells raised. Following admission to the children's ward, acute lymphoblastic leukaemia (ALL) was diagnosed. Mum and Dad were in shock but felt angry that the diagnosis was delayed and that they were not listened to.

- Using knowledge of the physiology of blood, explain each of Belle's symptoms.
- As well as FBC, what other investigations would be carried out?
- What might parental feelings be following the diagnosis?

ACTIVITY 31.1: REFLECTIVE PRACTICE

Remember, parents know their children. Professionals should hear and listen to their concerns. Think about how this could be applied to your practice.

SAFEGUARDING STOP POINT

Remember, children with low platelet counts in blood conditions such as leukaemia may present with bruising.

PSYCHOSOCIAL IMPACT OF CHILDHOOD CANCER

Communicating the news of the diagnosis is the point where the relationship with the team caring for the child commences and often continues over years.

SEE ALSO
CHAPTER 2

Belle's case and the parent voice (Aimee) below demonstrates how diagnosis of childhood cancer leads to profound emotional distress for families (Carlsson et al., 2019). Practical chaos/disruption also occurs – for example, the immediate need to take time off school/work and reorganise routines around treatment. Such disruption instigates a change in the life of the child and also family functioning, including reallocation or reorienting of roles (Jibb et al., 2018).

> "Family life was turned upside down. We were faced with the prospect of death of our precious child. There was nothing we could do. It was out of our control."
>
> **Aimee, parent**

WHAT'S THE EVIDENCE?

Read: Roser, K., Erdmann, F., Michel, G., Falck Winther, J. and Mader, L. (2019) 'The impact of childhood cancer on parents' socio-economic situation – a systematic review'. *Psycho-Oncology*, 28 (6): 1207-26.

List the impact on the family of childhood cancer diagnosis and treatment and consider how this evidence could be applied in your practice.

Reorganisation often involves the 'split family' (McCubbin et al., 2002) with, for example, one parent assuming responsibility for siblings while the other focuses on the sick child. This can be even more challenging for single parents or parents who may not have additional family to offer support.

> "Having other children at home and having to leave them sometimes for 2–3 weeks at the start of Jack's treatment was really hard."
>
> **Astrid, parent**

Parenting the sick child becomes the parents' 'master status', influencing every aspect of life and somewhat overshadowing other roles. 'Master status' is described in sociological literature by Hughes (1945). The parent voice below demonstrates this effect.

> "Everything we did and everywhere we went revolved around Greg's leukaemia and the restrictions and effects it had on him."
>
> **Aimee, parent**

ACTIVITY 31.2: CRITICAL THINKING

What social roles may become secondary for parents when caring for their child with cancer becomes their master status?

Treatment and hospital become part of family life as families strive to create some sort of normality in an abnormal situation (Jibb et al., 2018), alongside trying to 'battle' cancer (Price et al., 2012). Parents can feel isolated from their usual support networks (Jordan et al., 2015) and suffer exhaustion from juggling often competing demands of living through the uncertainty of their child's diagnosis and treatment (Molinaro and Fletcher, 2018).

WHAT'S THE EVIDENCE?

Thoitis (1986) argued that social support helped families 'keep going' through cancer treatment, providing them with the practical resources, as well as the emotional sustenance, to keep strong amidst sustained uncertainty. Types of social support have been identified (for example, Kaplan et al., 1977; Gottlieb, 1978; House, 1981). Commonalities indicate three types are discernible:

- Informational – provision of advice, suggestions and information that a person can use to address problems
- Instrumental – involving the provision of tangible assistance and services that directly assist the person in need
- Emotional – involving the provision of empathy, love, trust and caring

ACTIVITY 31.3: CRITICAL THINKING

Chart the type of support needed to address each issue below:

- Mother becomes emotionally distressed during her child's first chemotherapy
- A sibling asking questions about cancer; the parent is uncertain how to respond
- Parents do not feel ready to learn how to flush their child's central line
- A young person feels isolated during treatment
- Parents express concern about the financial implications of losing a salary due to their child's cancer treatment

Now consider how the charity Young Lives vs Cancer can support families when a child or YP is being treated for cancer www.younglivesvscancer.org.uk/life-with-cancer/support-whenever-you-need-it/your-young-lives-vs-cancer-intro/

Remember that parents require support at different stages of their child's cancer journey, including on the completion of therapy and during the following months and years (Hill and Gubi, 2020).

> "The end of treatment period can be fraught with emotions for parents: relief that treatment is over, gratitude to the team, anxiety that support is waning and fear that disease may return."
>
> **Kirsty, ward manager**

TREATMENT OF CHILDHOOD CANCER

Treatment takes the form of one or more of the following: chemotherapy, radiotherapy and surgery. For some children, high-dose chemotherapy followed by a haematopoietic stem cell transplant may be required. Immunotherapy is developing for certain conditions, for example neuroblastoma. Tests are required pre treatment to ascertain organ function for toxicity monitoring. These will be repeated at regular intervals during/after treatment in order to establish any toxicity development, which may in turn require the adaptation of drugs or dosages or additional supportive care. The child/YP will have a central line inserted (under general anaesthetic), enabling administration of drug therapy and supportive care. The disease and response to treatment is monitored at regular intervals.

Chemotherapy

Malignant conditions require cytotoxic chemotherapy, drugs which are toxic to cells and work by interfering with normal reproductive processes and cell division. Cytotoxic chemotherapy can be administered via oral and intravenous routes (bolus, short or continuous infusion) and occasionally intrathecally (given into the CSF). Children/YP may require hospital admission for treatment or attend a day unit/outpatient department. Occasionally, chemotherapy is delivered at home; for example, children with ALL have ongoing oral medication.

The cell cycle is the process that cells undergo in order to reproduce; including active stages where cells are dividing, and a resting phase. To discover more about the cell cycle and cell division, please see the video link at: www.youtube.com/watch?v=Q6ucKWIIFmg.

Cytotoxic drugs have different mechanisms, being active in different parts of the cell cycle. Consequently, several cytotoxic drugs are usually combined in treatment protocols to complement each other's action. Standardised protocols have been developed, meaning that a child/YP with a specific cancer would receive the same treatment regardless of their UK location.

As childhood cancer is rare, gaining insight into successful therapies is vital; thus, research conducted through clinical trials is incorporated into many treatment protocols.

ACTIVITY 31.4: TEAM WORKING

Go to www.cclg.org.uk. What is CCLG's role in working collaboratively in treating children/YP with cancer?

WHAT'S THE EVIDENCE?

Woodgate and Yanofsky (2010) uniquely examined parent perspectives (*n* = 31) through qualitative interviews about decision-making and clinical trials when their child was diagnosed with cancer. Analysis highlighted participation in decisions about clinical trials as a difficult experience, identifying six themes:

1. living a surreal event
2. wanting the best for my child
3. helping future families of children with cancer
4. coming to terms with my decision
5. making one decision among many
6. experiencing a sense of trust

In practice, how might parents' needs be addressed given the Woodgate and Yanofsky (2010) study findings?

Side effects of chemotherapy

Side effects experienced can vary, and as several drugs are usually used, the number of potential complications is increased.

Cytotoxic drugs cannot differentiate between healthy and malignant cells, so normal fast reproducing cells within the body are also affected, resulting in some commonly seen and complex side effects (Figure 31.2).

Side effects may be short term, lasting a number of days or weeks, or long term, continuing for a significant period of time, including after the completion of cancer treatment. While many are reversible, some may be lifelong (Table 31.3). Remember that with all symptoms the child/YP/parents need information and reassurance.

> "Dealing with some of the side effects of chemotherapy can be quite hard, but having the nurses and other people makes it a little easier to handle."
>
> **Astrid, parent**

Children/YP experiencing side effects may require significant levels of supportive care with further hospitalisation. Close monitoring and assessment are required to anticipate and identify problems and subsequently provide appropriate management. The production of healthy blood cells is also disrupted temporarily following many chemotherapy agents, leaving the child/YP at risk of related side effects – anaemia, thrombocytopenia and neutropenia. While transfusions of red cells and platelets can be given to help manage the first two complications, neutropenia cannot be addressed as easily and the child/YP will require antibiotics should infection be suspected or confirmed. As long-term immunity can be affected they are at risk of opportunistic infections that can cause significant morbidity and occasional mortality.

Infection (confirmed or suspected) in the immunocompromised child/YP should be treated as a medical emergency.

Long-term follow-up clinics continue for varying periods of time depending upon the presence or risk of complications.

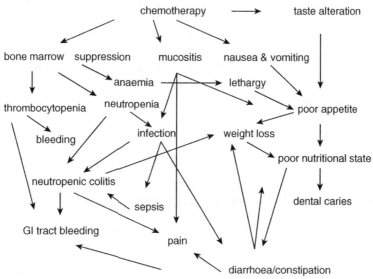

Figure 31.2 Complex effects of treatment

Table 31.3 Side effects of chemotherapy

Period	Potential symptoms	Supportive care
Immediate	Nausea/vomiting	Antiemetics pre-chemotherapy
	Allergic/sensitivity reactions	Pre-meds for agents known to increase risk of reaction; close monitoring
Short term	Alopecia	Provision of wig if desired
	Myelosuppression	Blood product support; treatment of suspected/identified infection
	Immunosuppression	Avoidance of infection risk factors and managing individual symptoms; use of prophylactic antibiotics and antivirals in certain protocols
	Nausea/vomiting	Antiemetics during and post-chemotherapy with adaptation if required; close monitoring
	Mucositis (painful inflammation and ulceration of the gastrointestinal tract)	Oral hygiene, analgesia, nutritional support
	Diarrhoea/constipation	Fluid and nutritional support, laxatives
	Organ toxicity	Close monitoring; adaptation of drug doses; additional intravenous fluids; oral/IV supplementation for altered blood chemistry (e.g., potassium)
	Haemorrhagic cystitis (blood in urine – certain cytotoxic agents)	Additional intravenous fluids and mesna to reduce irritation from cytotoxic drugs
	Fatigue	Change daily routine, enabling sleep and rest

(Continued)

Table 31.3 (Continued)

Period	Potential symptoms	Supportive care
Long term	Myelosuppression and immunosuppresssion	Avoidance of infection risk factors and manage individual symptoms
	Infertility	Involvement of reproductive specialists, sperm banking may be available for boys (post-puberty)
	Organ toxicity/failure	Close monitoring, involvement of specialist teams; organ transplant in rare cases
	Growth and development complications	Close monitoring via endocrine specialists
	Secondary cancers	Treat malignancy as appropriate
	Cardiomyopathy	Monitoring closely via cardiac specialists; transplant in rare cases

SAFETY WORKING WITH CHEMOTHERAPY

Given the hazardous side effects, precautions are required to protect handlers of cytotoxic chemotherapy, including staff and parents handling waste (i.e., urine, vomit). The Nursing and Midwifery Council Code of Professional Conduct (NMC, 2018) centres round four key areas, one being that we must 'preserve safety'.

"Preserving the safety of the child or young person, family and staff in the cytotoxic environment is crucial and requires a safe approach.

Spillage prevention

Administration guidelines

Follow protocol on correct disposal of waste including bodily fluids

Extravasation recognition"

Ward sister

ACTIVITY 31.5: CRITICAL THINKING

Click on the link to the Health and Safety Executive website to read about the safe use of cytotoxic drugs.

Safe handling of cytotoxic drugs in the workplace - Health and Social Care (hse.gov.uk)

How would you, as a children's nurse, ensure safety was maintained in relation to handling of cytotoxic drugs and waste?

Surgery

Surgery is often used in the treatment of solid tumours, the timing of which is dependent on the position and size of the tumour and its response to any earlier chemotherapy. If the tumour is too large or intricately involved with other organs or major blood vessels, chemotherapy is given first to shrink the tumour to make surgery less risky. In other situations, for example brain tumours, the tumour is often removed first and chemotherapy and/or radiotherapy given afterwards.

SEE ALSO
CHAPTER 16

Radiotherapy

Radiotherapy is the therapeutic application of radiation from high energy X-rays targeted at a tumour site in order to damage DNA, causing cells to die or be unable to divide (Bailey and Skinner, 2010). This localised treatment is used with some solid tumours, especially brain tumours, and is administered daily over several weeks, usually as an outpatient. Tissue and organ damage can occur as radiation passes through to reach the target. Consequently, radiotherapy of the developing brain – under 3 years of age – is generally avoided.

Proton beam therapy uses protons instead of X-rays, the risk of long-term side effects may be reduced but it is only suitable for certain groups of patients.

HAEMATOPOIETIC STEM CELL TRANSPLANT

For some children/YP the best hope of long-term survival is to receive very high-dose chemotherapy to eradicate any remaining disease. As this obliterates their bone marrow they then require haematopoietic stem cells – in the form of their own pre-harvested stem cells, a donor's bone marrow, or umbilical cord stem cells – to enable them to recover their own bone marrow function.

Side effects post stem-cell transplant are magnified due to the complete destruction of the child/YP's bone marrow. During this time the child/YP will be in protective isolation and require intense supportive care.

Immunotherapy

Immunotherapy involves using agents to enable the body's immune system and natural killer cells to recognise and attack cancer cells. Biological response modifiers are drugs, for example monoclonal antibodies, that work with the immune system to bring about malignant cell death in a number of ways: by attacking cancer cells, blocking signals that tell malignant cells to divide, blocking molecules that prevent the immune system from working correctly and by carrying cytotoxic drugs or radiation to cancer cells. The role and use of immunotherapy drugs in treatment protocols is increasing.

CASE STUDY 31.1: BELLE (2)

Belle has undergone her first block of chemotherapy and is being discharged home. Her parents are anxious about her medications and central line, being fearful about her risk of infection.

*   What is the role of the nurse in discharge preparation?
*   What are their likely needs for instrumental, informational and emotional support?
*   Which members of the team may be involved in Belle's care?

SEE ALSO
CHAPTER 28

SEE ALSO
CHAPTER 5

Care of children/YP with cancer is increasingly being carried out in the home. Parents usually take the lead in caring and often report feeling anxious and overwhelmed, and so require information, teaching and support, particularly following the first discharge (Flury et al., 2011). Some parents may be from medical backgrounds but they are parents first and foremost.

"The ward and clinic staff were very supportive knowing we were both 'medical' and understanding the added worries we had with extra medical knowledge but still treating us like the scared parents we ultimately were."

Aimee, parent

TEAM WORKING

Given the nature and duration of childhood cancer, care teams can be large, exist across care settings and members of the team can change over time. Such issues can cause problems to streamlined and quality care (NHS England, 2021).

Many professionals and organisations provide care for children/YP with cancer and their families, with each bringing their own individual expertise to ensure the physical needs of the child/YP are met alongside the emotional, social and spiritual needs of the child/YP and family. Charitable organisations have an important role to play, for example Young Lives vs Cancer and Make A Wish.

"His schoolteachers were fantastic, ensuring he could still go to school by making sure he had a one-to-one support worker to help him cope when on steroids, which made him very emotional and unpredictable."

Aimee, parent

Play and education are central as the child is continuing to grow and develop during treatment and associated care. Young people too are continuing to develop and have specific needs/requirements; the support of peers can be important with this group.

When everyone is using their abilities towards a common goal, i.e. the best care for each child/YP and family, the results are greater than those achieved by a single person.

These are viewed as pivotal for team working within childhood cancer care:

Trust and respect for child/YP and family also within team

Empathy and human approach

A focus on high standard individualised care

Meetings of team regularly

Well coordinated care straddling hospital/community

Organisations from statutory and voluntary sector working together

Recognition that consistency/continuity are important

Key worker to coordinate care

Information available re team roles and contacts

Negotiation with parents as experts

Good communication (within and across teams)

The role of the children's nurse

The children's nurse is the professional who spends the most amount of time with the child/YP and family, so they have a multifaceted role. The children's nurse is supporter/facilitator, leader/manager, and advocate for the child, YP and family, teacher/educator and team player, in addition to being the provider of physical care to the child/YP.

"It's much better if the nurses are a little crazy and are willing to play with me."

Salisu, child

Within the nurse's role as educator/teacher the nurse must educate the child/YP and/or family about many aspects, ensuring optimum health is promoted for the child/YP and the family. Health education/promotion opportunities are wide ranging and remembering these elementary ABCDEs of health promotion is helpful:

Avoid busy, crowded public areas

Be careful to handle body fluids safely whilst the child/YP is undergoing chemotherapy

Care of central line and infection control management/recognition

Discussion about vaccination status – no live vaccines when on treatment

Education regarding neutropenia, e.g. steps when child/YP's temperature rises

Sun safety – some chemotherapy drugs make children particularly sensitive to the sun

SEE CHAPTER 33

Despite improved survival rates, childhood cancer can lead to the death of some children/YP.

Nursing students often express some anxiety about going to specialised cancer units or areas where children/YP with cancer are cared for. Lack of certainty can exist about the type of care they can be involved in and the learning opportunities available.

CHAPTER SUMMARY

This chapter has highlighted the main principles of caring for a child/YP with cancer and their family:

- Care provision must be individualised and all-encompassing, addressing bio, psycho, social and spiritual elements of CYP and family
- Quality care for CYP with cancer and their families must be underpinned by the best available evidence
- Interdisciplinary approach involving statutory and voluntary services across care settings is essential
- Cure rates have increased over recent years but cure with least cost to the CYP is an essential consideration
- Long-term follow-up is an important part of childhood cancer care and continues for many years following completion of treatment

---

BUILD YOUR BIBLIOGRAPHY

Books

FURTHER
READING

- Caron, H.N., Biondi, A., Boterberg, T. and Doz, F. (eds), (2020) *Oxford Textbook of Cancer in Children* (Oxford Textbooks in Oncology, 7th edn). Oxford: Oxford University Press.

  A comprehensive textbook offering update clinical guidance on care of children with cancer and their families. A good reference book.

- Eiser, C. (2015) *Children with Cancer: The Quality of Life*. Abingdon: Routledge.

  Text examining how to ensure good quality of life for children with cancer and their families.

- Gibson, F. and Soanes, L. (eds) (2008) *Cancer in Children and Young People*. Chichester: John Wiley & Sons.

  A comprehensive book examining the principles of treatment and care of childhood cancer.

Journal articles

FURTHER
READING:
ONLINE
JOURNAL
ARTICLES

- Crane, S., Haase, J.E. and Hickman, S.E. (2019) 'Parental experiences of child participation in a phase i pediatric oncology clinical trial: "We don't have time to waste"'. *Qualitative Health Research*, 29 (5): 632–44.

  This study examines parents' decision-making, feelings, thoughts and experiences in participating in phase 1 clinical trials.

- Enskär, K., Darcy, L., Björk, M., Knutsson, S. and Huus, K. (2020) 'Experiences of young children with cancer and their parents with nurses' caring practices during the cancer trajectory'. *Journal of Pediatric Oncology Nursing*, 37 (1): 21–34.

This study examines and makes recommendations for the nurse caring for the child with cancer across the illness trajectory in partnership with the family.

- Mant, J., Kirby, A., Cox, K.J. and Burke, A. (2019) 'Children's experiences of being diagnosed with cancer at the early stages of treatment; an interpretive phenomenological analysis'. *Clinical Child Psychology and Psychiatry,* 24 (1): 3-18.

  This study examines the thoughts, feelings and perspectives of children when diagnosed and commencing treatment for childhood cancer, offering recommendations into addressing the needs of children.

- Van Schoors, M., De Mol, J., Laeremans, N., Verhofstadt, L.L., Goubert, L. and Van Parys, H. (2019) 'Siblings' experiences of everyday life in a family where one child is diagnosed with blood cancer: a qualitative study.' *Journal of Pediatric Oncology Nursing,* 36 (2): 131-42.

  The study presented here examines the experiences of siblings when their brother or sister was being treated for childhood cancer. The findings guide parents and health/social care professionals in addressing the needs of siblings.

Weblinks

FURTHER READING: WEBLINKS

- Cancer Research UK, Monoclonal Antibodies (MAB) www.cancerresearchuk.org/about-cancer/cancer-in-general/treatment/biological-therapy/types/monoclonal-antibodies This website hosts four videos about immunotherapy drugs and monoclonal antibodies.
- Macmillan Cancer Support, Bone Marrow or Stem Cell Transplants for Children's Cancers www.macmillan.org.uk/cancerinformation/cancertypes/childrenscancers/treatingchildrenscancers/bonemarrowstemcelltransplant.aspx Read more about bone marrow transplantation.
- Macmillan Cancer Support, Radiotherapy for Children with Head and Neck Cancers www.macmillan.org.uk/cancerinformation/cancertypes/childrenscancers/treatingchildrenscancers/radiootherapyheadandneckcancers.aspx Read more about radiotherapy in children and young people.
- Children with Cancer UK, Patient Stories www.childrenwithcancer.org.uk/stories/patient-story-lucy Meet Lucy and consider how she presented with a brain tumour, and the impact of treatment on her and her family.

GO TO

---

www.teenagecancertrust.org/help-and-support

Consider the work of the Teenage Cancer Trust and highlight the support they provide for young people with cancer.

REFERENCES

Bailey, S. and Skinner, R. (2010) *Paediatric Haematology and Oncology.* Oxford: Oxford University Press.

Carlsson, T., Kukkola, L., Ljungman, L., Hove'n, E. and von Essen, L. (2019) 'Psychological distress in parents of children treated for cancer: an explorative study'. *PLoSONE,* 14 (6): e0218860.

Children with Cancer UK (2021) Childhood cancer facts and statistics. Available at: www.childrenwith cancer.org.uk/childhood-cancer-info/understanding-cancer/childhood-cancer-facts-figures/

Children's Cancer Leukaemia Group (2022) 'About childhood cancer'. Available at: www.cclg.org.uk/ Childhood-cancer (accessed 3 May 2022).

Children's Cancer Measures (2013) *Manual for Cancer Services (version 3.0). National Cancer Peer Review*. London: National Cancer Action Team.

Flury, M., Caisch, U., Ullmann-Bremi, A. and Spichiger, E. (2011) 'Experiences of parents with caring for their child after a cancer diagnosis'. *Journal of Pediatric Oncology Nursing*, 28: 143–53.

Gottlieb, B.H. (1978) 'The development and application of a classification scheme of informal helping behaviours'. *Canadian Journal of Behavioural Science*, 10: 105–15.

Hill, L. and Gubi, P.M. (2020) 'Factors that may continue to impact a mother's emotional well-being once her child's treatment for cancer has completed and their implications for ongoing support'. *Illness, Crisis & Loss*, 30 (2): doi:10.1177/1054137320919916.

House, J.S. (1981) *Work Stress and Social Support*. Reading: Addison–Wesley.

Hughes, E.C. (1945) 'Dilemmas and contradictions of status'. *American Journal of Sociology*, 50: 353–9.

Jibb, L.A., Croal, L., Wang, J., Yuan, C., Foster, J., Cheung, V. et al. (2018) 'Children's experiences of cancer care: a systematic review and thematic synthesis of qualitative studies'. *Oncology Nursing Forum*, 45: 527–44.

Jordan, J., Price, J. and Prior, L. (2015) 'Disorder and disconnection: parent experiences of liminality when caring for their dying child'. *Sociology of Health and Illness*, 37 (6): 839–55.

Kaplan, B.H., Cassel, J.C. and Gore, S. (1977) 'Social support and health'. *Medical Care*, 15: 47–58.

McCubbin, M., Balling, K., Possin, P., Frierdich, S. and Bryne, B. (2002) 'Family resiliency in childhood cancer'. *Family Relations*, 51: 103–11.

Molinaro, M.L. and Fletcher, P.C. (2018) 'The balancing act: mothers' experiences of providing care to their children with cancer'. *Journal of Pediatric Oncology Nursing*, 35 (6):4 439–46.

National Cancer Registration and Analysis Service (NCRAS) (2021) 'Children, teenagers and young adults UK cancer statistics report 2021'. Available at: http://ncin.org.uk/cancer_type_and_topic_specific_work/ cancer_type_specific_work/cancer_in_children_teenagers_and_young_adults/ (accessed April 2021).

NHS England (2021) Children's cancer services: Principal treatment centres service specification. Available at: www.england.nhs.uk/publication/childrens-cancer-services-principal-treatment-centres-service-specification/ (accessed 20 June 2023).

NICE (National Institute for Health and Clinical Excellence) (2005) Improving outcomes in children and young people with cancer. Cancer service guideline [CSG7]. Available at: www.nice.org.uk/ guidance/csg7 (accessed 20 June 2023).

NICE (National Institute for Health and Care Excellence) (2014) Cancer services for children and young people. Quality standard [QS55]. Available at: www.nice.org.uk/guidance/qs55 (accessed 20 June 2023).

Nursing and Midwifery Council (NMC) (2018) *The Code: Professional Standards of Practice and Behaviour for Nurses, Midwives and Nursing Associates*. London: NMC. Available at: www.nmc.org. uk/standards/code/.

Price, J., Jordan, J., Prior, L. and Parkes, J. (2012) 'Comparing needs of families of children dying from malignant and non-malignant disease: an in-depth qualitative study'. *British Medical Journal Supportive and Palliative Care*, 2 (2): 127–32.

Thoitis, P.A. (1986) 'Social support as coping assistance'. *Journal of Consulting and Clinical Psychology*, 54: 416–23.

Woodgate, R. and Yanofsky, R. (2010) 'Parents' experiences in decision making with childhood cancer clinical trials'. *Cancer Nursing*, 33 (1): 11–18.

CARE OF CHILDREN AND YOUNG PEOPLE WITH LIFE-LIMITING ILLNESS

32

ANTOINETTE MENEZES, TRACIE LEWIN-TAYLOR AND JAYNE PRICE

THIS CHAPTER COVERS

- An exploration of what constitutes life-limiting illness in children
- The palliative care needs of children with life-limiting illnesses and their families
- The role of children's hospices in care provision
- Transition of young people supported by children's palliative care services to adult services.

> "At that point we could not change what was going to happen to our family and most especially to Anouk. However, we were able to choose who was going to support us and to a certain extent how we were going to live during that time. We wanted to identify areas of our lives we did have some control over, to find partners who would empower us to make difficult choices, to enable us to be the best parents we could be to our daughters, to facilitate us to continue to live normal lives, and to permit us to continue to live our family life the way we wanted to."
>
> **Catherine, parent**

INTRODUCTION

The quote above comes from a mother describing the moment they received the devastating news that their daughter had a life-limiting condition and would only live a few months or perhaps a year. Her words highlight the family need for support in making choices, guidance to navigate unchartered territory, help to create some normality for the child and the whole family unit.

When a child is diagnosed with a life-limiting illness families like Anouk's need high-quality, integrated responsive, flexible support designed to meet their individual needs (Fields et al., 2021). Community-based, interprofessional support is vital, and to achieve the desired goal professionals have to work collaboratively, ensuring the child and family are at the centre of everything they do.

This chapter examines the high-quality individualised care of babies, children and young people with life-limiting conditions in partnership with their families. The needs of children and families are illustrated through two case studies, encouraging you to think critically from the child and family's perspectives.

You do not need prior knowledge to read the chapter although you may find useful the Together for Short Lives (TfSL) website (www.together for shortlives.org.uk) and their *A Guide to Children's Palliative Care* (2018), which has a glossary of terms in Appendix 1 which will help to clarify terms you may not be familiar with or terms that are often used interchangeably.

What are life-limiting illnesses?

Life-limiting illnesses are sometimes referred to as life-shortening illnesses and are those conditions for which there is no reasonable hope of cure and from which children are likely to die before they reach adulthood. Experts indicate that although the numbers of children in the UK with life-limiting illnesses are increasing, they have found it difficult to estimate the exact numbers. Recent work suggests a future prevalence of life-limiting conditions ranging from 67.0 to 84.22 per 10,000 by 2030 (Fraser, 2021). It is important to also consider life-threatening conditions which are those conditions for which curative treatment is possible but may not be successful, for example childhood cancer.

The different conditions that render children requiring a palliative approach to care can be understood by examining the categorisation below (Together for Short Lives, 2018). Four categories of life-threatening/life-limiting conditions in children are:

1. Life-threatening conditions for which curative treatment may be feasible but can fail Access to palliative care services may be necessary when treatment fails or during an acute crisis, irrespective of the duration of threat to life. On reaching long-term remission or following successful curative treatment there is no longer a need for palliative care services. *Examples:* cancer, irreversible organ failures of heart, liver, kidney.
2. Conditions where premature death is inevitable There may be long periods of intensive treatment aimed at prolonging life and allowing participation in normal activities. *Examples:* cystic fibrosis, Duchenne muscular dystrophy.
3. Progressive conditions without curative treatment options Treatment is exclusively palliative and may commonly extend over many years. *Examples:* Batten disease, mucopolysaccharidoses.
4. Irreversible but non-progressive conditions causing severe disability, leading to susceptibility to health complications and likelihood of premature death Children can have complex healthcare needs, a high risk of an unpredictable life-threatening event or episode, health complications and an increased likelihood of premature death. *Examples:* severe cerebral palsy, multiple disabilities, such as following brain or spinal cord injury.

(Together for Short Lives, 2018)

A number of issues make caring for children with life-limiting conditions and their families complex. First, many rare life-limiting illnesses can affect children, some so unusual that only a handful of children are affected in the UK or the world. Second, in some cases the conditions in childhood are inherited, so more than one child can be affected in the family. Further, the unpredictable nature of the conditions involved mean that many of the children have complex needs and require constant, complete care, punctuated by long tiring journeys to care and treatment centres. Such life-limiting illnesses can cause progressive deterioration, so the child becomes increasingly dependent on parents and carers.

ACTIVITY 32.1: CRITICAL THINKING

Have you cared for a child with a life-limiting condition? Use a reflective model such as McNeilly et al. (2022) to reflect on how you felt during this experience or on any concerns you have if you have not cared for a child or family in this situation. Even if you have not yet cared for a child with a life-limiting condition, consider how you would feel and what anxieties you might experience.

The needs of children and families

Babies, children and young people affected by life-limiting illnesses have a spectrum of physical/emotional/social and spiritual needs, as do their families (Aidoo and Rajapakse, 2019). Asessment of such needs is not a one-off but rather a continuous process responsive to the ever-changing needs of the child and family. In relation to symptom management, a study of 198 children (Hoell et al., 2019) found that gastrointestinal and neurological symptoms were most prevalent across all four TfSL categories. Other symptoms identified included fatigue, lack of appetite, nausea and sleep changes, dyspnoea, fear, myoclonus, seizures and spasticity.

Some children and young people have a clear understanding of their condition but suffer from declining physical abilities. Others have complex learning difficulties and very limited insight into their own situation. Rasmussen and Grégoire (2015) and Hoell et al. (2019) describe the range of neurological symptoms which can occur, discussing evaluation and management. Some of the children communicate non-verbally and sensory support can enable them to explore their world and express themselves.

Each child and family has individual needs, which must be accurately assessed and provided for. Sometimes different family members – for example, fathers (Nicholas et al., 2016; Postavaru, 2019), mothers, grandparents (Tatterton and Walshe, 2019) and siblings (Malcolm et al., 2014; Fullerton et al., 2017).

SEE ALSO
CHAPTER 2

ACTIVITY 32.2: CRITICAL THINKING

Think about the needs of children with a life-limiting condition before you read on. Create a mind map of the needs of life-limited children that you can think of with branches for these headings:

- Physical needs
- Emotional needs
- Spirituality (Here we refer to spirituality as related to being human, how you nurture yourself as an individual - for example, some people do yoga, others go for a walk in the countryside (Llewellyn et al. [2015] and Crisp [2016] discuss these issues)
- Social needs and interaction with peers

Siblings need particular care and support as highlighted in the parent voice below:

"We prepared Matthias and his three brothers every step of the way by being open and honest ... We felt strongly that the children were to know everything but felt it was important for the siblings to know and understand after Matthias had been told and had the chance to share his thoughts and emotions first with my husband and myself. In my experience parent led/guided care was imperative, by a process of osmosis we were seeing and learning acceptance of our child's death.

Honesty, openness, freedom to speak, planning and preparation were key to the children's understanding of cancer diagnosis, treatment, palliative care and death."

Rosie, parent

THE ROLE OF CHILDREN'S HOSPICES

Children with life-limiting conditions and their families need support from hospitals and different community-based health, social and education providers. Children's hospices have a key role in the provision of care for this group of children and their families.

"In some ways it was [to] the rest of the extended family that the children's hospice gave invaluable assistance, not provided by any other service. The wonderful play therapist visited Neave weekly, ensuring she felt valued and important at a time in our lives when despite our best intentions life did revolve around our youngest daughter."

Catherine, parent

Children's hospices were first established in the UK in the early 1980s when Helen House opened in Oxford. Currently, there are over 50 services in the UK. Each provides a comparable but slightly different range of support.

ACTIVITY 32.3: REFLECTIVE PRACTICE

First search the web and locate your local children's hospice - jot down the range of services they offer. Then meet the children and families who use/have used children's hospice services (in the video links below):

- Shooting Star Children's Hospices gave us one last Christmas together - YouTube: www.youtube.com/watch?v=aUcVo5wPzlg
- Children's Hospice Care - Hugh's story - YouTube: www.youtube.com/watch?v=txw4a9sfCx4

Children's hospice care is generally provided by interprofessional teams which include for example doctors, nurses, counsellors, play and music therapists, physiotherapists and occupational therapists, family support workers as well as healthcare assistants. Some provide care in the child's home and some offer short breaks and symptom care as well as end-of-life care and post-bereavement support. Although some receive statutory funding they are primarily supported by charitable donations. Children's hospices adopt a child- and family-centred approach focusing on holistic care to meet the specific needs of each child and family. The voices of children with life-limiting illnesses are critical to enhance our understanding of their needs and experiences (Menezes, 2010).

SEE ALSO
CHAPTER 1

WHAT'S THE EVIDENCE?

Ling et al. (2016) found that families participating in their qualitative study most wanted support at home but also had concerns about the potential effects on family life and siblings of community care services and professionals visiting their home.

After reading the paper write a reflection about why you think families might want support in their own home, highlighting the specific concerns outlined in the findings.

Where referrals are made to the children's hospice close to diagnosis the child and family are offered support over long periods of time, perhaps years. The emphasis is on long-term support for families as well as symptom care, end-of-life care and bereavement support for families.

Together for Short Lives (2018) provide this definition:

Palliative care for children and young people with life-limiting conditions is an active and total approach to care, from the point of diagnosis or recognition, embracing physical, emotional, social and spiritual elements through to death and beyond. It focuses on enhancement of quality of life for the child/young person and support for the family and includes the management of distressing symptoms, provision of short breaks and care through death and bereavement. (TfSL, 2018)

Palliative care is therefore multifaceted and complex. The case studies below will help you unravel some of the components and complexities inherent in providing palliative care.

WHAT'S THE EVIDENCE?

Download the Together for Short Lives Core Care Pathway for children with life-limiting and life-threatening conditions at www.togetherforshortlives.org.uk/resource/core-care-pathway/

Identify the 3 stages and 6 standards.

Consider how you could use the Pathway to help you assess the unique needs of the children and families to draw up a care plan?

SEE ALSO
CHAPTER 33

CARE OF CHILDREN WITH A LIFE-LIMITING ILLNESS

Many children's hospices accept referrals pre-birth and the case below shows an example of an in-utero referral to a hospice service.

SEE ALSO
CHAPTER 30

CASE STUDY 32.1: JACK

Sarah was pregnant with Jack. She received an in-utero diagnosis of anencephaly early in her pregnancy. The local maternity and neonatal team referred Jack's mum to a hospice service at 36 weeks' gestation because his diagnosis was life limiting and met the hospice referral criteria.

Jack's parents visited the hospice supported by the community team and the specialist palliative care team. Lots of planning occurs in cases such as Jack's and these are really important to document and communicate well. Ahead of Jack's delivery, plans were put in place that involved decisions made collaboratively between professionals and parents. A symptom management plan was written; these can be used in any setting so if parents change their mind this plan can move with them ensuring medicines are available. Discussion around advance care planning occurred, and parents decided that they would like to donate Jack's heart valves. Importantly, this can occur in settings outside hospital so does not impact transfer of settings after death. Jack's parents were offered choice around care after delivery if Jack were to survive, and his parents decided that they wished for care to be provided within the hospital setting. Jack was born at 41 weeks' gestation and survived for 14 hours after delivery. The hospital team followed the individualised symptom care plan to manage Jack's end of life. Jack had access to a 24/7 children's specialist care team who would act as a central point to coordinate and lead his end-of-life care (NICE, 2016). Jack was transferred to the hospice for care after death. His parents were able to access bereavement support via the hospice.

- Think of a time when you have worked with a family that may not have been offered these choices. What do you think are the benefits of having open discussions with families?
- How do you think the needs of parents for an in-utero referral may differ from parents of a child?

It is often hard to predict what the future holds for babies and children requiring palliative care. Parallel planning is paramount within children's palliative care, to plan for life and death (TfSL 2018). It is important for families to be given choices; these include place of care, place of death, place of care after death, and emotional and bereavement support. Putting the child and family at the centre of decision-making is a priority in producing a plan of care that is right for them. The actual place of death may be less important than has been argued; the opportunity to place location of death may be a better proxy of high-quality end-of-life care than actual location (Mitchell et al., 2019).

SEE ALSO
CHAPTER 33

Communication is always paramount in providing the best care possible. Relationship building, demonstration of effort and competence, information exchange, availability, and appropriate level of child and parent involvement are valued by families (Hsiao et al., 2007).

Carr et al. (2022a) highlight how advance care planning (ACP) for life-limited children can improve care for the child and their family. The *End of Life Care Strategy* (Department of Health, 2008) clearly states that ACP and clarity about resuscitation decisions are essential to quality care. ACP may also lead to actions such as advance statements about wishes and preferences and withdrawal of treatment. For children and families this will include decisions relating to care in the case of acute deterioration and may also address preferences for organ and tissue donation (NICE, 2016). Initiating conversations with parents regarding making choices and planning in advance of their child's life although difficult, is recognised as important. However, practices vary and are unstandardised (Carr et al., 2022b).

WHAT'S THE EVIDENCE?

Review parental experiences of ACP from the evidence below:

Video at: www.youtube.com/watch?v=FysnNLEnQ-s

Carr, K., Hasson, F., McIlfatrick, S. et al. 'Parents' experiences of initiation of paediatric advance care planning discussions: a qualitative study'. *European Journal of Paediatrics*, 181: 1185-96. doi.org/10.1007/s00431-021-04314-6.

Jot down three key pieces of learning from parents regarding advance care planning.

SAFEGUARDING STOP POINT

As a nursing student you will be in a unique position to observe signs of abuse, neglect or changes in behaviour which may indicate that a child is being abused or neglected. Safeguarding issues can arise for life-limited children and their families. Make sure you know whom to ask for help if you have safeguarding concerns wherever you are working.

TRANSITION OF YOUNG PEOPLE SUPPORTED BY CHILDREN'S PALLIATIVE CARE SERVICES TO ADULT SERVICES

The second case study will discuss a further scenario dealing with a young person who receives palliative care.

CASE STUDY 32.2: MATTHEW

Matthew is 18, and has been known to a children's hospice service for many years. He has a diagnosis of Duchenne muscular dystrophy with cardiac involvement. He receives respite care from the hospice service both in house and from the hospice at home team. Matthew has had issues with recurrent chest infections which led to a deterioration and admission to an adult ward via Accident and Emergency. The hospital team informed his foster mother that Matthew was entering end of life; his medicines were discontinued and a 'do not attempt resuscitation' (DNAR) order was completed. Due to Matthew's age he needs to transition to adult services. The DNAR was replaced with a ReSPECT form. The difference in these two documents is that there is discussion with families around best interest, including interventions that could be considered in an end-of-life event. The individualised symptom care plan can be helpful in managing anticipated symptoms. These plans were shared with all settings that Matthew uses or may use. He also had access to a 24/7 paediatric specialist care team (see NICE, 2016). The challenges for Matthew and his mother moving forward into adult services include whether services will be funded to support the family and the provision available to provide respite care to a young man like Matthew.

Think about transition from childhood to adulthood and the need for young people to move from children's to adult services. What challenges do you think families face?

Most children and young people with life-limiting conditions are cared for mainly in the community, with hospice care being a lifeline for respite care or more urgent supportive care beyond hospital or education settings. Sadly, these families who are transitioning into adult settings face limited and under-resourced services due to limited funding and inexperience in working with young people with such complex needs. You may have experience yourself of an adult hospice and have seen the difference from children's hospices. Adult hospices are currently able to offer limited, if any, respite for families. This may see a change in the future.

Planning improves care; ACP and Resuscitation plans (ReSPECT) enabled Matthew to have discussion around management of both reversible and non-reversible aspects of his condition that can be supported in any care setting. Care is integrally intertwined with other clinical, social, educational, therapeutic and voluntary services to ensure that families receive the care required throughout their journey. Matthew attends education and liaison between all services involved is important so that a clear plan can be put in place in partnership with families.

Children's services will plan and support the family as much as possible to achieve a seamless transition. Every young person should be appropriately supported in adult services, with a multi-agency team fully engaged in facilitating care and support. There should be confidence from the young person, family and professional perspective in future planning and provision of care (Chambers, 2015). Activity 32.4 will help you reflect on learning from Matthew's case study.

ACTIVITY 32.4: CRITICAL THINKING

If you created a mind map about the needs of children with life-limiting illnesses at Activity 32.2, use a new colour and add to each branch one or two things you think a young person might need.

WHAT'S THE EVIDENCE?

The *Moving to Adult Services: What to Expect* guide (Together for Short Lives, 2016) is downloadable from:

Together for Short Lives Transition to Adult Services Pathway (togetherforshortlives.org.uk) and shows evidence to support this case study and to help you to review Activity 34.4.

CHAPTER SUMMARY

- Life-limiting illness reduces the child's life expectancy to childhood or young adulthood and brings sustained uncertainty for the child and family
- Children's hospice and palliative care agencies provide child- and family-centred interprofessional support, often over years
- Children, young people and their families have diverse and often very complex needs
- Good communication with the family and between agencies is critical
- Symptom management and planning for emergencies are very important aspects of care

BUILD YOUR BIBLIOGRAPHY

Books

- Downing, J. (ed.) (2020) *Children's Palliative Care: An International Case-Based Manual.* Cham: Springer.
- Mancini, A., Price, J. and Kerr Elliot, T. (2020) *Neonatal Palliative Care for Nurses.* Cham: Springer.

FURTHER
READING

  The above books are both useful texts in exploring different aspects of palliative care for babies, children and young people.

Journal articles

- Fields, D., Fraser, L.K., Taylor, J. and Hackett, J. (2023) 'What does "good" palliative care look like for children and young people? A qualitative study of parents' experiences and perspectives'. *Palliative Medicine*, 37 (3): 355–71.

FURTHER
READING:
ONLINE
JOURNAL
ARTICLES

  A study examining parents' experiences of quality palliative care for children and young people.
- Mendizabal-Espinosa, R.M. and Price, J.E. (2021) 'Family centred neonatal palliative care in children's hospices : a qualitative study of parents' experiences'. *Journal of Neonatal Nursing*, 27 (2): 141–6.

  A research study which demonstrated the value of children's hospices to parents whose baby was diagnosed with a life-limiting condition.
- Price, J., Hurley, F. and Kiernan, G. (2022) 'Managing an unexpected life – a caregiver's career': parents' experience of caring for their child with a non-malignant life-limiting condition'. *Journal of Child Health Care*, Oct 12; 13674935221132920.

  A research study examining parents' experiences of the often all-encompassing care of their child diagnosed or recognised as having a life-limiting condition.

Weblinks

- Together for Short Lives www.togetherforshortlives.org.uk UK charity representing life-limited children and their families. The website includes many resources for professionals.
- Hospice UK www.hospiceuk.org National charity for hospice care offering information about courses, conferences and policy.
- Contact a Family www.cafamily.org.uk National charity for families with disabled children including an A-Z of medical conditions, some life-limiting.

FURTHER
READING:
WEBLINKS

REFERENCES

Aidoo, E. and Rajapakse, D. (2019) 'Overview of paediatric palliative care'. *BJA Education*, 19 (2): 60–4.

Carr, K., Hasson, F., McIlfatrick, S. and Downing, J. (2022a) 'Initiation of paediatric advance care planning: cross-sectional survey of health professionals reported behaviour'. *Child Care Health Development*, 48 (3): 423–34.

Carr, K., Hasson, F., McIlfatrick, S. et al. (2022b) 'Parents' experiences of initiation of paediatric advance care planning discussions: a qualitative study'. *European Journal of Pediatrics*, 181: 1185–96.

Chambers, L. (2015) *Stepping Up: A guide to enabling a good transition to adulthood for young people with life-limiting and life-threatening conditions.* Bristol: Together for Short Lives.

Crisp, C.L. (2016) 'Faith, hope, and spirituality: supporting parents when their child has a life-limiting illness'. *Journal of Christian Nursing*, 33 (1): 14–21.

Department of Health (2008) *End of Life Care Strategy*. London: Department of Health.

Fields, D., Fraser, L.K., Taylor, J. and Hackett, J. (2023) 'What does "good" palliative care look like for children and young people? A qualitative study of parents' experiences and perspectives'. *Palliative Medicine*, 37(3): 355–71.

Fraser, L.K., Gibson-Smith, D., Jarvis, S., Norman, P. and Parslow, R.C. (2021) 'Estimating the current and future prevalence of life-limiting conditions in children in England'. *Palliative Medicine*, 35(9): 1641–51.

Fullerton, J.M., Totsika, V., Hain, R. and Hastings, R.P. (2017) 'Siblings of children with life-limiting conditions: psychological adjustment and sibling relationships'. *Child: Care Health and Development*, 43 (3): 393–400.

Hoell, J.I., Webber, H., Warfsmann, J. et al. (2019) 'Facing the large variety of life-limiting conditions in children'. *European Journal of Pediatrics*, 178: 1893–902.

Hsiao, J.L., Evan, E.E. and Zeltzer, L.K. (2007) 'Parent and child perspectives on physician communication in pediatric palliative care'. *Palliative & Supportive Care*, 5 (4): 355–65.

Ling, J., Payne, S., Connaire, K. and McCarron, M. (2016) 'Parental decision-making on utilisation of out-of-home respite in children's palliative care: findings of qualitative case study research – a proposed new model'. *Child: Care, Health and Development*, 42: 51–9.

Llewellyn, H., Jones, L., Kelly, P., Barnes, J., O'Gorman, B., Craig, F. and Bluebond-Langner, M. (2015) 'Experiences of healthcare professionals in the community dealing with the spiritual needs of children and young people with life-threatening and life-limiting conditions and their families: report of a workshop'. *BMJ Supportive and Palliative Care*, 5 (3): 232–9.

Malcolm, C., Gibson, F., Adams, S., Anderson, G. and Forbat, L. (2014) 'A relational understanding of sibling experiences of children with rare life-limiting conditions: findings from a qualitative study'. *Journal of Child Health Care*, 18 (3): 230–40.

McNeilly, P., McCloskey, S., Peacock, V. and Price, J.E. (2022) 'Reflecting on palliative care for children, young people and their families: a revised model'. *International Journal of Palliative Nursing*, 28 (10): pp. 482–90. ISSN (print) 1357-6321.

Menezes, A. (2010) 'Moments of realization: life-limiting illness in childhood – perspectives of children, young people and families'. *International Journal of Palliative Nursing*, 16 (1): 41–7.

Mitchell, S., Spry, J.L., Hill, E., Coad, J., Dale, J. and Plunkett, A. (2019) 'Parental experiences of end of life care decision-making for children with life-limiting conditions in the paediatric intensive care unit: a qualitative interview study'. *BMJ Open*, 9 (5): e028548.

NICE (National Institute for Health and Care Excellence) (2016) End of life care for infants, children and young people with life-limiting conditions: planning and management. NICE guideline [NG61]. Available at: www.nice.org.uk/guidance/ng61 (accessed 21 June 2023).

Nicholas, D.B., Beaune, L., Barrera, M., Blumberg, J. and Belletrutti, M. (2016) 'Examining the experiences of fathers of children with a life-limiting illness'. *Journal of Social Work in End-of-Life and Palliative Care*, 12 (1–2): 126–44.

Postavaru, G (2019) 'A meta-ethnography of parents' experiences of their children's life-limiting conditions', *Qualitative Research in Psychology*, 16 (2): 253–75.

Rasmussen, L.A. and Grégoire, M.C. (2015) 'Challenging neurological symptoms in paediatric palliative care: an approach to symptom evaluation and management in children with neurological impairment'. *Paediatrics and Child Health*, 20 (3): 159–65.

Tatterton, M.J. and Walshe, C. (2019) 'Understanding the bereavement experience of grandparents following the death of a grandchild from a life-limiting condition: a meta-ethnography'. *Journal of Advanced Nursing*, 75 (7):1406–17.

Together for Short Lives (2018) *A Guide to Children's Palliative Care: Supporting babies, children and young people with life-limiting and life-threatening conditions and their families*, 4th edn. Bristol: Together for Short Lives. Available at: www.togetherforshortlives.org.uk/resource/a-guide-to-childrens-palliative-care/.

CARE OF CHILDREN AND YOUNG PEOPLE AT THE END OF LIFE

33

JAYNE PRICE AND MELISSA HEYWOOD

THIS CHAPTER COVERS

- Assessment and planning in end-of-life care
- Symptom management for a child at end of life
- Ethical issues when caring for a dying child
- The interdisciplinary approach inherent in caring for a child at the end of life and their family
- Self-care for professionals working with children at the end of life

> "Caring for a dying child is for me one of the most difficult parts of being a nurse but it is also the most rewarding. Having a family entrust the care of their child to you at this time is the greatest privilege and honour – there is a real pressure to get it right, there are no second chances."
>
> **Stephanie Minnis, staff nurse, neonatal intensive care**

INTRODUCTION

Death of a child defies the expected order of life. No parent expects to outlive their child and such a life-altering event leads to profound and long-lasting grief (Pohlkamp et al., 2019). Fortunately, childhood death is relatively rare. However, estimates indicate that 722 children aged between 1 and 9 died in 2018 in the UK (RCPCH, 2020). In England and Wales, 2226 infant deaths (under age of one) and 789 child deaths (between 1 to 15 years of age) occurred in England and Wales in 2020; these are the lowest numbers of infant and child deaths since records began in 1980. Whilst accidents are the most common cause of death, cancer is the illness most frequently leading to the death of a child (RCPCH, 2020).

End-of-life care is defined as:

> care that helps all those with advanced, progressive, incurable illness to live as well as possible until they die. It focuses on preparing for an anticipated death and managing the end stage of a terminal medical condition. This includes care during and around the time of death, and immediately afterwards. It enables the supportive and palliative care needs of both child/young person and the family to be identified and met throughout the last phase of life and into bereavement. It includes management of pain and other symptoms and provision of psychological, social, spiritual and practical support and support for the family into bereavement.
>
> (Together for Short Lives, 2018: 33)

The definition highlights the multifaceted and all-encompassing nature of such care involving physical, emotional, social and spiritual elements in partnership with the family. The way a child dies can impact on the parents' bereavement (Butler et al., 2019) and is another driving factor in ensuring that a good death is achieved.

Caring for a child at the end of life can provoke feelings of anxiety for nurses and other healthcare professionals, even those with experience. Such feelings may be partway attributed to professionals feeling pressurised that there is only one chance to 'get it right' for the child and family. The quote at the beginning of the chapter highlights that caring for the dying child can present enormous challenges for the nurse but if done well, has potential to bring lasting benefits to the nurse as well as the family. This chapter unravels some of the complexities associated with providing end-of-life care, drawing on best practice. If working through this chapter and associated activities proves emotionally difficult or raises specific issues, you must seek help – for example, from your personal tutor or practice assessor/supervisor. Remember also there are support/wellbeing services in your university.

ACTIVITY 33.1: REFLECTIVE PRACTICE

Please rate your confidence in providing end-of-life care to a child
   1 no confidence   10 very confident
Then reflect what would move you up the confidence scale

"One of the situations that most children's nursing students dread is encountering their first death. It is a difficult experience but ultimately teaches you new depths of compassion and caring which aid your professional growth. Every student copes with the death of a child differently."

Kate, 3rd-year children's nursing student

HOW DO YOU KNOW A CHILD IS NEARING END OF LIFE?

It is important to remember that uncertainty often exists around when a child may die and it is difficult to predict (NICE, 2016). However, the child's body goes through many changes as part of the dying process. Understanding physical and emotional changes may alleviate some of your fears and misconceptions about death. These are signs that may present when a child is approaching end of life (not an exhaustive list):

- Increased fatigue – the child may take to bed and/or sleeping increased
- Respiratory changes – such as decreased and laboured breathing and in the last hours noisy/rattly breathing may be present. Increase in secretions as coughing and swallowing reflex reduce
- Decreased appetite and fluid intake – absence of a desire to eat/drink. In some cases difficulty swallowing or managing food/fluids safely
- Skin colour from circulatory changes – the child may become pale, cool to the touch, bluish and/or mottled. Particularly in hands, feet and lips
- Organ failure – the body shutting down
- Agitation or decreased alertness

Concept of a 'good death'

The term 'good death' is one that has been used repeatedly relating to adults, yet often contested and/or lacks clarity in the literature in relation to children (Chong et al., 2021). Further debate centres around the individuality of a good death, suggesting it is difficult to define (Widdas et al., 2013). Hendrickson and McCorkle (2008), following a dimensional analysis, proposed a model for achieving a good death for children with cancer. The model proposes how aspects of care and quality of life come together to influence the dying process and are multidimensional in nature. Having someone present at the time of death was a component of the Hendrickson and McCorkle model (2008). In addition to 'being there', constituent properties of a good death included a peaceful death where the child was symptom-free, the need to be cared for by familiar, caring professionals and dying in a place of the child's or parents' choosing (Butler et al., 2019). Minimising suffering and avoiding a prolonged death, whilst acknowledging the individual child, was central to an evidence-based model developed by Chong et al. (2019) relating to the child and a good death.

ACTIVITY 33.2: REFLECTIVE PRACTICE

Consider what you feel constitutes a good death. Relate your thinking to a practice experience. Read the Chong et al. (2021) paper and compare the attributes highlighted to your own experiences.

PLANNING END-OF-LIFE CARE

Planning individualised care for a child at the end of life (EOL) is undoubtedly legally and emotionally complex (Verberne et al., 2021). Planning should be viewed as a collaborative ongoing process involving the child (where possible), parents/family and healthcare team in order to address the changing needs/wishes of the child and family (Heywood and Hynson, 2012). Much planning should be undertaken before an EOL crisis situation arises, i.e., advance planning, with a clear focus on ensuring the child's comfort/best interests (Mack and Joffe, 2014). Therefore, advance care planning (ACP) relates to ongoing conversations that enable goals, wishes and treatment plans for the child or young person (CYP) with life-limiting/life-threatening conditions to be discussed by parents, healthcare professionals (HCP) and, where appropriate, the CYP (Carr et al., 2022). Despite the importance of advance planning, at times there is a lack of a consistent approach or in some cases health professionals often find ways to delay these difficult conversations or avoid them altogether, often fearing that they might cause further pain to already suffering families. Such difficult conversations which form part of such planning/decision-making, may include resuscitation, organ donation, or location of end-of-life care (Papadatou et al., 2021). Confronting these decisions can be overwhelming for families who are experiencing a myriad of grief reactions so they will need time to process information, permitting decision-making to occur in stages: setting goals, gathering information, processing and making sense of the information, making choices and evaluation (Sharman et al., 2005). It is important that families know that such decisions can and should be revisited (Popejoy, 2015) and for health professionals to view these conversations as process rather than event.

CASE STUDY 33.1: JESS

Colin and Jill's 1-year-old daughter Jess has an undiagnosed life-limiting condition and is being cared for in the hospice at the end of life. They have three other children aged 9, 7 and 2. Colin's parents live abroad. However, Jill's parents live close by and have been helping with Jess and the other children.

- What benefits would hospice care potentially have for this family?
- Colin seems less engaged and often absent from family meetings and medical appointments – what ways would you do to try to ensure Colin is more involved?
- How could you as the nurse address the potential needs of Jill's parents (Jess's grandparents)?
- Jill is anxious about the other children being around Jess, wanting to protect them. How would you guide her?
- Consider how you would promote memory-making in this case.

WHAT'S THE EVIDENCE?

Malcolm and Knighting (2021) conducted a qualitative study examining parents' experiences of community service provision and their child's EOL care.

Findings highlighted the following being as valued by parents:

(1) ability to facilitate changes in preferred place of death; (2) trusted relationships with care providers who know their child and family; (3) provision of child- and family-centred care; (4) specialist care and support provided as and when required; (5) quality/compassionate death and follow up bereavement care.

Consider how these findings could influence your practice and if they have relevance to those providing EOL care in hospice or hospital?

A care pathway as in Figure 33.1 (Together for Short Lives, 2013) can be used to guide care. The pathway acts as a useful trigger to ensure care addresses the physical, emotional, social and spiritual needs of the child and family.

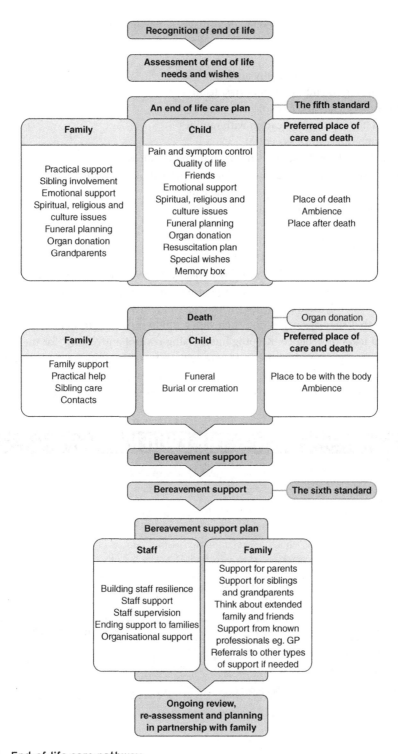

Figure 33.1 End-of-life care pathway

Widdas, D., McNamara, K. and Edwards, F. (2013) *A Core Care Pathway for Children with Life-limiting and Life-threatening Conditions*, 3rd edn. Bristol: Together for Short Lives. Reproduced with permission.

Planning must be centred round the needs and, where possible, wishes of the individual child and family:

- **C**ollaborative approach with family and team
- **A**dvance plan agreed and shared amongst team
- **R**egular review of plan and alteration as necessary
- **E**xplicit and honest communication with families
- **P**ain and symptom control as central
- **L**isten to child and family, supporting them in their choices
- **A**pproach which ensures emotional, social and spiritual needs are also addressed
- **N**ecessity to promote quality of life and make memories
- **S**ibling and grandparents' involvement is important

Parental coping

Parents living through the death of a child experience both emotional and practical chaos (Price et al., 2011). Parents can display a number of emotional responses, including disbelief, fear, anger, despair and hopelessness. Parents when caring for their dying child often experience guilt, particularly around their perception that they are neglecting their other children (Darlington et al., 2021) as caring for their dying child takes precedence. Keeping busy, taking control and 'doing' for their child in terms of providing care appears to enable parents to cope with some of their emotional responses (Price et al., 2011; Verberne et al., 2019). Continue to ask parents what they want to do for their child as death approaches; some parents may want to be with rather than do for – do not make any assumptions.

WHAT'S THE EVIDENCE?

The seminal work by Lazarus and Folkman (1984) identifies two different approaches to coping (which can be applied to parents coping with their child's end-of-life care):

- Problem-focused coping – a direct approach where the problem is evaluated and action is taken to avoid/change the situation
- Emotion-focused coping – a less direct approach, with the focus on reducing the emotional consequences of stressful or potentially stressful events

Considering Lazarus and Folkman's coping strategies, which do the following parental actions indicate? Jot these down.

Parental action	Lazarus and Folkman's approach
Organising grandparents to collect siblings from school	
Talking about feelings to staff nurse	
Surfing the net about symptom management	

Other family members

Within the ethos of family-centred care, the needs of siblings and grandparents as highlighted within the end-of-life pathway should be addressed (Widdas et al., 2013). Grandparents play important supportive roles and should not be forgotten during the end-of-life period. Grandparents suffer a double effect of loss in that they experience the pain of living through the loss of their grandchild, but in addition, they are watching their own child/family suffering (Gilrane-McGarry and O'Grady, 2011; Tatterton and Walshe, 2019). Parents can feel unsure about how to deal with the needs of their other children and often attempt to protect them from the truth around their sibling's death. In reality, siblings themselves indicate their need to be involved, and need for information, communication and reassurance (Lövgren et al., 2016; Eaton Russell et al., 2018).

Addressing the needs of siblings is essential. Consider how the children's nurse could work in partnership with parents to meet sibling need.

SYMPTOM MANAGEMENT

Children can experience a number of symptoms as they approach the end of life (Zernikow et al., 2019). Effective symptom management is vitally important and should include non-pharmacological strategies as well as pharmacological (NICE, 2016; Jassal, 2022). Symptom management differs significantly in children at the EOL and can be dependent on a number of factors, for example their diagnosis, age, cognitive and physiological developmental stage (Greenfield et al., 2020).

ACTIVITY 33.3: LEADERSHIP AND MANAGEMENT

The subcutaneous route of administration (via a syringe driver) is probably the most frequently used with children at EOL.

Consider the benefits of the subcutaneous route for children at the end of life.

Effective symptom management is about anticipating possible symptoms and preparing for their management to ensure comfort. As a child's death is not the end of the journey for their family, it is also about creating positive memories into bereavement. No one wants the last moments of a child's life to be of suffering and distress. Pivotal research demonstrated that parents of children who experienced 'a difficult symptom at end of life' were affected long into bereavement (Kreicbergs et al., 2005).

"Effective symptom management is about anticipating possible symptoms likely to occur for that child and preparing for their management to ensure comfort. As a child's death is not the end of the journey for their family, it is therefore also about creating positive memories as they begin the grieving process. No one wants the last moments of a child's life to be of suffering and distress."

Anne O'Reilly, specialist nurse, children's hospice

The more common symptoms encountered by children at EOL include pain, dyspnoea, nausea and vomiting, constipation, increased secretions, restlessness, anxiety and agitation, fatigue and seizures (Wolfe et al., 2015; Moresco and Moore, 2021). However, despite some challenges, the majority of symptoms can be adequately managed (Feudtner et al., 2011). Barriers that can contribute to lack of recognition of symptoms include the child's inability to report and describe their symptoms, the child denying symptoms to protect parents or failure of the clinicians to utilise appropriate assessment tools (Namisango et al., 2019). Nurses should proactively assess symptoms by observing the child, asking the child and/or the parents as well as using assessment tools available.

Challenges in pharmacological symptom management in children at the end of life include:

- Drugs may be unlicensed for use in children
- Conditions in childhood, and consequently symptoms, can be rare
- Limited research regarding symptom management in some non-malignant conditions
- Myths and fears about the use of certain drugs (e.g., morphine)
- Preparations may not always be suitable for use in children

---

ACTIVITY 33.4: REFLECTIVE PRACTICE

You are caring for a child at the end of life and the issue of starting a syringe driver with an opiod (morphine) for his pain relief has been raised. Mum is anxious that this will hasten death, so she wants to wait a few days.

Consider the management of this challenging issue.

Pain

Pain is the symptom most commonly associated with suffering at end of life. Children and parents often fear that pain will be unrelieved at this time (Bischoff et al., 2015; Friedrichsdorf et al., 2015).

Thorough assessment must:

SEE ALSO
CHAPTER 3

- Recognise the child's age and developmental stage
- Always use language appropriate to the child's developmental level
- Empower the child and family, by allowing choice and control where possible
- Involve investing time in developing trust with the child and family. This might mean spending some time drawing, reading or chatting with them

Of particular note is that a large percentage of children requiring EOL care have conditions that affect them cognitively, so their ability to communicate may be impaired. For this group of children observation is key. Observe the child's vocal sounds, facial expression, mood, eating, sleeping, movement and posture (Hunt, 2012). The Paediatric Pain Profile (see Figure 33.2) is a tool that is designed for assessing this particular group of children.

Paediatric Pain Profile
Baseline assessments

Pain Profile

Most troublesome pain (Pain A)

1. For each item please circle the number that best describes your child's behaviour when they have this pain.
2. Enter the number you have circled in to the "score" column.
3. Add up the numbers in the "score" column to give the total score.
4. Record the score on the Summary Graph

When my child has this pain, he or she...	Not at all	A little	Quite a lot	A great deal	Score
Is cheerful	3	2	1	0	
Is sociable or responsive	3	2	1	0	
Appears withdrawn or depressed	0	1	2	3	
Cries /moans/groans / screams or whimpers	0	1	2	3	
Is hard to console or comfort	0	1	2	3	
Self-harms e.g. biting self or banging head	0	1	2	3	
Is reluctant to eat / difficult to feed	0	1	2	3	
Has disturbed sleep	0	1	2	3	
Grimaces / screws up face / screws up eyes	0	1	2	3	
Frowns / has furrowed brow / looks worried	0	1	2	3	
Looks frightened (with eyes wide open)	0	1	2	3	
Grinds teeth or makes mouthing movements	0	1	2	3	
Is restless / agitated or distressed	0	1	2	3	
Tenses / stiffens or spasms	0	1	2	3	
Flexes inwards or draws legs up towards chest	0	1	2	3	
Tends to touch or rub particular areas	0	1	2	3	
Resists being moved	0	1	2	3	
Pulls away or flinches when touched	0	1	2	3	
Twists and turns / tosses head / writhes or arches back	0	1	2	3	
Has involuntary or stereotypical movements / is jumpy / startles or has seizures	0	1	2	3	
				TOTAL	

Please **tick the box** next to the word that best describes the severity of this pain

☐ None   ☐ Mild   ☐ Moderate   ☐ Severe   ☐ Very severe

© 2003. UCL/ICH and RCNI. This page is part of the Paediatric Pain Profile. It may be photocopied and used in the care of children with severe physical and learning disabilities.

7

Figure 33.2   Paediatric Pain Profile

Hunt, A., Goldman, A., Seers, K. et al. (2003) 'Clinical validation of thepaediatric pain profile'. *Developmental Medicine and Child Neurology*, 46 (1): 9-18. Reproduced with permission of UCLB. Available at https://xip.uclb.com/i/health care_tools/ppp.html

Other pain assessment tools include:

- FLACC – Face, Legs, Activity, Cry and Consolability – a behavioural assessment tool used in children from 2 months–8 years of age or up to 18 years for children with cognitive impairment
- Wong Baker FACES Scale – a self-reporting tool for children 3–18 years
- Visual analogue scale – a self-reporting tool for children 8-years and older

(www.rch.org.au/rchcpg/hospital_clinical_guideline_index/Pain_assessment_and_measurement/#Pain%20Assessment%20Tool, 2019)

ACTIVITY 33.5: CRITICAL THINKING

Which professionals may work collaboratively to assess and manage the pain of a child at the end of life?

Following an accurate assessment, a plan of care to manage the child's specific symptoms is formulated and implemented. These key principles should prevail:

1. Assess the pain – involve the parents
   Consider all factors contributing to the overall pain experience, e.g., anxiety, family stress
   Discuss the management strategy/plan – address potential parental anxieties
2. Use multimodal approaches – pharmacological and non-pharmacological, including massage, positioning, distraction
3. Utilise the least invasive route of medication administration – never intramuscular with children
4. Administer prescribed analgesics regularly
5. Minimise the number of doses
6. Plan ahead – try to anticipate exacerbations and potential crises
7. Prescribe regular laxatives (when using opioids)
8. Monitor the response (effectiveness and side effects), evaluate and reassess regularly

Other symptoms

In addition to pain, other symptoms may be experienced, also requiring assessment and management (see Table 32.2).

Table 33.1 Other symptoms and associated multimodal treatment/care (not an exhaustive list)

Symptoms	Explanation	Treatment options	Specific nursing care tips
Dyspnoea (shortness of breath)	Relatively common symptom in children Causes considerable anxiety in the child/ family if not controlled Very subjective sensation and reported symptoms may not match respiratory signs	Identify and treat underlying cause Opioids are very effective – e.g., morphine Benzodiazepines can be appropriate Some children find oxygen therapy helps alleviate dyspnoea	Dyspnoea is frightening for a child Provide reassurance - involve family Utilise a fan - a cool draft of air can be very helpful in reducing the feeling of breathlessness Utilise breathing exercises Appropriate positioning (upright) and relaxation may be useful
Secretions	A common symptom that children with a non-malignant diagnosis experience An increase in secretions is commonly experienced at EOL as the coughing and swallowing reflex reduce	Medications can be utilised to dry secretions but often have varying success e.g.,Glycopyrrolate and atropine	Gentle suction and physiotherapy can assist Nonpharmacological management strategies include regular positioning to allow secretions to drain, in combination with good mouth care

Symptoms	Explanation	Treatment options	Specific nursing care tips
Seizures	Experienced by children with: • primary or metastatic tumours of the brain • metabolic and genetic conditions	Anticonvulsant medications will be prescribed as maintenance treatment for seizures All families should have seizure management plan for emergency treatment of seizures including what medications should be administered and how long a seizure can be left before intervention	Maintaining child safety and dignity during seizure is essential
Restlessness, agitation and delirium	Not always an apparent cause but uncontrolled pain, hypoxia, anxiety and medications can be contributing factors	Use of medications to reduce symptoms where necessary – e.g., intranasal or buccal midazolam Midazolam is the sedation of choice and can be added into a syringe driver with other drugs	Nurse the child in a quiet and safe environment Reassure families that these symptoms can often be part of the dying process. Acknowledge it is very difficult to witness but that it is often not to the child
Nausea and vomiting	Identify the cause and then target anti-emetics according to their mode of action	Utilise anti-emetic medications as required – these can be added to drugs in the syringe driver (if the child has one) Identify causes that can be corrected and managed – e.g., pain, infection, drugs	Avoid strong smells and odours – e.g., perfume, foods Keep meals small and frequent if the child's appetite/condition allows Regular mouth care
Urinary retention	Some children with neurodegenerative disorders may experience difficulties with emptying their bladder Opiates can cause children to experience retention	Consider gentle bladder massage, warm baths or catheterisation	The family may value the opportunity to bath the child
Fatigue	A debilitating factor which can compromise quality of life Contributing factors – anaemia, depression, dehydration, malnutrition, insomnia and medications	Often a reflection of disease progression e.g., Attend school for shorter periods and at times of favourite classes/ subjects Planned activities can give the child a sense of wellbeing	Help child and family set realistic expectations and goals Encourage families to plan activities around the fatigue (when child has more energy)
Constipation	A number of factors can lead to constipation, including inactivity, weakness, poor food/fluid intake and reduced mobility; drugs such as opioids can cause constipation	Laxatives Rectal preparations should be avoided in children who are neutropenic/ thrombocytopenic	Provide privacy when using the toilet or, if the child wears a nappy, ensure appropriate hygiene and skin care

Information from: Children's Health Queensland Hospital and Health Service Paediatric Palliative Care Service (2014) and Jassal (2022)

CASE STUDY 33.2: DECLAN

Declan, a 4-year-old boy with metachromatic leukodystropy (MLD), is non-verbal, has global developmental delay, epilepsy and frequent muscle spasms. Declan receives his nutrition via gastrostomy and requires frequent oral suction. His mother carries out Declan's care at home with some input from carers.

In recent months Declan has had multiple admissions to hospital, mostly as a result of his increasing chronic lung disease and his susceptibility to chest infections.

Declan begins to experience an increase in his seizure activity. His secretions also have increased, becoming thick, green and difficult for him to cough up. He is more agitated, restless and irritable.

- How would you assess Declan's pain?
- How would you manage the other symptoms described?
- In what ways would you ensure Declan's care is child- and family-centred?
- What other care would you provide to ensure Declan is comfortable and that the complications of reduced mobility are recognised?
- What symptoms could you anticipate in the future?

ETHICAL ISSUES WHEN CARING FOR A DYING CHILD

Given the complexity of care at the end of life and the fact that many decisions are central to planning care, it is not surprising that a range of ethical issues can arise. The child's inability to act autonomously and the dependency on parents as surrogate decision-makers complicates the resolution of ethical dilemmas (see Table 33.2 and Case study 33.3).

Table 33.2 Potential ethical challenges

Ethical challenge	Example
Child as decision-maker	The child's ability to make choices – developmental level and life experience are major factors
Decision-making regarding treatment plan and goals	This includes:
	Life-sustaining inventions – ventilation, going to ICU Provision of hydration and nutrition Advance care planning
Treatment/procedure that appears to cause more burden to the child than benefit	Continuing chemotherapy in the last days of life
Parental refusal to utilise medication for symptom management	Morphine for pain relief and child is suffering
Parents refusing to tell CYP that they are dying	Anxious teenager asking questions about if they are dying

SEE ALSO
CHAPTER 8

CASE STUDY 33.3: RICHARD

Richard is 10 years old. He has Ewing's sarcoma and had a previous above-knee amputation. He has endured many years of treatments. Recently he has relapsed with no further treatment available. His parents do not want him to know he is dying and are keen to get him home as soon as possible.

As a registered nurse on night duty you check on him at 2 a.m. He is awake, says he is worried and asks, 'Am I going to die?'

- Applying ethical principles, how would you address this issue?
- Jot down the potential benefits of EOL care at home for Richard.

THE INTERDISCIPLINARY APPROACH

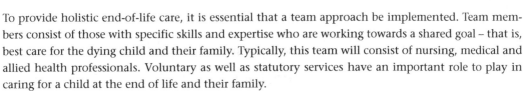

SEE ALSO
CHAPTER 5

To provide holistic end-of-life care, it is essential that a team approach be implemented. Team members consist of those with specific skills and expertise who are working towards a shared goal – that is, best care for the dying child and their family. Typically, this team will consist of nursing, medical and allied health professionals. Voluntary as well as statutory services have an important role to play in caring for a child at the end of life and their family.

For many families there are a multitude of services and individuals to liaise with across a range of care settings (see Figure 33.3). The identification of a key worker to coordinate care and ensure all services are working together is helpful (Heywood and Hynson, 2012; Lafci et al., 2021).

SELF-CARE FOR PROFESSIONALS WORKING WITH CHILDREN AT THE END OF LIFE

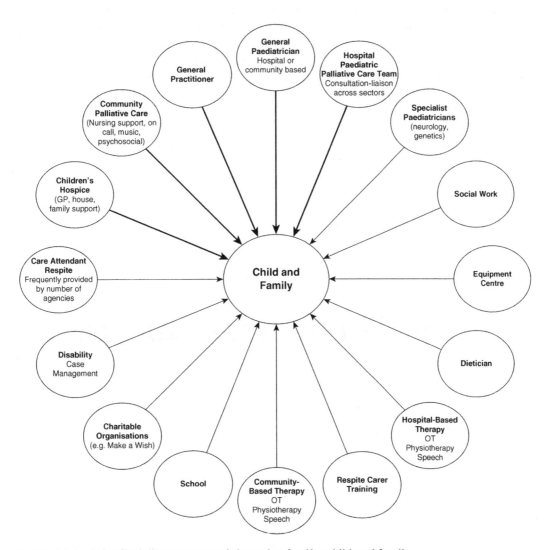

Figure 33.3   Interdisciplinary approach to caring for the child and family

"When my child died my world changed forever. Seeing the nurses who cared for us for 5 weeks in intensive care shed a tear provided us with such comfort at the most difficult of times. It helped us see that our son was important and loved by others too."

Leyla, parent

As caring for dying children and their families can be both emotionally and physically exhausting, it is essential to recognise that looking after yourself and your colleagues is integral to best practice for children and families (Morgan, 2009). Only when we look after ourselves and our colleagues can we continue to provide children and families with care and support at end of life on a regular basis. Self-awareness is crucial, and as professionals we need to have a clear knowledge of our own beliefs and needs (Furingsten et al., 2015).

Providing care to a dying child and their family can bring stress and anxiety for professionals providing care (Grimston et al., 2018). It is important to understand and acknowledge the impact that your work has on the personal and professional areas of your life (Beaune et al., 2018). Looking after oneself and developing self-care practices is imperative in ensuring best care is delivered to children and families (McCloskey and Taggart, 2010). Regular supervision, debriefing, access to professional expertise by staff in areas where EOL care is provided regularly, is necessary to minimise the risk of staff burnout.

A variety of strategies can be employed to ensure optimum health for all staff caring for dying children and their families. We need to 'rescue' ourselves and to look out for members of our team. Strategies for the self care of staff can include:

- **R**esources available within the organisation
- **R**eflect and debrief after the death of a child
- **R**espect and support the other members of the team
- **R**elevant training days may be useful
- **R**ealise your own ways of coping (including identifying your strengths)
- **R**emember to take care of yourself physically, mentally and spiritually

---

ACTIVITY 33.6: LEADERSHIP AND MANAGEMENT

As we come to this chapter's close, consider the findings below reflecting on how you could incorporate the wishes/needs of parents as a children's nurse leading and managing the care of a child at the end of life and their family.

Melin-Johansson et al. (2014) carried out an integrative literature review exploring parents' experiences and highlighted that parents' five main desires and goals when their child was at end of life were:

- Genuine communication
- Sincere relationships
- Respect as an expert
- Alleviation of the child's suffering
- Need for support

How could you incorporate the above evidence in your practice?

CHAPTER SUMMARY

To ensure that the principles of care for a child/family at the end of life highlighted in this chapter are addressed, remember your ABCDEFGs:

- **A**sk – ask the child and/or family what you can do for them (individualised care)
- **B**e – be there, be with and be available (and tell the parents/child you are available)
- **C**are – remember to care for the whole child, including physical, emotional, social and spiritual care. Be human and be empathetic
- **D**iscuss – discuss and explore arising ethical issues with sensitivity
- **E**nsure a team approach – recognise your limitations and draw on the expertise within the team
- **F**amily-centred care – be human and empathetic to parents, and remember siblings and grandparents
- **G**arner support strategies – ensure you develop your own self-care strategies
- **S**top, look and listen – reassess care plans regularly, while being flexible and responsive; child and family needs may change and this should be recognised and addressed

---
BUILD YOUR BIBLIOGRAPHY

Books

The chapters cited in each of these books give insights and guidance in caring for children after death.

- McNeilly, P. and Price, J. (2008) Chapter 44: 'Care of the child after death', in J. Kelsey and G. McEwing (eds), *Clinical Skills in Child Health Practice*. Oxford: Churchill Livingstone.
- Parry, M. (2022) Chapter 33: 'Care after death', in C. Delves-Yates (ed.), *Essentials of Nursing Practice*, 3rd edn. London: Sage.
- Chambers, L. (2019) Section 3: 'Care of a child after death', in *A Guide to End of Life Care*. Available at: Caring for the child at the end of life: A guide for professionals on the care of children and young people before death, at the time of death and after death (2nd edition) www.togetherforshortlives.org.uk/app/uploads/2019/11/TfSL-Caring-for-a-child-at-end-of-life-Professionals.pdf (accessed 8 July 2022).

FURTHER READING

Journal articles

- Barrett. L., Fraser, L., Noyes, J., Taylor, J. and Hackett, J. (2023) 'Understanding parent experiences of end-of-life care for children: a systematic review and qualitative evidence synthesis'. *Palliative Medicine*, 37 (2): 178–202.

  This paper gives useful insights in parents' experiences of EOL care through a systematic review.
- Malcolm, C. and Knighting, K. (2021) 'What does effective end-of-life care at home for children look like? A qualitative interview study exploring the perspectives of bereaved parents'. *Palliative Medicine*, 35 (8): 1602–11.

  This paper has useful insights into experiences of parents whose child had EOL care provided in the home.
- Snaman, J.M., Torres, C., Duffy, B., Levine, D., Gibson, D. and Baker, J. (2016) 'Parental perspectives of communication at the end of life at a pediatric oncology institution'. *Journal of Palliative Medicine*, 19 (3): 326–32.

  This paper gives useful insights into communication.

FURTHER READING: ONLINE JOURNAL ARTICLES

- van der Geest, I.M., van den Heuvel-Eibrink, M.M., van Vliet, L.M., Pluijm, S.M., Streng, I.C., Michiels, E.M., Pieters, R. and Darlington, A.S.E. (2015) 'Talking about death with children with incurable cancer: perspectives from parents'. *The Journal of Pediatrics*, 167 (6): 1320-6.

  Further examination of the complex issue of talking to children about death.
- Wender, E. and the Committee on Psychological Aspects of Child and Family Health (2012) 'Supporting the family after the death of a child'. *Pediatrics*, 130 (4): 1164-9.

  Bereavement care explored.

Podcasts

- Life, Love and Loss – A podcast for families caring for a child who is dying www.rch.org.au/podcasts/

Weblinks

FURTHER
READING:
WEBLINKS

- Jassal, S.S. (ed.) (2022) Symptom Management Guidelines, 10th edn. Bristol: Rainbows Children's Hospice. www.togetherforshortlives.org.uk/app/uploads/2022/05/Basic-Symptom-Control-in-Paediatric-Palliative-Care-2022.pdf This resource provides in-depth information on symptom management of children at the end of life. It is used by practitioners in practice reviewing management of a symptom.
- Winston's Wish www.winstonswish.org.uk A UK charity providing resources and support for bereaved children.

REFERENCES

Beaune, L., Muskat, B. and Anthony, S. (2018) 'The emergence of personal growth amongst healthcare professionals who care for dying children'. *Palliative and Supportive Care*, 16 (3): 298–307.

Bischoff, K., O 'Riordan, D., Fazzalaro, K., Kinderman, A. and Pantilat, S. (2015) 'Identifying opportunities to improve pain among patients with serious illness (S712)'. *Journal of Pain and Symptom Management*, 49 (2): 413.

Butler, A.E, Copnell, B. and Hall, H. (2019) 'When a child dies in the PICU'. *Pediatric Critical Care Medicine*, 20 (9): e447–e451.

Carr, K., Hasson, F., McIlfatrick, S. et al. (2022) 'Parents' experiences of initiation of paediatric advance care planning discussions: a qualitative study'. *European Journal of Pediatrics*, 181: 1185–96.

Children's Health Queensland Hospital and Health Service Paediatric Palliative Care Service (2014) *Practical Guide to Palliative Care in Paediatrics*. Available at: www.childrens.health.qld.gov.au/wp-content/uploads/PDF/brochures/palliative-care-in-paediatrics.pdf.

Chong, P.H., Walshe, C. and Hughes, S. (2019) 'Perceptions of a Good Death in children with life-shortening conditions: an integrative review'. *Journal of Palliative Medicine*, 22 (6): 714–23.

Chong, P.H, Walshe, C. and Hughes, S. (2021) 'A good death in the child with life shortening illness: a qualitative multiple-case study'. *Palliative Medicine*, 35 (10): 1878–88.

Darlington, A-S., Randall, D., Leppard, L. and Koh, M. (2021) 'Palliative and end of life care for a child: understanding parents' coping strategies'. *Acta Pediatrica*, 110 (2): 673–81.

Eaton Russell, C., Widger, K., Beaune, L., Neville, A., Cadell, S., Steele, R. et al. (2018) 'Siblings' voices: a prospective investigation of experiences with a dying child'. *Death Studies*, 42 (3): 184–94.

Feudtner, C., Hexem, K. and Rourke, M.T. (2011) 'Epidemiology and the care of children with complex conditions', in J. Wolfe, P.S. Hinds and B.M. Sourkes (eds), *Textbook of Interdisciplinary Pediatric Palliative Care*. Philadelphia: Elsevier Saunders.

Friedrichsdorf, S.J., Postier, A., Eull, D., Weidner, C., Foster, L., Gilbert, M. and Campbell, F. (2015) 'Pain outcomes in a US children's hospital: a prospective cross-sectional survey'. *Hospital Pediatrics*, 5 (1): 18–26.

Furingsten, L., Reet, S. and Forsner, M. (2015) 'Ethical challenges when caring for dying children'. *Nursing Ethics*, 22 (2): 176–87.

Gilrane-McGarry, U. and O'Grady, T. (2011) 'Forgotten grievers: an exploration of the grief experiences of bereaved grandparents'. *International Journal of Palliative Nursing*, 17 (4): 170–6.

Greenfield, K., Holley, S., Schoth, D.E., Harrop, E., Howard, R.F., Bayliss, J., Brook, L., Jassal, S.S., Johnson, M., Wong, I. and Liossi, C. (2020) 'A mixed-methods systematic review and meta-analysis of barriers and facilitators to paediatric symptom management at end of life'. *Palliative Medicine*, 34 (6): 689–707.

Grimston, M., Butler, A.E. and Copnell, B. (2018) 'Critical care nurses' experiences of caring for a dying child: a qualitative evidence synthesis'. *Journal of Advanced Nursing*, 74 (8): 1752–68.

Hendrickson, K. and McCorkle, R. (2008) 'Dimensional analysis of the concept: good death of a child with cancer'. *Journal of Pediatric Oncology*, 25 (3): 127–38.

Heywood, M. and Hynson, J.L. (2012) 'Paediatric palliative care: the challenging dimensions'. *Grief Matters*, 15 (2): 28–31.

Hunt, A. (2012) 'Pain assessment', in A. Goldman, R. Hain and S. Liben (eds), *Oxford Textbook of Palliative Care for Children*, 2nd edn. New York: Oxford University Press.

Jassal, S.S. (ed.) (UK) (2022) *Symptom Management Guidelines*, 10th edn. Bristol: Rainbows Children's Hospice. Available at: www.togetherforshortlives.org.uk/app/uploads/2022/05/Basic-Symptom-Control-in-Paediatric-Palliative-Care-2022.pdf

Kreicbergs, U., Valdimarsdóttir, U., Onelöv, E., Björk, O., Steineck, G. and Henter, J.I. (2005) 'Care-related distress: a nationwide study of parents who lost their child to cancer'. *Journal of Clinical Oncology*, 23 (36): 9162-71.

Lafci, D., Yildiz, E. and Pehlivan, S. (2021) 'Nurses' views and applications on palliative care'. *Perspectives in Psychiatric Care*, 57 (3): 1340–6.

Lazarus, R.S. and Folkman, S. (1984) *Stress, Appraisal and Coping*. New York: Springer.

Lövgren, M., Jalmsell, L., Eilegård Wallin, A., Steineck, G. and Kreicbergs, U. (2016) 'Siblings' experiences of their brother's or sister's cancer death: a nationwide follow-up 2–9 years later'. *Psycho-Oncology*, 25 (4): 435–40.

Mack, J. and Joffe, S. (2014) 'Parents communicating about prognosis: ethical responsibilities of pediatricians and parents'. *Pediatrics*, S24–9.

Malcolm, C. and Knighting, K. (2021) 'What does effective end-of-life care at home for children look like? A qualitative interview study exploring the perspectives of bereaved parents'. *Palliative Medicine*, 35 (8): 1602–11.

McCloskey, S. and Taggart, L. (2010) 'How much compassion have I left? An exploration of occupational stress among children's palliative care nurses'. *International Journal of Palliative Nursing*, 16 (5): 233–40.

Melin-Johansson, C., Axelsson, I., Jonsson Grundberg, M. and Hallqvist, F. (2014) 'When a child dies: parents' experiences of palliative care. An integrative literature review'. *Journal of Pediatric Nursing*, 29 (6): 660–9.

Moresco, B. and Moore, D. (2021) 'Pediatric palliative care'. *Hospital Practice*, 49 (Suppl 1): 422-30.

Morgan, D. (2009) 'Caring for dying children: assessing the needs of the pediatric palliative care nurse'. *Pediatric Nursing*, 35 (2): 86–90.

Namisango, E., Bristowe, K., Allsop, M.J. et al. (2019) 'Symptoms and concerns among children and young people with life-limiting and life-threatening conditions: a systematic review highlighting meaningful health outcomes'. *The Patient – Patient-Centred Outcomes Research*, 12: 15–55.

NICE (National Institute for Health and Care Excellence) (2016) End of life care for infants, children and young people with life-limiting conditions: planning and management. NICE guideline [NG61]. Updated July 2019. Available at: www.nice.org.uk/guidance/ng61.

Papadatou, D., Kalliani, V., Karakosta, E., Liakopoulou, P. and Bluebond-Langner, M. (2021) 'Home or hospital as the place of end-of-life care and death: a grounded theory study of parents' decision-making'. *Palliative Medicine*, 35 (1): 219–30.

Pohlkamp, L., Kreicbergs, U. and Sveen, J. (2019) 'Factors during a child's illness are associated with levels of prolonged grief symptoms in bereaved mothers and fathers'. *Journal of Clinical Oncology*, 38 (2): 137–44.

Popejoy, E. (2015) 'Parents' experiences of care decisions about children with life-limiting illnesses'. *Nursing Children and Young People*, 27 (8): 20–4.

Price, J., Jordan, J., Prior, L. and Parkes, J. (2011) 'Living through the death of a child: a qualitative study of bereaved parents' experiences'. *International Journal of Nursing Studies*, 48 (11): 1384–92.

RCPCH (Royal College of Paediatrics and Child Health) (2020) Child mortality. Available at: https://stateofchildhealth.rcpch.ac.uk/evidence/mortality/child-mortality/ (accessed 24 April 2023).

Sharman, M., Meert, K. and Sarnaik, A (2005) 'What influences parents' decisions to limit or withdraw life support?' *Pediatric Critical Care Medicine*, 6 (5): 513–18.

Tatterton, M.J. and Walshe, C. (2019) 'Understanding the bereavement experience of grandparents following the death of a grandchild from a life-limiting condition: a meta-ethnography'. *Journal of Advanced Nursing*, 75 (7):1406–17.

Together for Short Lives (2018) *A Guide to Children's Palliative Care: Supporting babies, children and young people with life-limiting and life-threatening conditions and their families*, 4th edn. Bristol: Together for Short Lives. Available at: www.togetherforshortlives.org.uk/resource/a-guide-to-childrens-palliative-care/.

Verberne, L.M., Fahner, J.C., Sondaal, S.F.V. et al. (2021) 'Anticipating the future of the child and family in pediatric palliative care: a qualitative study into the perspectives of parents and healthcare professionals'. *European Journal of Paediatrics*, 180: 949–57.

Verberne, L.M., Kars, M.C., Schouten-van Meeteren, A.Y.N., van den Bergh, E.M.M., Bosman, D.K., Colenbrander, D.A. et al. (2019) 'Parental experiences and coping strategies when caring for a child receiving paediatric palliative care: a qualitative study'. *European Journal of Paediatrics*, 178 (7): 1075–85.

Widdas, D., McNamara, K. and Edwards, F. (2013) *A Core Care Pathway for Children with Life-limiting and Life-threatening Conditions*, 3rd edn. Bristol: Together for Short Lives. Available at: www.togetherforshortlives.org.uk/assets/0000/4121/TfSL_A_Core_Care_Pathway__ONLINE_.pdf.

Wolfe, J., Orellana, L., Ullrich, C., Cook, E. F., Kang, T. I., Rosenberg, A. et al. (2015) 'Symptoms and distress in children with advanced cancer: prospective patient-reported outcomes from the PediQUEST study'. *Journal of Clinical Oncology*, 33 (17): 1928–35.

Zernikow, B., Szybalski, K., Hübner-Möhler, B., Wager, J., Paulussen, M., Lassay, L. et al. (2019) 'Specialized pediatric palliative care services for children dying from cancer: a repeated cohort study on the developments of symptom management and quality of care over a 10-year period'. *Palliative Medicine*, 33: 381–91.

CARE OF CHILDREN AND YOUNG PEOPLE WITH LEARNING DISABILITIES

34

TRISH GRIFFIN AND JANE LOPEZ

THIS CHAPTER COVERS

- Changing ideas and value base around children with learning disabilities
- The health, care and educational pathways that children with a learning disability follow
- The changing nature of learning disability
- Challenges to children's health and wellbeing

"
"Working alongside children with learning disabilities and their families is such a privilege. As a children's nursing student, I have learnt so much from spending time with children and their families. Their often complex and multifaceted health issues require a significant depth of knowledge and understanding to be able to provide high-quality care that is family focused."

Sarah, 3rd-year children's nursing student
"

INTRODUCTION

Every child, no matter what their individual and unique set of needs are, deserves the right to be cared for, supported, and treated with all aspects of their uniqueness met. Look past the disability and see the child. This chapter seeks to dispel misunderstandings by providing insights into children with learning disabilities and their families by explaining some of the key issues that shape their lives. Importantly, it seeks to enable you to focus on maximising the health and needs of the child and not their disability. Sarah's quote at the start of the chapter will tempt you to learn strategies you can adopt to support children with a learning disability across a range of settings and needs, including effective communication and inclusiveness (Beacock et al., 2015). Sarah in the quote above acknowledges the complex and multi-faceted health issues that shape the lives of children with learning disability and their families. With this in mind, the chapter that follows provides an examination of the diversity of issues. You will be inspired to extend your knowledge and understanding. This will empower you to deliver first-rate child-centred professional care based on your professional code of practice (NMC, 2018a) that ensures that the wishes and desires of the child lead to personalisation of support (Northway and Hopes, 2022: 35).

Changing ideas and value base around children with learning disabilities

Since the introduction of the NHS in 1948 significant influences have continued to shape the delivery of care and education services for children with learning disabilities. These changes gained momentum during the 1970s and 1980s with a dramatic move away from a medical model and segregated patterns of care based on the child's condition. The late 20th century heralded a cautious emergence of enlightened social policies focusing on child-centred approaches, developing each child to their fullest potential. Most notable were education, health and social care initiatives that began to implement a range of new health, education and social care policies and legislation including:

- Care Act 2014
- Children Act 1989
- Children Act 2004
- Children and Families Act 2014
- Disability Discrimination Act 1995
- Disability Discrimination (Northern Ireland) Order 2006
- Education Act 1981
- Education Act 1996
- Education Act 2011
- Education (Wales) Act 2014
- Education (Scotland) Act 2016
- Every Child Matters (Cm 5860; HM Treasury, 2003)
- Human Rights Act 1998
- National Health Service and Community Care Act 1990
- Special Educational Needs and Disability Act 2001
- The Equality Act 2010 (Northern Ireland)
- Valuing People: A New Strategy for Learning Disability for the 21st Century (Cm 5086, 2001)
- Working Together to Safeguard Children (HM Government, 2015, 2018) (all legislation accessisble at www.legislation.gov.uk/)`

The politicisation of ideas such as human rights, social role valorisation and integration alongside changes in terminology were perceived as moving service emphasis towards child rights. Innovative thinking concerning inclusion and the removal of disabling social, language, and environmental barriers challenged existing service provision. Labels previously used to categorise children such as 'mentally defective', 'subnormal' or 'mentally handicapped' were contested and seen as stigmatising. New terminology emerged – learning disability.

The USA, Republic of Ireland and Australia use the term 'intellectual disability'. The term 'global development delay' is recognised internationally. British social policy now uses 'learning disabled' and 'learning disability' with confusion arising as to how that differs from 'learning difficulties'. MENCAP (n.d.a) describes learning disability as 'a reduced intellectual ability and difficulty with everyday activities – e.g., household tasks, socialising, which affects someone for their whole life'. Most learning disabilities arise from a condition before, during or shortly after birth/childhood. It is estimated that 1.2 million people in England have a learning disability (Health Education England, 2023) although MENCAP (n.d.a) suggest this figure is 1.5 million people and who have 'significantly poorer health and increased age-adjusted mortality than their non-disabled peers' and therefore, greater health inequalities. Public Health England (PHE) stated that in 2014/2015, 70,065 children in England had a primary need associated with learning disability and had a statement of educational needs/education health and care plan (Barber, 2022: 15). There can also be associated issues such as:

- Cognitive ability – thinking and/or reasoning skills
- Communication strategies and skills
- Functional – practical, organisational skills
- Learning and educational development
- Memory
- Physical coordination, issues with mobility
- Physical and mental wellbeing
- Social behaviour

Whereas a learning difficulty constitutes a condition that creates an obstacle to a specific form of learning this does not affect the overall intelligence of an individual child. For example, a child with Rett syndrome is classed as having a learning disability but a child with dyslexia is classed as having a learning difficulty. There is obfuscation over both terms because the child is designated as having a statement of 'special educational needs/Education and Health Care Plan (EHC)'. This therefore signposts the formal provision of additional services. Children are further categorised by their ability within the range of learning disability – mild, moderate or severe. Additionally, a number of children can have more complex needs; these children are defined as having profound and multiple disabilities (PMLD) (Barr and Gates, 2019; Barber, 2022; MENCAP, n.d.a). Children with PMLD may also have:

- Profound, complex intellectual and multiple disabilities
- Severe communication problems
- Often extreme physical and/or sensory disabilities
- Complex health needs

It is important that you have an idea of the different terminology and (negative) 'labels' as these define the way both children (and adults) are not only perceived but also the care and services they receive; they are not meant to be negative constructs. Your strong value base strongly underpins your practice as a nurse.

———— TAKE A LOOK ————

MENCAP have produced many resources, including one explaining what a learning disability is. This short video can be found on YouTube:

https://youtu.be/9Tls8PyUVKc

THE CARE AND EDUCATIONAL PATHWAYS THAT CHILDREN WITH A LEARNING DISABILITY FOLLOW

Accessing services: The early years

Parents anticipate their baby reaching the early milestones. When this does not happen, it is a time of great anxiety for the family. Some babies born with more complex developmental and sensory problems may be identified at birth: parents are often the first to notice delays in their baby's progress and usually seek help via their friends, wider family, and professionals they trust, e.g., a health visitor (HV) or general practitioner (GP).

Valuing People Now (Department of Health, 2010) stated that best practice for children with a learning disability is access to a health service designed around their needs, delivered to a consistently high standard with additional support needed, early diagnosis and intervention are crucial. Currently, under section 23 of the Children and Families Act 2014, responsibility for early identification, assessment, diagnosis, intervention and review of the child's needs rests with the health service; the children's nurse plays a central role and to ensure that reasonable adjustments are made – this is a legal duty (PHE, 2020). Primary healthcare services include GPs, HVs, specialist nurses (e.g., community learning disability nurses, CLDN), speech and language therapists, dieticians, psychologists and physiotherapists. Often the professional most involved in the early years is the HV who has responsibility for checking the developmental achievements of the child as part of the universal Healthy Child Programme (Department of Health, 2009). Research from King's College London (Donetto et al., 2013) evidenced how the HV's coordination of care for the child contributed to parents being able to come to terms with and manage difficult circumstances.

HVs are well placed to advise parents about support. Charities such as MENCAP and the National Autistic Society (NAS) provide a wide range of resources and information. Others formed around specific conditions such as Down syndrome, Rett syndrome and mucopolysaccharide disorders, where families (and professionals) came together to enable research, share expert information and pool resources to improve their child's future outcomes.

During placement with a community-based nurse, you will have valuable learning opportunities to gain insight into the heath, social, educational, cultural and leisure aspects of both the child and family's life. Each insight will be unique and enable you to develop clinical, professional and communication skills (Beacock et al., 2015). *Strengthening the Commitment,* from the Scottish Government (2012), and subsequent documents, directs you to develop core knowledge and skills to work 'safely and appropriately' with people with learning disabilities. The Nursing and Midwifery Council also require that all nursing students and associate nurses are aware of the changing health and care needs of people (children and adults) and are expected to meet these as part of their education programme (NMC, 2018b).

CASE STUDY 34.1: JOANNA

You are on a placement with a health visitor. You have met Joanna, a single mother, her son Simon, aged 5, and her daughter Isabel, aged 2. The HV has arranged to undertake Isabel's health and development review. Isabel was diagnosed with Rett syndrome 2 months ago and is now having epileptic seizures and eating is proving very difficult for her. Joanna admits to being concerned about the impact Isabel is having on family life. Joanna also revealed that she finds Isabel's seizures absolutely terrifying. As you leave, Joanna argues with the HV that they – the professionals – must have got it wrong: Isabel will get better.

- Consider the psychosocial impact that a child with complex needs can have on family life.
- What professional skills do you think that the HV can use to establish a child-centred partnership with Joanna and her family?
- How can the HV help Joanna manage both Isabel's seizures and her own anxiety about the seizures?

Parents begin the difficult journey by establishing the nature of their child's unique issues, needs, and their 'diagnosis'. The ways in which parents and families learn (from professionals) can influence how they manage (or not) their child's unique circumstances and needs. Initially, parents may feel 'swamped' by facts and information, at times not given in a sensitive and understandable way by professionals who can use abbreviations and complex language. The HV and GP should remain a constant, enabling, for example, referral to the local authority's attention if they believe that the child has a disability, and may have special educational needs (SEN) (see Table 34.1).

Table 34.1 Special educational needs

Children will be considered to have a learning disability if any of the following conditions are met:

1. That they have been identified within education services as having a special educational need (SEN) associated with 'moderate learning difficulty', 'severe learning difficulty' or 'profound multiple learning difficulty' (Public Health England, 2016)

2. That they score lower than two standard deviations below the mean on a validated test of general cognitive functioning (equivalent to an IQ score of less than 70) or general development (ICD-11)

3. That they have been identified as having learning disabilities on locally held disability registers (including registers held by GP practices, community health services, e.g., through annual health checks (MENCAP, n.d.b) or at the local authority)

Since 1981 successive educational reforms have as their intent the ideal of all children attending mainstream schools, recognising that for some the need for an educational environment that provides an individualised learning environment where they can thrive is key. SEN or special schools were established where pupils can attend until they are 16 and, in England, until they are 18. Children and young people with a learning disability living in England and who have with a primary need associated with learning disabilities have a statement of special educational needs or an Education, Health and Care (EHC) plan (GOV.UK, n.d.; MENCAP, n.d.c).

In England in January 2022, the number of children and young people who had an EHCP was 473,300. This has increased each year since 2010. New EHC plans numbered 62,200 in 2021, this number is also rising. There were 93,300 initial requests for an EHC plan during 2021, up from 76,000 in 2020 (GOV.UK, n.d.).

There are approximately 1.2 to 1.5 million people living with learning disabilities and this number is likely to grow by 14% between 2001 and 2021.

For parents, meeting their child's needs becomes a paramount concern; it is vitally important that their concerns are heard by health professionals centrally placed to respond. The government continues to oblige the three major service providers to work together to meet the requirements and expressed wishes of the child and family. As previously mentioned, the Children and Families Act 2014 introduced the EHC plan, a carefully coordinated process to meet the assessed health, social and educational needs of the child. A child's EHC plan remains in place until they leave education and it is reviewed annually. Broadly speaking, Northern Ireland and Wales have similar systems and Scotland has articulated a clear commitment to support the child and their parents in removing barriers to services.

The school years

When a child with learning disabilities enters their school life, a key link for health and wellbeing is the school nurse. For a nursing associate or student nurse, a placement in a SEN school provides an opportunity to further gain professional, communication and clinical skills as well as working alongside nurses, therapists and teachers. School nurses (SN) work in partnership with the teaching team and support staff with children who require healthcare – e.g., medication. They play a major role in risk management (e.g., of epilepsy) and in health promotion, and can provide specific advice. SN work in partnership with other professionals, e.g., (CLDN), for expertise on, e.g., growing up, sexuality. Learning Disability nurses have a positive effect on meeting health outcomes for children (and adults) with learning disabilities (Scottish Government, 2012). This is an excellent opportunity for you to work closely with children who are not in a health setting and see first-hand how families, health, educational and community-based services work together in a child-first and family-centred approach.

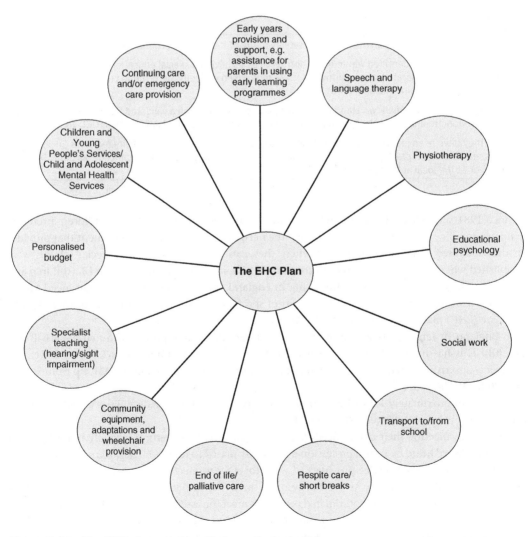

Figure 34.1 The EHC plan: services that may be included

Crucially, SNs can also identify emerging problems and make, in partnership with families, referrals to specialist services (e.g., Children and Young people's Mental Health (CYPMH) Services, Child and Adolescent Mental Health Services (CAMHS)). The prevalence rate of mental health needs amongst children with learning disabilities is thought to be much higher than amongst the mainstream school population, with 36% having a diagnosable mental health condition compared with 8% of those who do not have a learning disability (Foundation for People with Learning Disabilities, n.d.a) These figures are said to have increased greatly both during and post COVID-19, when children were isolated and social interaction and learning with peers and others was limited.

Parents play the major role in supporting their child's health and development although there are role tensions for parents and families, who need clear and easily understood health information. HVs, CLDNs and SNs are well placed to use their listening skills to hear, listen, and to learn from parents' stories and children's voices and to respect differences in families, e.g., cultural, diversity. This is an invaluable chance to observe skills and approaches that nurses use to establish clear two-way communication channels (e.g., school to home/home to school). The creation of opportunities for parents to share important aspects of their concerns and expectations are vital for their child's wellbeing and to begin to prepare them for the transition into adult services. As a student, you will have opportunity to both listen to and read at times, very personal yet insightful accounts into their lived experiences. These opportunities are most valuable as you learn from being *'in their shoes'*, which is a unique privilege.

THE TRANSITION FROM CHILDREN'S TO ADULT SERVICES

The transition from children's to adult services can be challenging, daunting and often unsettling for children and their families. Forward planning is crucial and ideally commences when the child is in their early teens. Planning for both health and educational transition is key. All children leave school and for children with learning disabilities, their school will have been a constant in their life since the age of 2. Parents may feel that the services that they have relied on will change or disappear as they move across to new, adult systems and provisions with their child. Person-centred planning with accessible information and honesty is both crucial and essential. When it is anticipated that a young person with an EHC plan will soon be leaving education or training, the local authority should agree in advance the support the young person might need to access and the support they might need to help them access it.

The Children's Commissioner for Wales in 2020 explored experiences and challenges that young people and families face transitioning to adult services. A number of good practices were highlighted, which included:

- Involving, listening to and hearing young people's desires and wishes
- Adequate support and access to appropriate support services
- Joined up working and planning together (Northway and Hopes, 2022: 159)

THE CHANGING NATURE OF LEARNING DISABILITY

Not only have services and attitudes changed, the children you meet are changing. Ground-breaking developments in healthcare alongside social change continue to impact on the nature of childhood learning disability. A hundred years ago, life expectancy for a child who had Down syndrome was under 10. In contrast, people with Down syndrome now live into older age, for example 70s. (See https://www.dailymail.co.uk/news/article-8823909/Britains-oldest-person-Downs-Syndrome-dies-aged-78.html)

Alongside care provision, legal changes in abortion laws and scientific developments in genetic screening have impacted on birth rates resulting in an acceptance of termination on detection of abnormalities – with some parents/mothers choosing to continue with their pregnancy whilst others not. Crucially, children who have difficulties arising from premature or very low birth weight have survived infancy due to advanced medical interventions. Inherited genetic conditions such as phenylketonuria and chromosomal abnormalities continue to result in children being born with a learning disability.

Improved public health measures have radically reduced the numbers of babies born to mothers who have had infections such as syphilis, toxoplasmosis or rubella during their pregnancy. Other children are identified as born with learning disabilities arising from lifestyle factors such as parental substance and alcohol misuse.

The disorders that result in a child being born with or developing a learning disability are too numerous to catalogue in this brief chapter. It is nonetheless an opportunity to provide you with more examples of conditions that illustrate the dimensions of a child's life that can be affected:

- Complications before, during or after birth
- Congenital/genetic abnormalities
- A debilitating illness or injury in early childhood affecting brain development – for example, meningitis or a road traffic accident
- Contact with damaging substances (e.g., alcohol, drugs, lead, toxins, or radiation) during pregnancy
- Neglect, physical abuse, and/or a lack of mental stimulation early in life (Barber, 2022; Foundation for People with Learning Disabilities, n.d.b)

In your practice, you are going to work with children, some of whom may have unique needs in addition to their learning disability. Here are some examples.

Children with cerebral palsy

Whilst not always resulting in a learning disability, cerebral palsy is a significant cause, and the resultant degree of learning disability varies greatly. Approximately 1 in 400 children are diagnosed with cerebral palsy, with the severity of symptoms varying greatly (SCOPE, n.d.). It is a lifelong condition affecting movement and coordination (NHS Scotland, 2017). Premature babies, especially those born before 26 weeks, are more likely to develop cerebral palsy. Cerebral palsy is not usually noticeable at birth, becoming more evident before 3 years of age.

Motor function problems are the distinguishing factor in cerebral palsy. Children may not reach milestones, be 'floppy or too stiff', have problems with sensory, communication and nutritional systems (particularly swallowing and aspiration) (Grayson et al., 2016) and may have a learning disability (NHS Scotland 2017). The National Institute of Health and Care Excellence (NICE, 2017) published guidance which will assist you when working with children with cerebral palsy, in particular regarding assessment and management.

To remind yourself of the relevant anatomy and physiology you can read chapters 12 and 16 in *Fundamentals of Children's Anatomy and Physiology: A Textbook for Nursing and Healthcare Students* (Peate and Gormley-Fleming, 2021).

Children with foetal alcohol spectrum disorder (FASD)

FASD is caused by exposure to alcohol prior to birth, directly attributable to the mother's consumption of alcohol. Alcohol is a teratogen and impacts on the growth and development of the embryo or foetus in the womb. Children may have a range of mild to severe intellectual and physical effects.

The number of children born each year with FASD is difficult to determine. Mothers may not disclose their drinking and professionals may misdiagnose. NICE in their briefing paper on FASD use data from Popova et al. (2017) which estimated a global prevalence of FASD of 7.7 per 1000 and in the UK, a prevalence of 32.4 per 1000 (NICE, 2019). It is important to note that whilst only a small proportion of these children will have learning disabilities, many will have neurocognitive defects that result in behavioural and learning difficulties.

ACTIVITY 34.1: CRITICAL THINKING

With the rate of children being born with FASD in the UK being more than three times higher than average across the world, do you consider that the government should take action to diminish the risks of foetal alcohol syndrome occurring and if so, how should public health agencies approach this? Discuss.

Children with Down syndrome

Down syndrome is most commonly caused by trisomy 21, an additional chromosome attached to chromosome 21 in every cell of the body. Children with Down syndrome resemble their parents and siblings but with some physical characteristics that are recognisable – for example, eyes with an epicanthic fold, broad hands with stubby fingers and a simian crease. The number of children born with Down syndrome, despite having declined since the introduction of screening, increased by 2009, which could be attributed to more people opting to start families later. Interestingly, an increasing number of mothers who were given results that indicated the risk following screening chose to go ahead with their pregnancies. Current estimates are that 1 in every 1000 babies (i.e., about 920) are born in the United Kingdom each year with Down syndrome (Down's Syndrome Association, n.d.a).

The Down's Syndrome Association (DSA) vision is to create conditions in which all people with Down syndrome live full and rewarding lives. They have spearheaded the 'Tell it Right® Start it Right' campaign from 2016 to ensure health professionals continue to provide information about Down syndrome in a non-biased manner – including non-invasive prenatal testing (NIPT) and addressing that prospective parents can feel pressurised into a termination when being given a very pessimistic view of the life chances of someone with Down syndrome, a view that is not always accurate.

SEE ALSO
CHAPTER 18

Children with Down syndrome are more prone to respiratory problems; they are more likely to breathe through their mouth. Between 40% and 60% of babies with Down syndrome have cardiac problems as a result of their congenital abnormality – for example, Fallot's tetralogy. Additionally, they are also at risk of hypothyroidism, atlanto-axial instability, leukaemia, delayed milk teeth and subsequent dental problems, ear and eye infections and lower white cell count.

The Down's Syndrome Association have developed a checklist as indicators of health issues that can be used during health checks with GPs and HVs (Down's Syndrome Association, n.d.b). Using this (and other checklists, e.g., hospital passports) will be an excellent learning opportunity for you whilst on placement with a HV or community nurse.

SEE ALSO
CHAPTERS 5,
9 AND 10

To remind yourself of the relevant anatomy and physiology please read the A&P link to *Fundamentals of Children's Anatomy and Physiology: A Textbook for Nursing and Healthcare Students* (Peate and Gormley-Fleming, 2021).

Children with autism

So what is autism? There are broad spectrums and diversities with definitions changing as we learn more about how autism can impact on our lives. Some need 24/7 support whilst others manage their lives without intervention and in their unique way. Children with (or without) learning disability are diagnosed/can be described as also being on the autistic spectrum, often experiencing difficulties making sense of their world and with their social imagination (National Autistic Society, n.d.). Because of these factors, children diagnosed with autism (and their families) can find their healthcare experience difficult. For children, an accurate autism assessment is required to determine the educational and healthcare (including psycho-social, visual, hearing, language, learning and culture) needs with interventions focusing on the context of their development. NICE has published guidance and recommendations for recognising and working with children who may be autistic (NICE, 2011).

As a healthcare professional, you will play an important role in helping parents improve their ability to communicate their concerns (however small these may seem) and to 'focus on the individual child, not their diagnosis' (Jones, 2015). This statement is echoed by the mother of Danny, a young person of 15 years with autism and who lives a full, unique life based on an individualised person-centred care package, especially relevant as Danny prepares transition to adult services in a few years' time.

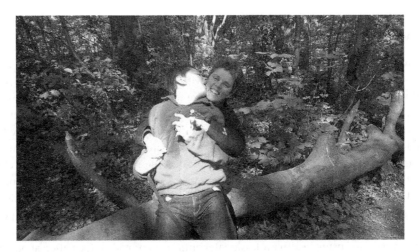

Figure 34.2 Danny

Autism spectrum disorder (ASD) is a developmental condition affecting the way the brain processes information. It occurs in varying levels, from minor to severe, is a lifelong condition with no single cause. About four times as many boys as girls are diagnosed (National Autistic Society, n.d.). ASD has a wide range of symptoms, often grouped into two main categories: problems with social interaction and communication, such as understanding other people's emotions and feelings, and restricted and repetitive patterns of thought, interests and physical behaviours (Jones, 2015). NICE suggest around half have an intellectual (learning) disability and approximately 70% have at least one other mental or physical health problem, often unrecognised, including eating and sleeping problems, epilepsy, anxiety, depression, attention deficit hyperactivity disorder and dyspraxia (Jones, 2015).

Signs of autism can be noticed in some children aged 2 (possibly earlier), becoming more noticeable as children grow. The role of the HV is crucial, as are nursery staff and teachers, to assist in assessment and an early, correct diagnosis. Appropriate support and interventions including social interaction, communication and cognitive skill development are key as well as access to key professional and educational provision via a specialist team (NICE, 2021). A key point for you is that effective and appropriate communication techniques are essential and that you listen to and hear parental and family concerns.

SEE ALSO
CHAPTER 2

ACTIVITY 34.2: CRITICAL THINKING

What communication skills and techniques do you need to communicate effectively with a child who is on the autistic spectrum? Where can you seek assistance in developing and refining these skills?

CHALLENGES TO CHILDREN'S HEALTH AND WELLBEING

Respiratory problems

Children with PMLD are more at risk of developing a respiratory problem because the nature of their disability may make them more prone to aspiration. The risk of this happening needs to be fully assessed by the multidisciplinary team. Dysphagia is also a problem Where children have difficulties swallowing this may be compounded by difficulty in coughing, which may lead to fluid and food entering the lungs. The number of children with learning disabilities who have enteral feeding to manage their nutritional needs has increased. A side effect of non-oral feeding is increased saliva production, which in turn may lead to aspiration.

An increase in enteral feeding has resulted in fewer hospital admissions for children with respiratory disease. Other physical abnormalities can also contribute to poor respiratory function; children with specific syndromes or birth defects, spinal problems such as kyphoscoliosis and neuromuscular defects can prevent the child breathing normally. Children can have asthma and allergies that impact on their ability to breathe with ease.

Nutrition

You may be working with children who have difficulties with their nutritional status. A common cause of malnutrition is insufficient dietary intake because of feeding/eating difficulties. Some may overeat as the result of an inherited condition, of which Prader–Willi syndrome is a good example. A defect in chromosome 15 disrupts the functioning of the hypothalamus, which plays a part in the production of hormones but, importantly, in regulating appetite.

Children may have their ability to consume and enjoy food impaired by several factors: these include physical, behavioural or possible autism. Physically, some conditions (e.g., foetal alcohol syndrome and Down syndrome) may result in the child having a deformity of their oral cavity or difficulties resulting in problems with sucking, chewing, swallowing, choking and aspiration. Detailed assessment by the multidisciplinary team of this may result in modifications, including how the child receives their nutrition.

You will need to be crucially aware of children's developing teeth and the condition of their gums and mouth. Certain medications can affect gums and cleaning teeth can for some children due to deformities or sensitivities, may be challenging. A speech and language therapist can advise as well as a dentist/dental nurse as to management techniques, use of electric toothbrushes, etc.

Children with physical disabilities may be unable to move themselves into a position that makes eating a comfortable and enjoyable process. Functionally and behaviourally some children may struggle or never develop the skills to eat by themselves unaided. There are a range of utensils and devices available to enable children to learn to eat independently or more independently.

Some children have problems with attention or proximity, or disruptive conduct (i.e., refusing to sit and refusal of food) that maintaining their mealtimes can be challenging. It is essential that you monitor children's food intake and are aware of over- and under-nutrition and closely monitor the child's nutritional status.

WHAT'S THE EVIDENCE?

Feeding children with cerebral palsy orally may encourage oral motor function, including language development skills. Enteral feeding may, however, be more effective in providing nutrition and hydration. Approaches to risk management for minimising the risk of aspiration is a key determinant in reaching a decision to provide an enteral intervention (Arvedson, 2013). However, evidence suggests that this is not always beneficial to family life, and the debate continues about giving children the opportunity for oral taste and the social aspects of feeding experiences.

- How can children's nurses help empower the child and their family to make difficult choices that involve discussions about risk management in this situation?

Epilepsy

The Epilepsy Society (n.d.a) estimate that around 1 in 5 people with learning (or intellectual) disability have epilepsy. Not only does it manifest much earlier in childhood, the more severe the learning disability the greater the incidence. Some children may have epilepsy as part of their syndrome – for example, Fragile X; some, resulting from their condition, for example, cerebral palsy. Seizures may be more difficult to manage until a management regime is in place. This is likely to include anticonvulsant medication, which needs to be carefully managed. The ketogenic diet (Epilepsy Society, n.d.b) may be tried when epilepsy does not respond to treatment, for example. Parents may be faced with administering emergency medication as well as managing regular medications. Enabling parents to make judgements and gain skills to manage their child's epilepsy requires you to be a skilled practitioner with advanced communication and education skills, and clinical knowledge in what could be a life-threatening situation.

CHILDREN WITH LEARNING DISABILITIES AND BEHAVIOURS THAT CAN CHALLENGE

All children require individual approaches. Parents and families can be adversely affected by the demands of physical care but more so by the level of behavioural problems Children who present with the most demanding behaviour problems can be referred to as having 'challenging behaviours or behaviours that can challenge'. This is broadly categorised in four ways: aggressive, destructive, or engaging in self-injurious behaviours or stereotypical behaviours. Some examples of behaviour that can challenge could include:

- Self-injuring, e.g., hurting themself and/or others, head banging, eye poking, biting, scratching themselves, head butting
- Destructive or aggressive behaviours, e.g., breaking or tearing things up
- Eating inedible objects, e.g., stones, pen tops, bedding, paper

- Making loud noises, screaming
- Spitting, smearing

NICE (2015) published clear recommendations and guidance around provisions of care for children whose behaviour challenges, including understanding of what the challenges are and providing child-centred interventions.

Developmental delays impede the ability to communicate and understand, and the learning disabled child may not progress to more 'acceptable behaviour/s'. It is essential to recognise that health and medical conditions can also be an underlying factor in behaviours that can challenge – for example, particularly painful are irritating inflammatory conditions such as earache and toothache. The child's means of communicating this to you could be to scream or lash out. This could be said for children showing other forms of behaviours that challenge, that it is a way of expressing themselves.

For parents, the impact on the quality of life of the family may be very distressing. For professionals, meeting the health, educational and social care needs of the child and family in a person-centred way demands a collaborative and effective approach. From the child's perspective it can put their personal safety at risk, disrupt home life and can lessen their ability to be included in ordinary social, educational, and recreational activities. In turn this can further affect their development by causing problems with their learning and attainment; their behaviour may be not only disruptive but put others at risk.

Interventions and management techniques are varied and too many to list in this chapter. However, the over-riding theme is consistency with the needs and rights of the child at the centre (United Nations, 1989), with interventions using non-restrictive practice.

CASE STUDY 34.2: RAVI

Ravi is currently on a children's ward whilst essential surgery is carried out to improve his bilateral cavovarous feet. Ravi finds the hospital environment very difficult. Ravi has severe learning disabilities and ASD. Ravi communicates with a few words and by PECS (Picture Exchange Communication System). Ravi shouts repetitively, slaps his face and furniture, then laughs loudly at the noise he makes. Ravi is constantly active, climbing out of his bed and onto the floor. When staff attempt to return Ravi to his bed he screams loudly and slaps his face. Ravi's mother suggests that the staff try wrapping Ravi tightly in his bedding as this is what she does at home.

- What might be the impact of Ravi's behaviour on the other children and parents in the ward?
- Why may children display enhanced problem behaviours in the clinical/hospital environment?

Suggest strategies that you could use to communicate with Ravi.

COMMUNICATION AND THE CHILD IN THE HEALTH SETTING

You are well placed to be supportive to both the child and the parents, by listening to them and to their concerns as well as assisting them to face the daunting challenge of providing multifaceted care over a protracted length of time. It can be difficult to help any child make sense of what is happening to them in a health setting; those with a learning disability face a greater challenge. They require nurses and other staff to use their extensive interpersonal skills to create a relationship that comforts the child (and their parents/family) and facilitates the care and interventions the child requires. Some children, for example those with ASD, will have a communication passport. It is crucial that you familiarise yourself with these as what you may see the child exhibiting may be the way that they communicate with you.

For many children with learning disabilities communicating can prove difficult. Parents and siblings often develop systems of understanding, picking up on cues of body language, using eye contact and facial expressions to interpret and convey meanings. Makaton and PECS are widely used as augmentative communication systems to assist children in finding their voice. Technological advances in Voice Output Communication Aids (VOCA) provide wonderful opportunities for most severely disabled children to express their needs and to interact. Books beyond Words have a range of health-related picture-only materials, including a selection for children with learning disabilities. Many apps are also available.

Many hospitals employ acute liaison nurses for children (and for adults) with learning disabilities. These are crucial roles and central to the navigation and communication of complex healthcare pathways that children can have. Acute liaison nurses enhance communication (and understanding) of the child's unique set of needs to both the child, their family and staff, and act as a link between the hospital, child/their family and community services. When on placement do seek out these nurses and shadow them to learn about the uniqueness of their role and skills.

Lessons learnt and good practice

Communication and coordination of care on every level are crucially important. Where this does not happen, the consequences can be devastating. Following successive investigations into avoidable deaths amongst patients with learning disabilities in acute hospital settings, service providers have been developing strategies to improve the care and communication experiences and review avoidable deaths. The Learning Disabilities Mortality Review (LeDeR) Programme commissioned by the Healthcare Quality Improvement Partnership (HQIP) on behalf of NHS England in June 2015, reviewed the deaths of people with learning disabilities aged 4 years and over, irrespective of whether the death was expected or not, the cause of death or the place of death. This identifies good practice and what has worked well, as well as where improvements to the provision of care could be made (NHS LeDeR, n.d.).

Oliver McGowan, a teenager with autism, died in hospital in 2016, as a result of being given antipsychotic medication against both Oliver's and his family's wishes. Oliver's mother, Paula, has tirelessly led a campaign for more training and education for health and social care staff to gain knowledge, skills and confidence to understand the needs and wishes of people who have learning disabilities and/or autism in their care. Paula's campaign has resulted in Health Education England (HEE) and Skills for Care developing a mandatory training package for health and social care staff, named and in honour of Oliver McGowan (HEE, 2021). Skills for Health and Skills for Care in 2019 updated the Core Capabilities Frameworks for (a) supporting people with learning disabilities and (b) supporting people with autism. As a nursing student, you will be expected to demonstrate skills and capabilities for effective partnership working and demonstrate the appropriate competencies in preparation for registration with the Nursing and Midwifery Council as part of the Standards for Education (NMC, 2018b).

There are many examples of good practice where 'alerts' are in place to raise staff awareness – in a sensitive way – that a child with learning disabilities is receiving care. Wales spearheaded the 'Care Bundle' which sets out the steps to be taken to ensure the safety of patients of all ages who have a learning disability in hospital or in an accident and emergency department. This is used countrywide. Derriford Hospital uses a system of NHS mail alerts that notify GPs, community teams for learning disabilities and other key liaison staff when a child or young adult with a learning disability is admitted. Great Ormond Street Hospital has developed a 'purple dot' added to the child's notes to denote that they have a learning disability. In addition, the expertise of specialist groups such as the NAS have helped develop communication and hospital passports that focus on individual needs – thus aiding communication with a child who, for example, does not like being touched – and gives their preferred name, how they eat, their health needs, etc.

ACTIVITY 34.3: REFLECTIVE PRACTICE

- Practise and learn eight Makaton signs that you consider essential to making a child feel reassured in an acute hospital setting
- Compile a list of questions that you consider essential to include in a communication or hospital passport for a young child with PMLD or ASD
- How could you reassure a young child who is on the autistic spectrum and does not like having people in close proximity or being touched?
- Explore how 'Books Beyond Words' can assist you in communicating with children (or their parents) who have a learning disability
- Reflect on your time with acute liaison nurses and list the benefits of their unique role

SEE ALSO
CHAPTER 9

SAFEGUARDING

It is suggested that children with disabilities are three times more at risk of physical, sexual and emotional abuse and neglect than their non-disabled peers, boys being more at risk than girls. Although a contentious issue, in some communities disabled children can be more at risk due to beliefs about 'evil spirits and witchcraft'. (For more information see Miller and Brown, 2014.) Children with learning disabilities are not a heterogeneous group; they manifest their needs and issues in many ways. Recognising that the children who are most at risk are children whose behaviours can be difficult or different to manage and challenge service provision helps to safeguard their welfare. The law differs in the four countries of the UK:

- England – https://learning.nspcc.org.uk/child-protection-system/england
- Northern Ireland – https://learning.nspcc.org.uk/child-protection-system/northern-ireland
- Scotland – https://learning.nspcc.org.uk/child-protection-system/scotland
- Wales – https://learning.nspcc.org.uk/child-protection-system/wales

---

As a student, you will need to be fully aware of safeguarding policy and procedures as they will differ depending on where you are in practice, e.g., in England, London has differences to neighbouring Surrey. Consider the whole picture and do raise any concerns that you may have with your practice assessors, practice supervisors or to the professionals you are in practice with (NMC, 2018b).

ACTIVITY 34.4: CRITICAL THINKING

In the previous case Ravi's behaviour is deemed to be causing problems and concerns on the ward. Ravi's mother sometimes secures him in his bed by wrapping him tightly in the bedding. These actions could be seen as a 'restrictive practice' which is unacceptable. The ward manager must ensure that the organisation's safeguarding protocols are followed.

Debate the issues here:

- Who is right and why?
- What strategies could be put in place to support Ravi and his mother during his stay in hospital?
- Who could provide specialist input and support and what could this be?

The Nursing and Midwifery Council (2018a) provide guidance for students and registrants in *The Code*.

For nursing students, the key requisite underpinning working with children who have learning disabilities is openness to learn about the whole child, extending both the child's communication skills and your own. Each child is unique and every encounter is different. This chapter has as its intent to motivate trainee nursing associates and nursing students to investigate the potential of the child with a learning disability notwithstanding their significant needs, problems, desires and wishes, and to design and deliver professional, competent nursing care and support.

CHAPTER SUMMARY

- Children with learning disabilities spend as much of their lives in an educational setting, where many of the child's needs are met, as in their home
- Effective communication is key to child-centred health, education and social care
- An extensive range of health, social and educational provision is available, delivered by experts with children's nurses at the centre – relationships become well established and knowledge is shared, problems are addressed and creatively resolved

BUILD YOUR BIBLIOGRAPHY

Books

FURTHER
READING

- Barr, O. and Gates, B. (2019) *Oxford Handbook of Learning and Intellectual Disability Nursing*, 2nd edn. Oxford: Oxford University Press.

  This new edition integrates a community-based approach with a greater focus the changing demography of the learning-disabled population i.e., on children and young adults with complex physical health needs as well as on older people.
- Norway, R. and Hopes, P. (2022) *Learning Disability Nursing*. St Albans: Critical Publishing.

  Well-reviewed text on learning disability nursing, suitable for pre and post registration nurses and with key themes of person-centred, values-based and multi-partnership working and learning.

Journal articles

FURTHER
READING:
ONLINE
JOURNAL
ARTICLES

- Evans, N. (2022) 'Abuse and neglect: what you can do to end bad practice'. *Learning Disability Practice*, 26 (1): 10–13. doi: 10.7748/ldp.26.1.10.s3.
- Golding, S. and Reynolds, E. (2022) 'Supporting a young person with autism and learning disability through transition from child to adult services'. *Learning Disability Practice*. doi: 10.7748/ldp.2022.e1964.
- Hennessy, T. and Doody, O. (2023) 'Taking blood from a person with learning disability: reflections on a parent's perspective'. *Learning Disability Practice*. doi: 10.7748/ldp.2023.e2204.
- Jarrett, S. and Tilley, E. (2022) 'The history of learning disability'. *British Journal of Learning Disabilities*, 50 (2): 132–42.
- Ridley, J. and Hopes, P. (2022) 'Reducing the use of restrictive paractices by applying a human rights based approach'. *Learning Disability Practice*. doi: 10.7748/ldp.2022.e2171.
- Wood, J. and Hartley-Smith, T-A. (2022) 'Supporting the mental health of children and young people with learning disabilities during Covid-19'. *Learning Disability Practice*. doi:10.7748/ldp.2022.e2195.

Weblinks

- NSPCC (Miller and Brown, 2014) *'We Have the Right to Be Safe*: Protecting Disabled Children from Abuse www.nspcc.org.uk/globalassets/documents/research-reports/right-safe-disabled-children-abuse-report.pdf
- NHS Choices, *Down's Syndrome* www.nhs.uk/Conditions/downs-syndrome/Pages/Introduction.aspx
- Children and Young People with Mental Health Needs, Autism or Learning Disability (2022) elearning for healthcare https://portal.e-lfh.org.uk/Component/Details/743132
- Makaton signs for nurses/doctors - Isabella signs https://www.youtube.com/watch?v=KMpqsnzy1P8

FURTHER
READING:
WEBLINKS

REFERENCES

Arvedson, J. C. (2013) 'Feeding children with cerebral palsy and swallowing difficulties'. *European Journal of Clinical Nutrition*, 67 Suppl 2.S2 (2013): S9–S12. Available at doi: 10.1038/ejcn.2013.22 (accessed 23 January 2023).

Barber, C. (2022) *Learning Disabilities A non-specialist introduction for nursing, health and social care.* Banbury: Lantern Publishing Ltd.

Barr, O., and Gates, B. (2019) *Oxford Handbook of Learning and Intellectual Disability Nursing*, 2nd edn. New York, NY: Oxford University Press.

Beacock, S., Borthwick, R., Kelly, J., Craine, R. and Jelfs, E. (2015) Learning Disabilities Meeting Educational Needs of Nursing Students. The UK Learning and Intellectual Disability Nursing Academic Network (LIDNAN) and the UK Council of Deans of Health (CoDH). Available at: www.councilofdeans.org.uk/wp-content/uploads/2015/01/LD-Nursing-report-Jan-15-Final.pdf (accessed 21 January 2023).

Beyond Words (n.d.) *Beyond Words empowering people through pictures.* Available at: booksbeyondwords.co.uk/ (accessed 13 July 2023).

Care Act 2014. Available at: www.legislation.gov.uk/ukpga/2014/23/contents accessed 19 January 2023).

Children Act 1989. Available at: www.legislation.gov.uk/ukpga/1989/41/contents (accessed 24 October 2023).

Children and Families Act 2014. Available at: www.legislation.gov.uk/ukpga/2014/6/contents/enacted (accessed 19 January 2023).

Communication Matters (n.d.) Types of AAC – Voice output communication aids. Available at: www.communicationmatters.org.uk/what-is-aac/types-of-aac/ (accessed 13 July 2023).

Department of Health (2009) *Healthy Child Programme: Pregnancy and the First Five Years of Life.* Available at: https://assets.publishing.service.gov.uk/government/uploads/system/uploads/attachment_data/file/167998/Health_Child_Programme.pdf (accessed 19 January 2023).

Department of Health (2001) *Valuing People: A New Strategy for Learning Disability for the 21st Century.* Norwich: Stationary Office. Available at https://assets.publishing.service.gov.uk/government/uploads/system/uploads/attachment_data/file/250877/5086.pdf (accessed 23 January 2023).

Disability Discrimination Act 1995. Available at www.legislation.gov.uk/ukpga/1995/50#:~:text=An%20Act%20to%20make%20it,establish%20a%20National%20Disability%20Council. (accessed 14 July 2023).

Donetto, S., Malone, M., Hughes, J., Morrow, E., Cowley, S. and Maben, J. (2013) Health visiting: the voice of service users - Learning from service users' experiences to inform the development of UK health visiting practice and services. London: National Nursing Research Unit, King's College London. Available at: www.kcl.ac.uk/archive/news/nmpc/2013/trusting-relationships-key-to-building-parental-confidence (accessed 13 July 2023).

Down's Syndrome Association (2018) Tell it Right ®. Available at www.downs-syndrome.org.uk/news/news-research/dsa-news/tell-it-right-update-may-2018/ (accessed 13 July 2023).

Down's Syndrome Association (2021) Annual health check information for GP's. Available at www.downs-syndrome.org/wp-content/uploads/2021/04/Annual-Health-Check-2021.pdf (accessed 23 January 2023).

Down's Syndrome Association (2023) About Downs Syndrome. Available at www.down-syndrome.org/en-gb/about-down-syndrome/ (accessed 23 January 2023).

Education Act 1981. Available at www.legislation.gov.uk/ukpga/1981/60/enacted (accessed 19 January 2023).

Education Act 1996. Available at www.legislation.gov.uk/ukpga/1996/56/contents (accessed 19 January 2023).

Education Act 2011. Available at www.legislation.gov.uk/ukpga/2011/21/contents/enacted (accessed 19 January 2023).

Education (Wales) Act 2014. Available at www.legislation.gov.uk/anaw/2014/5/contents/enacted (accessed 23 January 2023).

Education (Scotland) Act 2016. Available at www.legislation.gov.uk/asp/2016/8/enacted#~:text=An%20Act%20of%20the%20Scottish,to%20make%20provision%20in%20relation (accessed 23 January 2023).

Emerson, E. and Heslop, P,. (2010) *A Working Definition of Learning Disabilities.* Improving Health and Lives: Learning Disabilities Observatory. Available at www.researchgate.net/publication/265306674_A_working_definition_of_Learning_Disabilities#~:text=Children%20will%20be%20considered%20to%20have%20a%20learning,%E2%80%98severe%20learning%20difficulty%E2%80%99%20or%20%E2%80%98profound%20multiple%20learning%20difficulty%E2%80%99. (accessed 16 July 2023).

Epilepsy Society (2023a) *Learning Disabilities.* Available at https://epilepsysociety.org.uk/learning-disabilities (accessed 23 January 2023).

Epilepsy Society (2023b) *Anti-seizure Medication.* Available at https://epilepsysociety.org.uk/about-epilepsy/treatment/medication-epilepsy/anti-seizure-medication (accessed 13 July 2023).

Epilepsy Society (2023c) *Ketogenic diet.* Available at: https://epilepsysociety.org.uk/about-epilepsy/treatment/ketogenic-diet (accessed 13 July 2023).

Equality Act 2010. Available at www.legislation.gov.uk/ukpga/2010/15/contents (accessed 24 January 2023).

Equality Commission for Northern Ireland (2005) Disability Discrimination Code of Practice for Schools: Special Educational Needs and Disability (Northern Ireland) Order 2005. Available at www.equalityni.org/ECNI/media/ECNI/Publications/Employers%20and%20Service%20Providers/SENDOCoPforSchools2006.pdf (accessed 16 July 2023).

Every Child Matters (2003) Available at: https://assets.publishing.service.gov.uk/government/uploads/system/uploads/attachment_data/file/272064/5860.pdf (accessed 23 January 2023).

Foundation for People with Learning Disabilities (2023a) Learning Disability Statistics. Available at www.learningdisabilities.org.uk/learning-disabilities/help-information/learning-disability-statistics-/187699#~:text=For%20children%20and%20young%20people%2C%20the%20prevalence%20rate,those%20who%20did%20not%20have%20a%20learning%20disability (accessed 12 July 2023).

Foundation for People with Learning Disabilities (2023b) What causes learning disability? Available at: www.learningdisabilities.org.uk/learning-disabilities/a-to-z/l/learning-disabilities (accessed 23 January 2023).

GOV.UK (2023) Education, health and care plans Reporting year 2023. Available at https://explore-education-statistics.service.gov.uk/find-statistics/education-health-and-care-plans (accessed 13 July 2023).

GOV.UK (n.d. a) Education, health and care (EHC) plan. Available at www.gov.uk/children-with-special-educational-needs/extra-SEN-help (accessed 13 July 2023).

Grayson, R., Morling, E., Wing, J., Tusiine, H. and Oxtoby, G. (2016) *Supporting Children with Cerebral Palsy*, 2nd edn. London: David Fulton Publishers.

Health Education England (2021) The Oliver McGowan Mandatory Training in Learning Disability and Autism. Available at www.hee.nhs.uk/our-work/learning-disability/current-projects/oliver-mcgowan-mandatory-training-learning-disability-autism (accessed 13 July 2023)

Health Education England (2023) Learning Disability Available at hee.nhs.uk (accessed 19 January 2023)

HM Government (2018) *Working Together to Safeguard Children A guide to inter-agency working to safeguard and promote the welfare of children.* Available at: https://assets.publishing.service.gov.uk/media/5fd0a8e78fa8f54d5d6555f9/Working_together_to_safeguard_children_inter_agency_guidance.pdf (accessed 16 July 2023)

Human Rights Act 1998 Available at www.legislation.gov.uk/ukpga/1998/42/contents (accessed 19 January 2023).

International Classification of Diseases and Related Health Problems 11th Revision (2022) Available at ICD-11 (who.int) (accessed 13 July 2023).

Jones, S. (2015) 'Clinical update: Autism spectrum disorder'. *Nursing Standard,* 29 (38): 19–19 Available at http://journals.rcni.com/nursing-standard/autism-spectrum-disorder-ns.29.38.19.s20 (accessed 13 July 2023).

MENCAP (n.d. a) *What is a Learning Disability? Our Definition.* Available at: www.mencap.org.uk/learning-disability-explained/what-learning-disability (accessed 19 January 2023).

MENCAP (n.d. b) *Don't Miss Out – Annual Health Checks.* Available at: www.mencap.org.uk/advice-and-support/health/annual-health-checks (accessed 19 January 2023).

MENCAP (n.d. c) *Education, Health and Care Plan.* Available at www.mencap.org.uk/advice-and-support/children-and-young-people/education-health-and-care-plan (accessed 19 January 2023).

MENCAP (n.d. d) *Transition into adult services.* Available at www.mencap.org.uk/advice-and-support/children-and-young-people/transition-adult-services (accessed 12 July 2023).

Miller, D. and Brown, J. (2014) 'We have the right to be safe' protecting disabled children from abuse. NSPCC. Available at www.nspcc.org.uk/globalassets/documents/research-reports/right-safe-disabled-children-abuse-report.pdf (accessed 13 July 2023).

National Autistic Society (2023a) *What is Autism?* Available at: www.autism.org.uk/advice-and-guidance/what-is-autism (accessed 23 January 2023).

National Autistic Society (2023b) *The Picture Exchange Communication System, National Autism Resources.* Available at: https://nationalautismresources.com/the-picture-exchange-communication-system-pecs/ (accessed 13 July 2023).

National Institute for Health and Care Excellence (2015) Challenging Behaviour and Learning Disabilities: Prevention and interventions for people with learning disabilities whose behaviour challenges NICE guideline 11. Available at: www.nice.org.uk/guidance/ng11 (accessed 23 January 2023).

National Institute for Health and Care Excellence (2017a) Cerebral Palsy in under 25s: assessment and management NICE guideline [NG62]. Available at www.nice.org.uk/guidance/ng62#:~:text=It%20aims%20to%20make%20sure,and%20cerebral%20palsy%20in%20adults. (accessed 13 July 2023).

National Institute for Health and Care Excellence (2017b) Autistic spectrum disorder in under 19s: recognition, referral and diagnosis. Available at https://www.nice.org.uk/guidance/cg128 (accessed 13 July 2023).

National Institute for Health and Care Excellence (2021) Autism spectrum disorder in under 19s: support and management. Available at www.nice.org.uk/guidance/cg170 (accessed 25 January 2023).

National Health Service and Community Care Act 1990 Available at www.legislation.gov.uk/ukpga/1990/19/contents (accessed 19 January 2023).

NHS England (2023) The Oliver McGowan Mandatory Training on Learning Disability and Autism. Available at www.e-lfh.org.uk/programmes/the-oliver-mcgowan-mandatory-training-on-learning-disability-and-autism/ (accessed 13 July 2023).

NHS Health Scotland (2017) *People with Learning Disabilities in Scotland: 2017 Health Needs Assessment Update Report.* Available at www.healthscotland.scot/media/1690/people-with-learning-disabilities-in-scotland.pdf (accessed 13 July 2023).

NHS LeDeR (n.d.) LeDeR - Learning from lives and deaths. Available at https://leder.nhs.uk/about (accessed 28 January 2023).

Northway, R. and Hopes, P. (2022) *Learning Disability Nursing: developing professional practice*. St. Albans: Critical Publishing.

Nursing and Midwifery Council (2018a) *The Code. Professional Standards of Practice and Behaviour for Nurses and Midwives*. London: Nursing and Midwifery Council. Available at: www.nmc.org.uk/globalassets/sitedocuments/nmc-publications/nmc-code.pddf (accessed 11 January 2023).

Nursing and Midwifery Council (2018b) *The Standards of Proficiency for Registered Nurses*. London: Nursing and Midwifery Council. Available at https://www.nmc.org.uk/standards/standards-for-nurses/standards-of-proficiency-for-registered-nurses/ (accessed 11 January 2023).

Peate, I. and Gormley-Fleming, E. (eds) (2021) *Fundamentals of Children's Anatomy and Physiology: A Textbook for Nursing and Healthcare Students*, 2nd edn. Chichester: Wiley Blackwell.

Popova, S, et al. (2017) 'Estimation of national, regional, and global prevalence of alcohol use during pregnancy and foetal alcohol syndrome: a systematic review and meta-analysis.' *The Lancet global health*, 5.3 p.e290-e299 DOI: 10.1016/S2214-109X(17)30021-9

Public Health England (2016) *Learning Disabilities Observatory People with learning disabilities in England 2015: data tables*. Available at https://assets.publishing.service.gov.uk/government/uploads/system/uploads/attachment_data/file/613183/PWLDIE_2015_data_tables_NB090517.pdf (accessed 16 July 2023).

Public Health England (2020) *Reasonable Adjustments: a legal duty*. Available at www.gov.uk/government/publications/reasonable-adjustments-a-legal-duty/reasonable-adjustments-a-legal-duty (accessed 19 January 2023).

Public Health England (2023) *Learning Disability All Our Health* updated 2023. Available at www.gov.uk/government/publications/learning-disability-applying-all-our-health/learning-disabilities-applying-all-our-health#:~:text=The%20prevalence%20of%20learning%20disabilities,adults%20aged%2018%20or%20over. (accessed 16 July 2023).

SCOPE (2023) *Cerebral Palsy*. Available at www.scope.org.uk/advice-and-support/cerebral-palsy-introduction/ (accessed 13 July 2023).

Scottish Government (2012) *Strengthening the Commitment: The Report of the UK Modernising Learning Disabilities Nursing Review*. Available at: www.gov.scot/publications/strengthening-commitment-report-uk-modernising-learning-disabilities-nursing-review (accessed 19 January 2023).

Special Educational Needs and Disability Act 2001 Available at www.legislation.gov.uk/ukpga/2001/10/contents (accessed 24 January 2023).

The Disability Discrimination (Northern Ireland) Order (2006) Available at www.legislation.gov.uk/nisi/2006/312/made (accessed 24 October 2023).

The Makaton Charity (2023) *Learn Makaton*. Available at https://makaton.org/TMC/TMC/LearnMakaton.aspx (accessed 13 July 2023).

United Nations (1989) *The United Nations Convention on the Rights of the Child*. Available at: https://www.unicef.org.uk/wp-content/uploads/2016/08/unicef-convention-rights-child-uncrc.pdf (accessed 28 January 2023).

United Nations (n. d.) *Children with Disabilities*. Available at https://violenceagainstchildren.un.org/content/children-disabilities (accessed 13 July 2023).

Valuing People - A New Strategy for Learning Disability for the 21st Century (2001) Available at https://assets.publishing.service.gov.uk/media/5a7b854740f0b62826a041b9/5086.pdf (accessed 19 January 2023).

Valuing People Now (2010) Available at www.gov.uk/government/publications/valuing-people-now-summary-report-march-2009-september-2010 (accessed 19 January 2023).

CARE OF CHILDREN AND YOUNG PEOPLE WITH MENTAL HEALTH ISSUES

35

LAURENCE BALDWIN AND ANN COX

THIS CHAPTER COVERS

- Prevalence of some of the more common mental health problems in children and young people
- Recognition of some of the conditions, signs and symptoms of these mental health issues
- Initial treatment approaches and nursing skills in helping
- Identifying areas of concern, risk and safeguarding guidance when caring for children with mental health problems

"A girl had four birds. The first was named Depression, its wings vast, they could easily engulf her, trapping her in a suffocating embrace of feathers and keeping her there. The second was Anxiety, always flapping its wings and squawking, lodging its cries into the back of her head. The third was Stress, by being a parrot, it naturally repeats every worry the girl possesses. Nagging her until she cracks. The final being a woodpecker, named Hate. Hate taps venomous thoughts into her head, like jealously and doubt, until eventually she believes them. The girl loathed each bird! She wished they would stop encircling her, like vultures on the hunt. So, she took the advice of an old Peregrine, named Reason. 'Instead of be-ridding of your four birds, I will give you a fifth. A dove, named Forgiveness', said the Peregrine. The girl released the encaged dove. The dove broke the chains, which the girl was ignorant of, and sat proudly upon her shoulder. Astonished, the girl allowed herself to forgive the birds and they flew away freely. As Forgiveness broke her chains, she gained strength. Most importantly she forgave herself, for chaining the birds to her. She grew wings, learning to fly on her own. The girl became a bird. A bird named Positivity."

Eva Clarke, 13 years old, The Girl of Many Birds

INTRODUCTION

The opening quotation illustrates the feelings of Eva, a young person, regarding mental illness and is reproduced in this chapter with her consent. Sadly, the number of children and young people like Eva who experience mental health issues is growing steadily, and these children continue to present at a much earlier age than previously.

Whilst professional groups and individuals, alongside charities like Young Minds and Place2Be (with its royal patronage), have sought to highlight the importance of children and young people's mental health over the years, it remains a neglected and underfunded area. The recent pandemic has made worse the rates of anxiety, depression, eating problems and self-harm in this vulnerable group.

PREVALENCE OF SOME OF THE MORE COMMON MENTAL HEALTH AND BEHAVIOURAL PROBLEMS IN CHILDREN

Seventy per cent of children who experience mental health problems have not had appropriate interventions at a sufficiently early age. These are some of the most vulnerable people in our society (Green et al., 2005; Children's Society, 2008; Sempik et al., 2008; Bazalgette et al., 2015). Helping these children and recognising the impact their disability has on health and wellbeing and their educational and social progress is an ethical and professional imperative for all health and social care professionals in all settings.

The preferred current approach to caring for a child or young person with a mental health problem is to:

- Build resilience, capacity and inclusion
- 'Think family' and work in a systemic way
- Show respect
- Promote 'recovery capability' attitudes
- Minimise the stigma of mental illness
- Raise awareness of the importance and education of early detection, management and support for children who present with mental health issues
- Promote multi-agency working

The World Health Organization (WHO, 2015) estimate that, worldwide, 20% of adolescents in any given year may experience a mental health problem, with the origin of the difficulty starting at a young age. They have also (WHO, 2022) estimated a 25% increase in anxiety and depression, triggered by the COVID-19 pandemic, with women and young people particularly affected.

Data for Children and Young People's Mental Health (CYPMH, formerly known as CAMHS, Child and Adolescent Mental Health) is improving but is still incomplete. Surveys carried out by the Office of National Statistics (ONS) (Bazalgette at al., 2015) found that 10% of children (aged 5–16 years) already had clinically diagnosable mental health problems. More recently, the global pandemic has put additional pressure on the ability of young people to cope, and NHS Digital (2022) has a range of surveys which show increases in all areas of mental health issues, including eating problems. It is now thought as many as one in six young people are suffering from some form of mental difficulty at any given time.

The ONS survey, which comprised 7977 interviews with parents, children and teachers, found the prevalence of mental health problems in children (aged 5–16 years) to be: 4% for emotional problems (depression or anxiety), 6% for conduct problems, 2% for hyperkinetic (ADHD) problems, and 1% for less common problems (including autism, tic disorders, eating disorders and elective mutism). It is also important to note that most adult mental health problems have their onset in adolescence (Jones, 2018), so early intervention can prevent later development of chronic issues.

SEE ALSO
CHAPTER 11

RECOGNITION OF SOME OF THE CONDITIONS, SIGNS AND SYMPTOMS

According to Bazalgette et al. (2015), the rates of mental health problems rise steeply in mid to late adolescence. Fink et al. (2015) carried out a study of 3366 adolescents which found that, from 2009 to 2014, overall, adolescents experienced similar levels of mental health difficulties (i.e., emotional problems, peer problems, hyperactivity and conduct problems). There are also clear associations between childhood psychological problems and the ability of affected children to live, work and earn as adults. This is not what we desire for our young people and not how they can become happy healthy adults. It is also in opposition to the aspirations of the United Nations Convention on the Rights of the Child (United Nations, 1989).

SEE ALSO
CHAPTERS 11
AND 38

One in four adults and one in six children are likely to have a mental health problem in any year, which can have a profound impact on the lives of tens of millions of people in the UK, and can affect their ability to sustain relationships, work, and life. It is estimated that only about a quarter of people with a mental health problem receive ongoing treatment, meaning the rest deal with their mental health issues on their own (Mental Health Foundation, 2015).

Access *A National Service Framework for Children, Young People and Maternity Services* (Department of Health, 2004), a 10-year programme intended to stimulate long-term sustained improvement in children's health to ensure fair, high-quality integrated health and social care from pregnancy through to adulthood. For children and young people's mental health in England the CAMHS Taskforce in 2015 also produced the *Future in Mind* report which can be found here: www.england.nhs.uk/mental-health/cyp/. and *The Five Year Forward View for Mental Health* (Mental Health Taskforce to the NHS in England, 2016).

Contemporary issues in the field of children and young people's mental health epidemiology include: refinement of classification and assessment, inclusion of young children in epidemiologic surveys, integration of child and adult psychiatric epidemiology, and evaluation of both mental and physical disorders in children (Ries Merikangas et al., 2009).

Anxiety disorders

Anxiety is an umbrella term for a wide range of disorders. Whilst the mechanism of anxiety is the same, the presentation of the child will be very different depending on what difficulty the child is experiencing. Those experiencing disorders usually have recurring intrusive thoughts or concerns and may avoid certain situations out of worry. They may also have physical symptoms such as sweating, trembling, dizziness or a rapid heartbeat. Anxiety disorders are an extremely common form of mental illnesses defined by feelings of uneasiness, worry and fear. Anxiety is a normal response to when the brain perceives danger. We need anxiety to protect ourselves. For example, crossing a road, walking on a rocky path or walking down a dark alley, all of these situations will evoke an anxiety response and our bodies will release adrenaline and noradrenaline to try to manage the threat that it perceives. This sets off a catalyst of physiological responses and symptoms that we call anxiety. In normal situations, anxiety is a helpful response to a threat; however, at times our threat system becomes over-sensitive, we have increases over and above our normal anxiety response and anxiety becomes impactful in many different areas of life (Gilbert, 2018; Denefrio and Dennis-Tiwary, 2020).

Many people with an anxiety disorder do not realise they have a defined, treatable disorder and as a result anxiety disorders are thought to be underdiagnosed. The definition of an anxiety disorder also requires evidence of an impairment of day-to-day functioning. The child with an anxiety disorder often experiences a significantly reduced quality of life and anxiety disorders are also associated with other health-related issues (comorbidities).

Anxiety disorders are the most frequent conditions seen in children, followed by behaviour disorders, mood disorders (e.g., depression), and substance use disorders. A study conducted in 2020 of 2395 UK teenagers found that 27% of teenagers felt anxious most of the time (Mental Health Foundation, 2021). If this were generalisable across children in the UK, in 2019 there were 12.9 million children living in the UK, this would equate to 3.5 million children struggling with anxiety (Office of National Statistics (ONS), 2021a). This demonstrates the increase in anxiety disorders over recent years, exacerbated by the COVID-19 pandemic and its associated disruptions in education and communities.

Several types of anxiety disorders are identified in the *Diagnostic and Statistical Manual of Mental Disorders 5* (American Psychiatric Association (APA), 2013):

SEE ALSO
CHAPTERS 10, 11 & 13

- Obsessive-compulsive disorder (OCD)
- Generalised anxiety disorder (GAD)
- Panic disorder
- Post-traumatic stress disorder (PTSD)
- Agoraphobia
- Social phobia, also referred to as social anxiety disorder
- Specific phobia (also known as a simple phobia)
- Adjustment disorder with anxious features
- Acute stress disorder
- Substance-induced anxiety disorder
- Anxiety due to a general medical condition

Social phobia

This is the most common anxiety disorder and typically manifests before the age of 20. Specific, or simple phobias – such as a fear of snakes – are also very common, with more than 1 in 10 people experiencing a specific phobia in their lifetime. Social anxiety is a fear about being judged on performance. A performance can be contextualised as reading aloud, eating, walking, sitting an exam and speaking to others and any other behaviour that can be scrutinised by others. Read about Aidan's experience below.

CASE STUDY 35.1: AIDAN

Aidan is 18 years old and due to complete his final year of A levels at sixth form college. Aidan lives with his mum, Iris, a single mother and hotel manager, and a younger brother, Jonathan, aged 15.

Iris has observed a change in Aidan's behaviour since receiving results for his mock A level exams, in which he received good grades. Although his teachers report good progress, Aidan felt very disappointed with his results and has become very irritable. His brother complains that Aidan doesn't come out with him to play football any more and gives the excuse that he is too tired and has to study for getting into university. Aidan's peers say that he has become very distressed, he has started to hyperventilate and asks to be excused from class more frequently. One of his teachers has suggested he goes to see the school nurse to get 'checked over'.

- What are the key signs and symptoms Aidan presents with?
- How does this affect his family life and school life?

"When I was at school nobody spoke about it at school. When I tried to go and get help from many different places they said I was young and they didn't understand how I could possibly be suffering from mental health conditions. There was a lot of stigma around it. They said, 'you are young, you don't have anything to worry about'. Even after I was diagnosed I had people saying to me, 'you don't want people talking about it, you don't want people knowing about it'. There was no education about it and no discussion about it. It made me feel worse, and prevented me from seeking help.

[I got help] initially from my GP. She referred me to mental health services. I had cognitive behavioural therapy and I was prescribed medication. Once I started to speak about it, I got support from family and close friends; the biggest thing that changed my outlook was cognitive behavioural therapy.

Lynne, (Malik, 2016)"

What is the difference between fear and anxiety?

Fear is a physiological reaction to a specific threat in the present, such as being fearful of a snake or a spider in the same room. Anxiety on the other hand, although it presents with the same physiological reaction, is a response to what we think might happen in the future or having memories of distressing experiences from the past (Baton Rouge Behavioral Hospital, 2022).

Clinical depression

Clinical depression, also referred to as major depression, usually requires an occurrence of two or more episodes of significant depression. The number of young people aged 15–16 with depression nearly doubled between the 1980s and the 2000s (Beng Huat See and Gorard, 2013; Gorard and Beng Huat See, 2015).

In children, clinical depression needs to be distinguished from general 'growing pains', the emotions associated with child and adolescent development or normal everyday 'blues'. Depression can go unrecognised and untreated because it is passed off as the normal emotional and psychological experience of ongoing childhood growth and development.

Over 8000 children younger than 10 years old suffer from severe depression (Green et al., 2005). About 8700 children (0.2%) aged between 5 and 10 years old are seriously depressed. About 62,000 children (1.4%) between 11 and 16 years old are seriously depressed. Between 1 in 12 and 1 in 15 children self-harm (Mental Health Foundation, 2015), which is characterised by low mood and/or loss of interests or pleasure in life activities, continues for at least 2 weeks and includes five of the ten symptoms listed below:

- A low/depressed mood most of the day
- Diminished social interests or reduced pleasure in all or most activities
- Changes in appetite, e.g., significant or unintentional weight loss or gain
- Changes in sleep patterns, e.g., insomnia (lack of sleep) or sleeping too much
- Vocal angry outbursts or crying
- Agitation, irritability or psychomotor retardation noticed by others

- Physical complaints, e.g., stomach aches, headaches that do not respond to medical treatment
- Fatigue or loss of energy and vitality
- Feelings of worthlessness or excessive guilt
- Diminished ability to think or concentrate, or indecisiveness

Signs and symptoms of depression can be masked by other symptoms such as angry behaviour. Although this can occur in younger children, most children experience depression in very much the same way as adults, with feelings such as sadness, hopelessness and mood change.

Children may also begin using drugs and alcohol, particularly if they are over 12 years of age. If tearfulness or sadness become persistent or interfere with usual social activities, interests, schoolwork or family life, then a depressive illness may be indicated.

Self-harm and suicide

Self-harm and suicide is an increasingly serious and pervasive public health problem (see a selection of these websites: Samaritans, Papyrus, Mental Elf, YoungMinds, MindEd, Special Needs Jungle, NHS. uk/Livewell).

Early recognition and awareness of the likelihood of self-harm and suicide is important (at all ages) as early awareness may help the individual to have a voice and feel listened to and cared for at this darkest of times. Increasingly, help is being made available by routes such as social media and apps which are more readily accessed by young people. It is important to know the difference between these two things. Although people who self-harm are more at risk of completing suicide, most are not planning on ending their lives when they self-harm. Obviously, those who are thinking about ending their lives (have 'suicidal ideation') are high risk and need to have a risk management plan completed. This is now often called 'safety planning'. A simple tool for looking at the risk factors is called PATHOS (Kingsbury, 1996) which suggests looking at the following factors:

P_roblems longer than a month

A_lone when self harmed

T_hree hours planning or more

H_opelessness about the future

S_ad most of the time

If 'no' to a question score '0', if Yes score '1' – scores of 2 or more indicate the presence of significant suicidal thinking and the need to take action. Mental health professionals routinely use a more complex scoring system known as the Beck Suicide Intent Scale.

Self-harm

There has been a big increase in the number of young people being admitted to hospital or services because of self-harm which is done for other reasons (i.e., without intent to kill oneself). In recent years this figure has increased by 68% (YoungMinds), which indicates a crisis. Self-harm must be treated compassionately; young people often feedback that staff treated them differently as the harm is self-inflicted, but research indicates (Mental Health Foundation, 2006) that self-harm is a symptom of distress, not a condition in its own right. Nurses need to use their therapeutic relationships skills to engage young people and understand what the underlying issues are, and then ensure they get the treatment they need for those issues (Baldwin, 2020). NICE Guidelines for self-harm are complex and currently under revision, but still suggest routine admission to a paediatric ward or medical assessment unit (for older young people) until they can be fully assessed by CYPMHS staff, so children and young people's nurses will frequently be looking after this group in CED or on a ward, as well as advising in the community. As self-harm is such an emotive subject it can be difficult to deal with, but the crisis of attendance at hospital should be looked on as an opportunity to bring issues into the open and start planning with the young person and their family for better ways of coping with the distress that led to the self-harm.

IDENTIFYING AREAS OF CONCERN, RISK AND SAFEGUARDING GUIDANCE WHEN CARING FOR CHILDREN WITH MENTAL HEALTH PROBLEMS

SAFEGUARDING STOP POINT

Consider the role of the children's nurse in safeguarding children who may be considering suicide:

- How prepared would you be for having a discussion about a friend, family member or young person?
- Would you know how to contact assistance if you needed support/advice, at any hour of the day or night?

Role of the children and young people's nurse

First and foremost it is important to recognise that it is not possible to cover all mental and behavioural topics in such a short chapter, either in number or depth. The reader may therefore wish to explore some topics further. This includes issues around what to do if *you* have concerns about a child's mental health.

Please note that most mental and emotional disorders are likely to present either first, or early on with the children's nurse. It is therefore essential to be aware of key indicators and how to liaise with and refer children for appropriate professional assessment. This may be community-based or inpatient-based depending on the type of disorder, its severity and availability of services locally.

Many children's nurses are in an excellent position to detect children's behaviours that are concerning, but may also feel that they lack the knowledge and skills to manage or assess the situation alone. It is timely to remind ourselves that working with others in the team and other agencies should be the first step in raising your concerns. The Royal College of Nursing (2014) document *Mental Health in Children and Young People: A Toolkit for Nurses Who Are Not Mental Health Specialists* is updated at intervals and is an excellent resource for those who are not 'experienced' in mental health. A weblink is given in the resources listed at the end of the chapter.

Children and young people's nurses usually have excellent interpersonal skills across the developmental stages and an ability to connect through a wide range of communication and play techniques. These skills should not be underestimated. Rather, they should reassure you that you have an important part to play in early assessment and intervention. Working with and as part of the wider multidisciplinary team and across agencies and boundaries is part of what we do well.

It is essential to remember to act in the best interests of the child professionally, legally and proactively (NMC, 2018).

Responding in a non-critical way, listening actively and respecting the child's lived experience are important first steps in reducing the stigma which surrounds the topic of mental health and behavioural issues. Listening and risk assessment should precede formal intervention. Robbins and Mansfield (2020) talk about these things in more detail, and emphasise the importance of getting the environment right, which is particularly important if you are working in a ward which admits children and young people with mental health issues, even on a short-term basis (i.e., following self-harm).

This first step done well will go a long way to improving the child's experience of seeking help, and will have a far-reaching effect on the process of recovery. *Note*: Children with a high assessed risk of suicide need to be seen as an emergency and *should not* be treated as low risk of self-harm or suicide.

SEE ALSO
CHAPTERS 2
AND 8

CYPMHS and mental health expertise

For mental health practitioners to assess the signs and symptoms of any mental disorder, they will need to take time to gather information about the individual before confirming a diagnosis. Individual symptoms, such as sadness and worry, are not in themselves enough to indicate the presence of a clinical diagnosis. Equally important is the need to recognise how serious mental health disorders can be, and to ensure that child and family members know that these problems are treatable.

A mental health evaluation should be carried out sensitively with the child alongside parents or the primary caregiver. Additional psychological assessment may be needed and may include an assessment by a CYPMHS professional. Information will be gathered from teachers, friends and classmates to complete the mental health assessment. A diagnosis of a mental health disorder could increase the risk of suicide in children and young people in the short term, but leads to much better outcomes in the longer term.

Children who come from families with a history of severe mental health problems and or substance misuse are much more likely to suffer with mental health problems. This can also increase the risk of self-harm behaviours and suicide. Health practitioners need to ensure that parents and their children are aware of the side effects of psychiatric medication and what to do and who to call when unwanted side effects occur. Parents may deny the mental health difficulties their child is experiencing and delay accessing mental health services due to the social stigma of mental health difficulties – it is important to educate parents and other family members about the impact of mental health problems on their child and encourage them to access the support available from specialist mental health services. General awareness campaigns in media, schools, communities and in peer groups can help raise the profile of what is essentially an increasingly serious public health issue.

When assessing a child with mental health problems it is important to provide age-appropriate information in more than one format this will help the child understand the information more readily (Anderson and Montgomery, 1996) so that the child can understand the diagnosis and treatment options discussed. Children of any age can consent to treatment or an intervention if they can demonstrate competence and capacity. For children to consent under the age of 16 years, this will be guided by the Gillick Competency framework (*Gillick* v. *Norfolk and Wisbech Health Authority* [1985]) and those aged 16 years and over are guided by the Mental Capacity Act 2005. Involving children in decision-making and consent processes will improve the outcome of the intervention, improve the development of the child and will make them better decision-makers in adult life. The template below (Figure 35.1) (adapted from Cox, 2021) helps to demonstrate whether a child has the competence and capacity to make a decision. By completing each box with the child and the child being able to demonstrate the understanding of each aspect in each box, competence and capacity is proven. The template also provides opportunity for the nurse and the child to improve the competence and capacity of a child. For instance, if a child does not know some of the aspects about alternatives to the intervention being offered, the nurse can spend time with the child, developing their awareness and understanding of alternatives, therefore improving the child's competence and capacity (Cox, 2021). It is an ethical obligation for nurses to improve children's competence and capacity to make decisions (NMC, 2018).

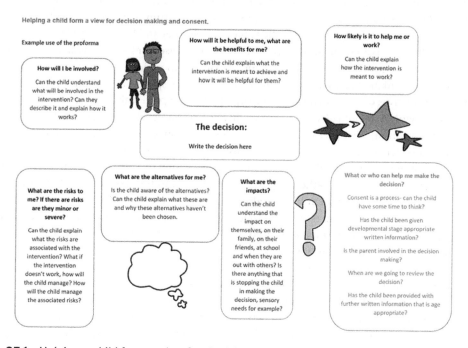

Figure 35.1 Helping a child form a view for decision-making and consent

If a child does not demonstrate competence or capacity, the child can collaborate with family and health professionals to their fullest ability, which respects the right of the child to be involved in decisions that affect their wellbeing and respects their autonomy and right to participate in their care (UNCRC, 1989; Children Act 1989).

> "My advocate made me feel like I am someone, and that I have the right to be listened to. I will never forget this."
>
> **Zoe, child, Coram Voice, 2017**

SEE ALSO
CHAPTER 34

Autism spectrum disorders

Autism is a lifelong, neurodevelopmental disorder, which is part of a group of disorders referred to as 'autism spectrum disorders' (ASD). In the *Diagnostic and Statistical Manual of Mental Disorders 5* (APA, 2013), ASD is characterised by two main areas of impaired development, namely (a) impaired social communication, e.g., unable to maintain a flow of conversation, and (b) fixated interests and repetitive behaviours, e.g., having a quite fixed knowledge base and repeating that knowledge (Lauritsen, 2013). Historically, autism was first recognised by Leo Kanner and Hans Asperger, and was ascribed many different names, from 'childhood schizophrenia', through classic and infantile autism to Asperger's syndrome. Other parts of what we now recognise to be a spectrum have been described variously as Pervasive Developmental Disorder, Semantic Pragmatic Disorder and Pathological Demand Avoidance Syndrome. DSM-5 classifies all these as 'Autism Spectrum Disorder', so this is the commonly used phrase, although it covers a very wide range of diversity from societal norms. Some see elements of strength in the thinking patterns which can emerge from this spectrum, and there is a movement to promote the positives of 'neurodiversity' compared to 'neurotypical' thinking (Silberman, 2016).

In children with ASD difficulty may arise in meeting social developmental milestones, e.g., problems with following another person's shift in gaze during a conversation. They are often described by their teachers as 'loners' and when they do socialise, focus on conversing with one person only – in a primary school setting, this could be a child who appears clingy to a teacher, and sees that teacher as the only focus of conversation, rather than the other children in the class or indeed other teachers.

In adolescence, ASD may present in the individual being unable to initiate and maintain meaningful conversation, demonstrating poor eye contact and limited gestures. This can negatively affect the development of social relationships with peers and others (Buxbaum and Hof, 2013). Young women with ASD are much better at adapting to social expectations and may appear to be coping well, when in fact they are 'masking', putting on a fake persona, but this is, in itself, emotionally exhausting. Young women can be much harder to diagnose because their symptoms are not so obvious.

One of the difficulties with the diagnosis of ASDs is that there is a high incidence of comorbidity with other mental health problems like anxiety, depression, obsessive compulsive disorder and ADHD to name a few. In addition, children and adolescents with autism may find it difficult to adapt to any change in environment, e.g., having to move desks in a classroom setting. For the more severe forms of autism there is also a high comorbidity with learning difficulties.

The development of ASD is unclear, but most theories point to links to genetics, some medical problems, complications of pregnancy and brain abnormalities (Buxbaum and Hof, 2013).

There is no treatment for the underlying issues of autism, but commonly helpful interventions, which fall into four main categories, include:

1. Social skills training where children and young people can be supported to develop speech and language skills, e.g., turn-taking during a conversation.
2. Cognitive Behaviour Therapy can be used to help develop learning techniques for problem-solving (although this needs to be adapted for people with ASD).
3. Drug therapy interventions tend to be used to manage some of the comorbid conditions, such as anxiety, obsessive compulsive disorder (OCD) and attention deficit hyperactivity disorder (ADHD), which often present alongside ASD.
4. Family-based approaches can help and support families/caregivers to cope with their child or young person who is diagnosed with autism.

The above approaches can be combined with specific educational interventions for use in a classroom environment and at home.

Attention deficit disorders

Attentional disorders can be called different things, but most commonly fall under ADHD (attention deficit hyperactivity disorder). There is also, for example, ADD, which is a variant that does not include hyperactive symptoms, and is more common in girls. The World Health Organization's classification system ICD-10 has a category which is more strictly defined, called hyperkinetic disorder, although the new ICD-11 changes this to ADHD, in line with what most people call the condition. Like ASD, it is a neurodevelopmental disorder, best understood as a deficit in the neurotransmitters which results in the core symptoms of:

Overactivity – which is persistent and present from an early age, and happens in all situations

Poor concentration – highly distractible, having difficulty filtering out external stimuli, so sticking to tasks is very difficult for more than very short periods of time

Impulsivity – living in the moment and being very reactive to distractions or whatever thoughts occur in an overactive mind

These symptoms need to be outside of developmental norms, so some of these presentations are common to very young children, for example, but change as they grow older. For children and young people with ADHD this can lead to poor peer relationships as their peers mature and become impatient with inability to carry out turn-taking in conversation, or the child/young person cannot complete longer activities like watching films, etc. Young people with ADHD, however, can be very good at online or video gaming, because the rapidly moving environment of most gaming suits their attentional span.

Assessment of ADHD should be completed by a community paediatrician, child and adolescent psychiatrist, or other 'suitably experienced healthcare professional' according to NICE Guidelines NG87 (2018), usually completed as part of a multidisciplinary assessment. This should include a developmental and family history as well as a mental health assessment (to exclude alternative diagnoses) and, if possible, a school observation, which might be done by a school nurse. Treatment may include behavioural advice, for mild to moderate cases, which is often done as group sessions using either '1-2-3 Magic' (Phelan, 2016) or New Forest (Daley et al., 2010) parenting programmes. For moderate to severe cases treatment will include medication which enables children and young people time to 'stop and think'. Medication for ADHD can be either stimulant or non-stimulant medication, although stimulants like methylphenidate are most commonly used. As these are Controlled Drugs they need careful titration and close supervision, as well as monitoring of physical development as lack of appetite is the most common side effect. Nurses, as independent prescribers and behavioural specialists, play an increasing role in neurodevelopmental clinics specialising in ADHD and ASD (which often present as comorbid conditions).

Some young people seem to develop better cognitive abilities to control their impulsive behaviour and learn to concentrate better as they get older, whilst some will continue to have these symptoms into adulthood.

CASE STUDY 35.2: MIKE AND TOM

Mike, a Clinical Nurse Specialist, regularly visits Tom (age 4) at home with his family to advise on behavioural management techniques. Tom is too young for medication, but has extreme hyperactivity, impulsivity and poor concentration, so keeping up with him, and keeping him safe, is an exhausting task for the family. When Tom is older Mike will continue to see him in the neurodevelopmental clinic to titrate his medication, monitor his growth and give ongoing behavioural advice as he grows older,

Eating problems and disorders

Although the specialist treatment of eating problems and disorders remains the domain of mental health staff there is a shortage of suitable in-patient facilities across the UK, and this group often find themselves on paediatric wards for physical healthcare whilst they wait for a specialist bed. Like the group who self-harm, it is important to be reflective whilst working with young people who restrict their eating because they can generate feelings of frustration and helplessness in healthcare staff.

There are several different forms of eating problems, which are well explained on the BEAT website, which also has a lot of support materials for young people: www.beateatingdisorders.org.uk/.

The principal ones with which people will be familiar are anorexia nervosa (AN) and bulimia nervosa (BN). Remember that 'anorexia' just means not eating, which may have a physical cause, whilst AN always has a mental health component. The restrictive eating of AN is accompanied by distorted thinking which means the young person (and it can be both young men as well as young women) does not see their size and image in the same way as other people, and may be striving for an impossible goal. AN has a high morbidity rate, both at the time of the illness, and later in life if severe damage to internal organs is done during the period of restricted eating. People with AN often talk about an internal 'voice of anorexia' which compels them to continue their restrictive eating patterns. Note that this is an internal voice, and different from the external voice hearing which characterises psychosis (Pugh and Waller, 2017).

Bulimia nervosa is characterised by binging and purging, so weight loss is not always a feature, but the underlying reasons for the disorder are often the same, usually centring around lack of self worth, and the thinking is similarly distorted and can be difficult to work with to achieve positive change.

Since the changes of DSM-5 (APA, 2013) an important change has been the inclusion of ARFID (avoidant/restrictive food intake disorder) as a diagnostic category. As the name suggest this condition is characterised by avoidance of, or severe restriction of certain foods in a manner which is severely impacting on their life. This may have a basis in sensory issues (so is common in ASD, for example), or may have a basis in a traumatic reaction or incident in relation to food (choking or food poisoning, for example), and can impact on physical health. As with all mental health conditions it is important to rule out a purely organic reason for this form of restrictive eating before treating ARFID as a psychological condition.

CASE STUDY 35.3: KATRINA AND KELLY

Katrina, an Eating Disorder Specialist Nurse, sees Kelly regularly in the CYPMHS Eating Disorder service to support her recovery from AN. Kelly is 14, and has been severely restricting her eating for several months, as well as exercising excessively, and has lost a considerable amount of weight. She still has a distorted body image and is convinced she is fat and ugly. The team closely monitor her weight and physical health as well as working with Kelly and her family to support her psychologically. As her thinking has been very fixed she is now on medication, which Katrina hopes will help her to think differently.

Hearing voices and psychosis

Many children hear voices that other people cannot hear. There are many reasons why children hear voices and they are not always related to more pervasive and serious mental illnesses such as psychosis and disorders such as schizophrenia. However, voice hearing in any context can be distressing to the child. In some circumstances a child hearing voices can be reassuring and self-soothing for them, and experienced as a comfort to them.

Children who have experienced significant trauma, have an autism spectrum disorder, have a learning disability, have eating disorders, have high levels of anxiety, have severe low mood and those children who are experiencing their psychosis are all known to experience voice hearing (DSM-5, 2013). Usually with those disorders that are not diagnosed as psychosis, the voices will be internal in the child's head, they will come and go depending on the level of stress the child is experiencing and the child can usually be distracted from the voices. However, in complex autism presentations, distraction from the voices can be more challenging. In psychotic presentations, there is usually a change in the sense of reality, the voices are external and distracting from the voices can be harder to do. It is important to eliminate any other reason for hearing voices such as substance misuse, and side effects of medication.

Voices can present in many different ways. The following list shares some of the different types of voices that can be heard by children:

- Command voices, where the voices are telling the child to do something
- Voices talking about the child, usually being hypercritical about the child
- Voices talking about others
- Children can hear music or singing
- Children can hear different sounds that are unrelated to the environment

(Rethink, 2022)

When a child experiences voices, it is important to understand the context of the voices, for example, are they exacerbated by stress? Finding patterns to the voices can be helpful in trying to manage them better (Mental Health Foundation, 2022). Using distraction techniques, such as listening to music, singing, or listening to podcasts, can be helpful. Most of the time voices will disappear by themselves if they are not related to a psychosis; however, Cognitive Behavioural Therapy can be helpful intervention to support those children that have more persistent voices (Hazell et al., 2016). If voices are severe, or it is expected that this is the onset of psychosis, then antispsychotic medication will be helpful for the child.

Spending time with the child and talking through their voice hearing experiences can be validating for the child. Providing a space for the child to discuss their difficulties and the nurse using their thereaputic skills to elicit the information from the child will help both the child and the nurse understand the context of the voices and how best to manage them (Cox, 2019).

——————— CHAPTER SUMMARY ———————

- This chapter looks at the prevalence of common mental and behavioural disorders in children and young people with a focus on anxiety, depression, autism or attentional disorders and recognising factors which may lead to self-harm and suicidal behaviour.
- Children and young people's nurses can often lack confidence when dealing with mental health problems, but usually have very good communication and engagement skills which are the things that children and young people value the most on those who are caring for them.

- Whilst other professionals may have more focused skills in helping children and young people in the long term it is vital to see this group as equally deserving of our care when they present in distress. General paediatric wards may not be the best place for them, but making them feel safe and inspiring hope that things can get better is part of nursing them back to full health.

———— BUILD YOUR BIBLIOGRAPHY ————

Journal articles

FURTHER
READING:
ONLINE
JOURNAL
ARTICLES

- Baranek, G.T., David, F.J., Poe, M.D., Stone, W.L., Linda, R. and Watson, L.R. (2006) 'Sensory Experiences Questionnaire: discriminating sensory features in young children with autism, developmental delays, and typical development'. *Journal of Child Psychology and Psychiatry*, 47 (6): 591–601.

  Provides a review of the sensory symptoms of autism and how these differ from sensory symptoms experienced in other healthcare problems – useful in assessment of autism spectrum disorders.

- Gondek, D., Edbrooke-Childs, J., Velikonja, T., Chapman, L., Saunders, F., Hayes, D. and Wolpert, M. (2016) 'Facilitators and barriers to person-centred care in child and young people mental health services: a systematic review'. *Clinical Psychology and Psychotherapy*, 24 (4): 870–86.

  Explores some of the essential skills required by mental health practitioners in caring for children and young people with mental health problems.

- Simmons, M.B., Hetrick, S.E. and Jorm, A.F. (2011) 'Experiences of treatment decision-making for young people diagnosed with depressive disorders: a qualitative study in primary care and specialist mental health settings'. *BMC Psychiatry*, 11: 194.

  Provides information on how 'partnership working' can be negotiated with both children and young people and their caregivers in the transition from primary care to specialist mental health settings.

- NICE, Autistic spectrum disorder in under 19s: recognition, referral and diagnosis. NICE guideline [CG128] ww.nice.org.uk/guidance/cg128 This document is useful for assessment of autism spectrum disorders.

- NICE, Autism spectrum disorder in under 19s: support and management. NICE guideline [CG170] www.nice.org.uk/guidance/cg170

- Place2Be and NAHT, *Children's Mental Health Matters: Provision of Primary School Counselling* www.place2Be.org.uk/media/10046/Children's_Mental_Health_Week_2016_report.pdf

- Department of Health, *Future in Mind: Promoting, Protecting and Improving Our Children and Young People's Mental Health* www.gov.uk/govern,ent/publications/improving-mental-health-services-for-young-people The report outlines a five-year vision for good mental health, recognising that everyone who works with children has a role in helping them to get the help they need.

- Royal College of Nursing, *Mental Health in Children and Young People: A Toolkit for Nurses Who Are Not Mental Health Specialists* www.rcn.org.uk/professional-development/publications/pub-003311

REFERENCES

American Psychiatric Association (APA) (2013) *Diagnostic and Statistical Manual of Mental Disorders*, Fifth edition *(DSM-5)*. Washington, DC: APA.

Baldwin, L. (2020) (ed.) *Nursing Skills for Children and Young People's Mental Health*. Cham: Springer.

Baton Rouge Behavioral Hospital (2022) Fear v Anxiety: Understanding the difference. [Online] Available at: https://batonrougebehavioral.com/fear-vs-anxiety-understanding-the-difference/#:~:text=Fear%20is%20an%20emotional%20reaction,with%20no%20trigger%20at%20all. (accessed 2 August 2022).

Bazalgette, L., Rahilly, T. and Trevely, G. (2015) *Achieving Emotional Wellbeing for Looked after Children: A Whole System Approach.* London: NSPCC.

Beng Huat See and Gorard, S. (2013) *What Do Rigorous Evaluations Tell Us about the Most Promising Parental Involvement Interventions? A Critical Review of What Works for Disadvantaged Children in Different Age Groups.* London: The Nuffield Foundation.

Buxbaum, J.D. and Hof, P.R. (2013) *The Neuroscience of Autistic Spectrum Disorders.* Oxford: Academic Press/Elsevier.

Children Act 1989. www.legislation.gov.uk/ukpga/1989/41/contents

Children's Society (2008) *Mental Health of Looked After Children in the UK: Summary The 2008 Survey.* Available at: www.childrenssociety.org.uk/what-we-do/research/initiatives/well-being/background-programme/2008-survey (accessed 25 April 2008).

Coram Voice (2017) *Mental Health Issues.* [Online] Available at: www.coramvoice.org.uk/professional-zone/mental-health-issues (accessed 15 November 2017).

Cox, A.M. (2019) 'Nurse or psychotherapist? Using nursing skills in therapeutic relationships and psychotherapies', in L. Baldwin (ed.), *Nursing Skills for Children and Young People's Mental Health.* Cham: Springer.

Cox, A.M. (2021) 'How can children aged 8-12 years be involved in decision-making and consent to processes in outpatient Child and Adolescent Mental Health Services (CAMHS)? An embedded case study'. D.Prof., University of Derby.

Daley, D., Sonuga-Burke, E.J.S., Laver-Bradbury, C., Thompson, M. and Weeks, A. (2010) *Step by Step for Children with ADHD: A self-help manual for parents.* London: Jessica Kingsley Publishers.

Denefrio, S. and Dennis-Tiwary, T.A. (2020) 'Threat sensitivity', in V. Zeigler-Hill and T. Shackelford, (eds), *Encyclopedia of Personality and Individual Differences.* Cham: Springer.

Department of Health (DH) (2004) *A National Service Framework for Children, Young People and Maternity Services: Core Standards.* London: DH. Available at: www.gov.uk/government/uploads/system/uploads/attachment_data/file/199952/National_Service_Framework_for_Children_Young_People_and_Maternity_Services_-_Core_Standards.pdf (accessed 4 June 2017).

Fink, E., Patalay, P., Sharpe, H., Holley, S., Deighton, J. and Wolpert, M. (2015) 'Mental health difficulties in early adolescence: a comparison of two cross-sectional studies in England from 2009 to 2014'. *Journal of Adolescent Health,* 56, (5): 502–7.

Gilbert, P. (2018) Introducing compassion focused therapy. [Online] Available at: www.cambridge.org/core/journals/advances-in-psychiatric-treatment/article/introducing-compassionfocused-therapy/ECBC8B7B87E90ABB58C4530CDEE04088 (accessed 2 August 2022).

Gillick v. Norfolk and Wisbech Health Authority [1985] 2 W.L.R. 413.

Gorard, S. and Beng Huat See (2015) *Do Parental Involvement Interventions Increase Attainment? A Review of the Evidence.* London: The Nuffield Foundation.

Green, H., McGinnity, A., Meltzer, H., Ford, T. and Goodman, R. (2005) *Mental Health of Children and Young People in Great Britain, 2004.* Newport: National Statistics.

Hazell, C.M., Hayward, M., Cavanagh, K., Jones, A-M. and Strauss, C. (2016) 'Guided self-help cognitive behavioral intervention for VoicEs (GiVE): study protocol for a pilot randomized controlled trial'. *Trials,* 17: 351.

Jones, P.B. (2018) 'Adult mental health disorders and their age at onset'. *British Journal of Psychiatry,* 202 (54): 5-10.

Kingsbury, S. (1996) 'PATHOS: A screening instrument for adolescent overdose: A research note'. *Journal of Child Psychology and Psychiatry*, 37 (5): 609-11.

Lauritsen, M.B. (2013) 'Autism spectrum disorders'. *European Journal of Child and Adolescent Psychiatry*, 22 (1): 37–42.

Malik, A. (2016) 'Suffering in silence: why the voices of young people on mental health must be heard'. *Commonspace* [Online]. Available at: www.commonspace.scot/articles/8829/suffering-silence-why-voices-young-people-mental-health-must-be-heard (accessed 10 November 2017).

Mental Capacity Act 2005. Available at: www.legislation.gov.uk/ukpga/2005/9/section/4.

Mental Health Foundation (2006) *Truth Hurts: A Report of the National Investigation into Self Harm amongst Young People*. London: MHF.

Mental Health Foundation (2015) *Fundamental Facts About Mental Health 2015*. London: Mental Health Foundation.

Mental Health Foundation (2022) *Hearing Voices*. [Online] Available at: www.mentalhealth.org.uk/explore-mental-health/a-z-topics/hearing-voices. (accessed 3 August 2022).

Mental Health Taskforce to the NHS in England (2016) *The Five Year Forward View for Mental Health*. Available at: www.england.nhs.uk/wp-content/uploads/2016/02/Mental-Health-Taskforce-FYFV-final.pdf (accessed 4 June 2017).

NHS Digital (2022) Mental Health of Children and Young People Surveys. [Online] Available at: https://digital.nhs.uk/data-and-information/publications/statistical/mental-health-of-children-and-young-people-in-england (accessed 22 June 2023).

NICE (National Institute for Health and Care Excellence) (2018) Attention deficit hyperactivity: diagnosis and management. *NICE guideline [NG87]*. Available at: www.nice.org.uk/guidance/ng87.

NMC (Nursing and Midwifery Council) (2018) *The Code: Professional Standards of Practice and Behaviour for Nurses, Midwives and Nursing Associates*. London: NMC. Available at: www.nmc.org.uk/standards/code/.

ONS (Office for National Statistics) (2021) Population estimates for the UK, England and Wales, Scotland and Northern Ireland: mid-2019. [Online] Available at: www.ons.gov.uk/peoplepopulationandcommunity/populationandmigration/populationestimates/bulletins/annualmidyearpopulationestimates/mid2019estimates (accessed 2 August 2022).

ONS (2021b) Suicides in the UK: 2018 registrations. [Online] Available at: www.ons.gov.uk/peoplepopulationandcommunity/birthsdeathsandmarriages/deaths/bulletins/suicidesintheunitedkingdom/2018registrations#suicide-patterns-by-age. (accessed 2 August 2022).

Phelan, T.W. (2016) *1-2-3 Magic: 3-step discipline for calm, effective and happy parenting*. Illinois: Soucebooks Inc.

Pugh, M. and Waller, G. (2017) 'Understanding the "anorexic voice" in anorexia nervosa'. *Clinical Psychology and Psychotherapy*, 24: 670–6.

Rethink (2022) Hearing voices. [Online] Available at: www.rethink.org/advice-and-information/about-mental-illness/learn-more-about-symptoms/hearing-voices/ (accessed 3 August 2022).

Ries Merikangas, K., Nakamura, E.F. and Kessler, R.C. (2009) 'Epidemiology of mental disorders in children and adolescents'. *Dialogues in Clinical Neuroscience*, 11 (1): 7–20.

Robbins, G. and Mansfield, S. (2020) 'Paediatric wards and children's wards: wrong place or right place for seeing distressed young people?', in L. Baldwin (ed.), *Nursing Skills for Children and Young People's Mental Health*. Cham: Springer.

Royal College of Nursing (RCN) (2014) Mental Health in Children and Young People: A Toolkit for Nurses Who Are Not Mental Health Specialists. Available at: www.rcn.org.uk/professional-development/publications/pub-003311 (accessed 9 February 2022).

Sempik, J., Ward, H. and Darker, I. (2008) 'Emotional and behavioural difficulties of children and young people at entry to care'. *Clinical Child Psychology and Psychiatry*, 13 (2): 221–33.

Silberman, S. (2016) *Neurotribes: The Legacy of Autism and How to Think Smarter about People who Think Differently*. London: Allen and Unwin.

United Nations (1989) *United Nations Convention on the Rights of the Child*. Available at: www.unicef.org.uk/what-we-do/un-convention-child-rights (accessed 6 June 2023).

World Health Organization (2015) World Health Statistics: Factsheet on Adolescent Health. Geneva: WHO.

World Health Organization (2022) Covid-19 pandemic triggers 25% increase in prevalence of anxiety and depression worldwide. Available at: www.who.int/news/item/02-03-2022-covid-19-pandemic-triggers-25-increase-in-prevalence-of-anxiety-and-depression-worldwide (accessed 22 June 2023).

PART 5   ON BEING A PROFESSIONAL CHILDREN'S NURSE

LEADERSHIP AND MANAGEMENT IN CHILDREN AND YOUNG PEOPLE'S NURSING

MELANIE HAYWARD

THIS CHAPTER COVERS

- Theories and models of leadership and management
- Importance of values-based and relational attributes
- The significance of emotional intelligence and its links to managing change, raising concerns and defusing conflict
- Managing and safeguarding care with children and young people

> "Leadership is not about titles, positions, or flowcharts. It is about one life influencing another."
>
> **(Maxwell and Dornan, 2018)**

INTRODUCTION

Effective and efficient leadership and management are central to high-performing healthcare services, to ensure the delivery of safe, compassionate, high-quality patient outcomes. The ever-increasing challenge of multifaceted organisational systems serving complex patients highlights the importance of inclusive, empowering, and caring nurse leaders and no more so than in children and young people's nursing. Some nurses aim for management or specialist positions, others want to remain in patient-facing roles solely focusing on the delivery of exceptional nursing care, yet indicated by the above quote, the reality of practice is that in any position, all nurses require leadership expertise to be effective.

Leadership and Management in Children and Young People's Nursing

---

ACTIVITY 36.1: REFLECTIVE PRACTICE – WHAT MAKES A 'GREAT LEADER'?

Spend time noting down and reflecting on the following:

- What characteristics and abilities makes someone a 'great leader'?
- Consider a leader you think highly of – why?
- Can you add anything further to what you think makes someone a great leader?

Leadership and management are terms that are often used interchangeably, and concerned with influencing and achieving identified objectives, they are both necessary for successful organisations (Ellis, 2021). Leaders do not need to be managers, but to be an effective manager, you need leadership expertise (Barr and Dowding, 2019). Fennell (2021) sees healthcare leadership as a two-way dynamic process which changes according to context and involves a leader being visionary and developing followers. Management in contrast organises and maintains resources and information (Gopee and Galloway, 2017).

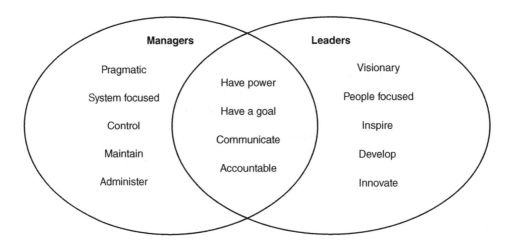

Figure 36.1 Commonalities and differences between leaders and managers

Leadership is a phenomenon which has progressed over time. As society has evolved there is increased recognition that leadership must relate to context and is an interpersonal activity which can be learned. The NHS Leadership Academy (2013) Healthcare Leadership Model is a reference point for nurses outlining required behaviours for a positive and effective 'NHS leadership style'. The evidence base for successful leadership, intelligence from service users, alongside the NHS constitutional values (Department of Health and Social Care, 2021) are incorporated into nine leadership dimensions to engage in and aspire to impact care at any career point, whether a pre-registration student or a Chief Nurse (Machon et al., 2019).

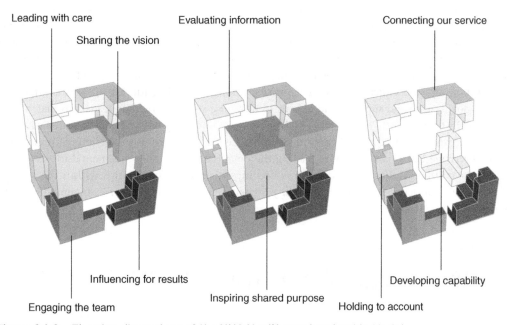

Figure 36.2　The nine dimensions of the NHS Healthcare Leadership Model

© NHS Leadership Academy. Reproduced with permission.

Traditional leadership behaviours may also be seen as:

Autocratic – is directive, controlling, makes decisions and expects compliance. This style can be useful in a crisis such as a paediatric respiratory arrest.

Democratic – favours working collaboratively through consultation. This is effective with most nursing teams and ensures team members feel valued.

Laissez-faire – is non directive and enables autonomy. This can be successful in specialist teams (complex community care, looked after children).

Bureaucratic – where individuals are in specific roles, undertaking particular duties, following established procedures often used, for example, in children's surgical units.

Situational – theories recognise that leaders and managers have to be flexible, analytical in their approach using a combination of behavioural styles, dependent on the context of the task. For environments with regular change (emergency department, or a team undergoing change) this style can be valuable (Cope and Murray, 2017; Barr and Dowding, 2019).

Adaptive – leadership supports progress and success and is often applied to patient-centred care (Long, 2020). It has been recognised as valuable in managing complex or shifting situations (COVID-19 pandemic), anticipating issues, articulating resultant need and empowering others to be part of the solution.

The literature identifies *relational styles*; focused on people and process using a values-based approach (James et al., 2021). This recognises the imperative of ethical, inclusive practice. *Transformational* leadership involves inspiring, trusting, supporting and empowering others by focusing on the higher purpose of their role and is extensively promoted in healthcare. *Servant* leadership advocates a symbiotic relationship with team members. Like transformational leadership, it empowers followers and recognises the importance of leaders also being followers. A selfless stance is taken where individual or team needs are prioritised, often leading by example. As with adaptive leadership, this style is recognised as being central to patient-centred care. *Authentic* leadership combines transformational with servant approaches, characterised by altruism and trusting relationships, this style employs compassion, honesty, and ethical behaviour (Giordano-Mulligan and Eckardt, 2019). This is important for high-quality care and supports individuals to recognise strengths helping leaders to match individuals' skills to solutions. This leads to a *collective* style of leadership where power is shared wherever motivation exists (West et al., 2014). Leadership is accepted as an inclusive, communal responsibility and everyone has a part to play in leading the organisation and are fundamental to its success (Nightingale, 2020). Collective leadership is contingent on the relationships within the system, focused on the principle that the responsibility lies with teams, within and across boundaries, rather than individuals (Timmins, 2015).

ACTIVITY 36.2: WHAT IS YOUR LEADERSHIP STYLE?

Diverse types of leadership exist because we all have distinct characteristics, skills, and knowledge due to our unique experiences, and certain styles are appropriate in specific situations and/or contexts.

- Undertake this quiz to help you identify your natural approach to leadership: www.mindtools. com/pages/article/leadership-style-quiz.htm
- Which do you think you are most like?
- Which style do you aspire to?

THE IMPORTANCE OF EFFECTIVE LEADERSHIP AND MANAGEMENT

The Care Quality Commission (2018) state that attributes of leadership and management practice significantly determine care outcomes. Inquiries, such as those of Laming (2003) and Kirkup (2015) and most recently Ockenden (2022) and the Child Safeguarding Practice Review Panel (2022), continually highlight the enormous negative influence of ineffective leadership and management on the welfare of children. Leadership and management necessitate a strong emphasis on 'no blame' when failures occur to maximise accountability, transparency and collective responsibility.

User satisfaction is a fundamental indicator of care which uses a culture of participation (Kennedy, 2010), involving young people in care decisions and valuing their voice. The You're Welcome Quality

Criteria (Office for Health Improvement and Disparities, 2023) embodies this for young people and the Berwick (2013) report recommends that the patient and carer voice should be 'heard constantly'.

SEE ALSO
CHAPTER 1

SAFEGUARDING STOP POINT: CHILD'S VOICE

A common criticism in Child Safeguarding Case Reviews is that professionals do not speak and listen to children enough. They should be seen as active partners in care, continually involved in decisions about them with information feedback which is developmentally appropriate to support any specific communication needs (HM Government, 2018; The National Institute for Health and Care Excellence, 2019).

Policy and guidance, alongside professional values all drive care excellence (World Health Organization, 2018), aiming to tackle health inequalities, prevent and treat acute illness/injury and support the management of long-term conditions, disease and disability (Department of Health and Social Care, 2004; Public Health England, 2016). However, the UK falls behind many countries when examining both child and young people's experiences and health and wellbeing outcomes (Hargreaves et al., 2019).

Comparcini et al. (2018) exploring children and young people's perceptions of care quality found kindness, honesty, and empathy to be most important and creating a caring culture is embedded within The Code of the Nursing and Midwifery Council (NMC, 2018), Healthcare Leadership Model (NHS Leadership Academy, 2013), the NHS Long Term Plan (NHS England and NHS Improvement, 2019) and the Nursing Strategy (NHS England, 2016).

The creation of integrated care systems is a significant step in supporting NHS leaders in using the above attributes to build effective relationships, cohesive systems and nurture innovation for progressive change (Department of Health and Social Care, 2022).

Whatever leadership styles are used, there are certain concepts primarily found within values-based and relational types (adaptive, transformational, servant, authentic, collective) which research indicates as beneficial for positive outcomes (Cummings et al., 2018; McCay et al., 2018). The Messenger and Pollard (2022) health and social care leadership report advocates this, which forms core competencies for children and young people's nurses.

Effective relational and values-based leadership has compassion at its centre (Dixon-Woods et al., 2014). Organisational culture is the 'way things are done around here', rooted in established practice and policy. According to Mannion and Davies (2018), there are three levels of healthcare culture:

- Visible manifestations – such as distribution of services, care pathways, staffing practices, management of risk and improvement
- Shared ways of thinking – values and beliefs on which the above are formed
- Deeper shared assumptions – instinctive practice that is often unquestioned

Culture is therefore both experienced and created; social justice and equity in compassionate relationships build trust, inclusion, and belongingness (Kline, 2019). Wise compassion balances authentic concern with the need to move the care plan forward with a final goal of individual and service outcomes, tackling the difficult things head on, but with genuine attention to people's emotions and wellbeing (West, 2021).

PRACTITIONER VOICE – BECOMING A NATIONAL NURSE LEADER

I am a nurse, fulfilling my childhood ambition, privileged to be within a profession which offers much opportunity, but as a nursing student *'being a leader'* was not on my radar. My values were shaped by my early career experience and those I have been privileged to care for. Compassion, integrity and dignity remain central to my work. Harnessing passion and learning fuelled the drive, strength, and confidence to take opportunities to work across organisational boundaries to influence and lead. Now as a national nurse leader, I work across government and globally with the World Health Organization, influencing and advocating nationally and internationally, being the voice for the profession and importantly for children and families. Being a leader requires resilience, humility, and authenticity, together with the ability to influence, negotiate and have vision. Importantly, leadership is about taking others with you and empowering their self-belief.

Wendy Nicholson MBE (RGN RSCN RNT) – Deputy Chief Nurse and Deputy Head of World Health Organization Collaborating Centre for Public Health Nursing and Midwifery, Office for Health Improvement & Disparities, Department of Health and Social Care

---

ACTIVITY 36.3: COMPASSIONATE LEADERSHIP VIDEO

Watch this video about collective compassionate leadership:

www.kingsfund.org.uk/audio-video/michael-west-leadership

Tips to support you to develop leadership qualities in practice are:

Attend – notice your own and others' challenges, reflect on yours and ask about theirs

Understand – be interested, question and consider what you and others can learn

Empathise – be aware of frequently shifting situations, sensitively listen and tune in to each other's emotions

Help – provide time and engage in actions that will be most helpful in lessening each other's distress

Emotional intelligence

To lead compassionately and effectively, all nurses need to also engage in self-compassion, which is central to emotional intelligence. Goleman (1999) delineated key domains of emotional intelligence as playing a significant role in supporting leadership, assisting to meet patient need. It is the ability to perceive, understand, manage and influence emotion to guide individual thinking, feeling and behaviours and through this recognise and attend to others.

Table 36.1 Summary of emotional intelligence characteristics

Self-awareness	Identifying own emotions and responses, and how these may impact others
Self-regulation	Controlling emotions and responses in a contextually appropriate way
Social awareness	Considering and seeking the perspective of, in order to motivate and/or empathise with, individuals and groups of people
Social skills	Suitably interacting and communicating with others to develop valuable relationships

SEE ALSO
CHAPTER 5

Evidence indicates that emotional intelligence is a predictor of individual and team performance in nursing, and parents and caregivers believe their children experience safer, higher-quality care when nurses demonstrate it (Wang et al., 2018; Gelkop et al., 2022).

Emotionally intelligent nurses are calm, rational, and successful in challenging situations, fulfilling professional standards and fulfilling their ethical obligation to care. They also foster teamwork through collaboration, promoting the need for all nurses to work together effectively.

According to West et al. (2015), successful teamwork is reliant on leadership which maximises the contributions of all team members. For this to happen, leaders need to understand the task, competencies and action required.

STUDENT VOICE – ROLE MODELS

During my time as a student, I have come across nurses who I am in awe of, hoping that one day, I too, might become like them. These people often leave you feeling valued, confident, and motivated. The inspirational nurses I have worked with were leaders who showed compassion, knowledge, and exceptional communication skills. They were respected and loved by their team because they were fair, hardworking, and kind. My advice to 3rd-year students attending their final placements is to find someone who displays these values, work closely with them, ask them questions, and find out why they do the things they do. Use them as a role model, because before you know it, you too will be a role model for others. Inspiration is powerful and contagious, so be the change you want to see.

Harrie Devlin (Children's Nursing Student).

Demonstrating professional values and behaviours, and supporting colleagues is a collective inter-professional responsibility that exists at all levels. Having effective role models, and being a role model help influence organisational culture. Healthcare organisations that are successful are flexible and adaptable, termed by Senge (1994) as 'learning organisations' where new models of thinking are encouraged, aspiration is welcomed, and people persistently discover and grow together.

Systems thinking is also crucial enabling effective leaders to collaborate in 'communities of practice' for joined-up thinking, risk management, and improved child and family nursing care. Leadership which understands unique circumstances, values difference and fosters psychological safety leads to inclusive and courageous teams. Empowering registered and pre-registered nurses to share anxieties, report concerns and support systems, promotes safe, compassionate high quality care.

ACTIVITY 36.4: CRITICAL THINKING – RAISING CONCERNS

Watch 'Raising concerns' video by Health Education England www.youtube.com/watch?v=zjau1EyOdi8

- As a nursing student, do you know how to raise any concerns regarding ineffective practice and/ or leadership that may lead to poor patient outcomes?
- See if you can find your placement area's Raising Concerns or Whistleblowing Policy, what do you think are the most important principles of the policy?

For further reading, look at: Nursing and Midwifery Council (2019) *Raising Concerns: Guidance for Nurses, Midwives and Nursing Associates*. Available at: www.nmc.org.uk/standards/guidance/raising-concerns-guidance-for-nurses-and-midwives/.

CHAPTER SUMMARY

- Every child and young people's nurse, no matter what level they work, role they hold or specialty they are in, is a leader for high-quality, safe care.
- Leadership and management are multifaceted, multicontextual and can be defined and examined in multiple ways.
- Leadership, which is values-based and relational, ensures children and young people's nurses can put their strengths to their best use and feel understood, valued and psychologically safe.
- Collectively, the nursing literature recognises key characteristics and competencies for effective leadership and management – compassion, emotional intelligence, role modelling, motivational skills, teamwork and courage.
- Children and young people's nursing teams and services need effective leadership and management at all levels to develop caring, transparent, learning cultures for staff to deliver continuous advancements for the health and wellbeing of patients and the wider population.
- Leadership is a professional responsibility and can be learned. It is a constant journey of personal and professional self-discovery and development and innovation for service improvement.

BUILD YOUR BIBLIOGRAPHY

Books

FURTHER
READING

- Ellis, P. (2021) *Leadership, Management and Team Working in Nursing*, 4th edn. London: Sage.

  Mapped to the NMC (2018) Standards, this book introduces nursing students to the principles and practice of leadership and management.

- Gopee, N. and Galloway, J. (2017) *Leadership and Management in Healthcare*, 3rd edn. London: Sage.

  Ideal reading when undertaking leadership modules and completing management placements. It has action points, case studies and strong practice guidelines to enable you to understand how leadership and management theory applies to care delivery.

- Barr, J. and Dowding, L. (2019) *Leadership in Health Care*, 4th edn. London: Sage.

  Supported by the NMC (2018) Standards, the need for leadership in an everyday context is highlighted throughout. There are activities to support you to engage in key leadership topics such as teamwork, communication, problem-solving, emotional intelligence, and critical self-reflection.

Journal articles

- Cummings, G.G., Tate, K., Lee, S. et al. (2018) 'Leadership styles and outcome patterns for the nursing workforce and work environment: a systematic review'. *International Journal of Nursing Studies*, 85: 19–60. doi:10.1016/j.ijnurstu.2018.04.016.

  A literature review providing evidence that relational leadership styles are associated with significantly improved outcomes for the nursing workforce and their work environments.

- James, A.H., Bennett, C.L., Blanchard, D. and Stanley, D. (2021) 'Nursing and values-based leadership: a literature review'. *Journal of Nursing Management*, 29 (5): 916–30. doi:10.1111/jonm.13273.

  A literature review exploring the understanding of values-based leadership in nursing for improved staff wellbeing, inter-professional practice, and patient outcomes.

- Lambert, S. (2021) 'Role of emotional intelligence in effective nurse leadership'. *Nursing Standard*, 36 (9). doi:10.7748/ns.2021.e11782.

  An easy-to-read article exploring emotional intelligence, its importance as a characteristic of effective nurse leaders and suggesting practical activities to develop related skills.

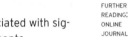

FURTHER READING: ONLINE JOURNAL ARTICLES

Weblinks

- The NHS Leadership Academy www.leadershipacademy.nhs.uk/ The academy exists to support NHS staff to develop their full leadership potential for high-quality care. There are lots of resources to discover and it is the home of the Healthcare Leadership Model.
- The Kings Fund www.kingsfund.org.uk/ An independent charity working to improve health and care in England. One of their four key topics that they produce resources for is Leadership, Systems and Organisations.
- NHS England – Leading Change, Adding Value www.england.nhs.uk/nursingmidwifery/ This section of the NHS England website holds relevant information to support nurses to engage and lead transformational change across health and care.

FURTHER READING: WEBLINKS

REFERENCES

Barr, J. and Dowding, L. (2019) *Leadership in Health Care*, 4th edn. London: Sage.

Berwick, D. (2013) *A Promise to Learn – a Commitment to Act – Improving the Safety of Patients in England*. London: Department of Health.

Care Quality Commission (2018) *Quality Improvement in Hospital Trusts: Sharing Learning from Trusts on a Journey of QI*. Gallowgate: Care Quality Commission. Available at: www.cqc.org.uk/publications/evaluation/quality-improvement-hospital-trusts-sharing-learning-trusts-journey-qi (accessed 3 June 2022).

Child Safeguarding Practice Review Panel (2022) *National Review into the Murders of Arthur Labinjo-Hughes and Star Hobson*. Available at: www.gov.uk/government/publications/national-review-into-the-murders-of-arthur-labinjo-hughes-and-star-hobson (accessed 3 June 2022).

Comparcini, D., Simonetti, V., Tomietto, M. et al. (2018) 'Children's perceptions about the quality of pediatric nursing care: a large multicenter cross-sectional study'. *Journal of Nursing Scholarship*, 50 (3): 287–95. Available at: https://doi.org/10.1111/jnu.12381.

Cope, V. and Murray, M. (2017) 'Leadership styles in nursing'. *Nursing Standard*, 31 (43). Available at: https://doi.org/10.7748/ns.2017.e10836.

Cummings, G.G., Tate, K., Lee, S. et al. (2018) 'Leadership styles and outcome patterns for the nursing workforce and work environment: a systematic review'. *International Journal of Nursing Studies*, 85: 19–60. Available at: https://doi.org/10.1016/j.ijnurstu.2018.04.016.

Department of Health (2011) *You're Welcome – Quality Criteria for Young People Friendly Health Services*. Available at: https://assets.publishing.service.gov.uk/government/uploads/system/uploads/attachment_data/file/216350/dh_127632.pdf (accessed 22 June 2023).

Department of Health and Social Care (2004) *National Service Framework: Children, Young People and Maternity Services*. Available at: www.gov.uk/government/publications/national-service-framework-children-young-people-and-maternity-services (accessed 10 April 2022).

Department of Health and Social Care (2021) *The NHS Constitution for England*. Available at: www.gov.uk/government/publications/the-nhs-constitution-for-england/the-nhs-constitution-for-england (accessed 23 March 2022).

Department of Health and Social Care (2022) *The Government's 2022–23 mandate to NHS England*. Available at: https://assets.publishing.service.gov.uk/government/uploads/system/uploads/attachment_data/file/1065713/2022-to-2023-nhs-england-mandate.pdf (accessed 4 June 2022).

Dixon-Woods, M., Baker, R., Charles, K. et al. (2014) 'Culture and behaviour in the English National Health Service: overview of lessons from a large multimethod study'. *BMJ Quality and Safety*, 23 (2): 106–15

Ellis, P. (2021) *Leadership, Management and Team Working in Nursing*, 4th edn. London: Sage.

Fennell, K. (2021) 'Conceptualisations of leadership and relevance to health and human service workforce development: a scoping review'. *Journal of Multidisciplinary Healthcare*, 14: 3035–51.

Gelkop, C., Kagan, I. and Rozani, V. (2022) 'Are emotional intelligence and compassion associated with nursing safety and quality care? A cross-sectional investigation in pediatric settings'. *Journal of Pediatric Nursing: Nursing Care of Children and Families*, 62: e98–e102. doi.org/10.1016/j.pedn.2021.07.020.

Giordano-Mulligan, M. and Eckardt, S. (2019) 'Authentic nurse leadership conceptual framework: nurses' perception of authentic nurse leader attributes'. *Nursing Administration Quarterly*, 43 (2): 164–74.

Goleman, D. (1999) *Working with Emotional Intelligence*. London: Bloomsbury.

Gopee, N. and Galloway, J. (2017) *Leadership and Management in Healthcare*, 3rd edn. London: Sage.

Hargreaves, D.S., Lemer, C., Ewing, C. et al. (2019) 'Measuring and improving the quality of NHS care for children and young people'. *Archives of Disease in Childhood*, 104 (7): 618–21.

HM Government (2018) *Working Together to Safeguard Children - A guide to inter-agency working to safeguard and promote the welfare of children*. Available at: https://assets.publishing.service.gov.uk/government/uploads/system/uploads/attachment_data/file/729914/Working_Together_to_Safeguard_Children-2018.pdf (accessed 22 June 2023).

James, A.H., Bennett, C.L., Blanchard, D. and Stanley, D. (2021) 'Nursing and values-based leadership: a literature review'. *Journal of Nursing Management*, 29 (5): 916–30.

Kennedy, I. (2010) *Getting It Right for Children and Young People: Overcoming cultural barriers in the NHS so as to meet their needs*. A review. Available at: www.gov.uk/government/publications/getting-it-right-for-children-and-young-people-overcoming-cultural-barriers-in-the-nhs-so-as-to-meet-their-needs (accessed 22 June 2023).

Kirkup, B. (2015) *The Report of the Morecambe Bay Investigation*. Norwich: TSO.

Kline, R. (2019) 'Leadership in the NHS'. *BMJ Leader*, 3 (4). doi.org/10.1136/leader-2019-000159.

Laming, Lord (2003) *The Victoria Climbié Inquiry*. CM5730. Norwich: TSO. Available at: http://dera. ioe.ac.uk/6086/2/climbiereport.pdf (accessed 9 April 2015).

Long, T. (2020) 'Effect of authentic leadership on newly qualified nurses: a scoping review'. *Nursing Management*, 27 (3). doi.org/10.7748/nm.2020.e1901.

Machon, M., Cundy, D. and Case, H. (2019) 'Innovation in nursing leadership: a skill that can be learned'. *Nursing Administration Quarterly*, 43 (3): 267–73.

Mannion, R. and Davies, H. (2018) 'Understanding organisational culture for healthcare quality improvement'. *BMJ*, 363: k4907. doi.org/10.1136/bmj.k4907.

Maxwell, J.C. and Dornan, J. (2018) *Becoming a Person of Influence: How to Positively Impact the Lives of Others*. Nashville: Thomas Nelson Publishing.

McCay, R., Lyles, A.A. and Larkey, L. (2018) 'Nurse leadership style, nurse satisfaction, and patient satisfaction: a systematic review'. *Journal of Nursing Care Quality*, 33 (4): 361–7.

Messenger, G. and Pollard, L. (2022) *Leadership for a Collaborative and Inclusive Future*. London: Department of Health and Social Care. Available at: www.gov.uk/government/publications/ health-and-social-care-review-leadership-for-a-collaborative-and-inclusive-future/leadership-for-a-collaborative-and-inclusive-future (accessed 9 June 2022).

NHS England (2016) 'Leading Change, Adding Value: A framework for nursing, midwifery and care staff'. NHS England. Available at: www.england.nhs.uk/wp-content/uploads/2016/05/nursing-framework.pdf (accessed 19 September 2021).

NHS England and NHS Improvement (2019) *The NHS Long Term Plan*. Available at: www.longtermplan. nhs.uk/wp-content/uploads/2019/08/nhs-long-term-plan-version-1.2.pdf (accessed 19 August 2021).

NHS Leadership Academy (2013) 'Healthcare Leadership Model'. NHS Leadership Academy. Available at:www.leadershipacademy.nhs.uk/wp-content/uploads/2014/10/NHSLeadership-LeadershipModel-colour.pdf (accessed 30 June 2017).

NICE (National Institute for Health and Care Excellence) (2019) Child abuse and neglect. Quality standard [QS179]. Available at: www.nice.org.uk/guidance/qs179/resources/child-abuse-and-neglect-pdf-75545669305285 (accessed 22 June 2023).

Nightingale, A. (2020) 'Implementing collective leadership in healthcare organisations'. *Nursing Standard*, 35 (5). doi.org/10.7748/ns.2020.e11448.

Nursing and Midwifery Council (NMC) (2018) *The Code: Professional Standards of Practice and Behaviour for Nurses, Midwives and Nursing Associates*. London: NMC. Available at: www.nmc.org.uk/standards/code/.

Ockenden, D. (2022) *Final Findings, Conclusions and Essential Actions from the Ockenden Review of Maternity Services at Shrewsbury and Telford Hospital NHS Trust*. Available at: www.gov.uk/ government/publications/final-report-of-the-ockenden-review (accessed 30 March 2022).

Office for Health Improvement and Disparities (2023) *'You're Welcome': establishing youth-friendly health and care services, GOV.UK*. Available at: https://www.gov.uk/government/publications/ establishing-youth-friendly-health-and-care-services/youre-welcome-establishing-youth-friendly-health-and-care-services (accessed 7 October 2023).

Public Health England (2016) *Health Matters: Giving Every Child the Best Start in Life*. Available at: www.gov.uk/government/publications/health-matters-giving-every-child-the-best-start-in-life/ health-matters-giving-every-child-the-best-start-in-life (accessed 10 April 2022).

Senge, P.M. (1994) *The Fifth Discipline Fieldbook: Strategies and Tools for Building a Learning Organization*. New York: Crown Business.

Timmins, N. (2015) *The Practice of System Leadership: Being Comfortable with Chaos*. London: The King's Fund. Available at: www.kingsfund.org.uk/publications/practice-system-leadership (accessed 13 March 2022).

Wang, L., Tao, H., Bowers, B.J., Brown, R. and Zhang, Y. (2018) 'When nurse emotional intelligence matters: How transformational leadership influences intent to stay'. *Journal of Nursing Management*, 26 (4): 358–65.

West, M.A. (2021) *Compassionate Leadership: Sustaining Wisdom, Humanity and Presence in Health and Social Care*. London: The Swirling Leaf Press.

West, M., Armit, K., Loewenthal, L., Eckert, R., West, T. and Lee, A. (2015) *Leadership and Leadership Development in Healthcare: The Evidence Base*. London: Faculty of Medical Leadership and Management. Available at: www.kingsfund.org.uk/publications/leadership-and-leadership-development-health-care (accessed 13 March 2022).

West, M., Eckert, R. and Pasmore, B. (2014) *Developing Collective Leadership for Health Care*. London: The Kings Fund. Available at: www.kingsfund.org.uk/publications/developing-collective-leadership-health-care (accessed 13 March 2022).

World Health Organization (WHO) (2018) *Standards for Improving the Quality of Care for Children and Young Adolescents in Health Facilities*. Geneva: WHO. Available at: https://apps.who.int/iris/handle/10665/272346 (accessed 10 April 2022).

LIFELONG LEARNING AND CONTINUING PROFESSIONAL DEVELOPMENT IN CHILDREN AND YOUNG PEOPLE'S NURSING

37

CLAIRE ANDERSON

THIS CHAPTER COVERS

- Examination of continuing professional development (CPD) for the children's nurse and why it is important
- Socio-political drivers for CPD
- The experience of nurses who have undertaken CPD
- Theories of learning and how they apply to CPD for the children's nurse

> "I have always been nervous about academic writing, lacking significantly in confidence … However, I did have a passion for learning and teaching and fully appreciated that lifelong learning is an essential part of not only my personal and professional development, but also that of others."
>
> **Judy, children's nurse**

INTRODUCTION

Once registered, nurses, shift by shift, gain more and more confidence in their ability to nurse. In contrast, many nurses lose confidence in their academic ability. The quotation above describes how one registered nurse feels about continuing her education. She is nervous and lacks confidence in her academic ability but at the same time recognises why continuing to learn as a nurse is so important. Continuing your development after you register as a nurse is referred to as 'continuing professional development' (CPD).

The Nursing and Midwifery Council (NMC) defines CPD as 'taking part in appropriate and regular learning and professional development activities that aim to maintain and develop your competence and performance' (NMC, 2017).

Nurses do need to know how to practise, and throughout their pre-registration education equal emphasis is placed on academic and practice achievement. After registering as a children and young people's nurse this balance between learning in practice and learning formally through academic study remains important. CPD is more than just academic development. While understanding the evidence that supports nursing practice is key, nurses also need to develop their nursing skills. This includes specific skills or updates that may be an employment or professional requirement.

In this chapter three nurses describe their CPD experience and it is clear that, while they have all achieved academic success, for some nurses the experience of CPD is not always easy.

EXAMINATION OF CPD FOR THE CHILDREN'S NURSE AND WHY IT IS IMPORTANT

Historically, there was an expectation that all nurses would maintain a portfolio that outlined all the different types of activities that they had undertaken as CPD. This process has been made more formal and in order to revalidate their registration with the NMC all nurses are required to provide evidence of their continuing practice and their continuing development (NMC, 2021):

- 450 practice hours over 3 years (or 900 hours if you have dual registration as a midwife and a nurse)
- 35 hours CPD, including 20 hours participatory learning
- A minimum of five pieces of practice-related feedback
- A minimum of five written reflective accounts on your CPD, and/or practice-related feedback, and/or an event or experience in your own professional practice and how this relates to The Code (NMC, 2018a)
- A reflective discussion with another NMC registrant covering your five written reflective accounts
- Health and character declaration
- Declaration that you have a professional indemnity arrangement
- Third-party confirmation that you have complied with the revalidation requirements

The NMC distinguishes between undertaking CPD by your self or with others which they describe as 'participatory learning': 'of those 35 hours of CPD, at least 20 must have included participatory learning' (NMC, 2021).

CPD can be done by yourself, for example searching and critiquing current evidence that relates to your practice. But, 20 hours of this CPD must be done in participation with others; this could be formal academic study or less formal, such as attending a conference. In both instances you need to provide evidence of this CPD for your re-validation.

The NMC has published standards for supervision and assessment (NMC, 2018b) which introduced three roles – Practice Supervisor, Practice Assessor and Academic Assessor. The roles of the Practice Supervisor and Practice Assessor replaced the previous student support and assessment roles of the mentor and sign-off mentor.

Preparation for these roles is less formal (although still counting as participatory CPD) and involves on-line resources along with local arrangements by healthcare providers, often in conjunction with Higher Education Institutions. The role of the Practice Supervisor is described as providing a 'role model' for students and it may be something that you undertake quite early in your career and preparing to become a Practice Supervisor may therefore be your first experience of CPD. The Practice Supervisor works with students and records feedback on their practice, knowledge and skills both to the student and the role of the Practice Assessor.

The Practice Assessor will also directly observe student practice but also considers the feedback from the Practice Supervisor. They use an objective and evidence-based approach to make decisions about assessment and progression of the student and work closely with the Academic Assessor to achieve this (NMC, 2018b).

It is important that you are aware of these roles because, as a registered nurse, you have a role in developing the future nursing workforce. As you grow more experienced in student supervision you will progress to taking on the role of the Practice Assessor. You may find the process of supporting students a little intimidating at first, but the CPD preparation will help. It is useful to remember your own experience as a student nurse when developing skills to become a Practice Supervisor/Practice Assessor. Rather than considering the roles challenging, remember how you were supported to develop your nursing skills; or perhaps you can remember a Practice Supervisor or Practice Assessor on whom you can model your own supervision and assessment styles.

SOCIO-POLITICAL DRIVERS FOR CPD

There are also many political drivers for developing the future workforce, which have some influence on CPD. This includes the NHS Long Term Plan (2019) and more recently the NHS Long Term Workforce Plan (2023), which identifies the need to educate the workforce who will deliver healthcare in the 21st century.

The case studies outline the personal opportunities and challenges the nurses had when undertaking CPD. The government has announced that frontline nurses, midwives and allied health professionals will be offered personalised development budgets of £1000 over 3 years (HM Treasury, 2019). However, it could be suggested that this reflects a reduction in the resources available to fund CPD. During the pandemic, the reliance on the nursing workforce was evident, as was the shortage of specialist skilled nurses to care for critically ill patients. It is acknowledged there is a global shortage of nurses, and the profession needs to be invested in (Catton and Iro, 2021). It is important that now, more than ever, developing the nursing workforce is a priority. Developing a workforce with the right skills often means developing specialist skills. As such, CPD needs to be more than mandatory training, it should represent developing nurses to be leaders of the profession and be able to deliver high-quality healthcare to the child and young person. The nurse undertaking CPD must value the experience and relate it to how it impacts on practice. The employing organisations need to value the nurse and recognise how their CPD achievements will enhance the care they deliver.

CPD is about taking the newly registered nurse on the journey from their graduation and forward throughout their career. It is also about recognising that there is an existing workforce of nurses who need to maintain their skills. There is an international shortage of nurses and the nurses who are in practice and specialised are an aging population (Griffith, 2012). CPD is about motivating this workforce to remain in nursing, valuing their existing knowledge and building on this knowledge to reflect and respond to the dynamic nature of nursing in the 21st century.

ACTIVITY 37.1: CRITICAL THINKING

Access the NHS Long Term Plan (2019) – which supports the use of digital technology in Chapter 5. The plan states that digitally enabled care will go mainstream across the NHS:

Technology will play a central role in realising the Long-Term Plan, helping clinicians use the full range of their skills, reducing bureaucracy, stimulating research and enabling service transformation. People will have more control over the care they receive and more support to manage their health, to keep themselves well and better manage their conditions, while assisting carers in their vital work.

www.longtermplan.nhs.uk/online-version/chapter-5-digitally-enabled-care-will-go-mainstream-across-the-nhs/

Just as the nature of nursing is a dynamic ever-changing process so is how we learn. One constant is that nurse education has always been about practice alongside knowledge and so the learning environment is not always in the classroom. It is important that nurses develop academically so that they are equipped with an understanding of the complexities of healthcare and that their contribution to this healthcare as a profession is valued and respected. However, alongside the formal learning there is a range of learning opportunities that are employed.

Simulation of clinical practice has been used in nursing studies for some time and it is particularly relevant to CPD. The approach has its foundations in Kolb's experiential learning theory – learning is achieved through expereince (Mitchell, 2020; Tolarba, 2021). The registered nurse often has to learn new skills and practise them competently. With simulated learning the student practises and is assessed in an environment that represents the clinical workplace, but not with real patients. While they are learning, the student can practise their skills without risk of harming the patient (Tolarba, 2021). There is some evidence that the student being assessed in a safe environment practising their clinical skills in cases using high-fidelity simulation is more likely to become confident and competent (Bradley, 2012).

During the COVID-19 pandemic much of CPD was delivered online or virtually and there have been some challenges and some benefits to this approach. The challenges sometimes related to the assumption or expectation that everyone had the technology required available to them at home (Bramer, 2020). Or that the student felt quite isolated and not fully supported by their lecturer in their development (Connolly et al., 2020). However, there were identified benefits such as the students were able to access the taught sessions both synchronously and asynchronously and that the approach was seen as more student-centred, allowing them to determine their progress through the learning process (Bramer, 2020).

ACTIVITY 37.2: CRITICAL THINKING

Read the NHS Long Term Plan and consider how it proposes to develop the workforce with the right skills to deliver healthcare in the 21st century.

www.longtermplan.nhs.uk/online-version/overview-and-summary/

Another relatively recent approach to learning is through social media sites. We live in a technological society and these sites offer a different mode of communication. The debate arises from when they are used without caution. Our priority must be the need to be professional when communicating via social media. When 'instagramming', tweeting, snapchatting or posting on Facebook we need to recognise the risk that these are public spaces and we must protect the confidentiality of children and their families, organisations and fellow professionals. Despite the cautionary advice (NMC, 2022), social media sites used in the right way are effective contemporary approaches to learning and offer the support of peer networks. Try using and participating the @WeCYPnurses X feed and joining @WeCommunities.

SAFEGUARDING STOP POINT

We need to protect the confidentiality of children and families when using social media sites, as per the NMC social networking guidance (2022).

- The principles of safeguarding should underpin our CPD:
- Health Education England must ensure that the principles of safeguarding are integral to education and training curricula for health professionals. (NHS England, 2015, p.21)

This chapter aims to identify why CPD is important for children's nurses and has begun by outlining socio-political drivers for this but will now explore the real-life experiences of nurses who have undertaken CPD. The case studies below refer to the three nurses mentioned earlier. They all undertook CPD to gain their degree as they had registered before all pre-registration courses were graduate level. Each of them describes the challenges of CPD but also how it has made them feel and how they will carry on in their CPD journey.

THE EXPERIENCE OF NURSES WHO HAVE UNDERTAKEN CPD

Below are three examples of registered nurses who are continuing their studies; two of them are completing their degree as they registered having completed a Diploma or Advanced Diploma in Nursing. This will not be the case for nurses completing their registering qualification today. All the examples relate to CPD and include what the nurses find challenging, how they feel and what they think they are achieving.

CASE STUDY 37.1: JUDY

Judy works as a practice educator and was completing a degree after qualifying as a children's nurse with a Diploma. She begins by describing her motivation to become a children's nurse:

'I knew from a very young age that I wanted to work with children and was very interested in the art of nursing. I grew up with a sibling who spent a lot of time as a child being cared for in hospital by children's nurses. I remember being fascinated with them, how hard they worked and how caring they were ... a true inspiration. I wanted to be just like them, making sick children's lives better in every way possible.'

(Continued)

As she reflects on her experience of CPD it is clear that she sees how it has impacted on her practice and how she will use the experience to influence other nurses.

'I want to specialise in practice education because by following this path, I am not only able to develop and influence my own practice for the better but am able to positively influence the care of many children and young people through the continued support, education, skills and knowledge of many nurses, parents and children and young people themselves, thus ensuring evidence-based practice and patient safety for all.'

- What motivated you to become a children and young people's nurse?

CASE STUDY 37.2: JON

Jon works in a clinical research facility and 'topped up' his non-honours degree. Like all nurses, he had to meet the professional requirements of maintaining his NMC status but was also under some pressure to complete his degree and work towards a Master's qualification.

'After working as a healthcare assistant with children with learning disabilities the move to study nursing seemed like the next logical career step after this, so I began my studies in 2005 at the age of 25 and I graduated with a non-honours degree. I have found that I am passionate about children's nursing and I have moved through the ranks and I have just moved from practice educator to a research facility.'

- In a healthcare climate where there are shortages of nurses and employers are finding it difficult to retain the nurses that they have, what would motivate you to remain in an organisation?
- What would motivate you to undertake CPD as a nurse?

CASE STUDY 37.3: HARPREET

Harpreet works in a bone marrow transplant specialist ward. She also talks about her motivation to become a children's nurse but is aware of the specialist nature of the type of nursing she does and the importance of developing practice with evidence.

'I was raised in a medical family and would often see the passion my parents had for their careers. I wanted to care for people and offer reassurance, kindness and support whilst they are experiencing some of the worst times of their lives. Unwell children along with their families need advocates and need to gain trust in care professionals. I wanted to be that for them and aim to make a horrible situation easier. I wanted to specialise in bone marrow transplants because the ongoing research and medication is the future to curing some of the worst conditions in the world.'

She refers to research that will change how the children in her specialty are being treated.

- Can you think of an example of evidence-based practice that has changed since you started nursing? This does not need to be specialist research; it could be something quite straightforward such as the research behind the importance of hand washing but still makes a big difference to how we practise.

THEORIES OF LEARNING AND HOW THEY APPLY TO CPD FOR THE CHILDREN'S NURSE

There are several theoretical approaches to learning that can be used in nursing.

Malcolm Knowles' andragogy model

The principles of andragogy, introduced by Malcolm Knowles in 1980 and developed further in 1984, emphasise the learning strategy of facilitating autonomous learning (Knowles et al., 2005). Rather than a passive approach to learning, the learner has to seek out the new knowledge for themselves. They may be aided in doing so by lecturers signposting their way but the responsibility is their own. In this approach the nurse makes sense of what they learn by applying this knowledge to their practice. Many nurses find it easier to learn if they can make sense of their learning. Their experience adds to the resources they have to draw from. The andragogical learner has to see the relevance and value in their learning experience.

WHAT'S THE EVIDENCE?

Malcolm Knowles (1984) describes five assumptions about the adult learner:

1. *Self-concept*: The adult learner differs from the child learner as they become more self-directed
2. *Adult learner experience*: The adult learner has more resources available to them through their own experiences
3. *Readiness to learn*: As a mature adult this relates their learning to the development of their social roles
4. *Orientation to learning*: The learner moves from focus on the subject to focus on a problem-solving approach
5. *Motivation to learn*: An adult learner motivates themselves to learn using an andragogical approach to learning, that is, using your own experience to inform but also as an autonomous learner seeking out the evidence you need

Answer the questions below:

- What does the evidence say about using antipyretics when a child is pyrexial?
- What is your experience of managing pyrexia in children?

Judy discusses how she initially lacked confidence but developed this during her studies, and not only gained in her own confidence but how she could use this to enable others to study.

"I have always been nervous about academic writing, lacking significantly in confidence. I also was not overly confident with teaching and assessing others and had not quite discovered my own teaching style or developed an appreciation for the different learning styles there are ..."

Judy, children's nurse

Harpreet also can see how by learning she is more confident in teaching:

"Since completing this module, I have continued to grow comfortable and confident in the art of teaching and assisting others, both patients, their families as well as my colleagues to learn new skills, assessing their understanding and competence as a progressive experience."

Harpreet, children's nurse

The constructionist or experiential approach

A different learning theory, the constructionist or experiential approach to learning, also recognises the value of experience. The learner uses their own experience and knowledge to develop and acquire more. Kolb's experiential learning style theory is typically represented by a four-stage learning cycle, as you can see in Figure 37.1.

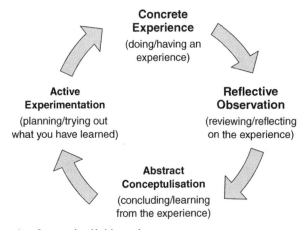

Figure 37.1 Kolb's cycle of experiential learning

www.simplypsychology.org/learning-kolb.html

An approach often used in constructionist learning is case-based learning or problem-based learning, where students work as a group or a team to explore a case or problem and which reflects the reality of the healthcare workforce. It is not without its challenges, as we can see from Harpreet's description of an experience when she was studying with a group of colleagues more senior to her:

"I found this module extremely challenging – especially the anatomy and physiology of the acutely ill. The classroom sessions were interactive but I was studying alongside some very senior staff members which made me self-conscious and unconfident in answering questions."

Harpreet, children's nurse

Anderson (2016) offers a helpful summary of different models of learning styles, while also acknowledging that there are limitations to aligning with a single approach. As an adult learner, the learning experience can be enhanced by using a range of styles to suit the learning experience. The models described styles that were often opposite from each other, so an active learner needs to apply their learning while a reflective learner needs to make sense of what is being learnt by thinking it through. A sensing learner needs accuracy and factual information while an intuitive learner learns through identifying possibilities or relationships between concepts.

Visual learners prefer images to learn from and verbal learners prefer written words. Sequential learners prefer to learn in steps each step adding to previous learning. While global learners prefer a more random approach. This is not a comprehensive list of learning styles, but it is meant to demonstrate the individual nature of learning. Being aware of the theory that supports learning and of our own preferred learning style helps to demystify the process and leads us to succeed in our CPD.

ACTIVITY 37.3: REFLECTIVE PRACTICE

Spend half an hour reflecting on something you studied in the last year and how this has changed how you practise as a nurse today - you might find this easier if you use a model such as John Driscoll's (2007). You can, however, use whatever model you are most familiar with.

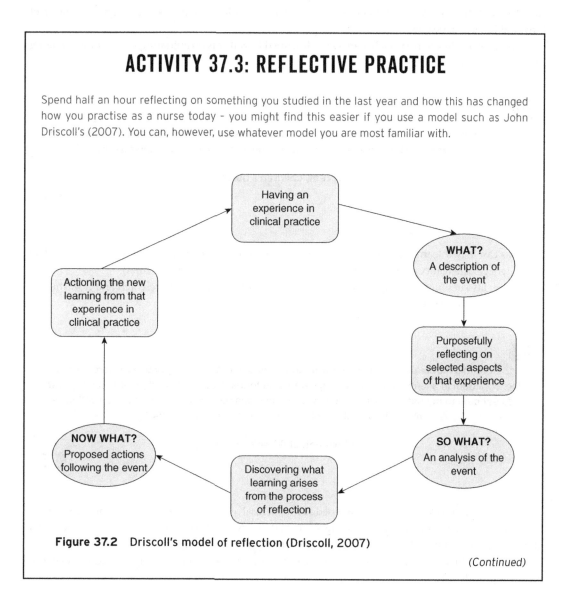

Figure 37.2   Driscoll's model of reflection (Driscoll, 2007)

(Continued)

- *What?* What did you study or, perhaps more accurately, what did you learn? What was the easiest thing about this learning experience or what did you enjoy the most during the time you were learning? Conversely, what was hardest or most challenging about the learning experience?
- *So what?* How are you using what you learnt in your practice today?
- *What next?* Have you shared the knowledge you learnt with anyone else – taught other students or perhaps the child or their family? How will you continue to develop and build on what you learnt?

Theory and practice

Here the case studies develop and demonstrate how the theories we have looked at apply to Harpreet, Judy and Jon's experiences.

Harpreet works in a very specialist area and described how it was intimidating when studying alongside her senior colleagues:

"The classroom sessions were interactive but I was studying alongside some very senior staff members which made me self-conscious and unconfident in answering questions."

Harpreet, children's nurse

This was case-based learning where students work as a group or a team to explore a case or problem, which reflects the reality of the healthcare workforce (constructionist/experiential).

Harpreet also describes her experience of undertaking a module related to research and how she now applies this knowledge to her practice:

"Before this module I was unfamiliar with how to find and critically appraise research. I now feel confident in searching and learning, being able to teach students and provide the highest, safest care to my patients. My clinical practice has benefited from the module as I will read routinely, search articles and discuss with colleagues."

Harpreet, children's nurse

The learner has to seek out the new knowledge for themselves. They may be aided in doing so by lecturers signposting their way but the responsibility is their own. In this approach the nurse makes sense of what they learn by applying this knowledge to their practice (andragogy).

Judy, in the first excerpt, was reflecting on her learning whilst undertaking a module related to mentoring students:

"I have always been nervous about academic writing, lacking significantly in confidence. I also was not overly confident with teaching and assessing others and had not quite discovered my own teaching style or developed an appreciation for the different learning styles there are. However, I did have a passion for learning and teaching and fully appreciated that lifelong learning is an essential part of not only my personal and professional development but also that of others."

Judy, children's nurse

The learner has to seek out the new knowledge for themselves. They may be aided in doing so by lecturers signposting their way but the responsibility is their own. In this approach the nurse makes sense of what they learn by applying this knowledge to their practice (andragogy).

Later, Judy describes their experience of undertaking a module exploring research methods and processes:

"Before completing this module, I really did not have a great knowledge base to enable me to confidently locate and interpret strong research to support my clinical practice. I knew the very basics of research interpretation, however this module enabled me to advance and build on those basic skills and knowledge. It really has, and will continue to have, a significant impact on every aspect of my nursing care, future study and role in practice development, strengthening my clinical judgement and confidence in passing this evidence-based knowledge and skill onto nursing students, parents/families and colleagues alike and most importantly keeping my clinical expertise as relevant as possible."

Judy, children's nurse

The learner uses their own experience and knowledge to develop and acquire more (constructionist/experiential).

Finally, Judy comments:

"The course gave me the confidence to start thinking about my own professional future and which direction to go."

Judy, children's nurse

The learner uses their own experience and knowledge to develop and acquire more (again, constructionist/experiential).

Jon was under pressure to gain an honours degree and also appears conscious of the professional requirements to study:

"They prove that I have continuously worked to further my knowledge and skills since qualification as well as complying with the minimum amount of study time needed every year to remain registered."

Jon, children's nurse

The learner has to seek out the new knowledge for themselves (andragogy).

There are many factors that motivate, but it is reassuring that Jon recognised that the learning experience was far more than simply meeting professional requirements:

"Together these three modules have given me a much wider and more comprehensive understanding in relation to surgical nursing as well as giving me the skills and knowledge to teach and assess students and junior nurses in the clinical setting."

Jon, children's nurse

The learner uses their own experience and knowledge to develop and acquire more (constructionist/experiential).

ACTIVITY 37.4: CRITICAL THINKING

What is your preferred learning style? Think about the last time you learnt something – this could be formally, such as a module at university, or it could be more applied, such as how to do a wound dressing. What learning styles did you use, and if you use these suggestions as examples of your own learning, did you use the same style each time?

CHAPTER SUMMARY

After reading this chapter you should:

- Be aware that CPD can enable you to inform and improve your practice, remembering that it is not only formal academic learning that counts as CPD
- Recognise that we work in a changing and complex healthcare system and this reflects the society that we live in

- Be aware that the way the children's nurse learns is informed and supported by learning theories such as andragogy and experiential learning theories. These are not abstract concepts – they help us make sense of how we learn

BUILD YOUR BIBLIOGRAPHY

Books

- Knowles, M.S, Holton, E.F., Swanson R.A. and Robinson, P.A. (2020) *The Adult Learner*, 9th edn. Abingdon: Routledge.

  Many nurses use Kolb's learning cycle but this text explains how it was developed and the principles of learning that underpin the learning cycle.

- Price, B. (2003) *Studying Nursing Using Problem-based and Enquiry-based Learning*. New York: Palgrave Macmillan.

  This is a seminal text on the process of problem-based learning. Not only does it explain the approach but also how to facilitate learning.

FURTHER
READING

Journal articles

- Stonehouse, D. (2020) 'Reflection and you'. *British Journal of Healthcare Assistants*, 14 (11): 572-4.

  This article outlines the importance of reflection and reflective practice, and introduces Gibbs' (1988) Reflective Cycle and Driscoll's (2007) Model of Structured Reflection.

- Burbach, B., Barnason, S. and Hertzog, M. (2015) 'Preferred thinking style, symptom recognition, and response by nursing students during simulation'. *Western Journal of Nursing Research*, 37 (12): 1563-80.

  This study explored the link between thinking styles rather than learning styles of students in a high-fidelity simulation case. They found that students' thinking was more rational rather than intuitive; that is, they would choose the most pragmatic solution rather than considering an instinctive response.

- Condon, B. (2015) 'Politically charged issues in nursing's teaching-learning environments'. *Nursing Science Quarterly*, 28 (2): 115-20.

  This paper explores the relationship between politics and education in the USA but has real relevance to the debate in the UK also.

- Rainey, D and Monaghan, C. (2022) 'Supporting newly qualified nurses to develop their leadership skills'. *Nursing Management*, 29 (5): 34-41.

  A personal skill that has been so important over the last few years is leadership – this helps nurses define their autonomy, role model good practice and develop their resilience.

FURTHER
READING:
ONLINE
JOURNAL
ARTICLES

Weblinks

- We Communities www.wecommunities.org This is an exciting online resource which allows you to contribute to the community of children's nurses. It has blogs and discussions which you are encouraged to participate in or you can ask questions and be offered support from your peers in this specialty of nursing.

FURTHER
READING:
WEBLINKS

- Nursing Times www.nursingtimes.net This is a valuable resource for the nursing profession and reports on breaking news developments for nurses. They are keen for nurses to write for them and there is guidance if you want to contribute to the journal.

REFERENCES

Anderson, I., (2016) 'Identifying different learning styles to enhance the learning experience'. *Nursing Standard*, 31 (7).

Bradley, C. (2012) The role of high-fidelity clinical simulation in teaching and learning in the health professions. Available at: www.researchgate.net/publication/319213058_High_Fidelity_Simulation_in_Nursing_Education (accessed 9 November 2021).

Bramer, C. (2020) 'Pre-registration adult nursing students' experiences of online learning: a qualitative study'. *British Journal of Nursing*, 29 (12): 677–83.

Catton, H. and Iro, E. (2021) 'How to reposition the nursing profession for a post-covid age'. *BMJ*, 373: n1105.

Connolly, M., Browne, F., Regan, G. and Ryder, M. (2020) 'Stakeholder perceptions of curriculum design, development and delivery for continuing e-learning for nurses'. *British Journal of Nursing*, 20 (17): 1016–22.

Driscoll, J. (2007) *Practising Clinical Supervision: A Reflective Approach for Healthcare Professionals*, 2nd edn. Edinburgh: Bailliere Tindall/Elsevier.

Griffith, M.B. (2012) 'Effective succession planning in nursing: A review of the literature'. *Journal of Nursing Management*, 20 (7): 900–11.

HM Treasury (2019) 'Career boost for almost half a million frontline NHS staff'. Available at: www.gov.uk/government/news/career-boost-for-almost-half-a-million-frontline-nhs-staff (accessed 19 February 2023).

Knowles, M. (1984) *The Adult Learner: A neglected species*, 3rd edn. Houston: Gulf Publishing.

Knowles, M., Holton, E. and Swanson, R. (2005) *The Adult Learner: The definitive classic in adult education and human resources development*, 6th edn. Burlington, MA: Elsevier.

Mitchell, A. (2020) 'Pandemic inspires innovative use of virtual simulation to teach practical skills'. *British Journal of Nursing*, 29 (20). doi.org/10.12968/bjon.2020.29.20.1214.

NHS England (2015) *Safeguarding Policy*. Available at: www.england.nhs.uk/wp-content/uploads/2015/07/safeguard-policy.pdf (accessed 19 September 2017).

NHS (2019) *The NHS Long Term Plan: Overview and Summary*. [Online] Available at: www.longtermplan.nhs.uk/online-version/overview-and-summary/ (accessed 9 November 2021).

NHS (2023) *NHS Long Term Workforce Plan*. Available at: www.england.nhs.uk/wp-content/uploads/2023/06/nhs-long-term-workforce-plan-v1.2.pdf

Nursing and Midwifery Council (NMC) (2017) *Standards for Competence for Registered Nurses*. Available at: www.nmc.org.uk/standards/additional-standards/standards-for-competence-for-registered-nurses (accessed 2 June 2017).

Nursing and Midwifery Council (NMC) (2018) *The Code: Professional Standards of Practice and Behaviour for Nurses, Midwives and Nursing Associates*. Available at: www.nmc.org.uk/standards/code/ (accessed 23 June 2023).

Nursing and Midwifery Council (2018) *Standards for Student Supervision and Assessment*. www.nmc.org.uk/globalassets/sitedocuments/standards-of-proficiency/standards-for-student-supervision-and-assessment/student-supervision-assessment.pdf (accessed 23 June 2023).

Nursing and Midwifery Council (2021) *Revalidation: What you need to do. Understand the revalidation requirements and how you can meet them.* Available at: www.nmc.org.uk/revalidation/requirements/ (accessed 9 November 2021).

Nursing and Midwifery Council (2022) *Social media guidance.* Available at: www.nmc.org.uk/standards/guidance/social-media-guidance (23 June 2023).

Tolarba, J.E.L., (2021) 'Virtual simulation in nursing education: a systematic review'. *International Journal of Nursing Education*, 13 (3).

DECISION-MAKING AND ACCOUNTABILITY IN CHILDREN AND YOUNG PEOPLE'S NURSING

38

LORRAINE HIGHE

THIS CHAPTER COVERS

- Decision-making in clinical practice
- Exploring who the decision-makers are in children and young people's healthcare
- Examining ways children's nurses improve their decision-making

"During my third year of training I worked on a burns unit. On one shift, a child came in for an outpatient dressing change and I assisted the nurse. Due to a miscommunication between myself and the nurse I brought her the wrong solution to irrigate the burn. I left the room and went to ask the nurse in charge why we used that solution instead of others. It was here that I realised my mistake and told the nurse in charge what had happened. Thankfully she was able to re-irrigate the wound and prevent any harm from occurring. This incident taught me the importance of being honest when I make mistakes and always double check when I am unsure. Moreover, I became more aware of my accountability to both my patients and colleagues. I learnt the importance of acting within my own limitations and that it is better to say when I cannot complete a task than for it to be administered in a potentially unsafe manner."

Sophie, 3rd-year children's nursing student

INTRODUCTION

Decision-making is arguably one of the most difficult and important processes a health professional has to undertake. The process requires skills in problem-solving, critical thinking, reflective practice and sound judgement, alongside knowledge of scientific evidence-based practice, ethical values and professional accountability. This chapter will discuss what we mean by clinical decision-making and how our clinical decisions display our professional accountability.

Pre-registration nursing courses as degree or masters programmes are designed to foster critical thinking and analytical reflection (NMC, 2023); however, the nature of the decisions made by a children's nursing student will depend upon the stage of the course they have reached, the clinical placement's culture and the preferences of the child or young person in their care. Throughout this chapter you will have the opportunity to identify who the decision-makers are in children's nursing and appraise theoretical models of decision-making in order to enable you to make decisions that promote safe and effective care.

DECISION-MAKING IN CLINICAL PRACTICE

Making decisions is something we do every day. Sometimes we make decisions that are not in our own best interests, but we choose to take a risk based on our judgement of a particular course of action. For example, I should have an apple for lunch, but I choose the chocolate biscuit, prioritising my mental wellbeing over my physical health. Professional decision-making involves the same process of balancing the pros and cons of a given situation, but crucially we are now making decisions that impact on children and we can be held accountable for those decisions

One of the most important factors in clinical decision-making is that of accountability. Accountability means being answerable to a higher authority for your actions. You may consider your actions are justifiable and in the best interests of your patient, but as a nurse, higher authorities can ask us to justify our actions.

Dimond (2019) identifies that there are four spheres of accountability in law for children's nurses:

- The profession through statute law
- Children and young people through tort law
- Society through public law
- The employer through the contract of employment

Profession

Our professional accountability is clearly outlined in The Code as set out by the NMC (2018) whose standards state we should: 'always practise in line with the best available evidence' (p.10); 'recognise and work within the limits of your competence' (p.15) and 'take measures to reduce as far as possible the likelihood of mistakes' (p.20). To be accountable, nurses must therefore have the ability to perform the care and accept this responsibility or alternatively have the authority to perform the care through appropriate delegation to another competent practitioner. The Code stresses that these standards also incorporate the expectations of our patients and the general public.

Students and newly qualified nurses can worry about the process of delegation. As the delegator of a caring task you remain responsible for the overall management of the child.

Watch a video by the NMC discussing the challenges nurses can experience when delegating care to other healthcare professionals available at:

www.nmc.org.uk/standards/code/code-in-action/delegation/

Children and young people

Nurses are also accountable to the individual patients and families under their care. The tort or civil law system allows a patient to seek compensation if they believe harm has been caused through negligence or a failure to uphold our duty of care. As a children's nurse it is important to be aware that a child who has suffered a personal injury has no time barrier to bringing an action against you, until they reach the age of 18 years. For example, you may need to rely on your nursing notes that are 21 years old because a newborn who suffers an injury has three years from their 18th birthday to present a civil action claim.

Society

Society holds you to account through public law. Examples for nurses would be the Medicine Act 1968 and the Mental Health Act 2007. It is possible to breach a public general act as a consequence of a decision you have made in your clinical practice. In these circumstances you would be asked to account for your actions in a criminal court of law.

Employer

Finally, a nurse who is employed by the NHS or another organisation is accountable to their employer through their contract of employment. The contract sets out the terms and conditions of employment and the standard of work expected of the employee. Nurses who breach NHS guidelines or local policies can expect to be held to account, through reasonable disciplinary procedures.

Professional judgement and decision-making is therefore open to scrutiny by a range of people, including children and young people, parents, colleagues, other professional staff and the public. My colleagues may comment on my poor choice of lunch, but this everyday decision will not be scrutinised by external criteria as outlined above through legal, clinical or procedural guidelines and standards.

WHO ARE THE DECISION-MAKERS IN CHILDREN AND YOUNG PEOPLE'S HEALTHCARE?

When decisions have to be made concerning a child's health, in the initial stages three parties are involved: the child, the parents and healthcare professionals. This section will discuss the role of each party and identify some of the challenges each party faces when contributing to healthcare decisions.

CASE STUDY 38.1: REENA

Reena is a 13-year-old girl with febrile neutropenia who refused to be transferred to the high-dependency unit (HDU) because the nurses in that ward are 'mean and uncaring'. Reena's parents are keen for her to be transferred where additional care and support can be obtained immediately. Following a long consultation with Reena and her parents the medical and nursing team respected Reena's wishes and agreed a treatment plan if Reena's condition was to deteriorate.

Two hours later Reena called over the nurse-in-charge to state that she had changed her mind, and agreed to be transferred to the HDU to 'satisfy her parent's wishes'.

- Who is the primary decision-maker in this case?
- What is your role as a nursing student?

Involving children and young people in decision-making

There are many reasons for involving children in decisions about their own healthcare and treatment. The ethical principle of autonomy or self-determination (Beauchamp and Childress, 2013) applies to children as well as adults. When children are given the opportunity to be part of the decision-making process this can give them a sense of control, which can in turn enhance their positive adjustment to the treatment plan. As illustrated in the case, Reena is unlikely to engage with the staff and care in the HDU as she does not agree with the transfer taking place.

The greatest challenge to involving children and young people in decision-making is their competence or ability to make a decision. Adults are assumed to be competent decision-makers, children are presumed to be incompetent and are therefore required to prove their competence. Reena's capacity to make a decision is not only a function of her age (as indicated by law) but also a reflection of her cognitive ability and personal experience. For example, Reena who has previous experience of hospitalisation and treatment is usually more competent to decide about a new treatment plan than less experienced children of a similar age and maturity.

"Having frequent operations throughout my life is frustrating and I hope things improve one day. Whilst my mum is very thorough questioning the doctors, she now encourages me to ask about my surgeries too and tries to explain afterwards things I'm not sure about. Some doctors can talk over me like I'm not there and forget I'm not a young child any more!"

Jordan, patient

SAFEGUARDING STOP POINT

Imagine a slightly different case, in which Reena refuses to remain in hospital for treatment due to her dislike of the hospital. As she is a competent child, what actions can be taken in such a situation?

The Children Act 1989, s 25 allows the use of secure accommodation to restrict the liberty of a child for 72 hours in any 28-day period. Secure accommodation is not specifically defined by the Children Act, but in practical terms the Act would advocate for locking the entrance to the ward (see Re B (A Minor) (Treatment and Secure Accommodation [1997]). Before restricting the liberty of a child or young person, the team must be satisfied that the child or young person has a history of absconding, is likely to suffer significant harm or that they are likely to injure themselves or other persons if they were to have their treatment in an alternative location.

Parents

Parents are used as proxies when their child is judged as not competent or does not have the legal right to make a decision. This parental responsibility is defined within the Children Act 1989, s 3(1) in which parents have a duty to act in the child's best interests. According to Beauchamp and Childress (2013), a surrogate decision-maker – in this case Reena's parents – must determine the highest net benefit among available options, assigning different weights to the interest Reena has in each option. Parents themselves must therefore have the ability to make reasoned judgements for which they require adequate knowledge and information, emotional stability and the ability to balance the best interests of their child or young person.

Parents are usually the most suited to judge what is in the best interests of their child. The assumption is based upon the premise that parents know more than anyone else about their children due to their constant, close proximity. However, as in the parent voice below, a parent's own distress regarding their child's condition or belief that they have to protect their child from upsetting information and decisions may prevent them from giving due attention to the child's needs and wishes. This does not mean that they are bad parents, just that they need support to make decisions at distressing times.

"As parents of a child with complex medical needs we are often faced with having to make difficult decisions on Matthew's behalf. Being kept fully informed is key, however upsetting the medical information is to receive, to help us prepare ourselves and Matthew to overcome the challenges ahead. We always seek professional advice where our knowledge is limited to ensure we can make informed decisions together with the medical professionals and Matthew now he is a teenager."

Gill, parent

WHAT'S THE EVIDENCE?

Read the article 'Children's participation in decision-making: balancing protection with shared decision-making using a situational perspective' by Coyne and Harder (2011).

This article provides a synopsis of the research, which identifies reasons why adults wish to protect children and provides a summary of children's competence to participate in decision-making. Whilst reading the article, consider the following:

- What are the possible barriers to shared situational decision-making?
- What are the possible consequences for children or young people's healthcare if they do not participate in shared decision-making?

Health professionals

Health professionals continue to self-regulate their standards of practice but as outlined earlier in this chapter, practitioners are increasingly held to account through public and employer scrutiny. As a result, the healthcare professional's role is to provide clinical judgements, decisions and interventions that are clearly explained, justified and defended when challenged either by children or young people and their parents. Children's nurses in particular are responsible for passing on healthcare information in a manner that can be understood and retained by children or young people and their family.

Judicial review

When a collaborative healthcare decision cannot be made, a fourth party involving our judicial system can be invited to make the final decision for a child or young person. The courts through their inherent jurisdiction exercise a supervisory role over healthcare decision-making. For example, in cases where those with parental responsibility strongly oppose the giving or withholding of treatment by a health professional the matter will be referred to the court for a decision. In a similar approach to parental responsibility, Lord Donaldson in the case of Re J (A minor) [1992] made it clear that the best interests of the child should always be sought when assessing any course of action to be taken.

WHAT'S THE EVIDENCE?

The test for determining the best interests of a child has developed over time as new cases have been brought to court. Thirty-five years ago, in the case of a child born with Down syndrome who needed urgent surgery for an intestinal blockage, the court limited its consideration of the best interest test to the life expectancy of the child [Re B (A minor) 1981]. Thirty-two years later Baroness Hale of Richmond in *Aintree University Hospitals NHS Foundation Trust v James* [2013] asserted that in considering the best interests, decision-makers must look at the child's welfare in the widest sense, not just medical but social and psychological; they must consider the nature of the medical treatment in question and try to put themselves in the place of the individual patient.

- What factors would you consider when determining the best interests of a child?

HOW CAN CHILDREN'S NURSES IMPROVE THEIR DECISION-MAKING?

To be accountable when making decisions you require knowledge and understanding, an ability to rationalise, the skills to carry out required actions and the ability to make decisions. This final part of the chapter will explore decision-making models, which can be utilised to facilitate effective decision-making in practice.

CASE STUDY 38.2: JOSHUA

Joshua is a 5-month-old infant who has been admitted to your ward for observation following a diagnosis of bronchiolitis. Currently his clinical observations are within normal parameters for his age, but his work of breathing has increased and the medical team are concerned he may deteriorate in the next few hours. The mentor you are working with appears concerned about Joshua, advising you to monitor his observations every 30 minutes. You ask your mentor about her decision-making process.

- Why do you think your mentor is concerned about Joshua?
- How do you determine the frequency of clinical observation monitoring for each child in your care?

Banning (2008) identified three models of clinical decision-making. All three models can be used when working in the clinical environment. The case of Joshua will be used to demonstrate these models in action.

The information-processing model

This model uses a scientific (hypothetical–deductive) approach to assist cognitive reasoning. The approach involves multiple stages:

- Cue recognition
- Hypothesis generation
- Cue interpretation
- Hypothesis evaluation (Tanner et al., 1987)

As a student nurse you may consciously use scientific information such as a protocol or guideline for bronchiolitis (cue interpretation) to enable you to recognise and interpret Joshua's vital signs and symptoms (cue recognition) to formulate a plan of care (hypothesis generation). By contrast, an experienced qualified children's nurse may work from the hypothesis (hypothesis generation) and then collect the information (cue recognition) to either confirm or refute the efficacy of the care decision (hypothesis evaluation). The way in which the decision-making stages are applied can therefore depend upon the nurse's knowledge and experience of caring for children with bronchiolitis.

The strength of the information-processing model is the certainty and reliability it can provide when clinical decisions are made. Decision-tree algorithms based upon this model have been found to significantly improve the decision-making ability of nurses (Aspiuynall, 1979). There are, however, significant drawbacks to this model as it assumes existing knowledge is available and accurate. In clinical practice the decisions we make often possess an element of uncertainty as nursing knowledge is not static but continuously advances with every decision and discovery we make.

ACTIVITY 38.1: REFLECTIVE PRACTICE

Can you identify a situation in which you have made a nursing decision using the information-processing model?

The intuitive–humanistic model

Benner (1984) describes a model where inexperienced nurses tend to use procedures and guidelines to make decisions, while the experienced nurse may use intuitive decision-making processes. The intuitive decision-making occurs when experienced nurses appear to make sense of a situation without relying on processing analytical principles. Through unconscious thought processing and pattern recognition a decision is often expressed as a 'gut feeling' or 'sixth sense'. For example, an experienced nurse, as in the case above, may decide to increase the monitoring of an infant like Joshua, due to a 'gut feeling' that they may tire and clinically deteriorate despite his clinical observations being within the normal range for his age.

ACTIVITY 38.2: CRITICAL THINKING

Now that you have read about two decision-making models, what factors can influence children or young people care-related decisions?

The clinical decision-making model

The use of intuitive knowledge for the purpose of decision-making has been challenged, as without analysis and evaluation it is more difficult to explain, justify and defend clinical judgements. This hybrid model (O'Neill et al., 2004) is based around a computerised decision-support system which uses hypothetical deduction (information-processing model) and pattern recognition (intuitive–humanistic model) as a basis of decision-making. Patient-specific data (e.g., case notes and clinical observations) are used as a tool to help the nurse anticipate health risks to their patients. The degree of risk of each potential problem is ranked and then the nursing action is implemented to reduce the most threatening of risks.

In the absence of a computerised decision-making system, the nurse caring for the infant with bronchiolitis can adopt the principles of this hybrid model by using both subjective and objective data to decide what actions are needed to prevent respiratory deterioration for Joshua. The knowledge, experience and the ability of the nurse to care for a child or young person whose condition can change rapidly are all elements that are considered in O'Neil et al.'s (2004) multidimensional model. As your nursing knowledge and clinical experience increase, your ability to make clinical decisions will become more refined and intricate.

CHAPTER SUMMARY

- We all make decisions every day, but professional decision-making has an additional element in that the decisions we make as nurses are open to scrutiny by a range of people, including children and young people, parents, professional colleagues and the general public
- Delivering understandable information and active engagement with a child or young person and their family in the decision-making process is essential
- There are several decision-making theories which attempt to capture the complexity of making decisions in clinical practice
- Theoretical knowledge and clinical experience impact on the decision-making strategies of children's nurses

BUILD YOUR BIBLIOGRAPHY

Books

- Standing, M. (2020) *Clinical Judgement and Decision Making in Nursing*, 4th edn. London: Learning Matters.

  Fully mapped to NMC standards and excellent for confidence in clinical decision-making.

FURTHER
READING

- Benner, P. (1984) *From Novice to Expert: Excellence and Power in Clinical Nursing Practice.* Menlo Park, CA: Addison-Wesley.

  This older but nevertheless seminal book is useful in assisting you to understand and appreciate your journey from a novice nurse to an expert practitioner. You will find examples of how nurses develop their decision-making skills through skill acquisition.
- Holland, K. (2020) *Understanding Decision Making in Nursing Practice.* London: Sage.

  An accessible and evidence-based introduction to decision-making in nursing practice using activities and case studies This book supports Future Nurse Standards of Proficiency and lessons learned from the COVID pandemic.

Journal articles

FURTHER
READING:
ONLINE
JOURNAL
ARTICLES

- Park, E.S. and Cho, I.Y. (2018) 'Shared decision-making in the paediatric field: a literature review and concept analysis'. *Scandanavian Journal of Caring Science*, 32 (2): 478–89.

  A literature review and concept analysis of shared decision-making.
- Maduermem, K. (2022) 'Shared decision-making.' Don't Forget The Bubbles. Available at: https://doi.org/10.31440/DFTB.51227 (accessed 13 February 2023).
- Boland, L., Graham, I.D., Légaré, F. et al. (2019) 'Barriers and facilitators of pediatric shared decision-making: a systematic review'. *Implemetation Science*, 14 (1): 7. doi: 10.1186/s13012-018-0851-5.

  Interesting review of decision-making in the area of pediatic medicine and care.
- The King's Fund, 'Make Shared Decision Making a Reality: No Decision About Me, Without Me' (Coulter and Collins, 2011) www.kingsfund.org.uk/sites/files/kf/Making-shared-decision-making-a-reality-paper-Angela-Coulter-Alf-Collins-July-2011_0.pdf www.kingsfund.org.uk/sites/files/kf/Making-shared-decision-making-a-reality-paper-Angela-Coulter-Alf-Collins-July-2011_0.pdf

  The Government wants shared decision-making to become the norm in the NHS. This report by the King's Fund clarifies the concept and outlines the actions needed.

CASES

Aintree University Hospitals NHS Foundation Trust v *James* [2013]
Re B (A Minor) (Wardship: Medical Treatment) [1981] 1 WLR 1421
Re B (Minors) (Residence Order) [1992] Fam 162
Re B (A Minor) (Treatment and Secure Accommodation) [1997] 1 FLR 618
Re J (A Minor) [1992] All ER 614@@

STATUTES

Children Act 1989
Medicine Act 1968
Mental Health Act 2007

REFERENCES

Aspiuynall, M. (1979) 'Use of a decision tree to improve accuracy of nursing diagnosis'. *Nursing Research*, 28: 182–5.

Banning, M. (2008) 'A review of clinical decision making: models and current research'. *Journal of Clinical Nursing*, 17 (2): 187–95.

Beauchamp, T. and Childress, J. (2013) *Principles of Biomedical Ethics*, 7th edn. Oxford: Oxford University Press.

Benner, P. (1984) *From Novice to Expert: Excellence and Power in Clinical Nursing Practice*. Menlo Park, CA: Addison Wesley.

Coyne, I. and Harder, M. (2011) 'Children's participation in decision-making'. *Journal of Child Health Care*, 15 (4): 312–19.

Dimond, B. (2019) *Legal Aspects of Nursing*, 8th edn. Harlow: Pearson Education.

Nursing and Midwifery Council (NMC) (2023) *Standards framework for Pre-registration Nursing Education Part 1*, London: NMC.

Nursing and Midwifery Council (NMC) (2018) *The Code: Professional Standards of Practice and Behaviour for Nurses and Midwives*. Available at: www.nmc.org.uk/standards/code/ (accessed 23 June 2023).

O'Neill, E., Dluhy, N., Fortier, P. and Howard, E. (2004) 'Knowledge acquisition, synthesis and validation: a model for decision support systems'. *Journal of Advanced Nursing*, 47 (2): 134–42.

Tanner, C., Padrick, K., Westfall, U. and Putzier, D. (1987) 'Diagnostic reasoning strategies for nurses and nursing students'. *Nursing Research*, 36 (6): 358–63.

INDEX

Page numbers followed by "f" and "t" refer to figures and tables, respectively.

Made in the USA
Middletown, DE
11 November 2024

64346934R00376